Cardiac Catheterization and Percutaneous Interventions

Cardiac Catheterization and Percutaneous Interventions

Edited by

I Patrick Kay MBChB PhD

Interventional Cardiologist
Cardiology Department
Dunedin Hospital
Dunedin
New Zealand

Manel Sabaté MD PhD FESC

Servicio de Cardiologia Intervencionista
Hospital Clinico Universitario San Carlos
Madrid
Spain

Marco A Costa MD PhD FSCAI

Assistant Professor of Medicine
Director of Research & Cardiovascular Imaging Core Laboratories
Division of Cardiology, University of Florida, Shands Jacksonville
Jacksonville, FL, USA

Foreword by **Patrick W Serruys** MD PhD FACC FESC

Taylor & Francis
Taylor & Francis Group

LONDON AND NEW YORK

A MARTIN DUNITZ BOOK

First published in the United Kingdom in 2004
by Taylor & Francis, an imprint of the Taylor & Francis Group, 11 New Fetter Lane, London EC4P 4EE

Tel.:   +44 (0) 20 7583 9855
Fax.:   +44 (0) 20 7842 2298
E-mail: info@dunitz.co.uk
Website: http://www.dunitz.co.uk

A CIP record for this book is available from the British Library.

Library of Congress Cataloging-in-Publication Data

Data available on application

ISBN 1 84184 230 3

Distributed in North and South America by
Taylor & Francis
2000 NW Corporate Blvd
Boca Raton, FL 33431, USA

Within Continental USA
Tel.: 800 272 7737; Fax.: 800 374 3401
Outside Continental USA
Tel.: 561 994 0555; Fax.: 561 361 6018
E-mail: orders@crcpress.com

Distributed in the rest of the world by
Thomson Publishing Services
Cheriton House
North Way
Andover, Hampshire SP10 5BE, UK
Tel.: +44 (0)1264 332424
E-mail: salesorder.tandf@thomsonpublishingservices.co.uk

Composition by EXPO Holdings, Malaysia

Printed and bound in Spain by Grafos SA

Contents

Contributors

Fernando Alfonso MD PhD FESC
Consultant Cardiologist
Interventional Cardiology
Cardiovascular Institute
San Carlos University Hospital
Madrid
Spain

Dominick J Angiolillo MD
International Cardiology Unit
Cardiovascular Unit
San Carlos University Hospital
Madrid
Spain

Theodore Adam Bass MD
Professor
Chief, Division of Cardiology
Medical Director, The Cardiovascular
Center at Shands Jacksonville
Director, Interventional Cardiology
Fellowship Program
FL, USA

Deepak L Bhatt MD
Interventional Cardiology
Director, Interventional Cardiology
Fellowship
Associate Director, Cardiovascular
Fellowship
The Cleveland Clinic Foundation
Department of Cardiovascular Medicine
Cleveland, OH, USA

Ad den Boer BSc
Technical Research Coordinator &
Project Leader
Thoraxcentre
University Hospital—Dijkzigt
Rotterdam
The Netherlands

Antonio Colombo MD
EMO Centro Cuore Columbus
Milan, Italy

Marco A Costa MD PhD FSCAI
Assistant Professor of Medicine
Director of Research & Cardiovascular
Imaging Core Laboratories
Division of Cardiology, University of
Florida, Shands Jacksonville
Jacksonville, FL, USA

Arthur W Crossman MD
The Cardiovascular Center at Shands
Jacksonville, FL, USA

Giuseppe De Luca MD
Interventional Cardiologist
Department of Cardiology
Isaka Kliniken
De Weezenlanden Hospital
Zwolle, The Netherlands

Carlo Di Mario MD PhD
Consultant Cardiologist
Royal Brompton Hospital
London, UK

Javier Escaned MD PhD FESC
Department of Interventional
Cardiology
Hospital Clinico San Carlos
Madrid, Spain

Paul S Gilmore MD
The Cardiovascular Center at Shands
Jacksonville, FL, USA

Richard Harper MBBS FRACP FACC
Professor
Department of Medicine
Monash University
Department of Cardiology and
Cardiovascular Research
Monash Medical Center
Clayton, VIC, Australia

Rosana Hernandez Antolín MD
PhD FESC
Interventional Cardiology Unit
Instituto Cardiovascular
Hospital Universitario San Carlos
Madrid
Spain

Sriram S Iyer MD
Director of Endovascular Therapy
Lenox Hill Hospital
New York NY, USA

I Patrick Kay MBChB PhD
Interventional Cardiologist
Cardiology Department
Dunedin Hospital
Dunedin
New Zealand

Ken Kozuma MD
Division of Cardiology
Department of Internal Medicine,
Teikyo University School of Medicine
Tokyo, Japan

Arun Kuchela MD FRCPC
Fellow in Interventional Cardiology
University of British Columbia,
Vancouver Health Sciences Center
Cardiac Catherization Laboratories
Vancouver, BC, Canada

Chi Hang Lee MBBS MRCP FAMS
Associate Consultant Cardiologist
Cardiac Department
National University Hospital
Singapore

Pedro A Lemos MD
Thoraxcenter
Department of Cardiology
Erasmus Medical Center
Rotterdam
The Netherlands

David McGaw MBBS (PhD)
Centre for Heart and Chest Research
Monash University and Monash Medical
Centre
Clayton
Melbourne, VIC, Australia

Koen Neiman MD
Thoraxcenter
Department of Cardiology
Erasmus Medical Center
Rotterdam
The Netherlands

Gishel New MBBS PhD FRACP FACC
Director of Cardiology
Box Hill Hospital
Monash University Department of
Medicine
Melbourne, Australia

John Ormiston FRACR, FRACP
Cardiac Investigation Rooms
Green Lane and Mercy Hospitals
Epsom
Auckland
New Zealand

Barbara O'Shaughnessy DSR BHSc
Mercy Angiography
Newmarket
Auckland
New Zealand

María José Pérez-Vizcayno MD
Interventional Cardiology
Cardiovascular Institute
San Carlos University Hospital
Madrid, Spain

Campbell Rogers MD FACC
Director, Cardiac Catheterization
Laboratory
Director, Experimental Cardiovascular
Interventional Laboratory
Brigham and Women's Hospital
Harvard Medical School
Boston, MA, USA

Gary S Roubin MBBS PhD FRACP
FACC FAHA
Director of Cardiology
Alfred Hospital
Monash University
Melbourne, Australia

Manel Sabaté MD PhD FESC
Interventional Cardiology Department
Cardiovascular Institute
San Carlos University Hospital
Madrid
Spain

Giuseppe M Sangiorgi MD
Interventional Cardiology
Emo Centro Cuore Columbus
Milan
Italy

Brett M Sasseen MD
Assistant Professor, Associate Director
Cardiovascular Disease Fellowship
Program and Associate Director,
Interventional Cardiology Fellowship
Program

Johannes Schaar MD
Erasmus MC
Thoraxcenter
Rotterdam, The Netherlands

Pieter C Smits MD PhD
Clinical Director
Department of Interventional
Cardiology
Erasmus Medical Center
Thoraxcenter
Rotterdam
The Netherlands

Goran Stankovic MD
Institute for Cardiovascular Diseases
Clinical Center of Serbia
Belgrade
Serbia and Montenegro

Harry Suryapranata, MD PhD
Interventional Cardiologist
Director of Clinical Research and
Catheterization Laboratory
Isala Klinieken
Hospital De Weezelanden
Department of Cardiology
Zwolle, The Netherlands

Glenn Van Langenhove MD PhD
Interventional Cardiology
Middelheim Hospital Antwerp
Antwerp
Belgium

Stefan Verheye MD FESC
Cardiovascular Translational Research
Institute
Antwerp
Belgium

Jiri J Vitek MD PhD
Lenox Hill Hospital
New York, NY, USA

Robert J Walker MBChB MD(Otago)
FRACP
Professor of Medicine
Consultant Nephrologist
Head of Department, Department of
Medical & Surgical Sciences
Dunedin School of Medicine
University of Otago
Dunedin
New Zealand

Mark Webster FRACP
Mercy Angiography
Newmarket
Auckland
New Zealand

Michael JA Williams MD FRACP
FACC
Cardiologist
Dunedin Hospital
Dunedin, New Zealand

Gerard T Wilkins MB ChB FRACP
Clinical Leader
Cardiology, Cardiothoracic Surgery,
Respiratory, Nephrology and
Endocrinology
Dunedin Hospital
Senior Lecturer in Medicine
University of Otago Medical School
Dunedin
New Zealand

Foreword

"The results of coronary angioplasty in patients with single vessel disease are sufficiently good to make the procedure acceptable for prospective randomised trials." So wrote Andreas Gruntzig in 1979, reporting the results of the first 50 patients treated with angioplasty. This paper represented the birth of one the major medical techniques of the 20th century.

Andreas Gruntzig pioneered and championed the new science of interventional cardiology. Since his time there has been a spiralling increase in technology and information. The transformation into an invasive or interventional cardiologist must account for these new technologies in a tactile and cognitive sense.

Drs Kay, Sabaté and Costa have created a book with both practical and scientific application, that will greatly assist the cardiologist. Chapters have been written by leading authors in their field and rising stars.

I congratulate the editors on their execution of their assignment. At last we have a text that is truly useful to the growth of the interventionalist.

Patrick W Serruys,
February 2004

Preface

Few fields of medicine have advanced at a more rapid rate than that of percutaneous intervention. Training and experience is the foundation on which an accomplished interventionalist stands. No text can profess to supplant this foundation, but in *Cardiac Catheterization and Percutaneous Interventions* we have created a practical text that will allay the fears of these early encounters and create confidence in performing percutaneous coronary and peripheral intervention.

We have created novel and exciting chapters addressing the basics (the things you wouldn't dare to ask), the pitfalls (the problems to avoid before you start), the proven approaches (the facts you are expected to know) and the new innovations (the techniques you will want to be first to perfect).

We would like to thank the contributors, all great practitioners and teachers who responded so willingly to our quest to create a current, practical and challenging text.

Special thanks should go to Alan Burgess and Abigail Griffin from Martin Dunitz Publishers whose expert guidance at critical moments allowed *Cardiac Catheterization and Percutaneous Interventions* to come to fruition.

I Patrick Kay, Manel Sabaté, Marco A Costa

1

Who should not go to the cathlab?

I Patrick Kay, Robert J Walker

General

Theoretically, there are few absolute contraindications to coronary angiography. Fortunately most people who are suitable for angiography will also be suitable for angioplasty. There are a few caveats that are relevant for patient selection, and we will discuss them in the next few pages. Some of these issues will be resolved over the next few years as non-invasive forms of coronary imaging become widely applicable. These imaging modalities may still involve the use of contrast, depending on whether they are based on computed tomography (CT) or magnetic resonance imaging (MRI). Despite these innovations, angioplasty will persist as the therapeutic intervention of choice for the majority of cases with coronary artery disease.

The first part of this chapter discusses areas that may cause concern, approaching the problem from the standpoint of a 'surgical sieve'. The second part discusses the very important area of renal disease.

Non-renal areas of concern

Cardiac issues

The following would constitute relative contraindications to catheterization:

- *Uncontrolled ventricular irritability.* Patients with ventricular arrythmia commonly require coronary angiography to rule out an ischemically mediated process. Indeed, coronary angiography with percutaneous

coronary intervention (PCI) may be the only way to control a persistent malignant arrythmia under such circumstances.

- *Severe electrolyte imbalance (potassium, sodium and calcium).* These derangements should be treated prior to presentation to the catheterization laboratory.
- *Uncontrolled hypertension.* Vigorous attempts should be made to control blood pressure prior to presentation to the catheterization laboratory. Poor control may lead to groin complications, increased coronary ischemia and stroke. The risk of stroke will also be increased should aggressive antiplatelet therapy be required in this context.
- *Uncontrolled left ventricular failure.* Unless left ventricular failure has been induced by an ischemically mediated event, in particular myocardial infarction with cardiogenic shock, the case should be deferred. In cases with ischemically mediated cardiogenic shock, intraaortic balloon pump insertion with angioplasty should be contemplated.
- *Drug toxicity (digitalis or overdose with other agents).* This situation may lead to or may be secondary to renal failure. Attempts should be made to decrease drug levels and provide cardiac support prior to coronary angiography. Cardiac pacing may be required.

Febrile illness

Cardiac catheterization is not absolutely contraindicated in patients with fever or infections. It would be wise, however, to contemplate the source of the infection, as substantial comorbidity could be associated even with a simple procedure such as angiography. A typical example is renal tract infection (see later in this chapter). The final decision will be placed in the hands of the physician, who will need to weigh up the risk of cardiac disease against that of the infection and its source.

Hematopoietic

Not infrequently, the physician will be confronted with marked abnormalities in hematological parameters. The most notable is likely to be thrombocytopenia. Most operators would be ill advised to consider cardiac catheterization on individuals with platelet counts less than 80 000. One would be even more reluctant to proceed if PCI were contemplated, given that antiplatelet therapy is still likely to be prescribed. A minimum platelet count of 100 000 is advised in those contemplating PCI. Similarly, severe neutropenia in patients (neutrophil count < 0.5) would be considered an absolute contraindication to either catheterization or PCI.

Severe anemia (Hb <80 g/l) may also be a contraindication to cardiac catheterization, particularly if PCI is contemplated. Appropriate transfusion of blood and gastrointestinal (GI) or bone marrow investigation should be contemplated. If urgent catheterization is required, then this can be performed with increased risk. Polycythemia, thrombophilia, and the leukemias are not absolute contraindications to cardiac catheterization. Instead, the medication used in the control of these illnesses may interact with those used at the time of catheterization/ PCI. Due consultation with a hematologist is advisable.

The final and of course most common cause of abnormal hematological finding is iatrogenic in origin – abnormal coagulation profiles secondary to the therapeutic ingestion of coumadin derivatives, or adverse reactions to other drugs. Generally speaking, this does not pose a major problem, as patients can be deferred until the international normalized ratio (INR) falls to lower levels (INR < 2.0). During this time, subcutaneous or intravenous heparin can be substituted if necessary. Alternatively, the femoral artery can be avoided and the radial approach used in preference if urgent therapy is necessary.

Gastrointestinal

Active gastrointestinal bleeding is generally a contraindication to cardiac catheterization and PCI. In individuals who develop GI bleeding prior to planned catheterization, the procedure should be deferred until appropriate upper or lower GI investigation has been completed. Urgent catheterization is only rarely required in those with active GI bleeding. Given that the procedure can be performed safely with little or no heparin, provided adequate consul-

tation occurs between cardiologist, gastroenterologist and surgeon, the procedure can be expeditiously and safely completed. If there is evidence of hemodynamic instability, then this will need to be promptly controlled, as it will clearly have implications for coronary ischemia and significant valvular disease.

Angioplasty is ill advised under circumstances of active bleeding or hemodynamic instability secondary to GI bleeding.

If bleeding occurs after stent implantation has been accomplished, then the physician will need to consider the risk/benefit profile of cessation of aspirin/clopidogrel. Published data from the CAPRIE study[1] suggests that the frequency of GI bleeding, including severe GI bleeding, was less with clopidogrel use than with aspirin. One could argue that, providing that active GI bleeding has stopped, then cessation of aspirin and continuation of clopidogrel may be reasonable as a means of minimizing the risk of subacute thrombosis. There are few published data concerning this problem, however, and each group will need to discuss the minimum requirements for antiplatelet therapy under such difficult circumstances.

Psychological/neurological

One of the most important contraindications to cardiac catheterization is the mentally competent patient refusing to undergo the procedure. The operator must be certain that the selected patient is able to give informed consent and that the risks and benefits of the procedure are well understood. Also, preexisting psychological complaints must be assessed and where possible a management pathway applied that will enable the patient to cope with the planned procedure.

One other concern here is with patients who have had a recent cerebrovascular accident, given the powerful antiplatelet agents that may be given during PCI. Angiography does not tend to cause problems unless there are rhythm disturbances or hemodynamic instability. There are reports of deterioration in neurological symptoms potentially caused by vasospasm, induced by contrast agents. These effects tend to last a matter of hours only. Naturally, the very process of performing cardiac catheterization can induce mechanical thromboembolism, which may lead to transient ischemic episodes or cerebrovascular accidents.

Other

The operator needs to be wary that there are weight limits to cardiac catheterization tables. Older units tend to permit only lighter frames (<140 kg), whereas current installations permit up to 200 kg.

Allergy to contrast agents is an important contraindication to proceeding with catheterization. Whether this contraindication is relative or absolute will depend on the severity of previous reactions and the nature of contrast agent to which the individual has reacted. Pretreatment with steroids/antihistamines may abort or diminish the reaction.

Renal considerations

The presence of renal impairment has been demonstrated to be a significant risk factor for subsequent morbidity and mortality in cardiac and general surgery.[2,3] It is also one of the most important risk factors for cardiac angiography. The presence of renal impairment should be considered initially as a potential contraindication to coronary angiography. However, in the majority of cases, the indication for coronary angiography and the impact that the underlying cardiac disease will have on the individual is such that the relative risk is justifiable. What must take place in the clinical assessment is the recognition of the renal impairment, its potential impact on subsequent outcome, and the institution of appropriate measures to minimize the risk related to renal impairment.

Cardiac catheterization and renal function

There are two major causes of renal dysfunction after cardiac catheterization:

- contrast media-induced nephrotoxicity;
- renal atheroemboli.

This chapter will deal with both of these potentially important complications, covering etiology, incidence, identification of risk, and management (including prevention).

Contrast-induced nephropathy

Contrast-induced nephropathy is now recognized as an important cause of iatrogenic acute renal impairment following the use of radiographic contrast media in diagnostic and interventional procedures. Mild transient decreases in glomerular filtration rate (GFR) after contrast administration occur in almost all patients.[4] In most studies, the definition of contrast-induced nephrotoxicity is an acute decline in renal function as measured as a rise in plasma creatinine of 25% or more, or 50%, or an absolute rise in plasma creatinine of 88 μmol/l above the

Table 1.1 Risk factors for contrast media-induced nephrotoxicity

- Preexisting renal impairment with a GFR <50 ml/min (plasma creatinine >200 μmol/l)
- Diabetic nephropathy with renal impairment
- Volume depletion.
- Congestive heart failure or other causes of reduced renal perfusion
- Multiple exposure to contrast media (short timeframe).
- Nephrotoxic drugs, especially nonsteroidal anti-inflammatory drugs (NSAIDs)

Adapted from Parfrey et al. J Am Soc Nephrol 2000;11:177–82.[5]

baseline value, within 48–72 hours following the administration of intravenous contrast media.[4,5] These changes are more likely to occur in patients with one or more of the risk factors listed in Table 1.1.

The incidence of contrast-induced nephrotoxicity is minimal in patients with normal renal function, including diabetics with normal renal function,[6,7] unless there is a significant intervening event associated with the procedure. In patients with mild to moderate renal impairment (plasma creatinine 130–200 μmol/l), the incidence is 4–11%,[6–8] but is increased with associated risk factors listed in Table 1.1. McCullough and colleagues[9] reported an incidence of acute renal failure (creatinine rise of >25% from baseline) of 14.5% in a series of 1826 consecutive patients undergoing coronary angiography. In the same study, 0.7% developed acute renal failure requiring dialysis.

Patients with marked renal impairment (plasma creatinine >200 μmol/l) have a much higher incidence of acute renal failure (5–11%). Diabetics with established renal impairment have an even higher incidence ranging from 9 to 33%.[6,8,10]

Clinical course

Typically, the rise in plasma creatinine occurs 24–48 hours following the procedure, peaking at 3–5 days before returning to the baseline value in most cases.[4] Although dialysis is infrequently required in the management of contrast-induced nephrotoxicity, it is not necessarily a benign condition. Up to as many as 30% of patients with contrast-induced nephropathy will be left with some degree of renal impairment.[11] The requirement for dialysis in contrast-induced nephrotoxicity most often occurs in high-risk patients undergoing coronary angiography.[9] In many cases, this is related to the severity of the underlying cardiac disease and cardiac dysfunction as well as other comorbidity, in particular diabetes with renal impairment. In addition, events related to the angiography/angioplasty procedure such as hypotension and atheroembolic disease (as discussed below) can contribute to the development of acute renal failure. The development of acute renal failure may be associated with a much higher risk of mortality.[9,12] Levy and colleagues[12] documented an increased mortality rate of 34%, compared with 7% in an age-matched, as well as matched for severity of comorbidity, control group. McCullough and colleagues[9] reported a similar incidence of mortality associated with contrast-induced acute renal failure requiring dialysis (36%) versus those with stable renal function (1%).

Pathogenesis

The mechanism of contrast-induced renal injury is not clearly established, but experimental studies suggest there are two main mechanisms. Contrast administration is associated with an intense (usually transient) renal vasoconstriction, which leads to a reduction in medullary blood flow. It is thought that the vasoconstriction is mediated in part by the release of endothelin.[13] Due to the associated atherosclerotic vascular disease, there is minimal release of the endogenous vasodilators nitric oxide and the prostaglandins.[14,15] If this is sustained or superimposed on impaired renal perfusion associated with renal atherosclerotic disease, and/or impaired cardiac function, then potentiation of medullary hypoxia and ischemia leading to acute tubular necrosis can occur.[16,17] Likewise, the concomitant administration of nonsteroidal anti-inflammatory drugs (NSAIDs), preventing the release of vasodilator prostaglandins, will potentiate the contrast-induced vasoconstriction.[18,19]

Experimental studies have demonstrated a direct toxic effect of contrast media on renal tubular epithelial cells in culture, which is enhanced under hypoxic conditions.[16] Tubular injury may also lead to the production of oxygen free-radicals, promoting further damage.[20] If there is pre-existing renal disease, there is a probable reduction in protective antioxidant enzymes, enhancing the risk of contrast-mediated injury. This may also explain in part the observed benefit of N-acetylcysteine administration in reducing contrast-induced toxicity[21,22] (see below).

Prevention and management

The most important aspect of management is prevention of contrast-induced nephrotoxicity. Clearly, the use of other imaging modalities, such as magnetic resonance angiography (MRA), where possible, in high-risk cases (Table 1.1) would avoid exposure to contrast. However, where coronary angiography is essential on the basis of clinical indication, there are a number of measures that can be implemented to minimize the development of contrast-induced nephrotoxicity.

- It is essential to optimize the patient's clinical status prior to exposure to contrast media.
- The patient's renal function needs to be known prior to the procedure. Given the inherent inaccuracy of

plasma creatinine alone as an estimate of renal function, determination of the GFR (creatinine clearance, CrCl) by estimation using the Cockcroft-Gault formula[23] should be undertaken:

$$CrCl \ (ml/min) = [(140 - age) \times weight \ (kg)]/$$
$$813 \times serum \ creatinine \ (mmol/l),$$
$$CrCl \ (female) = 0.85 \times CrCl.$$

- If GFR <50 ml/min, then the individual is at increased risk. The presence of renal impairment is the most significant risk factor for subsequent contrast-induced nephrotoxicity. At-risk patients should have their renal function monitored 48–72 hours after the procedure.[5]
- To minimize the effect of other adverse risk factors, the clinician should make sure that the patient is not on an NSAID or other potentially nephrotoxic agents where possible.
- Correction of intravascular volume depletion and avoidance of excessive doses of diuretics, which may produce intravascular volume depletion, is essential.
- Adequate hydration is necessary before and after coronary angiography (see below).
- Where possible, repetitive contrast studies closely spaced together should be avoided.

There have been a number of studies investigating the role of hydration and the use of diuretics. An excellent overview of recent studies has been published.[5] The use of intravenous fluids has reduced the likelihood of contrast-induced nephrotoxicity in a number of different studies. The rationale for this is correction of any underlying subclinical dehydration, but more importantly the maintenance of a high urine flow rate. This decreases the exposure time of the contrast to the tubular cells, as well as a reduction in active sodium reabsorption in the ascending limb of the loop of Henle. This, in turn, will reduce the oxygen requirements in the medulla, which are already reduced by the contrast-induced vasoconstriction of the vasa recta.

Mueller and colleagues[24] demonstrated a significant benefit of isotonic saline (0.9% saline) over half-isotonic (0.45% saline) in reducing the incidence of contrast nephrotoxicity in a randomized comparison in 1620 patients undergoing coronary angiography. Other studies have demonstrated the benefit of 0.45% saline for hydration protocols.[6,7,25] For outpatient procedures, oral hydration before the procedure and intravenous fluids for 6 hours afterwards has been shown to be as effective as inpatient hydration in reducing the risk of contrast nephrotoxicity in a series of patients undergoing cardiac catheterization.[26] Despite adequate fluid administration associated with the contrast procedure, it does not afford complete protection. Solomon and colleagues[25] found that 11% of patients with renal impairment still developed contrast nephrotoxicity despite intravenous saline beforehand.

Experimental studies suggested that furosemide or mannitol may provide protection against contrast-induced nephrotoxicity.[18] However, clinical studies do not support this. Solomon and colleagues[25] demonstrated that in patients undergoing coronary angiography who had renal insufficiency (serum creatinine > 180 μmol/l), hydration with 0.45% saline alone provided better protection against contrast-induced acute changes in renal function, than hydration plus mannitol or furosemide.

There was some evidence in this study that furosemide may be detrimental to renal function.[25] In addition, there is no good clinical evidence to support the use of low-dose dopamine, theophylline, calcium channel blockers, or atrial natriuretic peptide to prevent the development of contrast-induced nephrotoxicity (reviewed in reference 5).

The role of the type of contrast agent utilized – high-osmolar (ionic) versus low-osmolar (nonionic) – as a contributing factor to the development of contrast nephrotoxicity is still not clearly defined. In low-risk patients, randomized prospective studies do not support an enhanced benefit for the use of low-osmolar agents.[6,10,27] However, there is some supporting evidence from these studies that in high-risk patients, especially diabetics with renal impairment, low-osmolar contrast may reduce the risk of contrast nephrotoxicity.[5] It may be appropriate to

use the high-cost low-osmolar agents in the setting of high potential risk.

With the suggestion that contrast-induced nephrotoxicity may, in part, be mediated by oxidative injury, the use of N-acetylcysteine, a thiol-containing antioxidant, in combination with hydration has been used to reduce the risk of contrast-induced nephrotoxicity. Tepel and colleagues[21] demonstrated in a randomized controlled trial that there was less contrast-induced nephrotoxicity in the acetylcysteine treated group compared with control. Similar findings were demonstrated by Diaz-Sandoval and colleagues,[22] who also demonstrated a reduction in serum creatinine in the N-acetylcysteine-treated group. Upon closer inspection of the results, in both studies, the major finding was a reduction in the serum creatinine in the N-acetylcysteine-treated group rather than a major increase in the serum creatinine group in the placebo control group.[21,22] This would suggest that N-acetylcysteine may be having other effects on renal function, rather than protecting against contrast nephrotoxicity.

In another randomized study comparing N-acetylcysteine plus 0.45% saline hydration with 0.45% saline alone, before and after coronary angiography, Briguori

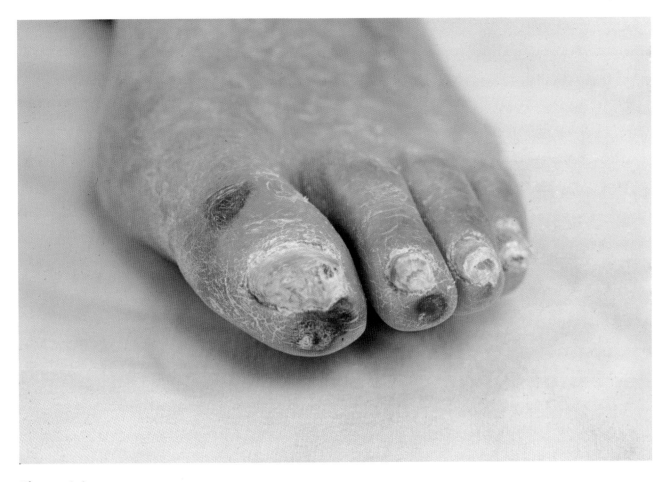

Figure 1.1
Cholesterol emboli precipitating areas of digital ischemia.

and colleagues[28] did not demonstrate a protective role for acetylcysteine. Clearly, larger studies with patients at greater risk are required to confirm a protective role for N-acetylcysteine.

Atheroembolic renal disease

This is an increasingly recognized complication from invasive vascular procedures such as angiography and angioplasty or vascular surgery. It can also occur following fibrinolytic therapy or anticoagulation.[29] It usually affects men over the age of 60 years with extensive atherosclerotic vascular disease, hypertension, and a history of smoking. In the past, the diagnosis was made primarily at postmortem;[30] however, a greater awareness of atheroembolic renal disease has led to an increased rate of diagnosis. The overall incidence still remains low. In one prospective series, the incidence of atheroembolic renal failure following coronary angiography was reported as less than 2%.[31]

The presence of a classic triad characterized by a precipitating event, acute or subacute renal failure, and evidence of peripheral cholesterol embolization strongly suggests the diagnosis[29] (Figure 1.1). The renal disease can present in several different ways. Atheroembolic disease associated with a procedure typically presents with acute symptoms suggestive of a systemic illness such as fevers, myalgias, arthralgias, livedo reticularis or discrete gangrenous lesions in the peripheries, emboli to other organs, and a rapid decline in renal function. In some cases, the diagnosis may initially be thought to be a vasculitis. The rapid decline in renal function helps differentiate the lesion from contrast-induced nephrotoxicity. The potentiating role of contrast cannot be excluded. Associated laboratory features include hypocomplementemia, eosinophilia, and raised inflammatory markers. Diagnosis can be confirmed on renal biopsy or skin biopsy in over 75% of cases.[32] The characteristic lesion involves extensive occlusion of small vessels with cholesterol emboli, especially in the arcuate and interlobular arteries. These are biconvex needle-shaped clefts remaining after dissolution of the cholesterol crystals during the histological preparation. The cholesterol emboli may set up a giant cell reaction[30,33,34] (Figure 1.2).

More frequently, the decline in renal function is progressive over several weeks after the vascular procedure, unlike contrast-induced nephrotoxicity, which usually resolves within 7–10 days. The reported mortality rate for atheroembolism is 73%.[32] Therapy is symptomatic and consists of the appropriate management of the renal failure. Renal function may or may not recover. The best approach to atheroembolic renal disease would be prevention, if possible, by exclusion of obviously high-risk patients.

Coronary angiography in high-risk individuals: a summary

Quite clearly, there is the potential to perform coronary angiography on a number of individuals who, by the nature of their atherosclerotic vascular disease, are at high risk of subsequent renal complications. For all situations, there has to be a thorough risk/benefit analysis involving the patient, cardiologist, and nephrologist. For high-risk

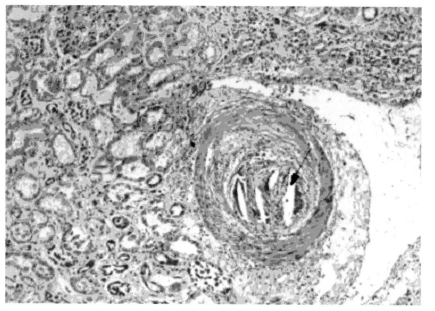

Figure 1.2
Renal atheroembolus. Light micrograph of an atheroembolus in a muscular renal artery showing cleft-like spaces (arrow) due to washout of the cholesterol crystals during histologic processing. (Reproduced from Rose BM. *UpToDate Clinical Reference Library, Release 10.3. Clinical Characteristics of Renal Emboli.* Wellesley, MA: UpToDate Inc.)

individuals, especially diabetics with established renal impairment, prior consultation with a nephrologist as part of the diagnostic workup should be undertaken. Then all possible options to minimize renal injury can be reviewed. In addition, a comprehensive explanation to the patient as to the risks of renal injury as well as the potential need for dialysis, which may follow coronary angiography in high-risk patients, can take place. It is imperative that patients with known renal impairment who need angiography have their procedure done in an institution where nephrological support is available. All patients require pre- and perioperative hydration and subsequent monitoring of their renal function.

References

1. CAPRIE Investigators. Lancet 1997;349:355–6.
2. Anderson RJ, O'Brien M, MaWhinney S. Renal failure predisposes to adverse outcome after coronary artery bypass surgery. Kidney Int 1999;55:1057–62.
3. O'Brien MM, Gonzales R, Shroyer AL, et al. Modest serum creatinine elevation affects adverse outcome after general surgery. Kidney Int 2002;62:585–92.
4. Solomon R. Contrast-medium-induced acute renal failure. Kidney Int 1998;53:230–42.
5. Murphy SW, Barrett BJ, Parfrey PS. Contrast nephrotoxicity. J Am Soc Nephrol 2000;11:177–82.
6. Parfrey PS, Griffiths SM, Barrett BJ, et al. Contrast material-induced renal failure in patients with diabetes mellitus, renal insufficiency or both. N Engl J Med 1989;320:143–9.
7. Rudnick MR, Berns JS, Cohen RM, Goldfarb S. Nephrotoxic risks of renal angiography: contrast media-associated nephrotoxicity and atheroembolism – a critical review. Am J Kidney Dis 1994;24:713–27.
8. D'Elia JA, Gleason RE, Alday M, et al. Nephrotoxicity from angiographic contrast material. Am J Med 1982; 72:719–25.
9. McCullough PA, Wolyn R, Rocher LL, et al. Acute renal failure after coronary intervention: Incidence, risk factors and relationship to mortality. Am J Med 1997;103:368–75.
10. Barrett BJ, Parfrey PS, Vavasour HM, et al. Contrast nephropathy in patients with impaired renal function: high versus low osmolar media. Kidney Int 1992;41:1274–9.
11. Porter GA. Contrast associated nephropathy. Am J Cardiol 1989;64:22E–6E.
12. Levy EM, Viscoli CM, Horwitz RI. The effect of acute renal failure on mortality: a cohort analysis. JAMA 1996; 275:1489–94.
13. Cantley LG, Spokes K, Clark B, et al. Role of endothelin and prostaglandins in radiocontrast-induced renal artery constriction. Kidney Int 1993;44:1217–23.
14. Brezis M, Heyman SN, Dinour D, Epstein FH. Role of nitric oxide in renal medullary oxygenation: studies in isolated and intact rat kidneys. J Clin Invest 1991;88:390–5.
15. Agmon Y, Peleg H, Greenfeld Z, et al. Nitric oxide and prostanoids protect the renal outer medulla from radiocontrast toxicity in the rat. J Clin Invest 1994;94:1069–75.
16. Heyman SN, Brezis M, Reubinoff CA, et al. Acute renal failure with selective medullary injury in the rat. J Clin Invest 1988;82:401–12.
17. Brezis M, Rosen S, Silva P, Epstein FH. Renal ischemia: a new perspective. Kidney Int 1984;26:375–83.
18. Heyman SN, Brezis M, Epstein FH, et al. Early renal medullary hypoxic injury from radiocontrast and indomethacin. Kidney Int 1991;40:632–42.
19. Walker RJ, Fawcett JP. Drug nephrotoxicity – cellular mechanisms. Prog Drug Res 1993;41:3–45.
20. Yoshioka T, Fogo A, Beckman JK. Reduced activity of antioxidant enzymes underlies contrast media-induced renal injury in volume depletion. Kidney Int 1992; 41:1008–15.
21. Tepel M, Van Der Giet M, Schwarzfeld C, et al. Prevention of radiographic contrast agent induced reductions in renal function by acetylcysteine. N Engl J Med 2000;343:180–4.
22. Diaz-Sandoval LJ, Kosowsky BD, Losordo DW. Acetylcysteine to prevent angiography-related renal tissue injury (the APART trial). Am J Cardiol 2001;89:356–8.
23. Cockcroft DW, Gault MH. Prediction of creatinine clearance from serum creatinine. Nephron 1976;16:31–41.
24. Mueller C, Buerkle G, Buettner HJ, et al. Prevention of contrast media-associated nephropathy: randomised comparison of 2 hydration regimens in 1620 patients undergoing coronary angiography. Arch Intern Med 2002;162:329–36.
25. Solomon R, Werner C, Mann D, et al. Effects of mannitol, and frusemide on acute decreases in renal function induced by radiocontrast agents. N Engl J Med 1994; 331:1416–20.
26. Taylor AJ, Hotchkiss D, Morse RW, McCabe J. PREPARED: preparation for angiography in renal dysfunction. A randomised trial of inpatient vs outpatient hydration protocols for cardiac catheterisation in mild to moderate renal dysfunction. Chest 1998;114:1570–4.
27. Schwab SJ, Hlatky MA, Pieper KS, et al. Contrast nephrotoxicity: a randomised controlled trial of a nonionic and an ionic radiographic contrast agent. N Engl J Med 1989; 320:149–53.
28. Briguori C, Manganelli F, Scarpato P, et al. Acetylcysteine and contrast agent-associated nephrotoxcity. J Am Coll Cardiol 2002;40:298–303.
29. Scolari F, Tardnico R, Zani R, et al. Cholesterol crystal embolism: a recognisable cause of renal disease. Am J Kidney Dis 2000;36:1089–109.
30. Thadhani RI, Camargo CA, Xavier RJ, et al. Atheroembolic renal failure after invasive procedures. Natural history based on 52 histologically proven cases. Medicine 1995; 74:350–8.
31. Saklayen MG, Gupta S, Suryaprasad A, Azmeh W. Incidence of atheroembolic renal failure after coronary angiography. A prospective study. Angiology 1997;48:609–13.
32. Fine MJ, Kapoor W, Falanga V. Cholesterol crystal embolization: a reivew of 221 cases in the English literature. Angiology 1987;38:769–84.
33. Kazancioglu R, Erkoc R, Bozfakioglu S, et al. Clinical outcome of renal cholesterol crystal embolization. J Nephrol 1999;12:266–9.
34. Smith MC, Ghose MK, Henry AR. The clinical spectrum of renal cholesterol embolisation. Am J Med 1981;71:174–80.

2

Radiation safety in the catheterization laboratory

Ad den Boer

Introduction

Radiation safety in a cathlab starts with the planning and building of the department. During the construction, protective measures must be built in.

Persons in the investigation room will receive radiation from two sources: the patient (scattering) and the X-ray tube (leakage and scattering).

Personnel dose reduction can be achieved by creating greater distances, shortening the radiation time, using shielding and protection devices, and by extra collimation. Patient dose reduction can be achieved by the use of modern techniques, such as pulsed fluoroscopy with extra beam filtering and extra collimation. Entrance radiation monitoring can be employed to avoid patient skin damage, registration of radiation can be used to optimize the procedure, and the detector dose settings can be adjusted, keeping in mind the ALARA ('as low as reasonably achievable') principle.

The biological risk for investigator and patient, as well as ergonomics, perception, and level of expertise, are described in this chapter.

Room shielding[1-3]

With cardiological equipment, the X-ray beam is restricted to the intensifier or detector size, even when the collimator is fully opened, direct radiation is unable to enter the room. This is why the investigation room needs only be shielded for secondary, scattered, radiation.

Depending on the distance to the wall, 0.25 mm lead shielding should be adequate to meet regulations; however, 2 mm shielding is advised by most suppliers.

In most cathlabs, the position of the patient is determined by the isocenter, and the position of the (scattering) radiation source is known. This allows the room to be constructed in such a way that lead shielding in doors may not be needed, provided that they cannot 'see' the source.

Taken into consideration that there is no secondary backscatter in the diagnostic range, shielding may be omitted above 210 cm from the floor.

Windows between the investigation and control rooms may be provided with lead glass; however, this is manufactured only in a limited range of sizes and is expensive. Normal glass with a thickness of 9 mm gives the same shielding as 0.5 mm of lead, and is available in all sizes. In the Thoraxcenter, Rotterdam, we use 18 mm of float glass between the investigation and control rooms, ending at a height of 210 cm, so that there is an acoustic opening between the ceilings for better communication.

The amount of room shielding is dependent on the quality of the radiation, the absorption of the material used, and the distance to the source.

The half-value layer (HVL) for the quality of radiation in the cathlab for lead is 0.12 mm, for concrete it is 18 mm, and for steel it is 1.9 mm.

Most published data on shielding are calculated with the assumption that direct radiation with a quality of 125 kV is entering the room.

The efficacy of materials in preventing scattered radiation in the catheterization laboratory can be estimated from the density of material (Table 2.1).

For cardiological investigations, one can see the patient as the radiation source with a dose rate of 0.1 mSv/h 1 meter distance from the isocenter. The maximum dose outside the room should not exceed 1 mSv/yr and that outside the building 0.1 mSv/yr.

Table 2.1   Densities of various materials

Material	Density (kg/dm³)	Material	Density (kg/dm³)	Material	Density (kg/dm³)
Mercury	13.5	Water	0.998	Aluminum	2.70
Copper	8.96	Iron	7.87	Lead	11.36
Concrete	1.5–2.4	Brownstone	3.4	Plaster	2.32
Glass (normal)	2.6	Glass (flint)	3.1–3.9	Granite	2.6–2.7
Sand	1.6	Street stone	1.5–2.0	PMMA	1.2

Additional shielding between the patient and the investigator is for the protection of personnel and is essential in interventional cathlabs (see the subsection below on 'Personnel protection').

Personnel dose reduction[1,4–10]

Scattered radiation

The radiation levels using digital cine mode (DCM) are about five times higher than during fluoroscopic imaging. The use of flat panel technology will bring the DCM and fluoroscopy radiation levels closer. At present, flat panel technology needs high dose levels for fluoroscopy compared with vacuum image intensifiers with video chains.

A small source-to-image distance (SID) requires the smallest dose. The larger the field of view (FOV) image size, the lower the dose; however, with large fields, the patient's own absorption of scattered radiation is less, giving a higher occupational dose. With flat panel technology, a larger FOV requires not a lower dose.

Extra collimation always reduces the doses for patient and operator. Scattered radiation levels from 0.2 to 4 mGy/h have been reported.[11]

For each diagnostic procedure, the investigator may receive a dose of 0.1–1.5 mGy, depending on the distance to the patient and the gantry angulation. The use of an extra screen between the investigator and the patient may reduce the head/neck dose by a factor of 10.[12]

In our practice, the scattered radiation levels at the investigator's cornea are less than 1 mSv/h (using 12.5 frame/s pulsed fluoroscopy, standing at the right side of the patient, at the groin); see Figure 2.1, in which three fluoroscopic techniques are compared.

Using the maximum dosages indicated on personal dosimeters (years 1996–2000), we calculated that the maximum dose received by an interventional cardiologist, based on 150 working days per year and four interventions per day, is 60 mSv/yr. The effective dose, wearing a special procedure apron (0.25 mm lead equivalent) and a thyroid protector and regularly using an extra screen between the patient and investigator, is less than 5 mSv/yr.

Tube leakage radiation

According to regulations, the X-ray tube leakage radiation level of 1 mSv/h must be measured at 1 m distance from the focal spot during fluoroscopy with the maximum tube voltage and the maximum allowed continuous current. Modern tubes are capable of working with a continuous current of more than 30 mA (3600 W/s). Tubes used in cardiology meet this specification and have much lower values; however, during intervention, the physician is often standing at a distance of 10 cm from the tube. At this distance, the radiation level may theoretically be 1 Sv/h, which is too high. Radiation levels of more than 0.2 mSv/h measured against the tube, due to scattering from the patient, are not exceptional.

The allowable leakage radiation norms should be much less for tubes used in a room where personnel need to stand adjacent to the gantry during the investigation. While modern tubes are externally cooled, there is (from a heat capacity point of view) no problem in adding extra shielding. Equally, the extra weight of shielding does not create a mechanical problem. In our opinion, the industry should aim for a maximal leakage level of less than 0.01 mSv/h at the surface of the tube and collimator.

Extra shielding (Figure 2.2) with lead flaps mounted under the table to avoid an extra dose from tube leakage radiation is not necessary if the tube leakage is <0.01 mSv/h.

A simple test can be performed to see tube leakage radiation: place a film against the tube, perform fluoroscopy for 10 min with maximum tube load (place an amount of copper or lead between the tube and the intensifier until the maximum output is reached) and have the film processed. If there is visible leakage of radiation on the film, ask the radiation safety department to quantify the radiation level and have some extra lead added (Figures 2.3–2.5). Adding extra shielding of 3 mm lead permits over 95% leakage radiation reduction.

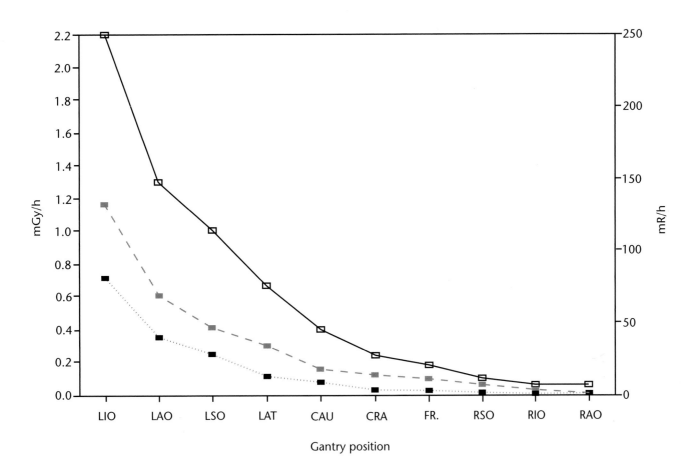

Figure 2.1
Cornea dose in air: radiation levels measured during continuous fluoroscopy with a 300 W/s tube (full line), during pulsed fluoroscopy with a 660 W/s tube (dashed line), and for a high-output (3600 W/s) grid switched tube with pulsed fluoroscopy and extra beam filtration (dotted line). Physician standing at right side of the table. LIO, left interior oblique; LAO, left anterior oblique; LSO, left superior oblique; LAT, lateral; CAU, caudal; CRA, cranial; FR, frontal; RSO, right superior oblique; RIO, right inferior oblique; RAO, right anterior oblique.

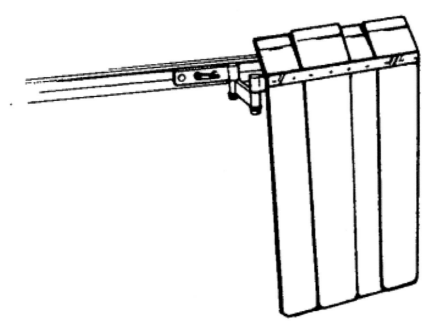
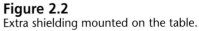

Figure 2.2
Extra shielding mounted on the table.

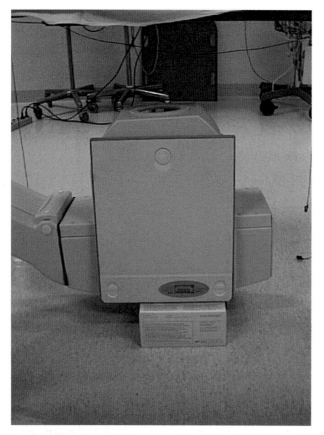

Figure 2.3
Placement of a film cassette against the tube.

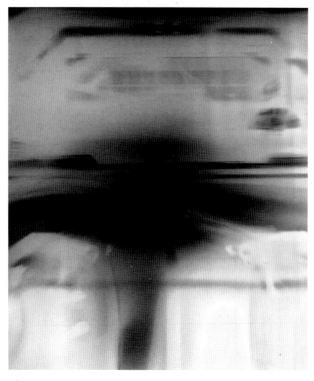

Figure 2.4
Leakage of radiation visible on film.

X-ray beam collimation

There are requirements regarding regulations for the collimator of the X-ray beam. The purpose of these requirements is to limit the X-ray beam to the image intensifier for safety reasons and to keep the amount of patient tissue being exposed to X-rays equal to the region being imaged. If the collimator blades are set too wide, additional patient tissue will be unnecessarily irradiated.

The regulatory requirements state that the X-ray beam must be restricted to (not larger than) the image intensifier phosphor size or detector size when the collimator is fully opened. These conditions are met if the collimator blades are visible on the television monitor during fluoroscopy. On changing to a smaller FOV must implicate that the beam size automatically becomes smaller. Changing to a larger FOV automatically results in a wider beam size; disabling of this function is dose-saving – one then widens the beam size manually, resulting in a beam as large as needed and not as large as possible. Extra collimation is not only dose-saving for the patient but also for the operator, with less tissue being irradiated and less scattering occurring. The patient is the first absorber for the scattered radiation, and more tissue around the radiated part will absorb scattering. Extra collimation increases the image quality, while there is less scattered radiation that creates gray fog on the detector.

Modern collimators are provided with a built-in ionization chamber, measuring the kerma × area product (KAP), the amount of radiation delivered during investigation (kerma = kinetic energy released in matter). Due to different gantry settings, the KAP value is not an indicator of the patient's entrance dose.

With the use of this dosimeter, the geometrical gantry, and patient position, a system has been developed that can monitor the actual entrance dose to avoid possible skin damage due to radiation.[13]

Personnel protection

Lead aprons in the cathlab must give adequate shielding. Special procedure aprons wrapped around the person in order to provide protection over 360° are advised. For optimal protection, a correct fit is essential – oversize armholes and a low collar decrease the efficiency of protection. An equivalency of 0.25 mm lead is sufficient using special procedure aprons; the front is double, giving 0.5 mm protection at the sternum and gonads. Careful handling is important; the best way to achieve this is to provide personnel with their own apron (stitch on names), tailored for a correct fit. The added hygeinic advantage is obvious – nobody likes to work in somebody else's sweaty wet apron. An apron needs cleaning; it may be cleaned in the shower and the inside and outside brushed. New composite materials such as Xenolite, Ergolite, and Ultraflex are lighter, lessening the physical weight on the shoulders and back. The use of a lum-

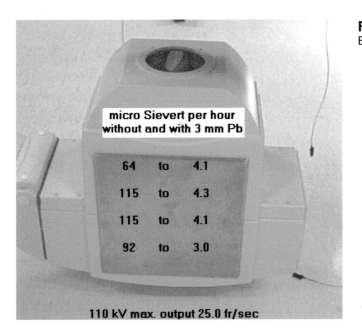

Figure 2.5
Extra shielding mounted and the effect.

bar support belt can take 50% of the weight off the shoulders as does the use of two piece aprons.

Lead-equivalency and attenuation of scattered radiation are related as follows:

* 0.25 mm: 70 kV = 97%, 105 kV = 90%;
* 0.35 mm: 70 kV = 98%, 105 kV = 94%;
* 0.50 mm: 70 kV = 99%, 105 kV = 97%.

To calculate the effective dose, one has to know which body parts are protected and the tissue-weighting factor:

gonads 20%	bone	lung 12%	colon 12%
stomach 12%	marrow 12%	liver 5%	bladder 5%
esophagus 5%	breast 5%	skin 1%	bone surface 1%
remainder 5%.	thyroid 5%		(the total is 100%)

From this list, the first nine items (read horizontally; totals 88) are protected using a special procedure apron; the effective dose is 12%. If a thyroid protector is used as well, the effective dose is 7%. The use of an extra screen between the patient and the operator can reduce the head/neck dose.[12] Measuring the scattered radiation dose per procedure, we found that over 75% of the personnel dose is received from the left projections (Figure 2.6). Using left gantry settings, an extra screen (Figure 2.7) can be placed between the operator (standing on the right side of the table) and the patient, resulting in dramatic dose reductions to the head and neck area (Figure 2.8).

Figure 2.6
Scatter diagram, for projections used.

Scattered radiation per investigation:

Scatter diagram; used projections

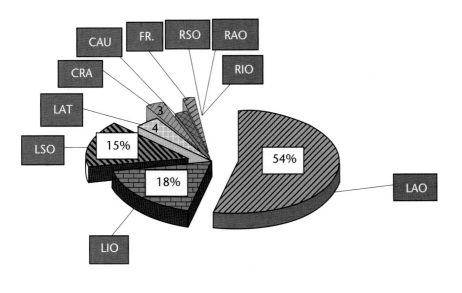

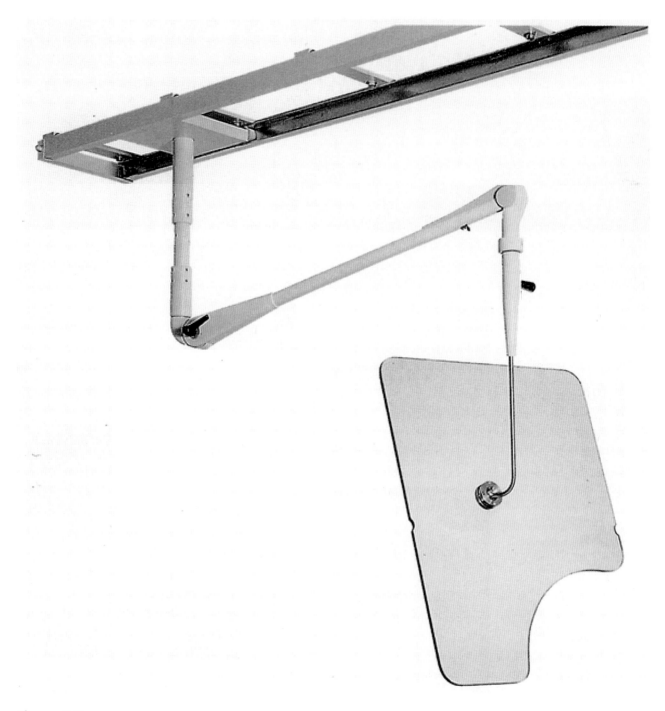

Figure 2.7
An extra screen can be placed between the investigator and patient.

Patient dose reduction

The maximum X-ray tube output during fluoroscopy is required to be 87 mGy/min (10 R/min) at 75 cm distance from the focal spot. In practice, the patient's skin is placed at 60 cm distance and the maximum dose rate is 0.136 Gy/min (15.6 R/min). The shorter the distance to the focal spot, the higher the dose rate. At 35 cm, the dose

rate is more than 43 Gy/min; one only needs a short time to cause severe skin damage to the patient. This is one of the reasons why radiological training is obligatory for investigators administering radiation – such short skin-to-tube placement could be defined as malpractice.

At 75 cm distance, an X-ray tube with a cooling capacity of 300 W/s (100 kV, 3 mA) delivers an output during fluoroscopy greater than 87 mGy/min. The industry is

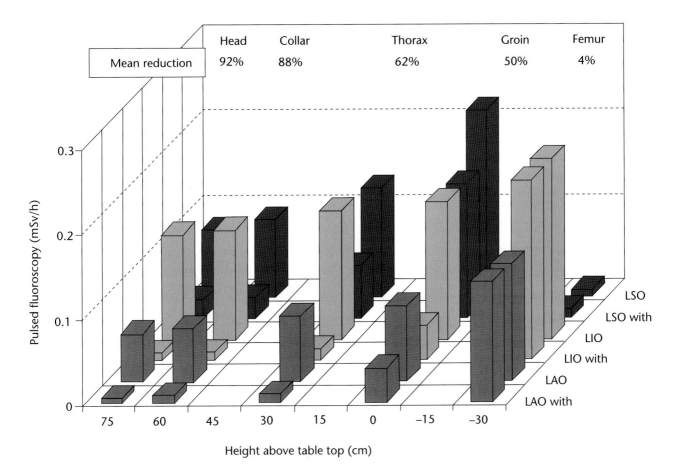

Figure 2.8
Scattered radiation levels with and without the use of an extra screen.

obliged to use a tube filtration of at least 2.5 mm aluminum to limit the output by filtering the low-energy components of the spectrum. Recently, X-ray tubes have been developed with an enormous cooling capacity (>3 kW/s), equivalent to a heat radiator.

Pulsed fluoroscopy, short (high-intensity) pulses to freeze motion, could be developed, due to these high-output tubes, but skin damage is easy to accomplish. The radiation created by an X-ray tube using 80 kV and three types of extra filtering is shown in Figure 2.9. The energy spectrum leaving the patient (20 cm water eqivalent) is shown in Figure 2.10. The difference between Figures 2.9 and 2.10 is the number of photons – over 90% are absorbed by the patient – it also illustrated that almost all photons with an energy less than 30 kV only contributes to absorption and not to image formation. The lowest curve in Figure 2.9 is best suited for imaging. Low-energy photons (<30 kV) only contribute to absorption. This is why extra filtering is very efficient in decreasing the entrance dose to the patient, while maintaining high-quality imaging.[11]

Extra filtering is only possible with high-output tubes, while the filters also weaken the total tube output. A factor of 5 or higher tube output is necessary to compensate

for an extra filter of 2 mm aluminum plus 0.4 mm copper. This is why extra filtering is not possible with 'old' (300–600 W/s) X-ray tubes, where there is insufficient output to allow fluoroscopy on adult patients. The patient entrance dose using different fluoroscopic techniques is shown in Figure 2.11. The entrance dose using high-output tubes with extra filtering may be a factor of 5 lower. Figure 2.11 also shows that removing the extra filters in modern installations with high-output tubes will give an unacceptable, dangerously high dose rate. In the Thoraxcenter, fluoroscopy is performed with an extra filter of 1 mm aluminum plus 0.2 mm copper and 1 mm aluminum plus 0.4 mm copper for DCM, on top of the obligatory 2.5 mm aluminum filter.

Lengthy X-ray guided interventions are increasingly being performed, even with low entrance dose rates, one may harm the patients' skin. Modern units are therefore equipped with X-ray tubes with a build-in ionization chambers, one can measure the amount of radiation used. When one considers the patient entrance dose, the use of X-ray units without pulsed fluoroscopy and X-ray tubes without extra filtering should be forbidden for electrophysiological and other lengthy fluoroscopic investigations and treatments.

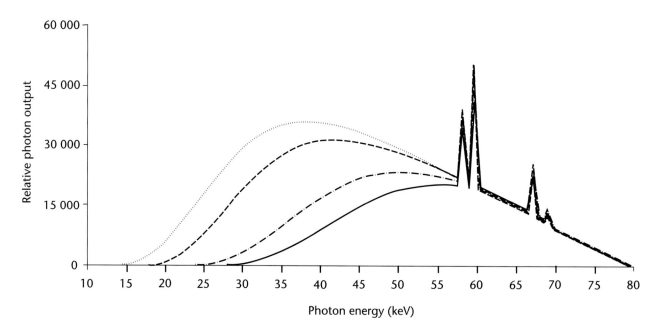

Figure 2.9
The energy spectrum entering the patient's skin at 75 cm skin-to-tube distance. ......, 2 mm Al; ---, 4 mm Al; ---, 4 mm Al + 0.2 mm Cu; ——, 4 mm Al + 0.4 mm Cu.

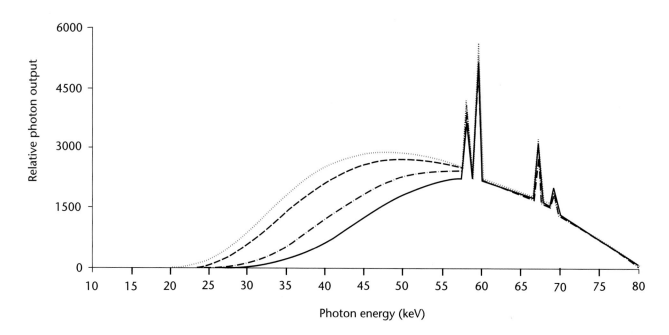

Figure 2.10
The energy spectrum entering the detector at 100 cm skin-to-detector distance (20 cm water equivalent). ......, 2 mm Al; ---, 4 mm Al; ---, 4 mm Al + 0.2 mm Cu; ——, 4 mm Al + 0.4 mm Cu.

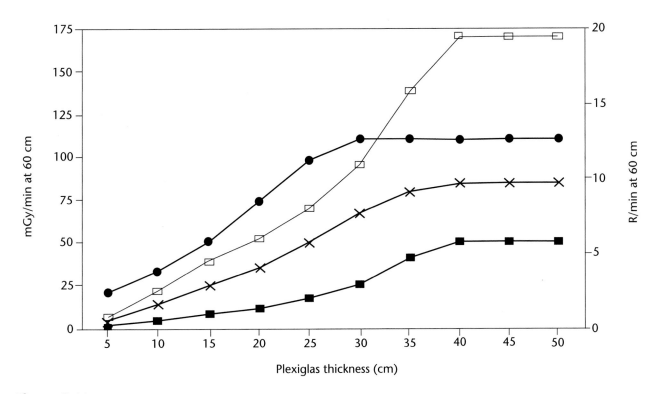

Figure 2.11
Entrance dose reduction using different techniques and extra filters. ●, continuous; ×, pulsed; □, high-output; ■, high-output pulsed plus filter. FFD = 100 cm; 7 inch entrance field.

Registration and monitoring

There is an obligation to record the dose during patient handlings where radiation is used. Modern units can create an X-ray report of an investigation. For the dose measured in the X-ray tube, the kerma × area product is an indicator that is especially useful during interventions.

A recently developed patient entrance dose monitoring system, using the geometrical settings of the gantry and table to calculate the skin dose per square centimeter, enables an investigator to prevent skin damage.[13] A graphical display of this system is shown in Figure 2.12. The actual irradiated skin area is marked as a square (even without fluoroscopy), enabling the physician to avoid overlap with previously irradiated skin parts by extra collimation or changing gantry settings. A dose report is integrated into the display, and the system gives an alarm if the dose at any part of the skin exceeds 1 Gy.

Detector dose settings

The manufacturers of imaging hardware each have different standard settings for their equipment. The higher the dose, the better the image quality. However, the question arises as to whether such quality is always necessary. The higher the dose settings, the greater the dose delivered to the patient and operator and the earlier an X-ray tube will deliver the maximum output. With low dose settings, the X-ray machine is able to penetrate larger objects and more obese patients. Modern equipment must be able to penetrate an amount of water of 40 cm with 110 kV during fluoroscopy before the maximum tube output is reached. Recently, X-ray tubes have been developed with a heat capacity over 3600 W/s, whereas 20 years ago tubes had a cooling capacity of only 300 W/s.

In cardiology, continuous fluoroscopy should no longer be used, since this technique provides a blurred image with moving objects and gives higher personnel dosages. Grid-switched pulsed fluoroscopy has been developed to freeze motion, with low pulse rates (15–12.5, 7.5–6.25 pulses/s) and electronic gap filling. In interventional cardiology, fluoroscopy is the most commonly used tool. Using the ALARA ('as low as reasonably achievable') principle, one has to optimize the X-ray unit in such a way that useful images are obtained with a minimum amount of radiation; one can use a low pulse frequency and accept a certain amount of noise. Of course, the signal noise must not be so high that it results in longer investigation times and the investigator tires.

When non-moving or slowly moving objects are investigated, electronic time filtering can be used to diminish noise; rapidly moving objects may exhibit ghost imaging.

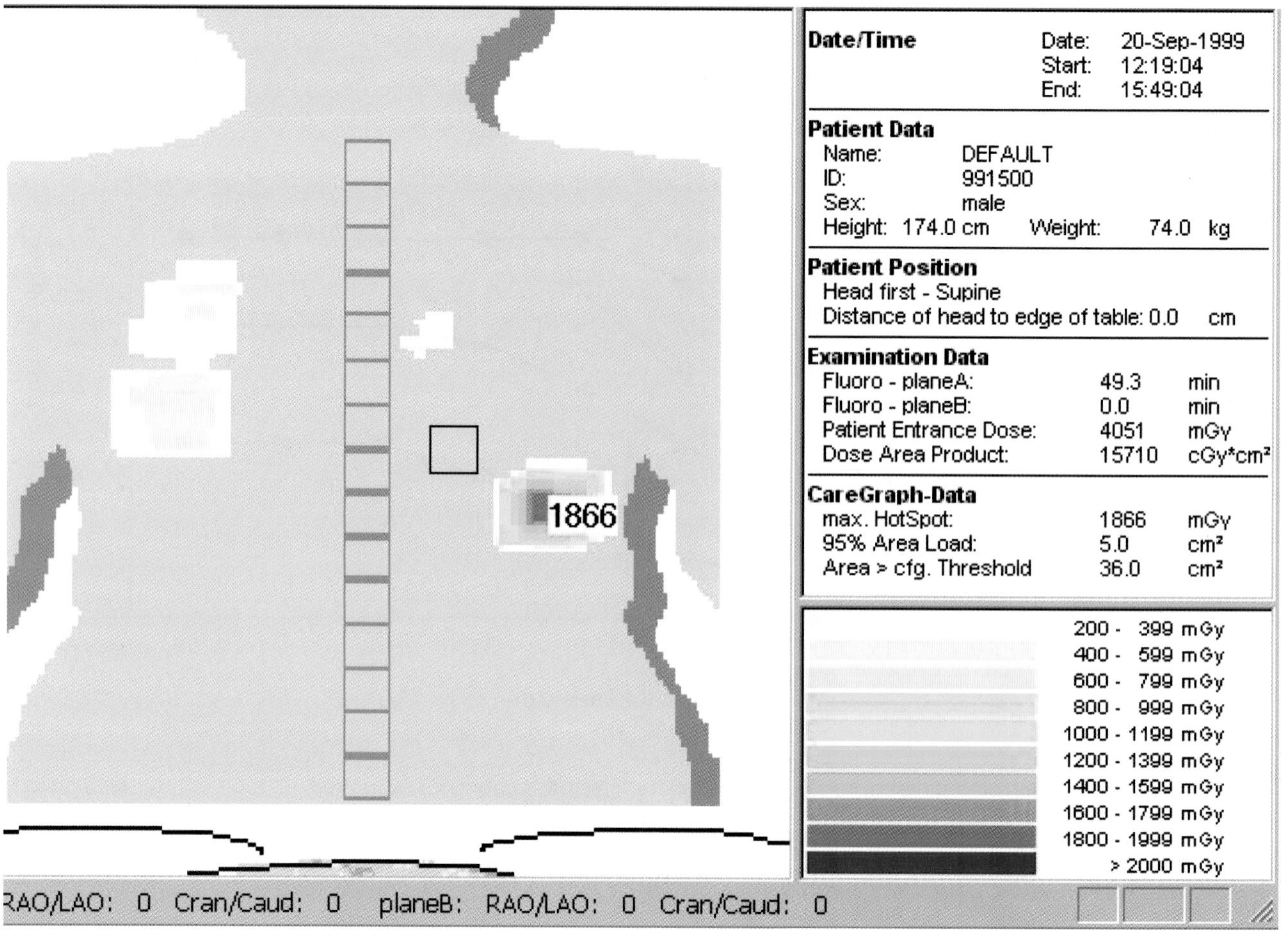

Date/Time		Date:	20-Sep-1999
Start:	12:19:04
End:	15:49:04

Patient Data
Name: DEFAULT
ID: 991500
Sex: male
Height: 174.0 cm   Weight: 74.0 kg

Patient Position
Head first - Supine
Distance of head to edge of table: 0.0   cm

Examination Data
Fluoro - planeA: 49.3   min
Fluoro - planeB: 0.0   min
Patient Entrance Dose: 4051   mGy
Dose Area Product: 15710   cGy*cm²

CareGraph-Data
max. HotSpot: 1866   mGy
95% Area Load: 5.0   cm²
Area > cfg. Threshold   36.0   cm²

200 - 399 mGy
400 - 599 mGy
600 - 799 mGy
800 - 999 mGy
1000 - 1199 mGy
1200 - 1399 mGy
1400 - 1599 mGy
1600 - 1799 mGy
1800 - 1999 mGy
> 2000 mGy

RAO/LAO: 0 Cran/Caud: 0   planeB: RAO/LAO: 0 Cran/Caud: 0

Figure 2.12
Skin dose monitoring can prevent injuries.

We are used to performing fluoroscopy with dose levels of 10/16/28 nGy per pulse on a 23/17/13 cm field size using standard image intensifiers and video chains. With a pulse frequency of 12.5 s^{-1} (normally used) the dose rates during fluoroscopy are 0.13/0.20/0.70 μGy/s. For the digital cine mode (DCM), the detector dose per image is a factor higher. The DCM mode is only used if quantification of images is desired. If the DCM mode is used for documentation (balloon and stent inflation) and no quantification is needed, the vendor should be asked about the possibility of storing fluoroscopic runs, decreasing the dose for patient and operator.

The use of outdated scattered radiation grids which are aluminium-covered and filled should be avoided; renewal of those grids with a carbon fiber-covered and -filled type saves 20% of the needed intensifier dose, due to less absorption, (Figure 2.13).

Modern equipment should be installed and fitted such that it is possible to work with very low dose settings for pulsed fluoroscopy. A detector dose of 10 nGy per image is technically possible using vacuum image intensifiers and modern imaging systems. The upcoming flat panel detectors show superior digital images, but while the detective quantum efficiency (DQE) is lower, one needs higher dose rates for fluoroscopy; future systems will have a higher DQE.

With low dose settings and modern tubes, one should be able to penetrate 40 cm water or polymethyl methacrylate (PMMA, i.e. Plexiglas/Perspex, during fluoroscopy, using a 17 cm (7 inch) field size. The higher the dose rate, the higher the kilovoltage used and the smaller the volume that can be penetrated (Figures 2.14 and 2.15). With low dose settings and the use of a 23 cm (9 inch) field of view, even 50 cm can be penetrated.

The higher the kilovoltage used, the more scattering will occur. A limitation of the highest X-ray energy to 110 kV during fluoroscopy is advisable. The scattered radiation coming from a large object is about 30% less compared with a 125 kV limitation (Figure 2.16). If radiating large objects, there is insufficient tube output at 110 kV, modern imaging chains shall increase the detector signal gain, resulting in a noisy but clear image. If no limitation (125 kV) is used one shall see a less noisy, but grey picture, due to more scattering.

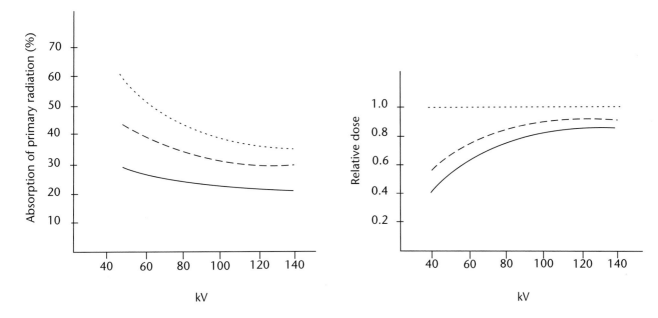

Figure 2.13
Scattered radiation grids and absorption......., aluminum-filled and covered (4 mm Al); –––, aluminum-covered, carbon fiber-filled (2 mm Al); ——, carbon fiber-filled and -covered (0.2 mm Al).

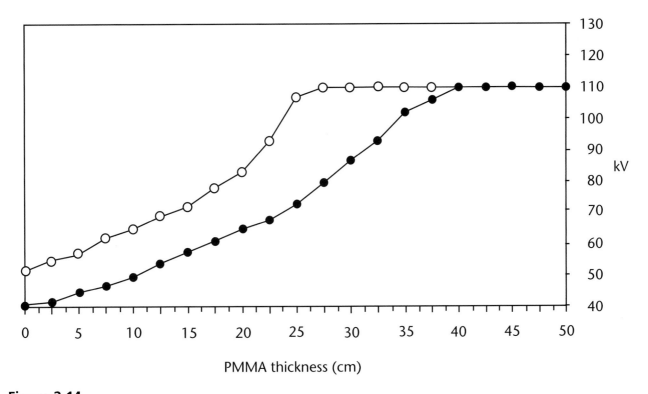

Figure 2.14
Fluoroscopy, penetration and kilovoltage used for different dose rates and an automatic exposure system with a fixed pulse width and coupled kV/mA values. ○, 4 μGy/s; ●, 0.12 μGy/s. 17 cm field size; FFD = 100 cm; 12.5 frames/s.

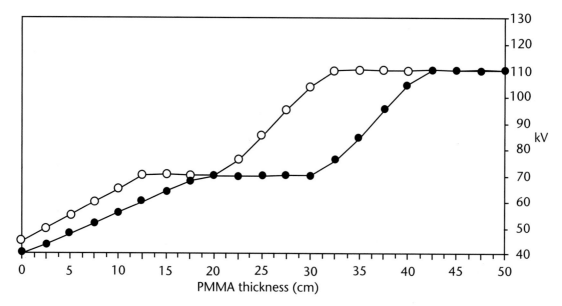

Figure 2.15
Fluoroscopy, penetration and kilovoltage used for different dose rates and an automatic exposure system with a kV plateau and with mA, kV, and pulse width regulation. ○, 4 μGy/s; ●, 0.12 μGy/s. 17 cm field size; FFD = 100 cm; 12.5 frames/s.

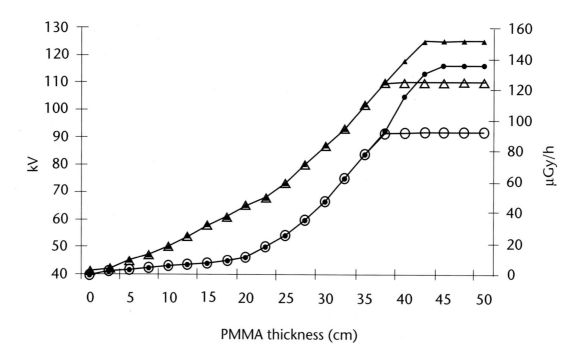

Figure 2.16
Fluoroscopy with and without kV limitation: a field size of 13 cm × 13 cm shows over 30% less scattering. ▲, 125 kV; △, 110 kV; ●, scatter 125 kV; ○, scatter 110 kV.

Biological risks[7,14–17]

Both patients and clinic staff are exposed to radiation during cardiac studies and interventions. Patients' radiation doses are considerably higher, since he/she is in the direct X-ray beam whereas staff are exposed to the scattered radiation, which is lower in magnitude. The personnel is exposed to a cumulative radiation dose from many different cardiac procedures, conducted over many years. Hence, both types of radiation exposure must be assessed for biological risks. Deterministic effects can be seen during a lifetime, mainly effected by cell killing. Stochastic effects are genetic effects and tumor induction.

Cancer risks and risk perception

The patient skin entrance exposure can be readily determined or measured with various types of radiation measurement devices attached directly to the X-ray equipment.[11]

To assess the potential cancer risks, the radiation doses to various organs in the patient's body must be obtained. The Center for Devices and Radiation Health (CDRH) of the US Food and Drug Administration (FDA) has published a Handbook of Selected Tissue Doses for Fluoroscopic and Cineangiographic Examinations of the Coronary Arteries.[18] This Handbook outlines procedures for estimating patient organ doses based upon the skin entrance radiation levels. The data were obtained from Monte Carlo calculations for a mathematical model of a person of a standard size and composition. Data are provided for 11 angiographic views and 6 different beam qualities. With this information, one can utilize NCRP Report 116[7] and NCRP Report 122,[19] can be used to calculate an effective dose equivalent (or effective dose) from radiation badge readings. From these values, the cancer risks can be estimated.

The probability of fatal cancer from exposure to ionizing radiation depends upon the organ dose involved, the type of radiation, and the fractionation of the radiation dose. The fatal cancer risks are quoted as:

- 0.005 per Sv for bone marrow;
- 0.002 per Sv for the breast;
- 0.0085 per Sv for lung tissue;
- 0.0008 per Sv for the thyroid;
- 0.0002 per Sv for the skin.

The most sensitive organs are the gastrointestinal tract, the lungs, the bone marrow, and the bladder.

The Cathlab: effects on the physician

We have calculated that the maximum dose received by an interventional cardiologist per year is 60 mSv. This (worst case) calculation was based on maximum dose measurements (150 working days per year and 4 interventions per day).[13] The effective dose, when wearing a special procedure lead apron (0.25 mm lead equivalent) and a thyroid protector and using an extra screen, is less than 5 mSv/yr. The maximum allowed dose is 20 mSv/yr, the received dosages will not show any deterministic or stochastic effect.

The probability of fatal cancer from exposure is acceptably small with respect to other daily risks.

The patient (Table 2.2)

Giving 1 Sv extra per 100 persons, 5 persons will develop cancer within the next 40 years. This means that the chance is about 0.025–0.033% for the next 40 years. This is negligible compared with the clinical risk of the primary disease process itself. The chance of developing fatal cancer due to

Table 2.2 Cancer risks according to carcinogen, exposure, and site					
Carcinogen	Exposure or circumstance				Cancer site(s)
	Occupational	**Medical**	**Social**	**Environmental**	
Benzene	+				Bone marrow
Asbestos	+			+/–	Lung, pleura, peritoneum
Arsenic	+				Lung, skin
Ionizing radiation	+	+			Marrow, bone, lung, others
Ultraviolet radiation	+		+		Lip, skin
Polycyclic hydrocarbons	+	+		+/–	Skin, scrotum, lung
Alkylating agents		+			Marrow, bladder
Steroids		+			Liver
Alcohol			+		Mouth, pharynx, esophagus, liver
Tobacco smoking			+		As above plus bladder
Overnutrition			+		Endometrium, gallbladder
Hepatitis B	+/–		+	+	Liver
Aflatoxin				+	Liver
Air pollution				+/–	Various
Sexual behavior (virus)			+		Cervix uteri
Population mixing (virus)			+		Marrow, Burkitt lymphoma

+, definite carcinogenic activity or circumstance; +/–, probable carcinogenic activity or circumstance.

the intervention is very small, especially with older patients. The benefit/risk analysis justifies cardiological intervention.

Heart and lungs

As the object of study, the heart receives the largest radiation dose of any internal organ, about 0.02 Gy for adult males undergoing a typical fluoroscopic and cine angiographic examination and over 0.08 Gy with percutaneous coronary intervention (PCI).[20]

Although the myocardium may be capable of enduring fractionated radiotherapy doses as high as 100 Gy without obvious clinical changes, pericarditis has been reported in 7% of patients who were treated for Hodgkin lymphoma and received a total dose less than 6 Gy. Changes seen in the pericardium include pericardial effusion, fibroses, and possibly subsequent constrictive pericarditis. Changes in small arteries, arterioles, and capillaries are most likely responsible for delayed radiation injury to the heart. Injuries to capillaries have been demonstrated after a single dose to the skin as low as 4 Gy. Injury to the microvasculature, and specific damage to endothelial cells, is apparently the most important factor in the delayed non-stochastic effects of radiation.[21]

The extent of radiation-induced damage from catheterization is not known, however, and would be difficult to assess since the myocardium is often already damaged prior to its radiation exposure in the catheterization laboratory.

The lung is a relatively radiosensitive organ, and will typically receive about a 0.01–0.02 Gy dose during percutaneous transluminal coronary angioplasty (PTCA).[20] A single dose of 6–7 Gy has been suggested as a clinical threshold for the development of radiation pneumonitis (inflammation of the lungs). A single dose of 10 Gy to both lungs will cause acute pneumonitis in 84% of patients.[21]

Breasts

Typical breast doses in adults undergoing PTCA are about 0.05 Gy, but in children undergoing lifesaving repairs for congenital abnormalities, the chest dose may vary from 0.01 to 0.025 Gy.[22] Radiation exposure of the infant breast in excess of 3 Gy may produce breast hypoplasia and later deformities.[23] In prepuberty, patient doses of 15–20 Gy delivered over a week as part of a radiation therapy course will impair development.

The cancer mortality risk rate for breast cancer in adult women is 0.0024 per Sv.

It should be noted that an over-table tube gives much higher doses to the breasts and that extra X-ray beam filtering during investigation is possible and worthwhile.

Hematopoietic tissues and gonads

Radiation sensitivity is more pronounced in tissues undergoing rapid reproduction, and thus hematopoietic bone marrow is highly sensitive to ionizing radiation. Bone marrow doses of about 0.02 Gy may be received during angioplasty procedures. Animal studies have shown that doses as low as 0.5 Gy can affect the hematopoietic system; however, the response is dependent on the amount of tissue irradiated.[21]

With the small imaging fields used in catheterization laboratories, hematopoietic radiation syndrome is not usually a concern. In young boys, 24 Gy has been suggested as the critical dose for severe impairment of Leydig cell function in the testes. However, menstrual irregularities may occur in females due to radiation exposures as low as 3 Gy.[24] Temporary sterility in males could occur at radiation doses to the gonads in the range of 1–5 Gy.

Thyroid

Typical thyroid doses are about 0.01 Gy for adults undergoing angioplasty, and are typically less in adults than for pediatric procedures.[25] The individual response to external radiation of the thyroid may be quite variable. Hyperthyroidism may be seen at doses as low as 10 Gy.[23] In adults, the thyroid cancer mortality risk rate is about 0.0008 per Gy.[26] Although exposure to radiation in childhood has been associated with the induction of thyroid tumors and hypothyroidism, most of these data are from children receiving doses for treatment of Hodgkin lymphoma.

Eyes

Cataracts are the most frequent delayed reaction to irradiation of the eyes. The lens of the eye is an avascular structure covered by a capsule. Single doses of 2 Gy or fractioned doses of 4 Gy may result in opacification. The latency period for the production of cataracts from the time of radiation exposure may range from 6 months to as long as 35 years. The typical latency period is 3–7 years. Absorbed doses to the lenses of the eyes exceeding 12 Gy give an almost 100% risk for the development of cataracts.

Skin (Table 6.3)

For complicated cardiac procedures, like PCI and electrophysiological studies, the patient skin entrance radiation

Table 2.3   Radiation effects on skin

Effect	Threshold	Onset	Peak	Comments
Epilation				
Temporary	~3 Gy	~2 wks		New hair is thinner
Permanent	~7 Gy	~2 wks		Protracted threshold, ~50 Gy
Erythema				
Early and transient	~2 Gy	Hours	~24 h	Not an indication for later response
Main effect	~6 Gy	~10 days	~2 wk	Reddening → pigmentation; pigment
	>10 Gy			may last for months
Desquamation				
and ulceration				
Dry desquamation	~10 Gy	~4 wks	~5 wks	
Moist desquamation	~15 Gy	~4 wks	~5 wks	Healing 2 wks to months; late atrophy
Secondary	~20 Gy	<6 wks		Dermal effect; ulceration secondary to
				sterilized basal cells; scarring

dose can range up to 5 Gy or more.[11,18] Radiation doses in this range may result in loss of hair (epilation) and skin reddening (erythema). These effects may occur at exposures as low as 2–3 Gy.[21,24,26] The sequence of radiation-induced skin burns can be described in three stages. Stage 1 (less than a week after exposure) is marked by a relatively prompt and transient erythema. This reddening is due to the release of histamine-like substances and proteolytic enzymes, which increase the permeability of the capillaries. This effect occurs within 1–2 days and then fades. Higher radiation doses result in more rapid identification of the erythema. Stage 2 of erythema is due to vessel damage. Reddening of the skin is followed by an increase in pigmentation due to activation of melanocytes (threshold about 5 Gy). This effect is an inflammatory reaction to depletion of basal cells in the epidermis. A dusky or mauve erythema develops to define stage 3 in 6–10 weeks or more following large radiation doses to the skin.

Healing can occur through repopulation from the edge of the burn if all clonogenic cells are sterilized. Above 18 Gy doses to the skin, vascular damage in the deep dermal plexus is thought to result in a rapid increase of dermal necrosis.

As doses are fractionated, the threshold for skin erythema rises. The smaller the radiated field, the better is the repair. The individual response to external radiation of the skin may be quite variable.

Using modern equipment, pulsed fluorosopy, with low (15 fr/s or less) pulse frequency with extra beam filtering and focal spot to skin distances more than 55 cm, no dermal effects are to be expected, even after a lengthy fluorosopic intervention.

Pregnancy (Table 2.4)

The fetal dose received is about 0.05 mSv for pregnant women undergoing angioplasty. Fluoroscopy in the groin area should be kept as low as possible. Almost all X-ray investigations are less than 30 mSv for the unborn child; most are less than 10 mSv.

The normal incidences of deformations of the fetus with prenatal radiation are shown in Table 2.5. The 8–15 weeks period is the most sensitive time for the fetus.

Patient information

Patients should be supplied with written information, if questions arise, remember to answer in layman's terms, and don't tell the patient what she/he cannot remember. Compare the risks to a fetus with natural incidence of deformation. Compare dose variations with the natural background, UV radiation and skin burn.

State the probability that no adverse effects are seen, place risks in perspective, use a positive approach; don't communicate by phone, but in person.

Table 2.4   Fetal dose and X-ray investigation (NCRP 98)

Investigation	Fetal dose (mSv)	
	Mean	Maximum
Abdomen	1.4	4.2
Colon	6.8	24
Thorax	<0.01	<0.01
CT thorax	0.06	0.96
CT abdominal	8	49
CT pelvis	25	79
PTCA	0.02	0.1

Calculation of dose to fetus

If necessary, the radiation safety department can calculate the fetal dose, using the following data: Fluoroscopy and cine time, the beam size and projections, the kilovoltage, the entrance dose (Gy-cm^2), the filtration, and the focal spot-to-skin distance. These data are available in X-ray and dosimetry reports from modern installations.

Conclusions

Pregnant nurses and technicians may do their normal work in the cathlab and in radiology departments. Pregnant physicians may continue their work; however, if the expected effective dose is more than 1 mSv/yr, then it may be preferable to decrease total exposure.

Local radiation protection regimes can be stricter, and may advise physicians not to perform interventions during pregnancy.

Under normal circumstances, radiological investigation should *not* exceed the deterministic threshold values.

The changes in stochastic effects are small.

Summary

The radiation doses from cardiac catheterization studies to patients and personnel are typically much lower than the levels thought to be necessary to produce significant biological effects in tissues exposed to radiation. However, suboptimal procedures, equipment malfunctions, frequently repeated studies, and/or difficult interventional procedures could easily drive patient radiation doses into the clinically relevant range.

Incidents of severe skin erythema in cardiac catheterization laboratories have been reported.[4,13,23,25,27–40] Moreover, radiation-induced cancer risk is a stochastic

process in which the relative magnitude of the risk increases with the cumulative radiation exposure.

It is therefore important to provide good quality assurance procedures in cardiac catheterization laboratories in order to optimize image quality while minimizing the levels of radiation to which patients and laboratory staff are exposed.

Ergonomics and perception
Physician comfort

The physician should adjust the investigating table to the optimal working height and the gantry position should be adapted to the correct isocenter. Unfortunately, few gantries are produced that allow elevation of the C or U arm. In biplane units, the isocenter is fixed, so that the table top has to be adjusted more than necessary. Placing the patient in a fixed isocenter means in general that the working height is suboptimal. Both situations are bad from an ergonomic point of view; the spinal column already has to deal with a lead apron, and moving the table top is an extra burden.

Patient comfort

Due to standardization of catheterization laboratories, fewer types of investigation tables are being produced, and these are not designed for patient comfort. Probably the best improvement with regard to patient comfort in the last decade or so is the use of temper foam mattresses. Better tables need to be developed; sedation of patients during long treatment should seldom be necessary.

Table 2.5   Radiation effects on the fetus

Period of exposure	Effect	Incidence (%)	Comments
Until 8 days	Spontaneous abortion	50–75	Rejection – all or nothing
9 days–8 weeks	Deformation of organs	6	Small change – a relatively high dose is needed
8–15 weeks	Mental retardation	0.5	0.5–1 Sv: brain damage, from lower IQ to severe incomplete development
After 15 weeks	Childhood cancer	0.1	0.5 Sv: delayed growth, mental retardation (3 IQ points per 100 mSv)

The (stochastic) effect of juvenile cancer, the chance of no incidence: to 13 weeks after conception: 0 mSv = 99.93%; 10 mSv = 99.75%; 50 mSv = 99.12%. After 13 weeks, 0 mSv = 99.93%, 10 mSv = 99.88%; 50 mSv = 99.70%.

A dose of 30 mSv from week 4; an extra chance of 0.5% of fatal tumor induction (An airplane flight from Atlanta to Amsterdam + return gives a dose of 0.04 mSv.)

Perception

Video screens used in cathlabs should be placed in one line with the working field so that one can see the X-ray image by simply changing eye direction. The room lights must be adjustable; the background light level around the monitors should be about the same as the mean intensity of the image for optimal perception. The monitor screens should be cleaned regularly and a test image should be viewed routinely to ensure that work is done under optimal conditions.

Expertise, competency, and ALARA[41]

Radiation can be harmful, and medical treatment should only be performed by a radiologically trained and qualified physician – 'no expertise is no performance'.

Medical X-ray exposure is the responsibility of a qualified physician. Justification, optimization, good medical practice, and medical investigation according to the ICRP 62 norms[41] are items that must be known by all qualified physicians. Training in radiation protection is a basic aspect of the optimization of medical exposures.

Safety considerations

In general, every European country has its own basic nuclear laws, which differ between countries. Radiation protection is basically determined by two principles: exposure must be justified by showing that it confers more benefit than harm, and exposure should be as low as reasonable achievable (the ALARA principle).

References

1. IEC Publication 407. Basic Safety Standards for the Health of Workers and the General Public Against the Dangers Arising from Ionization Radiation.
2. ICRP Publication 60. Recommendations of the International Commission on Radiological Protection. Ann ICRP 1991;22 (3):Nos 1–3.
3. Radiation Shielding for Diagnostic X-rays. Report of a Joint BIR/IPEM Working Party. British Institute of Radiology, February 2000.
4. European Directive 96/29 Euratom. Official Journal L 1996;159:0001–0114.
5. European Directive 84/446 Euratom. Official Journal L 1997;180:0022–0027.
6. NCRP Report 99, 1990. Distance Source to Patient, min. Source-to-Skin Distance.
7. NCRP Report 116, 1993. Limitation of Exposure to Ionizing Radiation.
8. NCRP Report 112, 1991. Calibration Of Survey Instruments Used in Rad. Protection.
9. ICRP Publication 59. The Biological Basis for Dose Limitation in the Skin. Ann ICRP 1991;20:No. 2.
10. Report No78, 1997. Institute of Physics and Engineering in Medicine. Catalogue of Diagnostic X-ray Spectra Book Spectrum and Other Data. ISBN 0904 1812 88X
11. den Boer A, de Feijter PJ, Hummel WA, et al. Reduction of radiation exposure while maintaining high-quality fluoroscopic images during interventional cardiology using novel X-ray tube technology with extra beam filtering. Circulation 1994;6:2710–14.
12. den Boer A, de Feijter PJ, Ruigrok P. Fluoroscopy during cardiac interventional procedures, an overview of radiological developments in the last decennium. Thoraxcenter J 1994;3:8–14.
13. den Boer A, de Feijter PJ, Serruys PW, Roelandt JRTC. Real-time quantification and display of skin radiation during coronary angiography and intervention. Circulation 2001; 104:1779–84.
14. AAPM Report No.70 (February 2001). Biological Risks Associated with Radiation Exposure in the Cathlab.
15. NCRP Report 115, 1993. Risk Estimates For Radiation Protection.
16. IAEA TECDOC 870, April 1996. Methods for Estimating the Probability of Cancer from Occupational Radiation Exposure.
17. Batter S, Shope TB (eds). Syllabus: A Categorical Course in Physics: Physical and Technical Aspects of Angiography and Interventional Radiology. Oak Brook, IL: Radiological Society of North America, 1995:167–70.
18. Stern SH, Rosenstein M, Renaud L, Zankl M. Handbook of Selected Tissue Doses for Fluoroscopic and Cineangiographic Examination of the Coronary Arteries. US Department of Health and Human Resources Publication FDA 95-8288, September 1995.
19. NCRP Report 122, 1995. Limitation of Exposure to Ionizing Radiation for Clinical Staff.
20. Pattee PL, Johns PC, Chambers RJ. Radiation risk to patients from percutaneous transluminal coronary angioplasty. J Am Coll Cardiol 1993;22:1044–51.
21. Mettler FA Jr, Upton AC. Medical Effects of Ionizing Radiation, 2nd edn. Philadelphia: WB Saunders, 1995.
22. Waldman JP, Rummerfield PS, Gilpin EA, Kirkpatrick SE. Radiation exposure to the child during cardiac catheterization. Circulation 1981;64:158–63.
23. Schueler BA, Julsrud PR, Gray JE, et al. Radiation exposure and efficacy of exposure techniques during cardiac catheterization in children. AJR 1994;162:173–7.
24. Scherer E, Streffer C, Trott KR (eds). Radiopathology of Organs and Tissues. New York: Springer-Verlag, 1991.
25. Martin EC, Olson AP, Steeg CN, Casarellas WJ. Radiation exposure on the pediatric patient during cardiac catheterization and angiography. Circulation 1981;64:153–63.
26. Pratt TA, Shaw AJ. Factors affecting the radiation dose to the lens of the eye during cardiac catheterization procedures. Br J Radiol 1993;66:346–50.
27. Scott NS. Reports on 69 cases of injuries associated with rays, 6 of which were caused by the patients conditions, but most of which were burns caused by X rays. Am X-Ray J 1897;1:57–66.
28. Calkins H, Niklason L, Sousa J, et al. Radiation exposure during radiofrequency catheter ablation of accessory atrioventricular connections. Circulation 1991;84:2376–82.

29. Cascade PN, Peterson LE, Wajszczuk WJ, et al. Radiation exposure to patients undergoing percutaneous transluminal coronary angioplasty. Am J Cardiol 1987;9:996–7.

30. Huda W, Peters KR. Radiation-induced temporary epilation after a neuroradiogically guided embolization procedure. Radiology 1994;193:642–4.

31. Kovoor P, Rieciardello M, Collins L, et al. Risk to patients from radiation associated with radiofrequency ablation for supraventricular tachycardia. Circulation 1998;15:1534–40.

32. Malkinson FD. Radiation injury to skin following fluoroscopically guided procedures. Arch Dermatol 1996;6:695–6.

33. Geise RA, Peters NE, Dunnigan A, Milstein S. Radiation dose during pediatric radiofrequency catheter ablation procedures. Pacing Clin Electrophysiol 1996;11:1605–11.

34. Karpinnen J, Parviainen T, Servomaa A, Komppa T. Radiation risk and exposure of radiologists and patients during coronary angiography and percutaneous transluminal coronary angioplasty (PTCA). Radiat Prot Dosim 1995;57:481–5.

35. Sovik E, Klow NE, Hellesnes J, et al. Radiation induced skin injury after percutaneous transluminal coronary angioplasty. Acta Radiol 1996;3:305–6.

36. Nahass GT. Acute radiodermatitis after radiofrequency catheter ablation. J Am Acad Dermatol 1997;5:881–4.

37. Lichtenstein DA, Klapholz L, Vardy DA, et al. Chronic radiodermatitis following cardiac catheterization. Arch Dermatol 1996;6:663–7.

38. D'Incan M, Roger H. Radiodermatitis following cardiac catheterization. Arch Dermatol 1997;2:242–3.

39. Shope TB. Radiation-induced skin injuries from fluoroscopy. Radiographics 1996;5:1195–9.

40. Knautz MA, Abele DC, Reynolds TL. Radiodermatitis after transjugular intrahepatic portosystemic shunt. South Med J 1997;3:352–6.

41. ICRP Publication 62. Protection in Biomedical Research. Ann ICRP 1991;22(3).

42. European Community Council Directive 96/29/EURATOM of 13 May 1996 laying down basic safety standards for the protection of the health of workers and the general public against the dangers arising from ionizing radiation. Official Journal L 159, 29/06/1996 P. 0001–0114.

43. European Community Council Directive 97/43/EURATOM of 30 June 1997 on health protection of individuals against the dangers of ionizing radiation in relation to medical exposure and repealing. Directive 84/466/Euratom Official Journal L 180, 09/07/1997 P. 0022–0027.

44. Handbook of health physics and radiological health. B. Shleien, LA Slaback and BK Birky. ISBN 0–683–18334–6.

Appendix A: Organizations

AAPM: American Association of Physicists in Medicine (www.aapm.org)
ARPS: Australian Radiation Protection Society (www.arps.org.au)
CDRH: Center for Devices and Radiation Health of the US Food and Drug Administration (www.fda.gov/cdrh/)
EURATOM: European Economic Community and the European Atomic Energy Community (http://europa.eu.int/abc/treaties_en.htm)
IAEA: International Atomic Energy Agency (www.iaea.org)
IRPA: Radiation Protection Association (www.irpa.net)
ICRP: International Committee of Radiological Protection (www.icrp.org)
IEC: International Electronical Commission (www.iec.ch)
NCRP: National Committee of Radiological Protection (www.ncrp.org)
RPB-HC: Radiation Protection Bureau – Health Canada (www.hc-sc.gc.ca/ehp/ehd/rpb)
UNSCEAR: United Nations Scientific Committee on the Effects of Atomic Radiation (www.unscear.org)
USEU: The United States Mission to the European Union (www.useu.be)

Appendix B: Nomenclature
International System of units (SI)

Exposure: 1 sievert (Sv) = 1 gray (Gy) = 1 J/kg = 100 roentgen (R)
Absorbed dose: Gy (previously rad ('radiation absorbed dose'): 1 rad = 0.01 Gy)
Equivalent dose: Sv (previously rem ('radiation equivalent man'): 1 rem = 0.01 Sv)
Effective dose: Sv
Collective effective dose: man Sv
Activity: Becquerel (Bq) (previously curie (Ci): 1 Ci = 3.7×10^{10} Bq)

Conversion factors

1 R = 0.258 mC/kg in air
1 R = 8.73 mGy in air and 9.2 mGy in muscle tissue
100 R = 1 Gy
1 Curie (Ci) = 37 Giga Becquerel (GBq);
1 mCi = 37 MBq
1 Bq = 2.7×10^{-11} Ci
1 Joule (J) = 1 Coulomb (C)

3

Current use of antiplatelet agents

Brett M Sasseen, Deepak L Bhatt

Introduction

Platelets play an important role in arterial thrombosis that leads to acute myocardial infarction (MI), stroke, and acute coronary syndromes.[1,2] Once endothelial disruption occurs, platelet adhesion, activation, and aggregation rapidly ensue, and a thrombotic event may then result.[3,4] Antiplatelet drugs may reduce the occurrence of arterial thrombosis. Current antiplatelet drugs include aspirin, the thienopyridines, and oral and intravenous glycoprotein IIb/IIIa inhibitors.

Oral antiplatelet agents

Aspirin

While the antipyretic and anti-inflammatory properties of salicylates were described more than 2400 years ago, acetylsalicylic acid was first introduced commercially in 1899. In 1948, Gibson[5] first proposed the use of salicylic acid for the treatment of coronary thrombosis. The critical role of aspirin became apparent with ISIS-2, which demonstrated a significant 21% reduction in mortality with its use in acute MI.[6]

Aspirin irreversibly acetylates prostaglandin H synthase, also known as cyclooxygenase (COX). The COX-1 isoform is expressed in most cells, including platelets, whereas COX-2 is rapidly induced only after exposure to inflammatory cytokines. Aspirin is a relative selective inhibitor of COX-1 and is 170-fold less potent in inhibiting COX-2.[7] Inhibition of COX-1 reduces levels of thrombox-ane A2, a potent vasoconstrictor and agonist of platelet aggregation, and also results in inhibition of endothelial cell production of prostacyclin, a vasodilator. Because mature platelets are anucleated and lack the ability to synthesize new COX, aspirin inhibits platelet function throughout its lifespan of 8–10 days.[8]

Aspirin is rapidly absorbed in the stomach and small intestine and can act on platelets with bioavailability close to 50% with single doses up to 1300 mg.[7] The inhibitory effects of aspirin are dose-dependent within the range of 5–100 mg daily. Daily doses of 75–100 mg produce almost-complete suppression of thromboxane synthesis within a few days. When 325 mg of aspirin is given orally, a maximal inhibition of thromboxane A2 occurs by 30 minutes.[9]

Secondary prevention trials

In ISIS-2, 17 187 patients with acute MI were randomized to intravenous streptokinase, oral aspirin (160 mg daily for 1 month), both, or neither. In addition to the 23% risk reduction in 5-week vascular mortality among patients receiving streptokinase, there was a 21% reduction among those receiving aspirin, and a 40% reduction among those receiving a combination of streptokinase and aspirin, which are all significant reductions.[6] This reduction in mortality also persisted at 15 months of follow-up. In this study, aspirin reduced the risk of non-fatal reinfarction by 49% and nonfatal stroke by 46%. Aspirin abolished the increased risk of early nonfatal rein-farction when streptokinase therapy was used alone (3.8% with streptokinase versus 1.3% with streptokinase plus aspirin).[6] This study demonstrated that short-term aspirin for acute MI decreases mortality and reinfarction,

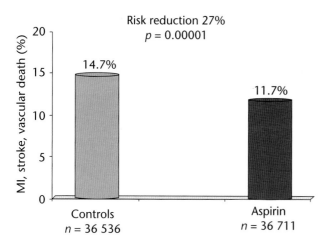

Figure 3.1
Antiplatelet trialists' meta-analysis demonstrating significant reduction in overall vascular events with aspirin. (Adapted from Antiplatelet Trialists' Collaboration. BMJ 1994;308:81–106.[11])

with benefits in addition to SK, and prevents the increase in reinfarction that is seen after thrombolytic therapy. Although aspirin was associated with an increased rate of minor bleeding from 1.9% to 2.5%, major bleeding, including hemorrhagic stroke, was not increased. Aspirin therapy, with a dose of 160–325 mg, is desirable for all patients with acute MI.[6,10]

The Antiplatelet Trialists' Collaboration meta-analysis included 145 randomized trials of prolonged antiplatelet therapy versus placebo in 70 000 patients with vascular disease and 30 000 low-risk patients from the general population (Figure 3.1).[11] In the high-risk patients, antiplatelet therapy reduced vascular mortality (risk reduction (RR) 18%; $2p < 0.0001$), nonfatal MI (RR 35%; $2p < 0.0001$), nonfatal stroke (RR 31%; $2p < 0.0001$), and combined vascular events (nonfatal MI, nonfatal stroke, and vascular death) (RR 27%; $2p < 0.0001$).[11] Among 20 000 patients who had acute MI, vascular events occurred in 10.6% receiving antiplatelet therapy versus 14.4% on placebo (RR 29%, $2p < 0.0001$). In this group, aspirin prevented 38 vascular events per 1000 treated for 1-month. This benefit extended out to 2 years. Aspirin should be administered indefinitely to all patients with vascular disease who do not have any contraindications (Figure 3.1).

Aspirin in unstable angina

In unstable angina, aspirin use was associated with a significant risk reduction in the rates of all-cause mortality or cardiac death and nonfatal MI. Aspirin reduced the risk of fatal or nonfatal MI by 71% at 7 days,[12,13] by 60% at 3 months,[14] and by 50% at 2 years.[15] In the Antiplatelet Trialists' Collaboration meta-analysis, aspirin use reduced

vascular events after 6 months in 4000 unstable angina patients from 14% to 9% ($p < 0.00001$). The risk of MI, stroke, or vascular death was reduced by greater than 25% in this patient group.[11]

Primary prevention

In the Physicians' Health Study, 22 071 male US physicians were randomized to aspirin 325 mg every other day or to placebo.[16] The primary outcome of cardiovascular death was not different between the aspirin group (0.23% per year) and placebo (0.24% per year). The total death rate was also similar between the two groups (aspirin, 0.4% per year, placebo 0.42% per year). However, the rate of MI was significantly reduced by 44% with aspirin (0.26% per year) as compared with placebo (0.44% per year; $p < 0.00001$). The observed overall stroke rate was slightly higher with aspirin (0.22% per year) as compared with placebo (0.18% per year; $p = 0.15$).[10,16] In addition, the rate of hemorrhagic stroke was also increased with aspirin (0.04% per year) versus the placebo group (0.02%; $p = 0.06$). The combined outcome of 'important vascular events' (nonfatal MI, nonfatal stroke, and death from a cardiovascular cause) was significantly reduced in the aspirin group (0.56% per year) as compared with the placebo group (0.68% per year, relative risk reduction 18%, $p = 0.01$).

The most appropriate dose of aspirin has not been clear until recently. Aspirin in such low doses as 40 mg daily has been shown to inhibit platelet cyclooxygenase irreversibly.[17] Higher doses impair endothelial prostacyclin production. Aspirin has been shown to reduce ischemic cardiac events in three of four primary prevention trials, the most beneficial effect being seen for nonfatal MI.[16,18–20] In the US Physicians' Trial and the UK Doctors' Trial, there was a trend toward increased total stroke and hemorrhagic stroke with aspirin, while there was a trend toward lower stroke with aspirin in the Thrombosis Prevention Trial (TPT) and the Hypertension Optimal Treatment (HOT) trial.[16,18–20] In the latter two trials, a much lower dose of aspirin (75 mg) was used daily. In addition, in a study of 2849 patients undergoing carotid endarterectomy who were randomized to either low doses (81 or 325 mg) or higher doses (650 or 1300 mg) of aspirin, the combined endpoint of risk of death, MI, or stroke was lower among patients receiving the two lower doses of aspirin at 30 days (5.4% versus 7.0%; $p = 0.07$) and at 3 months (6.2% versus 8.4%; $p = 0.03$).[21] Both for primary prevention and for chronic use in secondary prevention, the use of lower-dose aspirin (75–81 mg daily) may reduce the risk of ischemic events while minimizing the risk of hemorrhagic stroke and gastrointestinal bleeding.

In men with risk factors such as diabetes mellitus, hypertension, smoking, and older age, the reduction of ischemic cardiac and cerebrovascular events by the prophylactic use of aspirin probably outweighs the risk of hemorrhagic stroke and gastrointestinal and other bleeding.[10]

The Antithrombotic Trialists' Collaboration performed a meta-analysis of studies comparing antiplatelet therapy with placebo as well as different antiplatelet regimens in patients at high risk of occlusive vascular events.[22] Among these high-risk patients, antiplatelet therapy reduced the combined outcome of any serious vascular event by about one-quarter, nonfatal MI by one-third, nonfatal stroke by one-quarter, and vascular mortality by one-sixth. Similar reductions in vascular events were also seen in patients with diabetes mellitus, hemodialysis patients, patients with peripheral arterial disease, and those with carotid disease. In addition, aspirin at a dose of 75–150 mg daily produced a larger relative risk reduction in vascular events (32%) compared with higher doses. Consequently, this new evidence supports the view that aspirin should be used in daily doses of 75–150 mg for the long-term prevention of serious vascular events in high-risk patients, which should also include patients with diabetes mellitus, chronic renal failure or hemodialysis patients, and those with carotid disease.[22]

Use of aspirin in the cardiac catheterization laboratory

Two randomized trials comparing aspirin and dipyrimadole versus placebo showed significant reductions in ischemic complications in patients undergoing angioplasty.[23,24] One study demonstrated that Q-wave MI was significantly reduced, while the other showed that acute vessel closure occurred less frequently with the use of aspirin and dipyrimadole in patients undergoing angioplasty. Unless contraindicated, all patients undergoing percutaneous coronary interventions should receive aspirin.

Ticlopidine

Ticlopidine and clopidogrel are members of the class of thienopyridines (Figure 3.2). The structure of the molecules are similar; clopidogrel has an additional carboxymethyl side chain (Figure 3.2). Both drugs inhibit the binding of adenosine 5'-diphosphate (ADP) to the platelet ADP receptors, which prevents upregulation of the glycoprotein IIb/IIIa receptor and ultimately reduces binding of fibrinogen to the IIb/IIIa receptor.[25–27] These molecules also reduce thrombosis due to shear stress and increase the bleeding time by a factor of two.[28] These platelet effects are irreversible and last for the lifetime of the platelet. They do not affect the activated clotting time or the partial thromboplastin time.

Ticlopidine is a prodrug, and is metabolized to its active metabolite by the liver. The peak plasma level of the metabolite is 2 hours; however, it takes 5–7 days to achieve maximal platelet inhibition.[29] This delayed antiplatelet effect has been manifested as early subacute stent thrombosis.

Secondary prevention trials

In a meta-analysis by the Antiplatelet Trialists' Collaboration, ticlopidine compared with aspirin resulted in a non-significant 10% relative risk reduction in vascular death, MI, and stroke in patients with vascular disease.[11] However, ticlopidine compared with placebo resulted in a significant 33% relative risk reduction in vascular death, MI, and stroke in patients with vascular disease. In the Studio della Ticlopidinia nell'Angina Instabile Groupe, ticlopidine or placebo was administered to patients with unstable angina for 6 months. The ticlopidine group had a significant reduction in the combined endpoint of nonfatal MI or vascular death (7.3% versus 13.6%), for a relative risk reduction of 46% ($p = 0.009$).[30]

Use of ticlopidine in the cardiac catheterization laboratory

In two studies of patients not receiving aspirin undergoing angioplasty, ticlopidine significantly reduced the frequency of abrupt vessel closure.[24,31]

With the advent of coronary stenting, anticoagulation with warfarin and aspirin became the initial regimen, at a

Ticlopidine

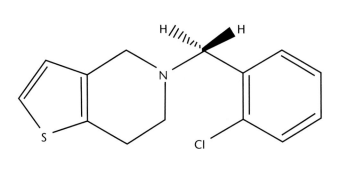

Clopidogrel

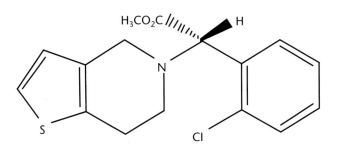

Figure 3.2
Structures of the thienopyridines ticlopidine and clopidogrel. (Adapted from Quinn MJ and Fitzgerald DJ. Circulation 1999;100:1667–72[41] with permission from Lippincott Williams & Wilkins.)

cost of increased bleeding and vascular complications. Five studies examined the use of ticlopidine plus aspirin, warfarin plus aspirin, or aspirin alone after coronary stenting to prevent acute and subacute thrombosis. All studies demonstrated equivalent or superior results with the combination of ticlopidine and aspirin, with a significant reduction in hemorrhagic complications.[32–36]

In the Full Anticoagulation versus Aspirin and Ticlopidine (FANTASTIC) study, 485 patients undergoing stenting were randomized to aspirin plus ticlopidine or aspirin plus warfarin. A primary endpoint of bleeding or peripheral vascular complications occurred in 33 patients (13.5%) in the antiplatelet group and 48 (21%) in the anticoagulation group (odds ratio 0.6; 95% confidence interval (CI) 0.36–0.98; $p = 0.03$).[36] Major cardiac-related events (death, infarction, or stent occlusion) in electively stented patients were less common (odds ratio 0.23, 95% CI 0.05–0.91; $p = 0.01$) in the antiplatelet group (3 of 123, 2.4%) than the anticoagulation group (11 of 111, 9.9%). Hospital stay was significantly shorter in the antiplatelet group (4.3±3.6 days versus 6.4±3.7 days; $p = 0.0001$). While no difference in stent occlusion was found between the two groups, acute stent thrombosis (within 24 hours) was more common in the antiplatelet arm (2.4%) compared with the anticoagulation arm (0.4%; $p = 0.06$). Subacute thrombosis was less frequent in the aspirin plus ticlopidine group (0.4% versus 3.5%; $p = 0.01$).

In the Stent Anticoagulation Restenosis Study Investigators (STARS) trial, 1965 patients who underwent coronary stenting were randomized to aspirin alone, aspirin plus warfarin, or aspirin plus ticlopidine. The primary endpoint of death, MI, target lesion revascularization, or angiographic thrombosis within 30 days was reduced in the combined antiplatelet group compared with the other two groups: 3.6% for aspirin alone, 2.7% for aspirin plus warfarin, and 0.5% for aspirin plus ticlopidine ($p < 0.001$).[35] Hemorrhagic complications occurred in 1.8% of the aspirin group, 6.2% of the aspirin plus warfarin group, and 5.5% in the aspirin plus ticlopidine group ($p < 0.001$ for the comparison).[35]

All five studies comparing aspirin, aspirin plus ticlopidine, and aspirin plus warfarin in patients undergoing stenting are represented in Figure 3.3.

The slow onset of action of ticlopidine may play a role in early stent thrombosis, as seen in the FANTASTIC study. Schömig, et al[37] examined the role of anticoagulation and antiplatelet therapy in their first 2833 patients undergoing coronary stent implantation. Stent thrombosis was as likely to occur in the first day after stent placement in patients treated with heparin while warfarin was being initiated as it was in patients treated with aspirin and ticlopidine. The subsequent rate of stent thrombosis decreased after the first day with antiplatelet therapy. If more complete platelet inhibition by a thienopyridine occurred prior to stent placement, then the risk of stent thrombosis might be reduced by a greater degree.

Steinhubl et al[38] examined the role of pretreatment with ticlopidine prior to stenting in the Evaluation of Platelet IIb/IIIa Inhibitor for Stenting (EPISTENT) study. In the placebo group of patients, ticlopidine pretreatment was associated with a significant decrease in the incidence of the composite endpoint of death, myocardial infarction, or target vessel revascularization at 1 year (adjusted hazard ratio 0.73; 95% CI 0.54–0.98; $p = 0.036$) (Figure 3.4). This endpoint was predominantly due to a reduction in periprocedural MI (8.4% versus 12.5%, $P = 0.048$). While abciximab further reduced the frequency of adverse events among pretreated patients, the risk reduction from ticlopidine pretreatment was approximately equal to the risk reduction seen with abciximab. Ticlopidine pretreatment did not significantly influence the risk of death or myocardial infarction in patients randomized to abciximab (Figure 3.4).

Side-effects

Ticlopidine is associated with such side-effects as nausea, diarrhea, and rash, which may require discontinuation in as many as 20% of patients.[39] Neutropenia occurs in 1–3% of patients, and this may rarely be life-threatening.

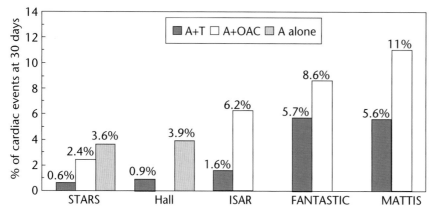

Figure 3.3
Five randomized studies of aspirin plus ticlopidine (A + T) versus aspirin plus oral anticoagulation (A + OAC) versus aspirin (A) alone in patients undergoing coronary stenting demonstrate reduced cardiac events at 30 days with ticlopidine plus aspirin. (Adapted from Bertrand ME et al. Circulation 2000;102:624–9[49] with permission from Lippincott Williams & Wilkins.)

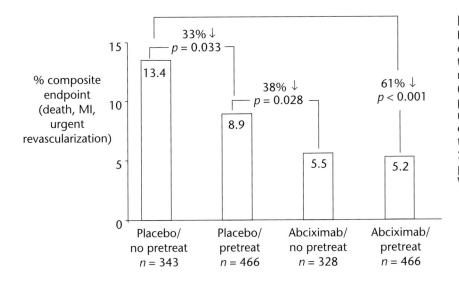

Figure 3.4
Data from the EPISTENT study demonstrating that pretreatment with ticlopidine was associated with a risk reduction of 33% at 30 days (predominantly from a reduction in periprocedural MI). Abciximab further reduced this risk of events by 38%, even among patients pretreated with ticlopidine. (Adapted from Steinhubl SR et al. Circulation 103:1403–9[38] with permission from Lippincott Williams & Wilkins.)

Thrombotic thrombocytopenic purpura (TTP) occurs very rarely with ticlopidine, with a frequency of 0.03%; however, TTP may be fatal in 25% of cases. TTP must be promptly treated with plasmapheresis.[40] Due to these rare but potentially life-threatening side-effects, blood counts must be serially examined in the first few months of ticlopidine use.

Clopidogrel

Clopidogrel bisulfate is a thienopyridine, similar in structure and function to ticlopidine, but different in a number of ways. Clopidogrel is also a prodrug, which is metabolized in the liver to other compounds that account for its activity. All metabolites of clopidogrel contain a carboxymethyl side-group.[27] The plasma half-life is approximately 8 hours; however, peak levels of the metabolites that account for the antiplatelet effects are achieved in approximately 1 hour. Similar to ticlopidine, it takes approximately 5 days to achieve maximal platelet inhibition from clopidogrel when no loading dose is administered.[41]

Secondary prevention

In the trial of Clopidogrel versus Aspirin in Patients at Risk of Ischemic Events (CAPRIE), 19 185 patients with peripheral vascular disease, cerebrovascular disease, or coronary artery disease were randomized to receive clopidogrel 75 mg daily or aspirin 325 mg daily.[42] At 3 years of follow-up, the patients randomized to clopidogrel had a statistically significant 8.7% reduction in the combined endpoint of vascular death, MI, or ischemic stroke ($p = 0.043$). Much of the beneficial effect of clopidogrel was due to a significant reduction in the incidence of fatal and nonfatal MI. MI occurred in 3.6% of the aspirin group and 2.9% of the clopidogrel group, accounting for a 19.2% relative risk

reduction in favor of clopidogrel. The side-effects of clopidogrel were very similar to those of aspirin, with rash occurring slightly more frequently and gastrointestinal complications occurring less frequently. Consequently, clopidogrel was discontinued slightly less often than aspirin.[42]

A subsequent analysis of the CAPRIE study found that rehospitalization for ischemic and bleeding events was also significantly reduced with clopidogrel versus aspirin.[43] Additionally, the benefit of clopidogrel over aspirin appears to have been amplified in patients at higher risk, such as those with diabetes mellitus or prior revascularization.[44,45]

In the Clopidogrel in Unstable angina to prevent Recurrent Events (CURE) trial, 12 562 patients with acute coronary syndromes (unstable angina or non-Q-wave MI) who presented within 24 hours of chest pain and had either new ischemic ECG changes (without ST-segment elevation) or an elevation of serum cardiac markers were randomized to clopidogrel 300 mg loading dose followed by 75 mg daily or placebo, both in combination with aspirin 75–325 mg daily.[46] The combination of clopidogrel and aspirin resulted in a significant decrease in the combined primary endpoint of cardiovascular death, nonfatal MI, or all-cause stroke compared with the aspirin-alone group (9.3% versus 11.4%; odds ratio 0.8; 95% CI 0.72–0.9; $p < 0.001$). When refractory ischemia was added to this combined endpoint, the clopidogrel plus aspirin group also had a reduced endpoint (16.5% versus 18.8% in placebo; odds ratio 0.86; 95% CI 0.79–0.94; $p < 0.001$). During hospitalization, there was a 32% reduction in severe ischemia ($p = 0.007$), an 8% reduction in revascularization procedures ($p = 0.03$), and an 18% decrease in heart failure ($p = 0.026$). No difference was seen in refractory ischemia after discharge. With long-term clopidogrel and aspirin use, there is a small but significantly increased risk of major, but not life-threatening, bleeding (3.7% versus 2.7%; hazard ratio (HR) 1.38; 95% CI 1.14–1.67; $p = 0.001$).[46] When clopidogrel was stopped within 5 days of bypass surgery, an increased risk of major bleeding or transfusion occurred (9.6% versus 6.3% in placebo; $p = 0.06$). This increased risk of bleeding was not observed when the clopidogrel was stopped for a period of greater than 5 days prior to surgery.

Based on these data, the American College of Cardiology/American Heart Association (ACC/AHA) formulated a change in the guidelines for antiplatelet therapy in acute coronary syndromes. The use of clopidogrel together with aspirin in patients in whom an early interventional approach is planned, along with the continuation of clopidogrel for at least 1 month and up to 9 months, is now a class I recommendation (conditions for which there is evidence that a treatment is useful and effective).[47]

Use of clopidogrel in the cardiac catheterization laboratory

Clopidogrel at 75 mg daily takes many days to achieve maximal platelet inhibition. Unlike ticlopidine, large loading doses are much better tolerated. When a 375 mg loading dose of clopidogrel is used, 60% platelet inhibition (as assessed by 5 μmol ADP) is achieved within 90 minutes, and maximal platelet inhibition occurs within 6 hours.[48]

Coronary artery stenting

In the Clopidogrel Aspirin Stent International Cooperative Study (CLASSICS), 1020 patients undergoing coronary stent implantation were randomized to clopidogrel 300 mg loading dose followed by 75 mg every day with aspirin 325 mg every day, clopidogrel 75 mg every day and aspirin 325 mg every day, or ticlopidine 250 mg twice daily with aspirin 325 mg every day.[49] The primary endpoint of major peripheral or bleeding complications, neutropenia, thrombocytopenia, or early discontinuation of study drug occurred in 9.1% of patients in the ticlopidine group and 4.6% of patients in the combined clopidogrel group (relative risk 0.50; 95% CI 0.312–0.81; $p = 0.005$). Overall rates of major adverse cardiac events (cardiac death, MI, and target lesion revascularization) were low and comparable between treatment groups (0.9% with ticlopidine, 1.5% with clopidogrel 75 mg daily, and 1.2% with the clopidogrel loading dose; $p = $ NS for all comparisons). In this study, clopidogrel was administered within 6 hours of the coronary intervention. This study demonstrated a superior safety profile for clopidogrel. The safety advantage of clopidogrel results from a lower frequency of noncardiac adverse events, with significantly fewer cases of skin disorders (0.7% versus 2.6%), gastrointestinal disorders (1.3% versus 2.6%), and allergy (0% versus 1.2%). Since clopidogrel is better tolerated, the risk of subacute thrombosis from early discontinuation of the drug, as with ticlopidine, should be reduced.[49]

In the Ticlid or Plavix Post Stent Study (TOPPS), 1016 patients undergoing stenting were randomized to clopidogrel with 300 mg loading dose followed by 75 mg every day for 14 days along with aspirin 325 mg every day or ticlopidine 500 mg loading dose followed by 250 mg twice daily along with aspirin 325 mg daily.[50] The primary endpoint was failure to complete 2 weeks of therapy, which occurred in 3.64% of the patients treated with ticlopidine and in 1.62% of the patients treated with clopidogrel ($p = 0.043$). The combined secondary endpoints of thrombocytopenia, major bleeding, cardiac death, Q-wave MI, stent thrombosis, and target vessel revascularization occurred in 4.60% of patients receiving ticlopidine and in 3.85% of patients receiving clopidogrel ($p = 0.551$). Within 30 days, stent thrombosis occurred in 1.92% of the patients in the ticlopidine group and in 2.02% of the clopidogrel group ($p = 0.901$).[50]

In the PCI–CURE study, 2658 patients undergoing percutaneous coronary intervention (PCI) in the CURE study were randomized to clopidogrel 300 mg loading dose followed by 75 mg daily along with aspirin ($n = 1313$) or placebo with aspirin ($n = 1345$).[51] All patients were pretreated with study drug for a median of 6 days before PCI during the initial hospital admission, and for a median of 10 days overall. After PCI, most patients received open-label thienopyridine for about 4 weeks, after which the study drug was restarted for a mean of 8 months. The primary endpoint, a composite of cardiovascular death, MI, or urgent target vessel revascularization within 30 days of PCI occurred in 4.5% of patients in the clopidogrel group as compared with 6.4% in the placebo group (relative risk 0.70; 95% CI 0.50–0.97; $p = 0.03$). Long-term administration of clopidogrel after PCI was associated with a lower rate of cardiovascular death, MI, or any revascularization ($p = 0.03$), and of cardiovascular death or MI ($p = 0.047$). Overall (including events before and after PCI), there was a 31% reduction in cardiovascular death or MI ($p = 0.002$). The lower rate of cardiovascular death, MI, or urgent revascularization in the clopidogrel group was seen as early as 2 days after PCI, and continued through 30 days. Most patients received open-label thienopyridine after PCI (>80% in both groups), suggesting that the benefit was mainly due to the effects of clopidogrel pretreatment. From the time of PCI to the end of follow-up (a mean of 8 months after PCI), there were significantly fewer cardiovascular deaths or MIs with clopidogrel than placebo ($p = 0.047$) (Figure 3.5).

In the clopidogrel group, glycoprotein IIb/IIIa inhibitors were used less frequently. ($p = 0.001$). At follow-up, there was no significant difference in major bleeding between the groups; however, the rate of minor bleeding was increased in the clopidogrel group at follow-up several months later (3.5% versus 2.0%; $p = 0.03$).[51] Repeat revascularizations were also lower in the clopidogrel group than the placebo group (14.2% versus 17.1%; relative risk 0.82; 95% CI 0.68–1.00; $p = 0.049$), mainly

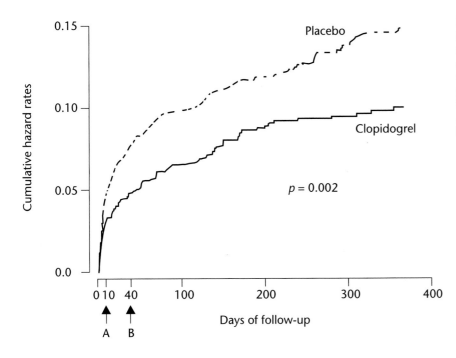

Figure 3.5
Kaplan–Meier curves in the PCI–CURE trial demonstrating significant early and long-term benefits of treatment with clopidogrel prior to and after percutaneous intervention. (Adapted from Mehta SR et al. Lancet 2001;358:527–33[51] with permission from Elsevier.)

because of a reduced need for a repeat PCI (10.7% versus 12.9%; relative risk 0.83; 95% CI 0.66–1.03).

The significant reduction in death or MI at 8 months in patients receiving clopidogrel strongly supports the long-term use of dual antiplatelet therapy after PCI.[47,51] Two registry analyses also support the value of pretreatment with clopidogrel in patients undergoing PCI, even if glycoprotein IIb/IIIa inhibitors are used at the time of the procedure.[52,53]

In a meta-analysis of three randomized trials and seven registries including a total of 13 955 patients that compared ticlopidine with clopidogrel in patients undergoing elective coronary stenting, the combined 30-day endpoint of major adverse cardiac events (defined differently in the trials) was 2.10% in the clopidogrel versus 4.04% in the ticlopidine group.[54] After adjustment for heterogeneity, the odds ratio of having an ischemic event with clopidogrel, as compared with ticlopidine, was 0.72 (95% CI 0.59–0.89; $p = 0.002$). The overall mortality rate was also lower in the clopidogrel group as compared with the ticlopidine group (0.48% versus 1.09%; odds ratio 0.55; 95% CI 0.37–0.82; $p = 0.003$) (Figure 3.6). All of the individual components of the composite endpoint favored clopidogrel over ticlopidine (Figure 3.7). These findings may have been due to a more rapid onset of antiplatelet action with the loading dose of clopidogrel, which was used in many of the studies, or to better compliance with clopidogrel.

The results of the randomized trials as well as the meta-analysis of clopidogrel versus ticlopidine in elective stenting suggest that the combination of clopidogrel and aspirin is a superior regimen to that of ticlopidine and aspirin. The side-effect profile is much improved with

clopidogrel, since its use is associated with significantly lower rates of rash, nausea, and vomiting, as well as a significantly reduced rate of neutropenia and TTP. Approximately 11 patients out of 3 million treated with clopidogrel have been reported to develop TTP, as compared with 250 cases per million treated with ticlopidine.[55] In addition, the frequency of major adverse cardiac events appears to be reduced with clopidogrel.[50,51,54] Therefore, clopidogrel with a loading dose of 300–375 mg, ideally at least 6 hours prior to the procedure, followed by 75 mg every day along with aspirin 75–325 mg every day for a total of 28 days, is the minimum recommended antiplatelet regimen after elective stenting.

However, the recently completed Clopidogrel for Reduction of Events During Observation (CREDO) trial may alter the minimum duration of clopidogrel and aspirin after stenting.[56] This trial of over 2000 patients undergoing PCI compared a clopidogrel loading dose versus placebo prior to PCI and compared 1 year of clopidogrel versus 1 month following PCI, with aspirin in all patients. Those patients with clopidogrel pretreatment had a nonsignificant reduction in the combined endpoint of death, MI, or urgent revascularization at 28 days (6.8% versus 8.3%; relative risk reduction 18.5%; $p = 0.23$). Those patients pretreated with clopidogrel greater than 6 hours prior to PCI had a larger reduction in the primary endpoint (absolute reduction 3.6% versus 0.9% in the group with less than 6 hours pretreatment; $p = 0.05$).[56] The 1-month results support the value of pretreatment with clopidogrel, even in patients receiving glycoprotein IIb/IIIa inhibitors. The 1-year results should provide valuable guidance regarding the duration of dual antiplatelet therapy after elective PCI.

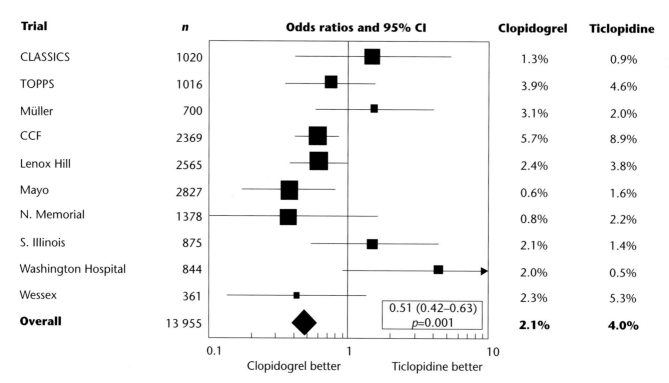

Figure 3.6
Odds ratio plots with 95% confidence intervals (CI) of 30-day major adverse cardiac events in all trials comparing clopidogrel with ticlopidine in patients undergoing coronary artery stenting. Estimates to the left indicate that clopidogrel is superior; estimates to the right indicate that ticlopidine is superior. CCF, Cleveland Clinic Foundation; CLASSICS, Clopidogrel Aspirin Stent International Cooperative Study; TOPPS, Ticlid or Plavix Post Stent. (Adapted from Bhatt DL et al. J Am Coll Cardiol 2002;39:9–14[54] © 2002 with permission from the American College of Cardiology Foundation.)

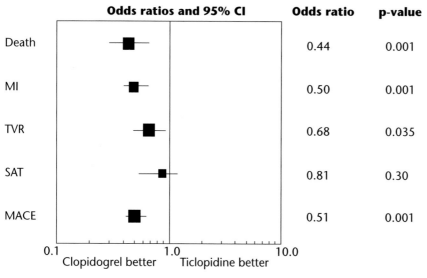

Figure 3.7
Odds ratios with 95% confidence intervals (CI) of individual components of the composite endpoint in the meta-analysis of trials comparing clopidogrel with ticlopidine. MI, myocardial infarction; TVR, target vessel revascularization; SAT, subacute thrombosis; MACE, major adverse cardiac events. (Adapted from Bhatt DL et al. J Am Coll Cardiol 2002;39:9–14[54] © 2002 with permission from the American College of Cardiology Foundation.)

Oral glycoprotein IIb/IIIa inhibitors

The role of platelet membrane glycoproteins (GPs) in platelet adhesion and aggregation, together with the action of their inhibitors, are discussed below in the section on intravenous GP IIb/IIIa inhibitors. The oral GP IIb/IIIa inhibitors all have longer half-lives than their intravenous counterparts, so they can be dosed one to three times daily with the ability to achieve significant inhibition of platelet inhibition. Similar to the intravenous GP IIb/IIIa inhibitors, two groups of oral platelet inhibitors exist. One group exhibits competitive inhibition that moves rapidly on and off the receptor (short 'off time'), in which a high level of drug is necessary to achieve adequate inhibition of platelet inhibition. The other class exhibits very tight binding affinity for the receptor, with most of the drug being found in the bound state, which might avoid low levels of platelet inhibition.[58] The first group constitutes the first-generation inhibitors of the platelet receptor, such as orbofiban, sibrafiban, and xemilofiban.

The Orbofiban in Patients with Unstable Coronary Syndromes (OPUS–TIMI-16) trial randomized 10 288 patients with acute coronary syndromes to placebo, 50 mg of orbofiban twice daily (50/50), or 50 mg of orbofiban twice daily for 30 days followed by 30 mg twice daily (50/30).[59] All patients received 150–162 mg of aspirin. The trial was stopped prematurely due to an increase in 30-day mortality in the orbofiban 50/30 group. At 10 months, the mortality was 3.7% in the placebo group, 5.1% in the 50/30 group ($p = 0.008$), and 4.5% in the 50/50 group ($p = 0.11$). No differences were found in the primary endpoint of death, reinfarction, recurrent ischemia, urgent revascularization, or stroke at 30 days between the groups. Major or severe bleeding was increased in the orbofiban groups. Interestingly, the subgroup of patients who underwent PCI who received orbofiban had a lower mortality and a significant reduction in the composite endpoint.[59]

In the Evaluation of Oral Xemilofiban in Controlling Thrombotic Events (EXCITE) trial, 7232 patients were randomized to placebo, or to 10 or 20 mg of xemilofiban 90 minutes prior to percutaneous coronary revascularization, and were maintained on 10 or 20 mg three times daily for 6 months.[60] All patients received aspirin and those who underwent stenting received ticlopidine. No significant difference in the composite endpoint of death or nonfatal MI at 6 months was found; however, severe bleeding occurred more frequently in the xemilofiban groups. Mortality at 30 days was increased in the xemilofiban 10 mg group (0.8% versus 0.3% in the placebo group; $p = 0.02$), which persisted at 6 months.

In the Sibrafiban versus Aspirin to Yield Maximum Protection from Ischemic Heart Events Post-Acute Coronary Syndromes (SYMPHONY) trial, 9233 acute coronary syndrome patients were randomized to aspirin, low-dose sibrafiban, or high-dose sibrafiban. No differences were seen in the primary composite endpoint of death, nonfatal MI or reinfarction, or severe recurrent ischemia at 90 days between the three groups.[61] Major bleeding was significantly more common with both low-dose (5.2%) and high-dose (5.7%) sibrafiban, compared with aspirin (3.9%).

In the second SYMPHONY trial, 6671 patients with acute coronary syndromes were randomized to aspirin alone, low-dose sibrafiban with aspirin, or high-dose sibrafiban with aspirin. Again, no differences were seen in the primary endpoint of death, MI or reinfarction, or severe recurrent ischemia at 90 days: 9.3% in the aspirin group, 9.2% in the low-dose sibrafiban plus aspirin group, and 10.5% in the high-dose sibrafiban plus aspirin group.[62] However, mortality was significantly higher in the high-dose sibrafiban group (2.4%; odds ratio 1.83; 95% CI 1.17–2.88) compared with the low-dose sibrafiban (1.7%) or aspirin (1.3%; $p = 0.05$ versus aspirin alone) groups. The combination of death or MI was also significantly greater in the high-dose group compared with the other two groups. Major bleeding was significantly more frequent in the low-dose group (5.7%) versus aspirin alone (4.0%), but not in the high-dose group (4.6%).

Several explanations for the failure of current oral GP IIb/IIIa inhibitors in clinical trials have been postulated. Important pharmacokinetic and pharmacodynamic differences may exist between the oral and intravenous routes of administration. Intravenous compounds achieve high levels of platelet inhibition, while the lower levels achieved with the oral agents (ranging from 30% to 60% for low doses and from 50% to 80% for high doses) may not be optimal in protecting against events. In addition, peaks and troughs exist in the level of platelet inhibition with the oral agents. Bioavailability differences between patients may result in substantial variability in the level of platelet inhibition achieved. Also, these agents may need to be administered with aspirin or clopidogrel.[17,58,62] Some data suggest that the agents may be prothrombotic. Orbofiban increases platelet surface P-selectin, a marker of increased platelet activation.[63] One investigation demonstrated that orbofiban is both an antagonist and a partial agonist of the GP IIb/IIIa inhibitor.[64] Conformational changes in the GP IIb/IIIa receptor occur when binding to a GP IIb/IIIa inhibitor takes place. However, after these drugs dissociate from membrane receptors, the conformational changes persist, and platelets may actually be more likely to bind fibrinogen than before exposure to the GP IIb/IIIa receptor antagonist.[65]

In December 2000, the Blockade of the IIb/IIIa Receptor to Avoid Vascular Occlusion (BRAVO) trial of the oral GP IIb/IIIa blocker lotrafiban was terminated early because of concerns about both safety and efficacy. Patients receiving lotrafiban had a higher mortality rate than placebo (2.7% versus 2.0% for placebo; $p = 0.022$), and the lotrafiban group also had an increased incidence of serious thrombocytopenia (2.2% versus 0.5%) and major bleeding (4.2% versus 1.3%; $p < 0.0001$). As a result of these findings, development of lotrafiban was discontinued.[57]

In a meta-analysis of four oral GP IIb/IIIa inhibitor trials, a significant increase in mortality was observed with oral GP IIb/IIIa therapy (odds ratio 1.37; 95% CI 1.13–1.66; $p < 0.001$) (Figure 3.8).[66] This effect was present despite aspirin use and treatment with either low-dose or high-dose therapy. Although a reduction in urgent revascularization was observed with oral GP IIb/IIIa inhibition, no significant increase in MI was found. These observations suggest a direct toxic effect of the oral agents rather than a prothrombotic effect of the drugs in patients.

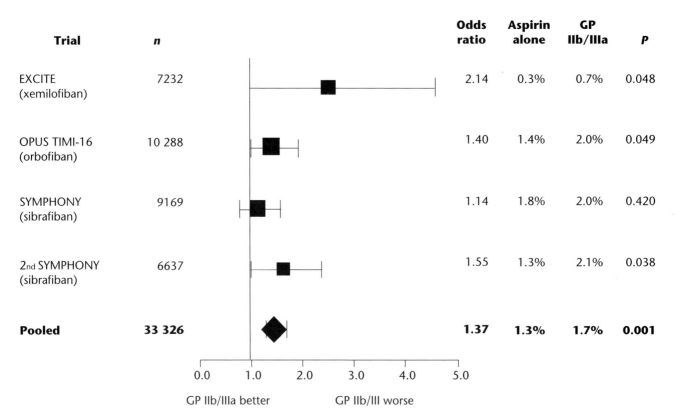

Trial	n		Odds ratio	Aspirin alone	GP IIb/IIIa	P
EXCITE (xemilofiban)	7232		2.14	0.3%	0.7%	0.048
OPUS TIMI-16 (orbofiban)	10 288		1.40	1.4%	2.0%	0.049
SYMPHONY (sibrafiban)	9169		1.14	1.8%	2.0%	0.420
2nd SYMPHONY (sibrafiban)	6637		1.55	1.3%	2.1%	0.038
Pooled	**33 326**		**1.37**	**1.3%**	**1.7%**	**0.001**

Figure 3.8
Odds ratios and 95% confidence intervals for risk of death in oral GP IIb/IIIa inhibitor trials. (Adapted from Chew et al. Circulation 2001;103:3240–9[66] with permission from Lippincott Williams & Wilkins.)

Utilizing intravenous glycoprotein IIb/IIIa inhibitors

Platelet glycoprotein receptors

The role of the platelet membrane glycoproteins was elucidated from Nurden and Caen and by Phillips, who identified deficiencies of two different platelet membrane glycoproteins (designated GP IIb and GP IIIa) in several patients with Glanzmann's thrombasthenia, a hereditary disorder characterized by severe mucocutaneous hemorrhage, marked prolongation of bleeding time, and abnormal clot retraction.[67–69]

All of these receptors are composed of two chains, an α subunit and a β subunit, which are held together by noncovalent bonds (Figure 3.9). The α subunits have three or four divalent cation-binding domains, whereas β subunits contain many disulfide bonds. These two subunits are identified as GP IIb, a typical integrin subunit α_{IIb}, and GP IIIA, a typical β subunit (β_3). The GP IIb/IIIa receptor is platelet-specific and uniquely adapted for platelet function. GP IIIa (β_3) however, can form a complex with another α subunit, α_v, to form the $\alpha_v\beta_3$ vitronectin receptor, which is present on endothelial cells, osteoclasts, and other cells. Trace amounts of $\alpha_v\beta_3$ are

also present on platelets (approximately 50–100 receptors per platelet receptor).[70,71]

Many different ligands, such as von Willebrand factor (vWF), fibronectin, vitronectin, CD40, and thrombospondin are able to bind to platelet GP IIb/IIIa under appropriate conditions of platelet activation, and can be inhibited by peptides containing the RGD sequence (a three-amino-acid sequence: arginine–glycine–aspartic acid) (Figure 3.10). Hence, many small molecules that are RGD derivatives have been developed as potential GP IIb/IIIa inhibitors.[72]

Although many different proteins can bind to GP IIb/IIIa in vitro under appropriate conditions of platelet activation, during ex vivo platelet aggregation in normal plasma, fibrinogen appears to be the dominant protein binding to the receptor. Studies with ex vivo flow chambers designed to simulate better in vivo conditions, however, indicate that vWF plays a more important role than fibrinogen.[69]

Platelet adhesion and aggregation

Damage to a normal blood vessel or an atherosclerotic plaque results in exposure of adhesive glycoproteins such

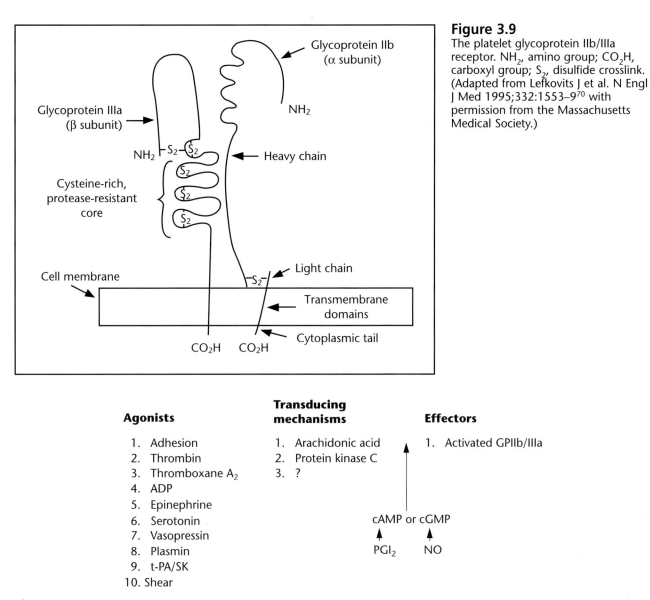

Figure 3.9
The platelet glycoprotein IIb/IIIa receptor. NH_2, amino group; CO_2H, carboxyl group; S_2, disulfide crosslink. (Adapted from Lefkovits J et al. N Engl J Med 1995;332:1553–9[70] with permission from the Massachusetts Medical Society.)

Agonists	Transducing mechanisms	Effectors
1. Adhesion	1. Arachidonic acid	1. Activated GPIIb/IIIa
2. Thrombin	2. Protein kinase C	
3. Thromboxane A_2	3. ?	
4. ADP		
5. Epinephrine		
6. Serotonin		
7. Vasopressin		
8. Plasmin		
9. t-PA/SK		
10. Shear		

cAMP or cGMP

PGI$_2$ NO

Figure 3.10
Agonists produce signals through the transducing mechanisms, ultimately activating the GP IIb/IIIa receptor. The GP IIb/IIIa receptor is the final common pathway in platelet aggregation. Prostacyclin (prostaglandin I$_2$, PGI$_2$) and nitric oxide (NO) inhibit activation by generating cyclic adenosine monophosphate (cAMP) or cyclic guanosine monophosphate (cGMP). t-PA, tissue-type plasminogen activator; SK, streptokinase. (Adapted from Collier BS. Coronary Artery Dis 1992;92:1016–29.[71])

as vWF and collagen. Platelets have receptors for these glycoproteins that result in platelet adhesion. These receptors are present on the surface of platelets in their active states, so they can affect adhesion immediately after vascular injury.[3,4,70] Thus, platelet adhesion is controlled by the normal endothelial lining 'hiding' the adhesive glycoproteins from the circulating platelets. After platelet adhesion, the platelet undergoes an activation process that produces a conformational change in the GP IIb/IIIa receptor so that it has a high binding affinity for fibrinogen, vWF, and perhaps other glycoproteins. Clustering and upregulation of platelet receptors in the membrane then ensues.[71,73] Because both fibrinogen and vWF are multi-valent molecules, they can bind to GP IIb/IIIa receptors on two different platelets simultaneously, resulting in platelet crosslinking and platelet aggregation[70] (Figure 3.11).

Platelet aggregation requires the presence of one or more platelet-activating agents, most of which are synthesized and released only at sites of vascular injury.[3,4] Activated platelets synthesize and release the platelet activators thromboxane A$_2$, ADP, and serotonin, and they facilitate thrombin formation. These factors promote further conformational changes in platelets and accelerate platelet aggregation significantly. The final common pathway for platelet aggregation, regardless of the agonist, is a conformational change in the GP IIb/IIIa receptor that

Adhesion and Activation

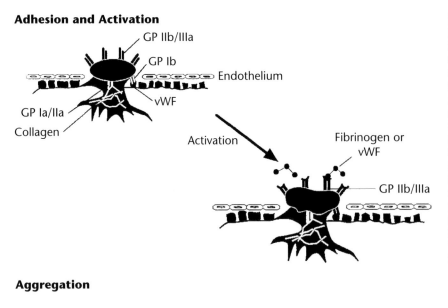

Aggregation

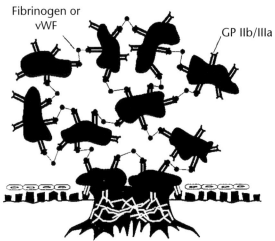

Figure 3.11
Platelet activation after exposure to tissue factor causes changes in the shape of platelets and conformational changes in GP IIb/IIIa receptors, transforming them into a ligand-receptive state. Release of ADP, serotonin, thromboxane A_2, and thrombin recruits more platelets to stimulate the same cascade. Circulating von Willebrand factor (vWF) and fibrinogen form cross-bridges between activated platelets with ligand-receptive GP IIb/IIIa receptors, facilitating platelet aggregation. (Adapted from Coller BS. Circulation 1995;92:2373–80[69] with permission from Lippincott Williams & Wilkins.)

results in it developing high affinity for its adhesive glyco-protein ligands.[69–71]

Intravenous GP IIb/IIIa inhibitors

The glycoprotein IIb/IIIa inhibitors in clinical use consist of antibodies, peptides, and small nonpeptide molecules that bind to the $\alpha_{IIb}\beta_3$ platelet receptor to inhibit platelet aggregation.[74]

Abciximab (Reopro, Lilly) is a murine–human chimeric Fab fragment of a 7E3 antibody that was derived from immunization of a mouse with human platelets.[74] Abciximab inhibits platelet function by blocking the GP IIb/IIIa receptor by steric hindrance, thereby preventing the binding of fibrinogen and vWF to activated platelets. It also binds with equivalent affinity to the vitronectin receptor ($\alpha_v\beta_3$), which is present on platelets, vascular

endothelial cells, and smooth muscle cells.[69] Abciximab is administered as a bolus of 0.25 mg/kg, followed by a 0.125 μg/kg/min infusion for 12 hours. While abciximab has a serum half-life of approximately 30 minutes, it has biologic effects for up to 15 days. The maximum inhibition was seen $\frac{1}{2}$ hour after administration of the bolus, followed by partial recovery from both GP IIb/IIIa receptor block-ade and inhibition of ADP-mediated platelet aggregation 12 hours after cessation of abciximab therapy.[75] Up to 13% of GP IIb/IIIa receptor blockade was observed at 15 days after administration. In addition, the drug appears to equilibrate onto new platelets entering the circulation. Consequently, reversibility of abciximab may be achieved with platelet transfusion.[74,76]

Binding of many physiologic ligands to GP IIb/IIIa receptors (and to the vitronectin receptor) requires the Arg-Gly-Asp (RGD) sequence. The active domain of many of the smaller GP IIb/IIIa antagonists usually contains this sequence or a structure designed to mimic it.[76] Tirofiban (Aggrastat, Merck) is small nonpeptide derivative of tyro-sine, based on the RGD sequence. Consequently, this molecule occupies the binding site of the GP IIb/IIIa pocket and competitively inhibits platelet aggregation as mediated by vWF or fibrinogen. The plasma half-life is approximately 2 hours, and the major route of excretion is renal. One commonly used dose is 0.4 μg/kg bolus infusion for 30 minutes followed by a maintenance infusion of 0.1 μg/kg/min. In patients with severe renal dysfunction (creatinine clearance <30 ml/min), the dose should be lowered significantly. For patients with a creatinine clearance less than 30 ml/min, both the loading dose and the infusion of tirofiban should be halved. Moderate reduction in plasma clearance of the molecule is also found in the elderly (>65 years).[76–78]

Eptifibatide (Integrilin, Cor Therapeutics) is a cyclic heptapeptide based on barbourin, a 73-amino-acid peptide isolated from the venom of the Southeastern pygmy rattlesnake, *Sistrurus m barbouri*.[76] This molecule has specificity for the GP IIb/IIIa integrin due to the Lys-Gly-Asp (KGD) sequence, a variation on the more common RGD sequence. Unlike abciximab, eptifibatide is specific for the GP IIb/IIIa integrin, without any appreciable binding to $\alpha_v\beta_3$. With the administration of doses of 90–180 μg/kg/min, maximal plasma doses are achieved within 5 minutes. The plasma half-life is approximately 2.5 hours, and the majority of the drug is eliminated through renal mechanisms, thereby requiring lower doses in patients with a creatinine clearance of less than 30 ml/min. The plasma concentration of free eptifibatide decreases rapidly after the drug is completed. Eptifibatide dosing has been less well studied in patients with renal insufficiency; however, a 135 μg/kg bolus followed by a 0.5 μg/kg/min infusion has been used in patients with serum creatinine levels between 2 and 4 mg/dL.[76,78]

Lamifiban is also a small molecule, nonpeptide, which is very specific for the binding sequence of the IIb/IIIa integrin. The plasma half life of the molecule is approximately 4 hours. The two highest doses studied (boluses of 600 and 750 μg followed by infusions of 4 and 5 μg/min) inhibited platelet aggregation (induced by ADP 10 μmol and by TRAP 100 μmol) by over 80%, but was associated with a significant increase in bleeding time at both doses.[79]

GP IIb/IIIa inhibition during coronary revascularization

The initial studies evaluating GP IIb/IIIa inhibitors occurred in the setting of percutaneous coronary intervention (PIC).

In the first of such trials, the Evaluation of 7E3 for the Prevention of Ischemic Complications (EPIC), patients with unstable angina, acute MI, or high-risk coronary morphologic characteristics underwent coronary angioplasty or atherectomy and were randomized to placebo, abciximab bolus (0.25 mg/kg i.v.), or abciximab bolus and infusion (10 μg/min) for 12 hours.[80] The patients receiving the abciximab bolus and infusion had a significant reduction in death, MI, unplanned revascularization, or use of a stent or

intraaortic balloon pump (IABP) at 30 days: 8.3% versus 12.8%, a relative risk reduction of 35% ($p < 0.0008$). No significant reduction in the combined endpoint occurred in the abciximab bolus-alone group. The predominant effects were the reduction in nonfatal MI (both Q-wave and non-Q-wave MI) and in emergency percutaneous transluminal coronary angioplasty (PTCA).[80] The beneficial effects of abciximab in this high-risk group occurred at a cost of significant increases in major bleeding: up to 14% compared with 7% in the placebo group ($p < 0.001$) Transfusions also occurred more frequently in the abciximab groups.

In this study, abciximab improved the composite outcome at 3 years: 41.1% versus 47.2% in placebo, a relative risk reduction of 19% ($p = 0.009$).[81] Unlike many other studies utilizing abciximab, the rates of repeat revascularization were also reduced significantly up to 3 years: 34.8% versus 40.1%, a relative reduction of 19% ($p = 0.021$).[81] These results suggest an additional role of abciximab, such as inhibition of the vitronectin receptor with a subsequent reduction in clinical restenosis.

In the Evaluation in PTCA to Improve Long-Term Outcome with Abciximab GP IIb/IIIa Blockade (EPILOG) trial, patients undergoing elective balloon angioplasty were randomized to heparin alone, abciximab with standard-dose heparin (bolus 100 U/kg, goal activated clotting time (ACT) > 300 s), or abciximab with low-dose heparin (70 U/kg, goal ACT > 200 s).[82] Both abciximab groups had significant reductions in the combined 30-day endpoint of death, MI, and urgent revascularization: 5.2% in the abciximab and low-dose heparin group, 5.4% in the abciximab and high-dose heparin group, and 11.7% in the heparin plus placebo group ($p < 0.001$ for both comparisons). Utilizing lower doses of heparin in addition to early removal of vascular access sheaths resulted in lower rates of major bleeding with abciximab plus low-dose heparin (3.1% heparin, 3.5% abciximab plus standard heparin, 2.0% abciximab plus low-dose heparin; $p = $ NS).[82]

In the c7E3 Fab Antiplatelet Therapy in Unstable Refractory Angina (CAPTURE) study, the combined 30-day endpoint of death, MI, or urgent revascularization for refractory ischemia was significantly reduced from 15.9% to 11.3% ($p = 0.012$) in the patients who were treated with 18–24 hours of abciximab prior to angioplasty and for 1 after the procedure.[83] In the 24 hours preceding angioplasty, the incidence of death or nonfatal MI was also significantly reduced in patients receiving abciximab: from 2.8% to 1.3% ($p = 0.032$).[84] The combined event rate was also significantly reduced during the first 48 hours after PCI in the abciximab group (2.8% versus 5.8% in placebo; $p = 0.009$).[84]

An elevated serum troponin T level is a marker for thrombus formation and for a group of patients at high risk for future cardiac events. In the CAPTURE study, the relative risk of death or MI was reduced by 77% (odds ratio 0.23; 95% CI 0.14–0.49; $p = 0.002$) in those patients with elevated troponin T levels who were treated with abciximab.[85] No benefit of abciximab treatment was seen in patients without elevated troponin T levels with respect to the relative risk of death or MI at 6 months (odds ratio 1.26; 95% CI 0.74–2.31; $p = 0.47$).

In the EPISTENT trial, patients were randomized to stent plus heparin, stent plus abciximab, or PTCA plus abciximab. The combined rate of death, MI, or urgent revascularization at 30 days was reduced significantly in both abciximab groups: from 10.8% to 5.3% in the stent plus abciximab group ($p < 0.001$) and to 6.9% in the PTCA plus abciximab group ($p = 0.007$).[86] These effects were maintained at both 6 months and 1 year. The overall mortality rate at 1 year was significantly reduced in patients receiving stent and abciximab compared with stent alone (1.0% versus 2.4%; $p = 0.037$).[87] Among patients with diabetes, those receiving stent and abciximab had a significant reduction in target vessel revascularization at 6 months compared with the stent-alone group (8.1% versus 16.6% in the placebo group; $p = 0.02$) or compared with the angioplasty plus abciximab group (8.1% versus 18.4%; $p = 0.008$).[88] This effect on target vessel revascularization was also maintained at 1 year.[87] The benefit of abciximab on reducing mortality was notable in diabetics, including those undergoing multivessel PCI.[89,90] The benefits of abciximab are also consistent across different percutaneous revascularization techniques, such as balloon angioplasty, elective stenting, 'bailout' stenting, and atherectomy.[91,92]

In the Randomized Efficacy Study of Tirofiban for Outcomes and Restenosis (RESTORE), high-risk patients (unstable angina or acute MI) who underwent angioplasty and were randomized to tirofiban 10 μg/kg bolus followed by a 36-hour infusion of 0.15 μg/kg/min had a trend toward a reduction in the combined endpoint of death, MI, and repeat angioplasty or stent placement at 30 days (10.3% versus 12.2%, a 16% risk reduction; $p = 0.160$).[93] However, 2 days after angioplasty, the tirofiban group had a 38% reduction in the combined endpoint (5.4% versus 8.7%; $p = 0.005$). At 7 days, there was also a 27% reduction in this same combined endpoint (7.6% versus 10.4%; $p = 0.022$). One criticism of this study is the lack of systematic collection of periprocedural creatine kinase (CK) enzymes at all sites.

In the Do Tirofiban and Reopro Give Similar Efficacy Trial (TARGET), 2398 patients were randomized to tirofiban (10 μg/kg bolus, followed by 0.15 μg/kg/min for 18–24 hours) or abciximab in patients undergoing elective stenting or angioplasty. Those patients receiving abciximab had a greater reduction in the 30-day combined endpoint of death, MI, or urgent target vessel revascularization (6.0% versus 7.6%; $p = 0.038$), demonstrating the superiority of abciximab over tirofiban.[94] Again, the predominant effect was the significant reduction in nonfatal MI. CK-MB elevations six times normal and higher were reduced to a greater degree in the abciximab group. However, by 6 months, there was no significant difference

between the two groups in the combined endpoint of death, MI, or any target vessel revascularization. While there was no significant difference in the rate of major bleeding or transfusions, tirofiban was associated with a lower rate of minor bleeding episodes and thrombocytopenia.[94]

In the Integrilin to Minimize Platelet Aggregation and Coronary Thrombosis-II (IMPACT-II) trial, patients undergoing elective, urgent, or emergent coronary intervention were randomized to placebo or eptifibatide 135 μg/kg bolus followed by either 0.5 or 0.75 μg/kg/min intravenous infusion for 20–24 hours. The composite endpoint of death, MI, revascularization, or stent implantation for abrupt vessel closure trended lower in each of the eptifibatide groups: 9.2% and 9.9% versus 11.4% ($p = 0.063$ for 135/0.5 dose; $p = 0.22$ for 135/0.75 dose).[95] Eptifibatide treatment did not increase rates of major bleeding or transfusion. Studies conducted after IMPACT-II showed that ex vivo measurements of the pharmacodynamics of eptifibatide were dependent on the blood anticoagulant; citrated anticoagulation removes Ca^{2+} from the GP IIb/IIIa inhibitor and enhances the apparent inhibitory activity of eptifibatide.[96] When Ca^{2+} is removed from blood, the fibrinogen-binding activity of platelets is reduced. With the doses of eptifibatide tested in IMPACT-II, only moderate values (about 50%) of GP IIb/IIIa receptor blockade occurred, resulting in only 50–60% inhibition of platelet aggregation.[96]

In the Platelet Glycoprotein IIb/IIIa in Unstable Angina: Receptor Suppression Using Integrilin Therapy (PURSUIT) trial, unstable angina patients were randomized to placebo or eptifibatide 180 μg/kg bolus with either 1.3 or 2.0 μg/kg/min for 72 hours. Approximately 23% of the patients underwent PCI during their hospital admission. Those patients receiving high-dose eptifibatide undergoing PCI had a 31% reduction in the incidence of the composite endpoint of death or MI at 30 days (11.6% versus 16.7%; $p = 0.01$).[97] Eptifibatide reduced the frequency of the composite endpoint both before and after the procedure among patients undergoing early revascularization.[84] Severe bleeding and packed red blood cell transfusions occurred more frequently in the eptifibatide group.[97]

In the Eptifibatide in Planned Coronary Stent Implantation (ESPRIT) trial, 2064 patients undergoing routine stent placement were randomized to eptifibatide, given as two 180 μg/kg boluses 10 minutes apart and a continuous infusion of 2.0 μg/kg/min for 18–24 hours, or placebo, along with aspirin, heparin, and a thienopyridine.[98] This dose was utilized to ensure platelet aggregation of 85–95%, with a second bolus to ensure no fall in the platelet inhibition level early in the periprocedural time period. Those patients receiving eptifibatide had a 37% reduction in the combined primary endpoint of death, MI, urgent target vessel revascularization, or bailout therapy for thrombotic complications at 48 hours: from 10.5% to 6.6% ($p = 0.0015$). In this patient group, eptifibatide demonstrated durable results. At 30 days, the patients

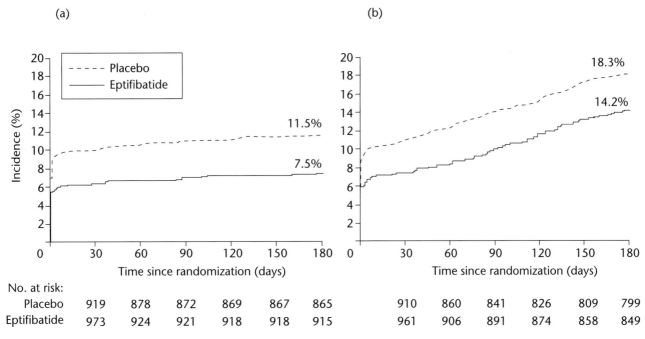

Figure 3.12
ESPRIT 6-month outcomes. (a) For the composite endpoint of death or MI, the hazard ratio (HR) is 0.63 (95% CI 0.47–0.84; p = 0.002). (b) For the composite endpoint of death, MI, or target vessel revascularization, HR = 0.75 (95% CI 0.60–0.93; p = 0.008). (Reproduced from O'Shea JC et al. JAMA 2001;285:2468–73[99] with permission from the American Medical Association.)

receiving eptifibatide had a similar reduction in the incidence of death, MI, or urgent target vessel revascularization: from 10.5% to 6.8% (p = 0.003).[98] Major bleeding occurred more frequently in the eptifibatide group (1% versus 0.4% in the placebo group; p = 0.027); however, there was no difference in the rates of transfusions between the two groups. By 6 months, death or MI was reduced 34% from 11.5% to 7.5% in the eptifibatide group (hazard ratio (HR) 0.63; 95% CI 0.47–0.84; p = 0.002).[99] Similarly, the composite of death, MI, or urgent target vessel revascularization was reduced from 18.3% to 14.2% (HR 0.75; 95% CI 0.6–0.93; p = 0.008) (Figure 3.12). Much of this benefit began early (within 48 hours after initiation of therapy) and was maintained throughout the 6 months. Again, as in many of the other trials, the significant component of these endpoints was the reduction in MI: from 10.4% to 7.0% (HR 0.65; 95% CI 0.48–0.88; p = 0.005). The 6-month mortality rate in the eptifibatide group was 0.8% versus 1.4% in the placebo group (p = 0.19), and the target vessel revascularization occurred in 8.6% of the eptifibatide group versus 9.4% of the placebo group (p = 0.51).[99]

In a meta-analysis of 17 788 patients undergoing any revascularization, treatment with any intravenous GP IIb/IIIa inhibitor was associated with a significant reduction in the risk of death or MI at 30 days by 38% (odds ratio 0.62; 95% CI 0.55–0.70; 2p < 0.00001) (Figure 3.13). These events occurred in 5.6% of patients in the treatment group and in 8.7% of controls. In absolute terms, an additional 31 patients will be prevented from dying or

having an MI for every 1000 patients treated with GP IIb/IIIa inhibitors at 30 days.[100]

However, in a meta-analysis of 12 trials with 17 469 patients who underwent any form of revascularization, treatment with intravenous GP IIb/IIIa inhibitors was associated with a significant increase in the risk of having severe bleeding (odds ratio 1.38; 95% CI 1.04–1.85; 2p = 0.03) (Figure 3.14). Major bleeding occurred in 4.2% of patients in the treatment group and in 3.2% of controls. The absolute rate difference indicates an excess of 10 severe bleeds for every 1000 patients treated with GP IIb/IIIa antagonists.[100]

Other considerations with the use of GP IIb/IIIa inhibitors

Care should be taken when these agents are used in patients who require surgical revascularization. Due to the increased risk of surgical bleeding, all agents should be stopped prior to coronary artery bypass surgery. Abciximab should be stopped as soon as surgery is contemplated, and platelet transfusion is strongly recommended if surgery occurs within the first 12–24 hours after its administration. Due to their shorter half-lives, tirofiban or eptifibatide should be stopped at least 4 hours prior to bypass surgery.[17,78] Patients who received GP IIb/IIIa inhibitors prior to coronary artery bypass surgery did not have increased bleeding rates in randomized trials.[101–103]

Study	Treatment	Control	Odds ratio (fixed), 95% CI	Weight (%)	Odds ratio (fixed), 95% CI
ADMIRAL	7 / 149	12 / 151		1.6	0.57 [0.22 – 1.49]
CAPTURE	30 / 630	57 / 635		7.8	0.51 [0.32 – 0.80]
EPIC 30 days	49 / 708	72 / 696		9.8	0.64 [0.44 – 0.94]
EPILOG	73 / 1853	85 / 939		15.7	0.41 [0.30 – 0.57]
EPISTENT 30 days	86 / 1690	83 / 809		15.1	0.50 [0.37 – 0.68]
ERASER	11 / 154	8 / 71		1.5	0.61 [0.23 – 1.65]
ESPRIT 30 days	67 / 1040	104 / 1024		14.2	0.61 [0.44 – 0.84]
IMPACT	3 / 101	2 / 49		0.4	0.72 [0.12 – 4.45]
IMPACT-II	190 / 2682	112 / 1323		20.2	0.83 [0.65 – 1.05]
ISAR-2	5 / 201	12 / 200		1.7	0.40 [0.14 – 1.16]
Kerelakes DJ	0 / 73	0 / 20		0.0	Not estimable
RAPPORT	11 / 241	14 / 242		1.9	0.78 [0.35 – 1.75]
RESTORE 30 days	54 / 1071	69 / 1070		9.5	0.77 [0.53 – 1.11]
Simoons ML	1 / 30	3 / 30		0.4	0.31 [0.03 – 3.17]
Total (95% CI)	587 / 10523	633 / 7264		100.0	0.61 [0.55 – 0.69]

Test for heterogeneity: chi-square=16.83, df=12, p=0.1562
Test for overall effect: Z=-8.05, p=0.00

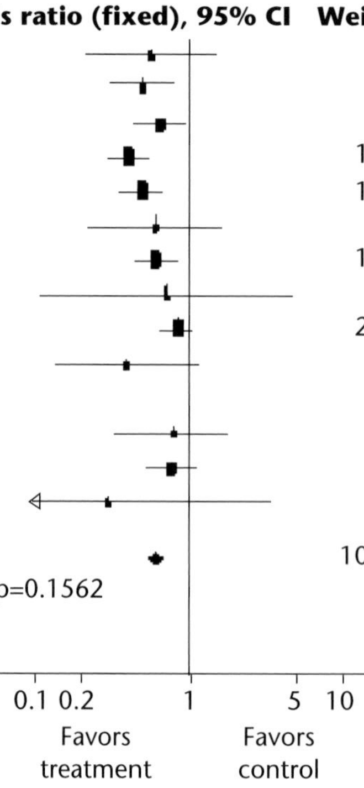

0.1 0.2   1   5   10
Favors   Favors
treatment   control

Figure 3.13
Meta-analysis of primary outcome of death or MI at 30 days in GP IIb/IIIa inhibitor trials in which any percutaneous revascularization occurred. (Reproduced from Bosch X and Marrugat J. Cochrane Database System Rev 2002;2:1–48.[100] Copyright Cochrane Library. Reproduced with permission.)

Study	Treatment	Control	Odds ratio (random), 95% CI	weight (%)	Odds ratio (random), 95% CI
ADMIRAL	1 / 149	0 / 151		0.8	3.06 [0.12 – 75.74]
CAPTURE	24 / 630	12 / 635		9.3	2.06 [1.02 – 4.15]
EPIC 30 days	99 / 708	46 / 696		15.4	2.30 [1.59 – 3.31]
EPILOG	51 / 1853	29 / 939		13.5	0.89 [0.56 – 1.41]
EPISTENT 30 days	2 / 1590	2 / 809		2.0	0.51 [0.07 – 3.61]
ESPRIT 30 days	13 / 1040	4 / 1024		5.0	3.23 [1.05 – 9.93]
IMPACT	5 / 101	4 / 49		3.7	0.59 [0.15 – 2.29]
IMPACT-II	132 / 2682	60 / 1328		16.5	1.09 [0.80 – 1.50]
ISAR-2	7 / 201	9 / 200		5.9	0.77 [0.28 – 2.10]
RAPPORT	40 / 241	23 / 242		11.9	1.89 [1.10 – 3.28]
RESTORE 30 days	57 / 1071	40 / 1070		14.5	1.45 [0.96 – 2.19]
Simoons ML	1 / 30	3 / 30		1.5	0.31 [0.03 – 3.17]
Total (95% CI)	432 / 10 296	232 / 7173		100.0	1.38 [1.04 – 1.85]

Test for heterogeneity: chi-square = 23.41, df = 11, p = 0.0154
Test for overall effect: Z = 2.19, p = 0.03

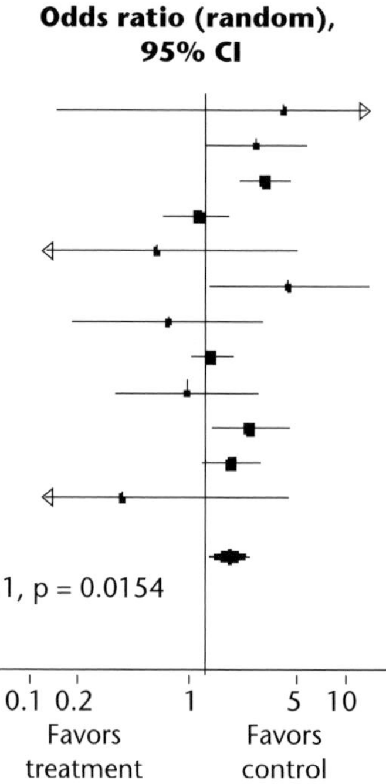

0.1 0.2   1   5   10
Favors   Favors
treatment   control

Figure 3.14
Meta-analysis of secondary outcome of major bleeding at 30 days in GP IIb/IIIa inhibitor trials in which any percutaneous revascularization occurred. (Reproduced from Bosch X and Marrugat J. Cochrane Database System Rev 2002;2:1–48.[100] Copyright Cochrane Library. Reproduced with permission.)

Heparin therapy may be required during treatment both with eptifibatide and with tirofiban.[104] In the PRISM–PLUS study, the tirofiban-alone group was stopped early due to an excess of deaths.[105] In the setting of PCI, an appropriate dose of heparin is necessary to avoid excessive bleeding rates, as seen in the EPIC study.[80] Heparin should be dosed at 70 U/kg, with a goal ACT of 250 s, or a target activated partial thromboplastin time (PTT) of 50–70 s.[80,106] After PCI, the heparin should generally be discontinued, with removal of the access sheath when the ACT reaches 180 s, while the GP IIb/IIIa inhibitor infusion is continued. These measures will help reduce bleeding at the vascular access site.

GP IIb/IIIa inhibitors during acute coronary syndromes

Six large trials have examined the role of GP IIb/IIIa inhibitors in patients presenting with unstable angina or non-ST-segment elevation MI.

In the PURSUIT trial, the acute coronary syndrome patients who were randomized to eptifibatide had a 1.5% absolute reduction in death or MI at 30 days (14.2% versus 15.7% for placebo; $p = 0.04$).[97] Eptifibatide reduces both the size and incidence of MI in patients with unstable angina or non-ST-segment elevation MI.[107] This benefit was maintained at 6 months as well.[108]

In the Platelet Receptor Inhibition in Ischemic Syndrome Management (PRISM) trial, 3232 patients with unstable angina were randomized to tirofiban 0.6 μg/kg intravenous bolus for 30 minutes followed by 0.15 μg/kg/min for 48 hours or unfractionated heparin. The composite endpoint of death, MI, or refractory ischemia at 48 hours was reduced 32%, from 5.6% to 3.8% ($p = 0.01$).[109] Both refractory ischemia and MI were reduced by approximately one-third in the tirofiban group. The tirofiban group had a trend toward a reduction in the composite endpoint both at 7 days (10.3% versus 11.2% for placebo; $p = 0.33$) and at 30 days (15.9% versus 17.1% for placebo; $p = 0.34$). The overall mortality rate was significantly reduced in the tirofiban group at 30 days: from 3.6% to 2.3% ($p = 0.02$). In addition, the patients undergoing percutaneous revascularization had a significant reduction in the overall endpoint at 30 days, from 27.3% to 21.6% (HR 0.72; 95% CI 0.53–0.98).[109]

Heeschen et al[110] determined that patients with elevated levels of troponin I and T had significantly greater rates of death or myocardial infarction in the PRISM study (Figure 3.15). In addition, those troponin I-positive patients who received tirofiban had a lower rate of death (1.6% versus 6.2%; HR 0.25; 95% CI 0.09–0.68; $p = 0.004$) and MI (2.7% versus 6.8%; HR 0.37; 95% CI 0.16–0.84; $p = 0.01$) at 30 days than those in the heparin group. The risk of death or MI at 30 days of the troponin-positive patients treated with tirofiban was similar to that of troponin-negative patients in the tirofiban group (4.3%

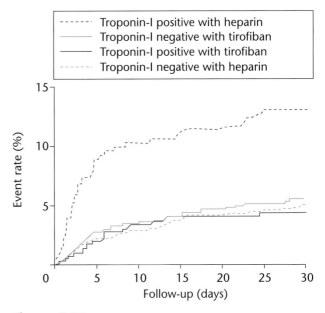

Figure 3.15
Reduction in death or myocardial infarction in troponin-positive patients who received tirofiban. Tirofiban reduced the event rates to those with negative troponin levels. (Adapted from Heeshen et al. Lancet 1999;354:1757–62[110] with permission from Elsevier.)

versus 5.7%; $p = 0.56$). The benefit of tirofiban treatment for troponin-positive patients was independent of whether patients continued with medical treatment or underwent coronary revascularization after 48 hours of treatment. At 30 days, the decrease in mortality or myocardial infarction remained significant in both groups (HR for medical therapy 0.30; $p = 0.004$; HR for revascularization 0.37; $p = 0.02$).[110] Tirofiban had similar effects in reducing death or MI at 30 days in patients with elevated troponin T levels.

The PRISM in Patients Limited by Unstable Signs and Symptoms (PRISM–PLUS) study randomized 1915 patients with unstable angina or non-ST-segment elevation MI to tirofiban with heparin or heparin alone for 48–72 hours.[105] The tirofiban-alone group was stopped prematurely due to an excess of mortality at 7 days (4.6%, as compared with 1.1% for the heparin group). The primary endpoint of death, MI, or refractory ischemia at 7 days was reduced 32%: from 17.9% in the heparin group to 12.9% ($p = 0.004$) in the tirofiban and heparin group. The reduction was due primarily to a 47% decrease in MI ($p = 0.006$) and a 30% reduction in refractory ischemia ($p = 0.02$). This endpoint was also significantly reduced at 30 days (HR 0.78; 95% CI 0.63–0.98; $p = 0.03$) and at 6 months (HR 0.81; 95% CI 0.68–0.97; $p = 0.02$). Major bleeding and transfusions were slightly more frequent with the combination therapy than with heparin alone.[105]

In the Global Use of Strategies to Open Occluded Coronary Arteries (GUSTO)-IV trial, over 7800 acute coronary syndrome patients were randomized to placebo, abciximab bolus and 24-hour infusion, or abciximab bolus and 48-hour infusion. All patients received aspirin and

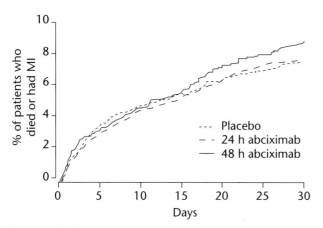

Figure 3.16
Composite primary endpoint of 30-day death or MI in the GUSTO-IV study. (Reproduced from The GUSTO-IV ACS Investigators. Lancet 2001;357:1915–1924[111] with permission from Elsevier.)

either unfractionated or low-molecular-weight heparin. No differences were seen in the 30-day combined death or MI rates between the groups: 8% for placebo, 8.2% for 24-hour abciximab, and 9.1% for 48-hour abciximab[111] (Figure 3.16). The lack of benefit with abciximab was consistent in most subgroups. Mortality at 48 hours while on therapy was significantly higher in patients receiving abciximab than in those on placebo, but by 7 days, event rates in all groups were similar. Major bleeding and blood transfusions were increased in the abciximab 48-hour infusion group. One explanation for these results may be a decline in the antithrombotic effect with the dose and duration of abciximab used. Kereiakes et al[112] observed that during the continuous infusion of abciximab, a large variation in the inhibition of platelet aggregation occurred. Incomplete blockade of GP IIb/IIIa receptors may be associated with enhanced expression of CD40 ligand and subsequently a prothrombotic and proinflammatory effect.[113,114]

The GP IIb/IIIa inhibitors demonstrate early benefits during medical therapy as well as protecting against myocardial damage following percutaneous intervention. A meta-analysis of CAPTURE, PURSUIT, and PRISM–PLUS demonstrated a 34% relative risk reduction in death or nonfatal MI in this early period prior to intervention in the GP IIb/IIIa group (2.5% versus 3.8% in the placebo group; $p < 0.001$) (Figure 3.17).[84] The event rate during the first 48 hours after PCI was also significantly lower in the GP IIb/IIIa group (4.9% versus 8.0%; 41% reduction; $p < 0.001$).

In a meta-analysis of six trials, 31 402 acute coronary syndrome patients randomized to a GP IIb/IIIa inhibitor had an absolute 1% reduction in 30-day death or MI rate (10.8% versus 11.8% for placebo, odds ratio 0.91; 95% CI 0.84–0.98; $p = 0.015$).[115] The greatest benefit was seen in patients with elevated troponin levels; a 15% reduction in the 30-day death or MI rate occurred with the use of GP IIb/IIIa agents in this patient group (10.3% versus 12% for placebo; HR 0.85; 95% CI 0.71–1.03). Overall, major bleeding complications were increased in the GP IIb/IIIa

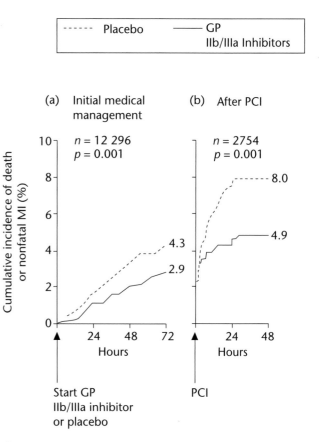

Figure 3.17
Reduction in death or nonfatal MI (a) prior to and (b) after PCI with GP IIb/IIIa inhibition. (Adapted from Boersma E et al. Circulation 1999;100:2045–8[84] with permission from Lippincott Williams & Wilkins.)

group (2.4% versus 1.4%; $p < 0.0001$). Intracranial bleeding was not increased with the use of GP IIb/IIIa inhibitors compared with the placebo group.[115]

Lamifiban, a small-molecule nonpeptide GP IIb/IIIa inhibitor, was evaluated in a dose-ranging study, Platelet IIb/IIIa Antagonism for the Reduction of Acute Coronary Syndromes Events in a Global Organization Network (PARAGON). In this study, 2282 unstable angina and non-ST-segment elevation MI patients were randomized to placebo, low-dose lamifiban, or high-dose lamifiban, with or without heparin. The composite of death or nonfatal MI occurred in 10.6% of the low-dose lamifiban, 12.0% of the high-dose lamifiban, and 11.7% of the placebo group at 30 days ($p = 0.67$).[116] However, by 6 months, the rate of death or MI was lowest in the low-dose group (13.7% versus 17.9% for placebo; $p = 0.027$) and intermediate in the high-dose group (16.4%; $p = 0.45$). Bleeding events were increased in the high-dose group.

In PARAGON-B, lamifiban did not significantly reduce the primary endpoint of death, MI, or severe recurrent ischemia at 30 days in acute coronary syndrome patients (Figure 3.18).[117] However, in the subgroup of patients with an elevated troponin T, who had a much higher event rate, lamifiban significantly reduced the 30-day composite

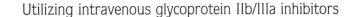

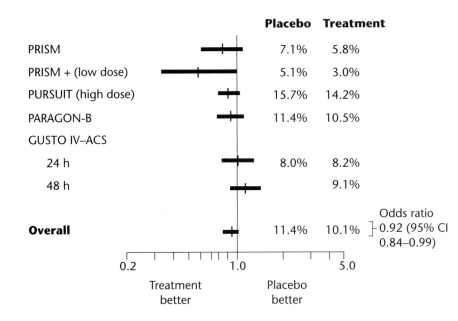

		Placebo	Treatment
PRISM		7.1%	5.8%
PRISM + (low dose)		5.1%	3.0%
PURSUIT (high dose)		15.7%	14.2%
PARAGON-B		11.4%	10.5%
GUSTO IV–ACS			
24 h		8.0%	8.2%
48 h			9.1%
Overall		11.4%	10.1%

Odds ratio 0.92 (95% CI 0.84–0.99)

0.2   1.0   5.0

Treatment better   Placebo better

Figure 3.18
Combined endpoint of 30-day death or MI in major trials using parenteral GP IIb/IIIa inhibitors in acute coronary syndrome patients. (Adapted from Boersma E et al. Circulation 1999;100:2045–8[84] with permission from Lippincott Williams & Wilkins.)

primary endpoint from 19.4% to 11.0% ($p = 0.01$).[118] Due to the limited sample size of troponin-positive patients, the investigators did not show a statistically significant interaction of troponin status with treatment. However, as seen below, the combined odds ratio of three studies, including PARAGON-B, show a highly significant benefit of GP IIb/IIIa antagonists in reducing combined death or MI in patients with elevated troponin levels (odds ratio 0.33; 95% CI 0.19–0.57), along with a significant interaction between positive troponin status and glycoprotein use (Figure 3.19).[118] Patients with positive troponins have more extensive coronary disease, more complex lesions, and more often thrombus at the culprit lesion.[119,120] Therefore, the mechanism for the positive treatment effects of GP IIb/IIIa inhibitors in patients with elevated troponin levels likely reflects their ability to prevent or minimize microvascular embolization. Despite

these results, further development of lamifiban has been halted.

GP IIb/IIIa inhibitors during acute myocardial infarction

Although fibrinolytic therapy became the standard of care for acute MI in the mid-1980s, no further reduction in mortality has been achieved with this therapy since the introduction of front-loaded alteplase in the GUSTO-I trial.[121] Fibrinolytic therapy is complicated by reocclusion with subsequent reinfarction, inadequate myocardial perfusion, and intracranial hemorrhage.

The Thrombolysis In Myocardial Infarction (TIMI)-14 investigators examined the role of abciximab with varying doses of alteplase along with heparin in patients with acute

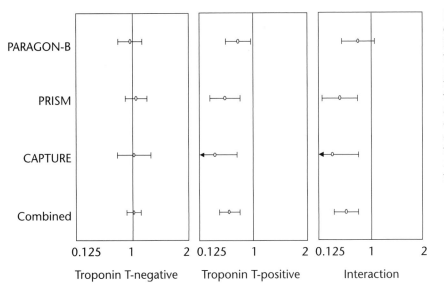

PARAGON-B, PRISM, CAPTURE, Combined

0.125   1   2   0.125   1   2   0.125   1   2

Troponin T-negative   Troponin T-positive   Interaction

Figure 3.19
Odds ratios with 95% confidence intervals for death or MI among troponin-negative and -positive patients and for interaction of troponin status with treatment effect for PRISM, CAPTURE, PARAGON-B, and combined trials. Values to the left of the centerline (1) indicate a benefit of GP IIb/IIIa inhibitors. (Adapted from Newby KL et al. Circulation 2001;103:2891–6[118] with permission from Lippincott Williams & Wilkins.)

MI. They determined that abciximab with 50 mg alteplase and low-dose heparin resulted in a 77% TIMI grade 3 flow rate at 90 minutes, without an increase in the risk of bleeding.[122] Similarly, in Strategies for Patency Enhancement in the Emergency Department (SPEED), abciximab added to reteplase 5+5 U and heparin (60 U/kg) resulted in the highest TIMI grade 3 rates at 60 minutes in acute MI patients.[123] These studies provided the basis for much larger phase III studies utilizing combination reduced-dose fibrinolytic and GP IIb/IIIa inhibitor therapy.

Another angiographic study used a combination of eptifibatide and alteplase for patients with acute MI. In the Integrilin and Low Dose Thrombolysis in Acute MI (INTRO AMI) study, a dose-finding study, a combination of double-bolus eptifibatide (administered within 10 minutes of each other) with infusion in addition to low-dose alteplase produced the greatest TIMI grade 3 flow and the most optimal myocardial perfusion as measured by corrected TIMI frame count.[124] The combination eptifibatide and alteplase group had an absolute 16% improvement in TIMI grade 3 flow over alteplase alone at 60 minutes. It is unclear whether the angiographic superiority of this com-

bination group will translate into a survival benefit or a reduction in recurrent ischemic events.

In the Enoxaparin as Adjunctive Antithrombin Therapy for ST-Elevation Myocardial Infarction (ENTIRE)/TIMI-23 study, 483 patients with acute MI were randomized to full-dose tenecteplase with unfractionated heparin, tenecteplase with enoxaparin, or half-dose tenecteplase with abciximab and either unfractionated heparin or enoxaparin. When compared with full-dose tenecteplase, combination therapy with half-dose tenecteplase plus abciximab was associated with a similar TIMI grade 3 flow at 60 minutes and a trend toward more complete ST-segment resolution at 180 minutes. This therapy resulted in a reduction of the combination of death and MI at 30 days at the cost of an increase in major hemorrhage.[125]

In GUSTO-V, 16 588 patients with ST-segment elevation MI were randomized to open-label half-dose reteplase (5+5 U) with abciximab (0.25 mg/kg bolus and 0.125 µg/kg/min for 12 hours) or full-dose reteplase (10+10 U) with either unfractionated heparin or low-molecular-weight heparin in a superiority study. The primary endpoint of 30-day mortality rate did not differ

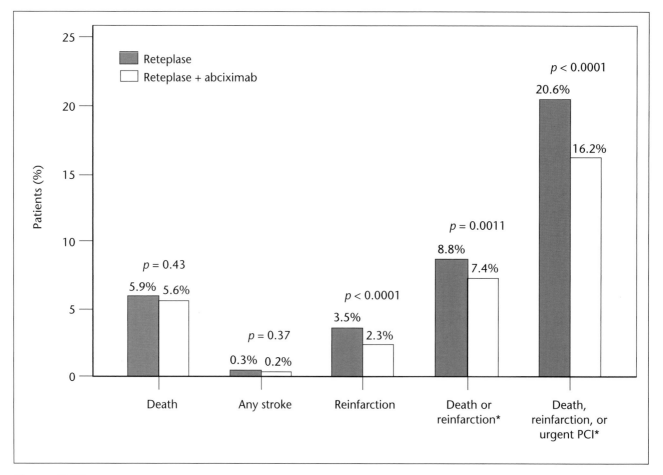

Figure 3.20
Primary and secondary endpoints at 30 days in GUSTO-V. *indicates at day 7 or at discharge, whichever occurred earlier. (Adapted from Chan AW and Moliterno DJ. Curr Opin Cardiol 2001;16:375–83.[127])

between the two groups (5.6% in the combined group versus 5.9% in the reteplase group; $p = 0.43$) (Figure 3.20).[126,127] However, the composite of death or nonfatal reinfarction was significantly reduced in the combined group (7.4% versus 8.8% in the reteplase group; $p = 0.0011$) The use of percutaneous interventions by 7 days was also significantly reduced from 27.9% in the reteplase group to 25.4% in the abciximab group ($p = 0.013$). The frequencies of major cardiac complications, such as ventricular arrhythmias, asystole, ventricular septal defect, or ventricular rupture, were reduced with the combined regimen. The overall combined rate of stroke was similar in the two groups, however, there was a trend towards an increase in intracranial hemorrhage in patients older than 75 years treated with the combination of reteplase and abciximab (2.1% versus 1.1%; $p = 0.07$). As expected from other studies, the rate of moderate or severe nonintracranial bleeding was significantly increased in the combined group (4.6% versus 2.3%; $p < 0.0001$). In addition, the use of any transfusion or thrombocytopenia was also greater in the abciximab groups.[126]

In the Assessment of the Safety and Efficacy of a New Thrombolytic Regimen (ASSENT)-3 study, 6095 acute ST-elevation MI patients were randomized to one of three regimens: full-dose tenecteplase with unfractionated heparin for 48 hours, half-dose tenecteplase with abciximab and low-dose unfractionated heparin, or full-dose tenecteplase and enoxaparin for a maximum of 7 days. The composite 30-day endpoint of death, in-hospital reinfarction, or in-hospital refractory ischemia was significantly reduced in the enoxaparin group (11.4%) and in the abciximab group (11.1%), compared with the unfractionated heparin group (15.4%; $p = 0.0001$) (Figure 3.21).[128] The combined efficacy and safety endpoint (death, reinfarction, refractory ischemia, intracranial hemorrhage, or major bleeding) was also reduced in the enoxaparin and abciximab groups (13.8% and 14.2%, versus 17.0% in the unfractionated heparin group; $p = 0.0081$). The rates of

in-hospital death or reinfarction were also lower in the enoxaparin and abciximab groups than in the unfractionated heparin group (6.8% and 7.3%, versus 9.1%; $p = 0.0198$). Both the enoxaparin and abciximab groups underwent significantly fewer urgent PCIs in hospital than the unfractionated heparin group. No significant differences in total stroke or intracranial hemorrhage were found between the three treatments. However, the rate of major bleeding complications was three times higher in patients older than 75 years and in diabetic patients receiving abciximab compared with unfractionated heparin.[128] Similar to GUSTO-V, bleeding episodes and transfusions occurred more frequently in the combined treatment groups.

The results of these studies demonstrate that a combination of abciximab and reduced-dose fibrinolytic agent yields similar reductions in 30-day mortality as compared with fibrinolytic therapy alone, with a greater reduction in reinfarction, recurrent ischemia, and in-hospital urgent PCI.[126,128] Such a regimen may be an alternative to standard fibrinolytic therapy in certain patient groups, such as younger patients with larger anterior infarctions who may be eligible to undergo urgent percutaneous coronary revascularization. However, in patients 75 years and older, primary percutaneous revascularization or fibrinolytic therapy alone would be the optimal treatment, given the increased risk of intracranial hemorrhage and other major bleeding episodes with the combination therapy in this age group.

GP IIb/IIIa inhibitor facilitated MI and adjunctive therapy

Primary stenting for acute ST-segment elevation MI is associated with a reduction in TIMI grade 3 flow as well as a trend towards increased mortality in the first 6 months compared with angioplasty alone, despite a reduced rate

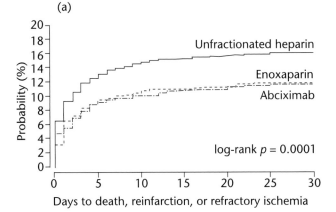

(a)

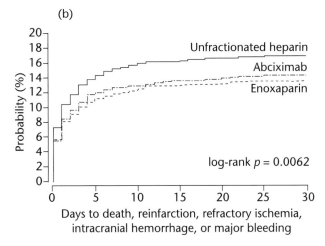

(b)

Figure 3.21
Kaplan–Meier curves for primary efficacy endpoint (a) and for combination efficacy and safety endpoint (b) in ASSENT-3. (Adapted from ASSENT-3 Investigators. Lancet 2001;358:605–13[128] with permission from Elsevier.)

of restenosis and target vessel revascularization.[129] These findings may result from distal embolization associated with stent placement. The GP IIb/IIIa inhibitors are effective in reducing this microvascular embolization, which is usually associated with platelet activation and aggregation.[78]

Neumann et al[130] examined the role of abciximab in 200 patients undergoing primary stenting for acute MI. The patients randomized to abciximab had an increased peak flow velocity in the culprit vessel, reduced wall motion abnormalities, and had a higher global left ventricular ejection fraction than the heparin-alone group at 14-day follow-up.

In addition to improving myocardial blood flow, abciximab prior to revascularization improves infarct artery patency at 60 or 90 minutes in the setting of acute MI. In SPEED, TIMI grade 3 flow was 27% at 60–90 minutes, while in TIMI-14, TIMI grade 3 flow was 32% at 90 minutes in the abciximab-alone arms (Figure 3.22).[123] In the Glycoprotein Receptor Antagonist Patency Evaluation (GRAPE) pilot trial, abciximab was administered to acute MI patients in the emergency department. TIMI grade 3 flow was present in 18% of patients, while TIMI grade 2 or 3 flow was found in 40% of patients – both at a median time of 45 minutes from abciximab administration to angiography (Figure 3.22).[131] These results are higher than in acute MI patients treated with only heparin and aspirin, in which the TIMI grade 3 flow does not exceed 10% after 60 minutes.[132]

Of the 2099 patients enrolled in EPIC, 64 underwent primary or rescue angioplasty for acute MI. The primary composite endpoint of death, reinfarction, repeat intervention, or bypass surgery at 30 days was reduced by 83% with the use of abciximab in this group (26.1% placebo versus 4.5% abciximab bolus and infusion; $p = 0.06$). At 6 months, ischemic events were reduced from 47.8% with placebo to 4.5% with abciximab bolus and infusion

($p = 0.002$), particularly MI ($p = 0.05$) and repeat revascularization ($p = 0.002$).[133]

In the ReoPro and Primary PTCA Organization and Randomized Trial (RAPPORT), patients with acute MI of less than 12 hours duration who were undergoing primary angioplasty were randomized to placebo or abciximab. Abciximab significantly reduced the combined endpoint of death, reinfarction, or urgent target vessel revascularization at 6 months (11.6% for abciximab versus 17.8% for placebo; $p = 0.05$) at a price of increased risk of major bleeding, primarily at the access site (16.6% versus 9.5%; $p = 0.02$).[134]

These small studies encouraged the use of GP IIb/IIIa inhibitors in larger acute MI studies. Schömig et al.[135] randomized 140 acute MI patients to front-loaded alteplase with unfractionated heparin or primary stenting with abciximab. The stent plus abciximab group had a smaller infarct size and a greater salvage index, compared with the alteplase group approximately 10 days later. In addition, the cumulative incidence of death, reinfarction, or stroke at 6 months was lower in the stent plus abciximab group than in the alteplase group (8.5% versus 23.2%; relative risk 0.34; 95% CI 0.13–0.88; $p = 0.02$).

In the Abciximab before Direct Angioplasty and Stenting in Myocardial Infarction Regarding Acute and Long-Term Follow-up (ADMIRAL), 300 patients with acute MI were randomized to abciximab plus stenting or placebo plus stenting. The primary endpoint of death, reinfarction, or urgent revascularization of the target vessel at 30 days was significantly reduced from 14.6% in the placebo group to 6.0% in the abciximab group ($p = 0.01$) (Figure 3.23).[136] This composite endpoint was also reduced in the abciximab group at 6 months (15.9% placebo versus 7.45%; $p = 0.02$).

One important finding from ADMIRAL is that the TIMI grade 3 flow was significantly higher in the abciximab

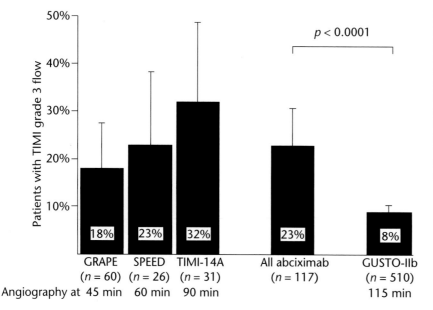

Figure 3.22
Preangioplasty Thrombolysis in Myocardial Infarction (TIMI) grade 3 flow with 95% confidence interval in emergency room-initiated abciximab patency trials (GRAPE and SPEED) compared with TIMI flow grades prior to PCI in the angioplasty arm of GUSTO-IIb. (Adapted from van den Merkhof LF et al. J Am Coll Cardiol 1999;33:1528–32[131] with permission from the American College of Cardiology Foundation.)

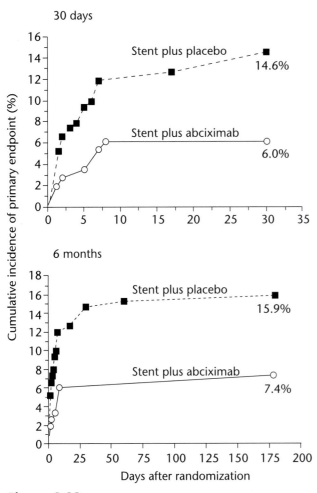

Figure 3.23
Kaplan–Meier curves showing cumulative incidence of the primary endpoint: death, reinfarction, or urgent target vessel revascularization, at 30 days and 6 months in ADMIRAL. At 30 days, there was a 59% relative risk reduction in the primary endpoint in the abciximab group ($p = 0.01$). At 6 months, there was a 53% risk reduction in the primary endpoint in the abciximab group ($p = 0.02$). (Adapted from Montalesot G et al. N Engl J Med 2001;344:1895–903.[136])

group than in the placebo group at angiography (16.8% versus 5.4% for placebo; $p = 0.01$) and the combination of TIMI grade 2 or 3 flow was also greater in the abciximab group (25.8% versus 10.8%; $p = 0.006$).[136] Consequently, the rate of procedural success was higher with abciximab than with placebo (95.1% versus 84.3%; $p = 0.01$). At 6 months, the frequency of TIMI grade 3 flow remained higher in the abciximab group than in the placebo group (94.3% versus 82.8%; $p = 0.04$). In addition, culprit vessel reocclusions occurred less frequently in the abciximab group (2.9% versus 12.1%; $p = 0.04$). Left ventricular ejection fraction was significantly greater in the abciximab group both at 24 hours and at 6 months. However, the improvement in the combined endpoint at 30 days and at 6 months was confined to the 26% of patients who received abciximab well in advance of revascularization.[136]

One study evaluated the use of abciximab in both primary angioplasty and stenting for acute MI. In the Controlled Abciximab and Device Investigation to Lower Late Angioplasty Complications (CADILLAC), 2082 patients with acute MI were randomized to PTCA alone or with abciximab or to stenting alone or with abciximab. At 6 months, the primary endpoint of death, stroke, reinfarction, or any revascularization of the target vessel occurred in 20% after PTCA alone, 16.5% after PTCA and abciximab, 11.5% after stenting alone, and 10.2% after stenting plus abciximab ($p < 0.0001$).[137] There were no significant differences in the rates of death, stroke, or reinfarction between the groups. The difference in the primary endpoint occurred due to a significant reduction in target vessel revascularization rates (ranging from 15.7% after PTCA to 5.2% after stenting plus abciximab; $p < 0.001$). The rate of angiographic restenosis was reduced from 40.8% after PTCA to 22.2% after stenting ($p < 0.001$). In addition, the rates of reocclusion of the infarct-related artery were 11.3% after PTCA and 5.7% after stenting ($p = 0.01$).

In CADILLAC, the routine use of stenting in acute MI resulted in higher event-free survival and better angiographic outcomes than PTCA. The clinical benefits of stenting were consistent in all subgroups, due primarily to lower rates of early and late restenosis and reocclusion of the infarct-related artery. Both the clinical benefits and the angiographic findings were all independent of abciximab use. However, abciximab did reduce the rate of subacute thrombosis and recurrent ischemia leading to repeat revascularization of the target vessel several weeks after primary PTCA or stenting. Unlike previous studies, abciximab did not improve TIMI flow rates or reduce the rates of angiographic restenosis, late reocclusion of the infarct artery, or late cardiac events after PTCA or stenting. No differences were found in left ventricular ejection fraction among the groups.[137] One criticism of this study is the lack of power to detect a difference in the abciximab groups, given the relatively low event rates seen in this trial.

Contraindications to the use of GP IIb/IIIa inhibitors

GP IIb/IIIa inhibitors should not be used in patients with active bleeding. Recent major surgery (last 3 months), stroke (within 6 months), thrombocytopenia (platelets $< 100 \times 10^9/l$), trauma, or uncontrolled hypertension are all relative contraindications to the use of these agents.[78]

Bleeding complications

In EPIC, the rate of major bleeding with abciximab bolus and infusion was significantly increased (14% compared with 7% in the placebo group; $p < 0.001$).[80] This rate of bleeding may be minimized with low-dose heparin as well as early sheath removal in the setting of PCI.[82] Clinical factors that may increase the risk of bleeding complications with the use of GP IIb/IIIa inhibitors include female sex, older age, lower weight (<70 kg), acute MI, type C lesions, and coronary intervention.[138] Procedural risk factors that may increase the risk of bleeding with the use of these agents include procedural failure, large sheath size, use of a venous sheath, and urgent coronary artery bypass grafting (CABG) surgery.[139] Recent modifications, which have been shown to reduce the incidence of major bleeding when using GP IIb/IIIa inhibitors, include the use of reduced dosing-weight base-adjusted heparin (70 U/kg) with lower target ACT (200–250 s) values during percutaneous revascularization, avoidance of postprocedural heparin, early removal of vascular access sheaths, and development of protocols for vascular access site management and transfusion.[82,139] Additionally, the decreased rate of emergency CABG surgery after unsuccessful angioplasty may also have contributed to the lower rate of bleeding.[139] With these advances, the rate of major bleeding in PCI using these agents has been reduced to nearly that of placebo.

In the event that emergency CABG surgery is necessary, the infusion of the GP IIb/IIIa inhibitor should be stopped as soon as possible. An excess of bleeding complications with CABG surgery after treatment with the shorter-acting small-molecule GP IIb/IIIa inhibitors has not been demonstrated.[139] However, abciximab has been associated with increased bleeding in emergency CABG by two groups.[140,141] Tirofiban or eptifibatide should be stopped at least 4 hours prior to surgery.[78] With abciximab, the infusion should be discontinued as soon as possible and surgery should be delayed as long as possible, for up to 12–24 hours, to allow recovery of platelet function. In the operating room, ACT should be monitored to guide heparin use during bypass. Platelet transfusions should be administered if abciximab is still active or if bleeding complications occur.[140]

Thrombocytopenia is uncommon with any of the IIb/IIIa antagonists, and platelet counts less than 100×10^9/l occur in less than 5% of all patients treated. Severe thrombocytopenia with abciximab (platelets $< 20 \times 10^9$/l) occurs in approximately 0.4–1.0% of patients.[142] Thrombocytopenia usually manifests within the first 24 hours, with the most severe form occurring within 1 hour. Platelet counts should be assessed within the first 4 hours and again on a daily basis when a GP IIb/IIIa antagonist is utilized.[78] In the abciximab registry, no cases of hypersensitivity, major bleeding, or death were reported in over 500 patients treated with repeated administration of abciximab. While the overall rate of thrombocytopenia in these patients was consistent with first abciximab treatment (4.6%), the rate of severe thrombocytopenia (platelets $< 20 \times 10^9$/l) was increased to 2.4% with readministration.[143] Delayed thrombocytopenia, after hospital discharge, occurred in four patients (0.8%), including two who developed profound thrombocytopenia. Human antichimeric antibodies (HACA) developed in about 5% of all patients within 1 month after the administration of abciximab. After readministration, an additional 82 of 432 patients (19.0%) became HACA-positive. HACA did not neutralize the in vitro inhibition of platelet aggregation by abciximab or correlate with clinical events. Finally, no patients receiving repeat administration of abciximab developed heparin-induced thrombocytopenia.[143]

Conclusions

The past decade has seen several advances in antiplatelet agents. Aspirin remains the backbone of antiplatelet therapy. The ADP receptor antagonist clopidogrel has been demonstrated to be superior to aspirin, although the combination of aspirin and clopidogrel appears particularly promising for a wide variety of indications. The intravenous GP IIb/IIIa antagonists are important to improve the results of PCI, particularly in patients with acute coronary syndromes, acute MI, or diabetes; they also have a role in the initial medical management of high-risk patients with acute coronary syndromes. The exact role of the GP IIb/IIIa inhibitors in combination with fibrinolytics and PCI for acute MI remains to be elucidated.

References

1. Bhatt DL, Topol EJ. Antiplatelet and anticoagulant therapy in the secondary prevention of ischemic heart disease. Med Clin North Am 2000;84:163–79.
2. Bhatt DL, Kapadia SR, Yadav JS, et al. Update on clinical trials of antiplatelet therapy for cerebrovascular diseases. Cerebrovasc Dis 2000;10 (Suppl S5):34–40.
3. Fuster V, Badimon L, Badimon JJ, Chesebro JH. The pathogenesis of coronary artery disease and the acute coronary syndromes (Part 1). N Engl J Med 1992;326:242–50.
4. Fuster V, Badimon L, Badimon JJ, Chesebro JH. The pathogenesis of coronary artery disease and the acute coronary syndromes (Part 2). N Engl J Med 1992;326:310–18.
5. Gibson PC. Salicylic acid for coronary thrombosis? Lancet 1948;1:965.
6. ISIS-2 Collaborative Group. Randomised trial of intravenous streptokinase, oral aspirin, both, or neither among 17,187 cases of suspected acute myocardial infarction: ISIS-2. Lancet 1988;ii:349–60.
7. Pedersen AK, FitzGerald GA. Dose-related kinetics of aspirin. Presystemic acetylation of platelet cyclooxygenase. N Engl J Med 1984;311:1206–11.
8. Fitzgerald DJ, Roy L, Catella F, FitzGerald GA. Platelet activation in unstable coronary disease. N Engl J Med 1986;315:983–9.
9. Feldman M, Cryer B. Aspirin absorption rates and platelet inhibition times with 325 mg buffered aspirin tablets (chewed or swallowed intact) and with buffered aspirin solution. Am J Cardiol 1999;84:404–9.
10. Cairns JA, Theroux P, Lewis HD, et al. Antithrombotic agents in coronary artery disease. Chest 2001; 119:228S–52S.

11. Antiplatelet Trialists' Collaboration. Collaborative overview of randomized trials of antiplatelet therapy. Prevention of death, myocardial infarction, and stroke by prolonged antiplatelet therapy in various categories of patients. Antiplatelet Trialists' Collaboration. BMJ 194;308:81–106.

12. Theroux P, Ouimet H, McCans J, et al. Aspirin, heparin, or both to treat acute unstable angina. N Engl J Med 1988;319:1105–11.

13. Theroux P, Waters D, Qui S, et al. Aspirin versus heparin to prevent myocardial infarction during the acute phase of unstable angina. Circulation 1993;88:2045–8.

14. Lewis HD, Davis JW, Archibald DG, et al. Protective effects of aspirin against acute myocardial infarction and death in men with unstable angina. Results of a Veterans Administration Cooperative Study. N Engl J Med 1983; 309:396–403.

15. Cairns JA, Gent M, Singer J, et al. Aspirin, sufinpyrazone, or both, in unstable angina: results of a Canadian multicenter clinical trial. N Engl J Med;313:1369–75.

16. Steering Committee of the Physicians' Health Study Research Group. Final report on the aspirin component of the ongoing Physicians' Health Study. N Engl J Med 1989; 321:129–35.

17. Berger PB. Oral antiplatelet agents: aspirin, ticlodipine, clopidogrel, cilostazol, and the oral glycoprotein IIb/IIIa inhibitors. In: (Topol EJ, ed). Acute Coronary Sydromes. New York: Marcel Dekker, 2001;453–98.

18. Medical Research Council. Randomized trial of low intensity oral antiocoagulation with warfarin and low-dose aspirin in the primary prevention of ischemic heart disease in men at increased risk: the Medical Research Council's General Practice Research Framework Thrombosis Prevention Trial. Lancet 1998;351:233–41.

19. Peto R, Gray R, Collins R, et al. Randomized trial of prophylactic daily aspirin in British male doctors. BMJ 1988;926:313–16.

20. Hansson L, Zanchetti A, Carruthers SG, et al. Effects of intensive blood-pressure lowering and low-dose aspirin in patients with hypertension: principal results of the Hypertension Optimal Treatment (HOT) randomized trial. Lancet 1998;351:1755–62.

21. Taylor DW, Barnett HJ, Haynes RB, et al. Low-dose and high-dose acetylsalicylic acid for patients undergoing carotid endarterectomy: a randomized controlled trial. ASA and Carotid Endarterectomy (ACE) Trial Collaborators. Lancet 1999;353:2179–84.

22. Antithrombotic Trialists' Collaboration. Collaborative meta-analysis of randomized trials of antiplatelet therapy for prevention of death, myocardial infarction, and stroke in high risk patients. BMJ 2002;324:71–86.

23. Schwartz L, Bourassa MG, Lesperance J, et al. Aspirin and dipyrimadole in the prevention of restenosis after percutaneous transluminal coronary angioplasty. N Engl J Med 1988;318:1714–19.

24. White CW, Chaitman B, Knudson ML, Chisholm RJ, and the Ticlopidine Study Group. Antiplatelet agents are effective in reducing the acute ischemic complications of angioplasty but do not prevent restenosis: results from the ticlopidine trial. Coronary Artery Dis 1991;2:757–67.

25. Savi P, Herbert JM. ADP receptors on platelets and ADP-selective antiaggregating agents. Med Res Rev 1996;16:159–79.

26. Mills DC, Puri R, Hu CJ, et al. Clopidogrel inhibits the binding of ADP analogues to the receptor mediating inhibition of platelet adenylate cyclase. Arterioscler Thromb 1992;86:479–91.

27. Coukell AJ, Markham A. Clopidogrel. Drugs 1997; 54:745–50.

28. Yang LH, Fareed J. Vasomodulatory action of clopidogrel and ticlopidine. Thromb Res 1997;3:437–502.

29. Puri RN, Colman RW. ADP-induced platelet activation. Crit Rev Biochem Mol Biol 1997;3:437–502.

30. Balsano F, Rizzon P, Violi F, et al. Antiplatelet treatment with ticlopidine in unstable angina. A controlled multicenter clinical trial. The Studio della Ticlopidina nell'Angina Instabile Group. Circulation 1990;82:17–26.

31. Bertrand ME, Allain H, LaBlanche JM, on behalf of the Investigators of the TACT study. Results of a randomized trial of ticlopidine versus placebo for prevention of acute closure and restenosis after coronary angioplasty (PTCA): the TACT study. Circulation 1990;82(Suppl III):190.

32. Hall P, Nakamura S, Maiello L, et al. A randomized comparison of combined ticlodipine and aspirin therapy versus aspirin therapy alone after successful intravascular ultarasound-guided stent implantation. Circulation 1996; 93:215–22.

33. Urban P, Macaya C, Rupprecht HJ, et al. Randomized evaluation of anticoagulation versus antiplatelet therapy after coronary stent implantation in high risk patients: the Multicenter Aspirin and Ticlopidine Trial after Intracoronary Stenting (MATTIS). Circulation 1998; 98:2126–32.

34. Schomig A, Neumann FJ, Kastrati A, et al. A randomized comparison of antiplatelet and anticoagulant therapy after the placement of coronary stents. N Engl J Med 1996;334:1084–9.

35. Leon MB, Baim DS, Popma JJ, et al. A clinical trial comparing three anti-thrombotic-drug regimens after coronary artery stenting. Stent Anticoagulation Restenosis Study Investigators. N Engl J Med 1998;339:1665–71.

36. Bertrand ME, Legrand V, Boland J, et al. Randomized multicenter comparison of conventional anticoagulation versus antiplatelet therapy in unplanned and elective coronary stenting. The Full Anticoagulation versus Aspirin and Ticlopidine (FANTASTIC) study. Circulation 1998; 98:1597–603.

37. Schomig A, Kastrati A, Schuhlen H, et al. Risk factor analysis for stent occlusion within the first month after successful coronary stent placement. J Am Coll Cardiol 1998; 31(Suppl A):99A.

38. Steinhubl SR, Ellis SG, Wolski K, et al. Ticlopidine pretreatment before coronary stenting is associated with sustained decrease in adverse cardiac events: data from the Evaluation of Platelet IIb/IIIa Inhibitor for Stenting (EPISTENT) trial. Circulation 2001;103:1403–9.

39. Yosipovitch G, Rechavia E, Feinmesser M, David M. Adverse cutaneous reactions to ticlopidine in patients with coronary stents. J Am Acad Dermatol 1999;41:473–6.

40. Steinhubl SR, Tan WA, Foody JM, Topol EJ, for the EPISTENT Investigators. Incidence and clinical course of thrombotic thrombocytopenic purpura due to ticlopidine following coronary stenting. JAMA 1999;281:806–10.

41. Quinn MJ, Fitzgerald DJ. Cardiovascular drugs: ticlopidine and clopidogrel. Circulation 1999;100:1667–72.

42. CAPRIE Steering Committee. A randomized, blinded, trial of Clopidogrel versus Aspirin in Patients at Risk of Ischaemic Events (CAPRIE). Lancet 1996;348:1329–39.

43. Bhatt DL, Hirsch AT, Ringleb PA, et al. Reduction in the need for hospitalization for recurrent ischemic events and bleeding with clopidogrel instead of aspirin. Am Heart J. 2000;140:67–73.

44. Bhatt D, Marso S, Hirsch A, et al. Amplified benefit of clopidogrel versus aspirin in patients with diabetes mellitus. Am J Cardiol 2002;90:625–8.

45. Bhatt DL, Chew DP, Hirsch AT, et al. Superiority of clopidogrel versus aspirin in patients with prior cardiac surgery. Circulation 2001;103:363–8.

46. Yusuf S, Zhao F, Mehta SR, et al, for the CURE Trial Investigators. Effects of clopidogrel in addition to aspirin in patients with acute coronary syndromes without ST-segment elevation. N Engl J Med 2001;345:494–502.

47. Braunwald E, Antman EM, Beasley JW, et al. ACC/AHA 2002 guideline update for the management of patients with unstable angina and non-ST-segment elevation myocardial infarction: a report of the American College of Cardiology/American Heart Association Task Force on Practice Guidelines (Committee on the Management of Patients With Unstable Angina). J Am Coll Cardiol 2002;40:1366–74.

48. Savcic M, Hauerk J, Bachmann F, et al. Clopidogrel loading dose regimens: kinetic profile of pharmacodynamic response in healthy subjects. Seminars in Thrombosis and Hemostasis 1999;25(Suppl 2):15–19.

49. Bertrand ME, Rupprecht HJ, Urban P, Gershlick AH, for the CLASSICS Investigators. Double-blind study of the safety of clopidogrel with and without a loading dose in combination with aspirin compared with ticlopidine in combination with aspirin after coronary stenting. The Clopidogrel Aspirin Stent International Cooperative Study (CLASSICS). Circulation 2000;102:624–9.

50. Taniuchi M, Kurz HI, Lasala JM. Randomized comparison of ticlopidine and clopidogrel after intracoronary stent implantation in a broad patient population. Circulation 2001;104:539–43.

51. Mehta SR, Yusuf S, Peters RJG, et al, for the Clopidogrel in Unstable angina to prevent Recurrent Events trial (CURE) Investigators. Effects of pretreatment with clopidogrel and aspirin followed by long-term therapy in patients undergoing percutaneous coronary intervention: the PCI–CURE study. Lancet 2001;358:527–33.

52. Chew DP, Bhatt DL, Robbins MA, et al. Effect of clopidogrel added to aspirin before percutaneous coronary intervention on the risk associated with C-reactive protein. Am J Cardiol 2001;88:672–4.

53. Assali AR, Salloum J, Sdringola S, et al. Effects of clopidogrel pretreatment before percutaneous coronary intervention in patients treated with glycoprotein IIb/IIIa inhibitors (abciximab or tirofiban). Am J Cardiol 2001; 88:884–6, A6.

54. Bhatt DL, Bertrand ME, Berger PB, et al. Meta-analysis of randomized and registry comparisons of ticlopidine with clopidogrel after stenting. J Am Coll Cardiol 2002; 39:9–14.

55. Bennett CL, Connors JM, Carwile JM, et al. Thrombotic thrombocytopenic purpura associated with clopidogrel. N Engl J Med 2000;342:1773–7.

56. Steinhubl SR, Transcatheter Cardiovascular Therapeutics (TCT) 2002 oral presentation.

57. Heartwire. December 12, 2000/www.theheart.org.

58. Cannon CP. Platelet glycoprotein IIb/IIIa inhibition in acute coronary syndromes. In: Thrombosis and Thromboembolism (Goldhaber SZ, Ridker P, eds). New York: Marcel Dekker 2002;101–24.

59. Cannon CP, McCabe CH, Wilcon RG, et al, for the OPUS–TIMI 16 Investigators. Oral glycoprotein IIb/IIIa inhibition with orbofiban in patients with unstable coronary syndromes (OPUS–TIMI 16) trial. Circulation 2000; 102:149–56.

60. O'Neill WW, Serruys P, Knudtson M, et al, for the EXCITE Trial Investigators. Long-term treatment with a platelet glycoprotein-receptor antagonist after percutaneous coronary revascularization. N Engl J Med 2000;342: 1316–24.

61. The SYMPHONY Investigators. Comparison of sibrafiban with aspirin for prevention of cardiovascular events after acute coronary syndromes: a randomized trial. Lancet 2000;355:337–45.

62. The Second SYMPHONY Investigators. Randomized trial of aspirin, sibrafiban, or both for secondary prevention after acute coronary syndromes. Circulation 2001;103:1727–33.

63. Casey M, Fornari C, Bozovich GE, et al. Increased expression of platelet P-selectin in patients treated with oral orbofiban in the OPUS–TIMI 16 study. Circulation 1999;100(Suppl I):161.

64. Cox D, Smith R, Quinn M, et al. Evidence of platelet activation during treatment with a GP IIb/IIIa antagonist in patients presenting with acute coronary syndromes. J Am Coll Cardiol 2000;36:1514–19.

65. Peter K, Schwarz M, Ylanne J, et al. Induction of fibrinogen binding and platelet aggregation as a potential intrinsic property of various glycoprotein IIb/IIIa ($\alpha_{IIb}\beta_3$) inhibitors. Blood 1998;92:3240–9.

66. Chew DP, Bhatt DL, Sapp S, Topol EJ. Increased mortality with oral platelet glycoprotein IIb/IIIa antagonists: a meta-analysis of phase III multicenter randomized trials. Circulation 2001;103:201–6.

67. Nurden AT, Caen JP. An abnormal platelet glycoprotein pattern in three cases of Glanzmann thrombasthenia. Br J Haematol 1974;28:253–60.

68. Phillips DR, Jenkins CSP, Luscher EF, Larrieu MJ. Molecular differences of exposed surface proteins on thrombasthenic platelet plasma membranes. Nature 1975; 257:599–600.

69. Coller BS. Blockade of platelet GP IIb/IIIA receptors as an antithrombotic strategy. Circulation 1995;92:2373–80.

70. Lefkovits J, Plow EF, Topol EJ. Platelet glycoprotein IIb/IIIa receptors in cardiovascular medicine. N Engl J Med 1995;332:1553–9.

71. Coller BS Inhibitors of the platelet glycoprotein IIb/IIIa receptor as conjunctive therapy for coronary artery thrombolysis. Coronary Artery Dis 1992;3:1016–29.

72. Pytela R, Pierschbacher MD, Ginsberg MH, et al. Platelet membrane glycoprotein IIb/IIIa: member of a family of Arg-Gly-Asp-specific adhesion receptors. Science 1986: 231:1559–62.

73. Shattil SJ. Function and regulation of the β_3 integrins in hemostasis and vascular biology. Thromb Haemost 1995;74:149–55.

74. Topol EJ, Byzova TV, Plow EF. Platelet GP IIb–IIIa blockers. Lancet 1999;353:227–31.

75. Mascelli MA, Lance ET, Damaranju L, et al. Pharmacodynamic profile of short-term abciximab treatment demonstrates prolonged platelet inhibition with gradual recovery from GP IIb/IIIa receptor blockade. Circulation 1998;97:1680–8.

76. Kleiman NS. Pharmacokinetics and pharmacodynamics of glycoprotein IIb–IIIa inhibitors. Am Heart J 1999;138:S263–75.

77. Kereiakes DJ, Broderick TM, Roth EM, et al. Time course, magnetitude, and consistency of platelet inhibition of abciximab, tirofiban, or eptifibatide in patients with unstable angina pectoris undergoing percutaneous coronary intervention. Am J Cardiol 1999;84:391–5.

78. Bhatt DL, Topol EJ. Current role of platelet glycoprotein IIb/IIIa inhibitors in acute coronary syndromes. JAMA 200;284:1549–58.

79. Theroux P, Kouz S, Roy L, et al. Platelet membrane receptor glycoprotein IIb/IIIa antagonism in unstable angina. The Canadian Lamifiban study. Circulation 1996;94:899–905.

80. The EPIC Investigators. Use of a monoclonal antibody directed against the platelet glycoprotein IIb/IIIa receptor in high-risk coronary angioplasty. N Engl J Med 1994;330:956–61.

81. Topol EJ, Ferguson JJ, Weisman HF, et al. Long-term protection from myocardial ischemic events in a randomized trial of brief integrin β_3 blockade with percutaneous coronary intervention. JAMA 1997;278:479–84.

82. The EPILOG Investigators. Platelet glycoprotein IIb/IIIa receptor blockade and low-dose heparin during percutaneous coronary revascularization. N Engl J Med 1997;336:1689–96.

83. The CAPTURE Investigators. Randomised placebo-controlled trial of abciximab before and during coronary intervention in refractory unstable angina: the CAPTURE study. Lancet 1997; 349:1429–35.

84. Boersma E, Akkerhuis M, Theroux P, et al. Platelet glycoprotein IIb/IIIa receptor inhibition in non-ST elevation acute coronary syndromes. Early benefit during medial treatment only, with additional protection during percutaneous coronary intervention. Circulation 1999;100:2045–8.

85. Hamm CW, Heeschen C, Goldmann B, et al. Benefit of abciximab in patients with refractory unstable angina in relation to serum troponin T levels. N Engl J Med 1999;340:1623–9.

86. The EPISTENT Investigators. Randomised placebo-controlled and balloon-angioplasty-controlled trial to assess safety of coronary stenting with use of platelet glycoprotein-IIb/IIIa blockade. Lancet 1998;352:87–92.

87. Lincoff AM, Califf RM, Moliterno DJ, et al. Complementary clinical benefits of coronary artery stenting and blockade of platelet glycoptorein IIb/IIIa receptors. N Engl J Med 1999;341:319–27.

88. Topol EJ, Mark DB, Lincoff AM, et al. Outcomes at 1 year and economic implications of platelet glycoprotein IIb/IIIa blockade in patients undergoing coronary stenting: results from a multicenter randomized trial. Lancet 1999;354:2019–24.

89. Bhatt DL, Marso SP, Lincoff AM, et al. Abciximab reduces mortality in diabetics following percutaneous coronary intervention. J Am Coll Cardiol 2000;35:922–8.

90. Bhatt DL, Chew DP, Topol EJ. The importance of intravenous antiplatelet therapy with abciximab during percutaneous coronary intervention in diabetic patients. Cardiovasc Rev Rep 2001;21:161–4.

91. Bhatt DL, Lincoff AM, Kereiakes DJ, et al. Reduction in the need for unplanned stenting with the use of platelet glycoprotein IIb/IIIa blockade in percutaneous coronary intervention. Am J Cardiol 1998;82:1105–6, A6.

92. Bhatt DL, Lincoff AM, Califf RM, et al. The benefit of abciximab in percutaneous coronary revascularization is not device-specific. Am J Cardiol 2000;85:1060–4.

93. The RESTORE Investigators. Effects of platelet glycoprotein IIb/IIIa blockade with tirofiban on adverse cardiac events in patients with unstable angina or acute myocardial infarction undergoing coronary angioplasty. Circulation 1997;96:1445–53.

94. Topol EJ, Moliterno DJ, Herrmann HC, et al. Comparison of two platelet glycoprotein IIb/IIIa inhibitors, tirofiban and abciximab, for the prevention of ischemic events with percutaneous coronary revascularizations. N Engl J Med 2001;344:1888–94.

95. The IMPACT-II Investigators. Randomised placebo-controlled trial of effect of eptifibatide on complications of percutaneous coronary intervention: IMPACT-II. Lancet 1997;349:1422–8.

96. Phillips DR, Teng W, Arfsten A, et al. Effect of Ca^{2+} on GP IIb–IIIa interactions with integrilin. Enhanced GP IIb–IIIa binding and inhibition of platelet aggregation by reductions in the concentration of ionized calcium in plasma anticoagulated with citrate. Circulation 1997;96:1488–94.

97. The PURSUIT Trial Investigators. Inhibition of platelet glycoprotein IIb/IIIa with eptifibatide in patients with acute coronary syndromes. N Engl J Med 1998;339:436–43.

98. The ESPRIT Investigators. Novel dosing regimen of eptifibatide in planned coronary stent implantation (ESPRIT): a randomized, placebo-controlled trial. Lancet 2000;356:2037–44.

99. O'Shea JC, Hafley GE, Greenberg S, et al. Platelet glycoprotein IIb/IIIa integrin blockade with eptifibatide in coronary stent intervention. The ESPRIT trial: a randomized controlled trial. JAMA 2001;285:2468–73.

100. Bosch X, Marrugat J. Platelet glycoprotein IIb/IIIa blockers for percutaneous coronary revascularization, and unstable angina and non-ST segment elevation myocardial infarction. Cochrane Database System Rev 2002;2:1–48.

101. Raymond RE, Lincoff AM, Booth JE, et al. Coronary bypass surgery within 12 hours of administration of abciximab remains safe despite an increased risk of perioperative bleeding. Eur Heart J 1998;19:238.

102. Barr E, Thornton AR, Sax FL, et al. Benefit of tirofiban + heparin therapy in unstable angina/non-Q-wave myocardial infarction patients is observed regardless of interventional treatment strategy. Circulation 1998;98:1-504.

103. Marso SP, Bhatt DL, Roe MT, et al. Enhanced efficacy of eptifibatide administration in patients with acute coronary syndrome requiring in-hospital coronary artery bypass grafting. Circulation 2000;102:2952–8.

104. Lauer MA, Houghtaling PL, Peterson JG, et al. Attenuation of rebound ischemia after discontinuation of heparin therapy by glycoprotein IIb/IIIa inhibition with eptifibatide in patients with acute coronary syndromes: observations from the Platelet IIb/IIIa in Unstable Angina: Receptor

Suppression Using Integrilin Therapy (PURSUIT) trial. Circulation 2001;104:2772–7.

105. The Platelet Receptor Inhibition in Ischemic Syndrome Management in Patients Limited by Unstable Signs and Symptoms (PRISM–PLUS) Investigators. Inhibition of the platelet glycoprotein IIb/IIIa receptor with tirofiban in unstable angina and non-Q-wave myocardial infarction. N Engl J Med 1998;338:1488–97.

106. Chew DP, Bhatt DL, Lincoff AM, et al. Defining the optimal activated clotting time during percutaneous coronary intervention: aggregate results from 6 randomized, controlled trials. Circulation 2001;103:961–6.

107. Alexander JH, Sparapani RA, Mahaffey KW, et al. Eptifibatide reduces the size and incidence of myocardial infarction in patients with non-ST elevation acute coronary syndromes. J Am Coll Cardiol 1999;33(Suppl A):331A.

108. Harrington RA, Lincoff MA, Berdan LG, et al. Maintenance of clinical benefit at six-months in patients treated with the platelet glycoprotein IIb/IIIa inhibitor eptifibtide versus placebo during an acute ischemic coronary event. Circulation 1998;98:1-359.

109. The Platelet Receptor Inhibition in Ischemic Syndrome Management (PRISM) Study Investigators. A comparison of aspirin plus tirofiban with aspirin plus heparin for unstable angina. N Engl J Med 1998;338:1498–505.

110. Heeshen C, Hamm CW, Goldmann B, et al, for the PRISM Study Investigators. Troponin concentrations for stratification of patients with acute coronary syndromes in relation to therapeutic efficacy of tirofiban. Lancet 1999;354:1757–62.

111. The GUSTO-IV ACS Investigators. Effect of glycoprotein IIb/IIIa receptor blocker abciximab on outcome in patients with acute coronary syndromes without early coronary revascularization: the GUSTO-IV ACS randomized trial. Lancet 2001;357:1915–24.

112. Kereiakes DJ, Broderick TM, Roth EM, et al. Time course, magnitude, and consistency of platelet inhibition by abciximab, tirofiban, or eptifibatide in patients with unstable angina pectoris undergoing percutaneous coronary intervention. Am J Cardiol 1999;84:391–5.

113. Scarborough RM, Kleiman NS, Phillips DR. Platelet glycoprotein IIb/IIIa antagonists: What are the relevant issues concerning their pharmacology and clinical use? Circulation 1999;100:437–44.

114. Cohen M. Glycoprotein IIb/IIIa receptor blockers in acute coronary syndromes: Gusto IV–ACS. Lancet 2001;357:1899–900.

115. Boersma E, Harrington RA, Moliterno DJ, et al. Platelet glycoprotein IIb/IIIa inhibitors in acute coronary syndromes; a meta-analysis of all major randomized clinical trials. Lancet 2002;359:189–98.

116. The PARAGON Investigators. International, randomized, controlled trial of lamifiban (a platelet glycoprotein IIb/IIIa inhibitor), heparin, or both in unstable angina. Circulation 1998;97:2386–95.

117. The Platelet IIb/IIIa Antagonist for the Reduction of Acute Coronary Syndrome Events in a Global Organization Network (PARAGON)-B Investigators. Randomized, placebo-controlled trial of titrated intravenous lamifiban for acute coronary syndromes. Circulation 2002;105: 316–21.

118. Newby KL, Ohman EM, Christenson RH, et al, for the PARAGON-B Investigators. Benefit of glycoprotein IIb/IIIa inhibition in patients with acute coronary syndromes and troponin T-positive status. The PARAGON-B Troponin T Substudy. Circulation 2001;103:2891–6.

119. Wu AHB, Abbas SA, Green S, et al. Prognostic value of cardiac troponin T in unstable angina pectoris. Am J Cardiol 1995;76:970–2.

120. Heeschen C, van den Brand MJ, Hamm CW, et al. Angiographic findings in patients with refractory unstable angina according to troponin T status. Circulation 1999; 1827–34.

121. The GUSTO Investigators. An international, multicenter, randomized comparison of reteplase with alteplase for acute myocardial infarction. N Engl J Med 1997;337:1118–23.

122. Antman EM, Giugliano RP, Gibson CM, et al, for the TIMI 14 Investigators. Abciximab facilitates the rate and extent of thrombolyhsis. Results of the Thrombolysis in Myocardial Infarction (TIMI) 14 trial. Circulation 1999; 99:2720–32.

123. Strategies for Patency Enhancement in the Emergency Department (SPEED) Group. Trial of abciximab with and without low-dose reteplase for acute myocardial infarction. Circulation 2000;101:2788–94.

124. Brener SJ, Zeymer U, Adgey AA, et al. Eptifibatide and low-dose tissue plasminogen activator in acute myocardial infarction: the Integrilin and Low-Dose Thrombolysis in Acute Myocardial Infarction (INTRO AMI) trial. J Am Coll Cardiol 2002;39:377–86.

125. Antman EM, Louwerenburg HW, et al. Enoxaparin as adjunctive antithrombin therapy for ST-elevation myocardial infarction: results of the ENTIRE–Thrombolysis in Myocardial Infarction (TIMI) 23 trial. Circulation 2002; 105:1642–9.

126. The GUSTO-V Investigators. Reperfusion therapy for acute myocardial infarction with fibrinolytic therapy or combination reduced fibrinolytic therapy and platelet glycoprotein IIb/IIIa inhibition: the GUSTO V randomized trial. Lancet 2001;357:1905–14.

127. Chan AW, Moliterno DJ. Defining the role of abciximab for acute coronary syndromes: lessons from CADILLAC, ADMIRAL, GUSTO IV, GUSTO V, and TARGET. Curr Opin Cardiol 2001;16:375–83.

128. The Asessment of the Safety and Efficacy of a New Thrombolytic Regimen (ASSENT)-3 Investigators. Efficacy and safety of tenecteplase in combination with enoxaparin, abciximab, or unfractionated heparin: the ASSENT-3 randomised trial in acute myocardial infarction. Lancet 2001;358:605–13.

129. Grines CL, Cox DA, Stone GW, et al, for the Stent Primary Angioplasty in Myocardial Infarction Study Group. Coronary angioplasty with or without stent implantation for acute myocardial infarction. N Engl J Med 1999; 341:1949–56.

130. Neumann F-J, Blasini R, Schmitt C, et al. Effect of glycoprotein IIb/IIIa receptor blockade on recovery of coronary flow and left ventricular function after the placement of coronary-artery stents in acute myocardial infarction. Circulation 1998;98:2695–701.

131. van den Merkhof LFM, Ziljstra F, Olsson H, et al. Abciximab in the treatment of acute myocardial infarction eligible for primary percutaneous transluminal coronary angioplasty. Results of the Glycoprotien Receptor Antagonist Patency Evaluation (GRAPE) pilot study. J Am Coll Cardiol 1999;33:1528–32.

132. GUSTO-IIb Angioplasty Substudy Investigators. A clinical trial comparing primary coronary angioplasty with tissue plasminogen activator for acute myocardial infarction. N Engl J Med 1997;336:1621–8.

133. Lefkovits J, Ivanhoe RJ, Califf RM, et al, for the EPIC Investigators. Effects of platelet glycoprotein IIb/IIIa receptor blockade by a chimeric monoclonal antibody (abciximab) on acute and six-month outcomes after percutaneous transluminal coronary angioplasty for acute myocardial infarction. Am J Cardiol 1996;77:1045–51.

134. Brener SJ, Barr LA, Burchenal JEB, et al, on behalf of the ReePro and Primary PTCA Organization and Randomized Trial (RAPPORT) Investigators. Randomized, placebo-controlled trial of platelet glycoprotein IIb/IIIa blockade with primary angioplasty for acute myocardial infarction. Circulation 1998;98:734–41.

135. Schömig A, Kastrati A, Dirschinger J, et al, for the Stent versus Thrombolysis for Occluded Coronary Arteries in Patients with Acute Myocardial Infarction Study Investigators. Coronary stenting plus platelet glycoprotein IIIb/IIIa blockade compared with tissue plasmogen activator in acute myocardial infarction. N Engl J Med 2000;343:385–391.

136. Montalescot G, Barragan P, Wittenberg O, et al, for the ADMIRAL Investigators. Platelet glycoprotein IIb/IIIa inhibition with coronary stenting for acute myocardial infarction. N Engl J Med 2001;344:1895–903.

137. Stone GW, Grines CL, Cox DA, et al, for the Controlled Abciximab and Device Investigation to Lower Late Angioplasty Complications (CADILLAC) Investigators. Comparison of angioplasty with stenting, with or without abciximab, in acute myocardial infarction. N Engl J Med 2002;346:957–66.

138. Aguirre FV, Topol EJ, Ferguson JJ, et al, for the EPIC Investigators. Bleeding complications with the chimeric antibody to platelet glycoprotein IIb/IIIa integrin in patients undergoing percutaneous coronary intervention. Circulation 1995;91:2882–90.

139. Blankenship JC. Bleeding complications of glycoprotein IIb–IIIa receptor inhibitors. Am Heart J 1999;138:S287–96.

140. Gannie JS, Zenati M, Kormos RL, et al. Abciximab and excessive bleeding in patients undergoing emergency cardiac operations. Ann Thorac Surg 1998;65:465–9.

141. Alvarez JM. Emergency coronary bypass grafting for failed percutaneous coronary artery stenting: increased costs and platelet transfusion requirements after the use of abciximab. J Thorac Cardiovasc Surg 1998;115:472–3.

142. Schulman SP, Goldschmidt-Clermont PJ, Topol EJ, et al. Effects of integrelin, a platelet glycoprotein IIb/IIIa receptor antagonist, in ustable angina. Circulation 1996; 94:2083–9.

143. Tcheng JE, Kereiakes DJ, Lincoff AM, et al, for the ReoPro Readmistration Registry Investigators. Abciximab readministration: results of the ReoPro Readmistration Registration. Circulation 2001;104:870–875.

4

Complications and how to deal with them

Rosana Hernandez Antolín

Introduction

Visualization of cardiac chambers, great vessels and coronary arteries requires invasion of the cardiovascular system through an access site (arterial and/or venous), advancement of catheters inside major vessels up to left or right cardiac chambers/great vessels, selective cannulation of coronary ostia, and administration of contrast media for appropriate visualization on X-ray examination.

Complications[1–3] (Table 4.1) may occur at any level of the process, and include access site complications (excessive bleeding, pseudoaneurysms, fistulae, and dissections), complications anywhere in the vascular system (dissections, embolism, thrombosis, and occlusion of any vessel, including femoral, iliac, renal, mesenteric, subclavian, carotid, and coronary arteries), and general complications, including contrast media side-effects. The clinical consequences of these complications are excessive local

Table 4.1   Clinical complications of diagnostic and therapeutic procedures

Complication	Diagnostic procedures (%)	PTCA (%)	Valvuloplasty (%)
Death	0.1–0.5	0.5–2	0.1–1
Myocardial infarction[a]	0.1–0.2	2–5	0.05–0.1
Cardiac surgery[b]	0.01	0.5–1	0.5–2
Neurological events:			
Transient	0.3–0.5	0.3–0.5	0.2–1
Permanent	0.1–0.2	0.1–0.3	0.1–0.5
Cardiac perforation[c]	0.01–0.1	0.5–2	0.5–2
Arrhythmia:			
Defibrillation	0.1–0.2	0.1–1	0.01–0.2
PM insertion	0.05–0.1	0.1–1	0.05–0.1
Access site complications:			
Without surgery	1–5	1–10	1–10
With surgery	0.1–1	0.5–2	0.5–2
Vasovagal reaction[d]	1–4	1–4	1–4
Severe allergy	0.01–0.05	0.01–0.05	0.01–0.05

[a] Myocardial infarction defined as increase in CK, CK-MB, or troponin level.

[b] Cardiac surgery indicated for ischemia or perforation.

[c] Cardiac tamponade requiring pericardiocentesis.

[d] Vasovagal reaction requiring atropine and fluid administration.

bleeding and its hemodynamic consequences, ischemia or infarction in affected territories being particularly devastating, arrhythmia or conduction defects, impairment of cardiac or renal function, and even death if any of the above are severe enough, unrecognized, or not appropriately managed.

The risk of developing complications depends on the patient's condition[2] (Table 4.2), the type of procedure,[3] and the operator's skills. Patients with heart failure, acute myocardial infarction, severe valvular disease, pulmonary hypertension, left main or triple vessel coronary artery disease, or left ventricular dysfunction are at increased risk of developing severe heart failure, pulmonary edema, cardiogenic shock, and death.[2] Patients of advanced age, diabetics, hypovolemic patients, and those with previously impaired renal function are at high risk for post-catheterization renal failure. Patients who are overweight, or on antithrombotic/antiplatelet agents and those who are not compliant with strict bed rest after the procedure are at high risk for access site complications. Older

patients with diffuse atherosclerotic disease and significant aortic tortuosity are at increased risk of dissection, thrombosis, and ischemia in the affected territory that may result in transient or permanent neurological disability.

The type of procedure is a major determinant of complications. A diagnostic coronary angiogram is usually a quick procedure that can be performed in most cases in less than 20 minutes, and complications other than those at access sites are rare. In some patients, diagnostic catheterization may be a more complex procedure, as in cases of severe aortic stenosis or marked tortuosity in the aorta. In these cases, the intensive and prolonged manipulation of catheters and the use of straight/extra support wires are associated with a higher risk of complication (embolic events, coronary dissections, left ventricular perforation, and severe left ventricular failure). Therapeutic procedures have specific complications, such as coronary occlusion, vessel rupture, and cardiac tamponade, as detailed later.

The operator's experience and in-depth preparation of the case are also important issues in preventing com-

Table 4.2   Patients at increased risk for complications and ways to minimize risk

	Clinical setting	Prevention
Increased general risk	Age	—
	Obesity	Weight reduction
	Severe general disease	—
	Severe pulmonary disease	Compensation
	Renal failure	Hydration
	Previous contrast reaction	Premedication
Increased cardiac risk	Three-vessel coronary disease	—
	Left main disease	—
	NYHA class IV	Compensation
	Severe mitral or aortic disease	—
	Mechanical prosthesis	—
	Left ventricular dysfunction	Small amount of contrast
	Pulmonary hypertension	—
	Cardiac failure	Compensate
	High-risk exercise test	Be aware of left main disease
Increased vascular risk	Severe aortic tortuosity	Extra care with wires/catheters
	Aortic atherosclerotic plaques	Extra care with wires/catheters
	Severe vascular disease	Extra care with wires/catheters
	Recent stroke	Deferred catheterization if possible
	Uncontrolled hypertension	Hypertension control
Increased access site risk	Bleeding disorder	Platelets, vitamin K
	Anticoagulation	Discontinued
	Severe aortic insufficiency	—
	Uncontrolled hypertension	—
	No bedrest compliance	Sedation
	Psychological factors	Sedation
Increased renal risk	Age	—
	Diabetes	—
	Hypovolemia, dehydration	Hydration
	Renal failure	Optimize renal function
	Contrast given recently (<48 hours)	Delay for a few days

plications, and augment the speed, appropriateness, and efficiency of treatment to deal with complications upon occurrence. Procedures performed by skilful operators are associated with shorter procedural time, less radiation exposure, less contrast, and a lower complication rate. Although a prolonged procedural time may be related to the complexity of the case, procedural time is an independent predictor of the incidence and severity of complications. For this reason, intravascular procedures should be kept as short as possible in order to minimize contrast use and complications; occasionally, long-lasting diagnostic procedures should even be discontinued if the patient is tired or too much contrast has been used. The procedure can be safely continued at any time with a different vascular approach, using different catheters, or with a more experienced operator.

Avoiding unnecessary invasive intravascular procedures is another way of preventing complications. Even in low-risk patients, diagnostic cardiac catheterization should be carefully evaluated and only performed when procedural information may result in a different therapeutic strategy. In the case of therapeutic procedures, the potential benefit should be carefully weighed against the risk of complications.

Therefore, although they are infrequent during diagnostic intravascular procedures, complications may be life-threatening, and even mild complications will result in patient discomfort and a delay in recovery. A careful assessment of the indications for the procedure,[4,5] appropriate patient and operator preparation for the case, and optimal technique will minimize the incidence and severity of complications.

Complications common to diagnostic and therapeutic intravascular procedures

Access site complications

Access site complications are common, and include hematomas of any size, pseudoaneurysms, and arteriovenous fistulae.[6] Such complications are more frequent in older, female, overweight, or previously anticoagulated patients, and can be prevented by careful puncture (avoiding posterior puncture of the artery) and compression techniques, and appropriate bed rest (6–12 hours) after the procedure. *Small hematomas* are common (2–15%), and usually produce only mild discomfort for a few days. *Large hematomas* (>10 cm) are less frequent (1–2%), and are particularly prevalent in patients on antithrombotic, aggressive antiplatelet, and/or fibrinolytic therapy. Large hematomas may require prolonged rest, a delay in hospital discharge, and blood transfusions, and complete resolution may take 3–4 weeks. Diagnosis can be made based on

clinical features (no femoral murmur) and confirmed by a Doppler study performed with standard echocardiography equipment. Occasionally, large hematomas become infected, and any purulent collection should be surgically drained from a large cavity. This may take 2–3 months to heal. *Uncontrolled bleeding* (either evident or into the retroperitoneal space) with severe hemodynamic compromise requires aggressive fluid/blood replacement and ruling out bleeding of another origin (gastrointestinal). Although it can be managed medically in most cases, vascular surgery may sometimes be required. Other access site complications are *femoral pseudoaneurysms* and *arteriovenous fistulae*, which occur more frequently if femoral puncture is too low (>2 cm below the inguinal ligament). Diagnosis is based on clinical grounds (the presence of a hard, pulsatile mass and a systolic murmur in the case of a pseudoaneurysm and a continuous murmur in the case of an arteriovenous fistula) and confirmed by Doppler examination (Figure 4.1). In most cases, femoral pseudoaneurysms can be closed successfully[7] with femoral compression followed by bed rest for 12–24 hours after antithrombotic medication has been discontinued. Patients with unresolved pseudoaneurysm and those with large arteriovenous fistulae might require vascular surgery, as do those with uncontrolled persistent femoral bleeding.

The use of smaller catheters (5F or 4F) and other access sites such as the radial approach in properly selected patients (positive Allen maneuver) may decrease the incidence of access site complications. Several closure devices for femoral use have been developed in the last decade, based either on the delivery of a procoagulant agent (collagen) at the arterial puncture site or on the use of surgical sutures. All of these devices are convenient since they allow early ambulation, providing more comfort to the patient, but are quite expensive and require a perfect technique to be effective. Nevertheless, no device has been proven to decrease vascular complications in the general population, although they may be useful in patients at high risk for vascular complications.

Intravascular complications

Intravascular complications include *dissections, thrombosis,* and *embolisms*. Dissections of the aorta, femoral (Figure 4.2), iliac, carotid, and subclavian (Figure 4.3) arteries are rare (<1%) during invasive intravascular procedures. The dissection can be caused by the wire or the sheath at the access site and can extend retrogradely upwards into the vascular system. This occurs more frequently in older, hypertensive patients with marked aortic tortuosity. Gentle manipulation of wires is essential to prevent dissection. This complication should be suspected when the wire is entrapped and fails to progress. Early recognition of this condition will prevent further progression of the dissection; the wire should be withdrawn from the dissection

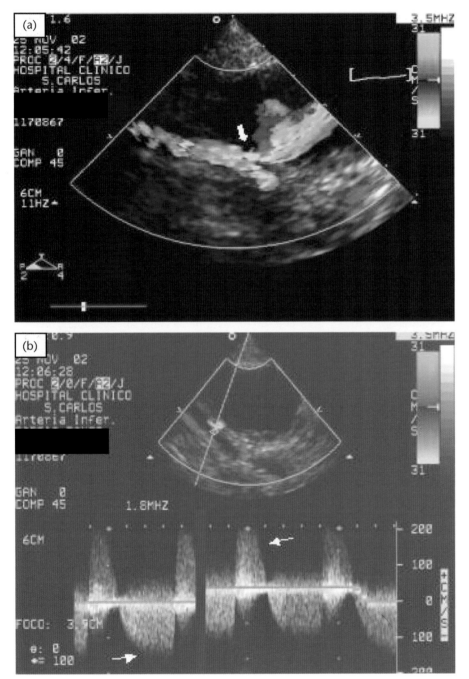

Figure 4.1
Doppler examination of a femoral pseudoaneurysm. (a) Color Doppler. The arrow indicates the neck of the pseudoaneurysm. (b) Continuous Doppler examination with systolic and diastolic flow (arrows).

site and the procedure should be performed through a different access site or deferred in elective cases. Small dissections usually do not impair flow, are asymptomatic, and seal off spontaneously in a few days. Occasionally, when dissection occurs in a severely obstructed femoral artery, the artery might occlude with or without clinical signs of acute ischemia. Large dissections, particularly when located in the ascending, descending, or abdominal aorta require careful clinical observation and imaging (usually with computed tomography (CT) or magnetic resonance (MRI)). The use of low-molecular-weight heparin is usually recommended in relatively small vessels (carotid, renal,

and subclavian arteries) with a significant risk of occlusion, but not in aortic dissections since it may preclude spontaneous thrombosis of the false lumen.

Dissection of the left or right coronary artery ostia, although rare (<1 in a 1000), can occur during selective cannulation of coronary arteries for diagnostic or therapeutic purposes. Wall damage may occur when the catheter tip is not coaxial with the coronary lumen or is against the arterial wall, or when contrast medium is injected too rapidly. Amplatz-type and 7–8 F guiding catheters are more dangerous than smaller, Judkins-type catheters. Dissection of the right ostium tends to occur in patients with angio-

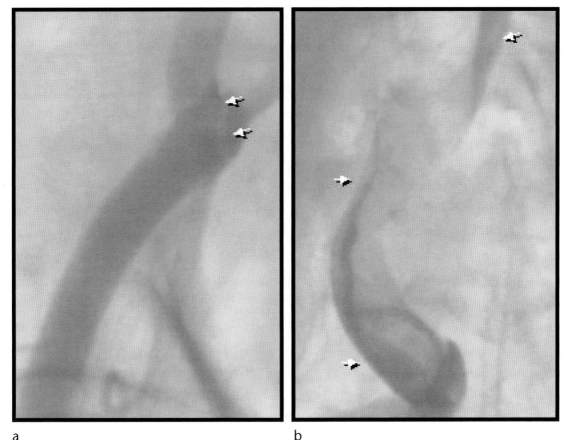

a   b

Figure 4.2
Femoral dissection during diagnostic cardiac catheterization. (a) Initiation of the dissection (arrows). (b) Dissection has progressed upwards (arrows).

graphically normal coronary arteries; such dissection frequently continues downwards to the distal portion or the vessel (crux cordis) and is associated with acute closure and ischemic changes in the inferior wall. Dissection of the left ostium may occur in patients with or without significant left main coronary artery disease (Figure 4.4). In either case, left main dissection is frequently associated with acute ischemic changes, cardiogenic shock, and cardiocirculatory arrest within a few minutes. Under these circumstances, emergency percutaneous transluminal coronary angioplasty (PTCA) is the only alternative, and although frequently successful from an angiographic point of view, the mortality rate is as high as 50% in most series.

Occasionally, ostial dissection may produce retrograde aortic dissection in either the right (Figure 4.5) or the left coronary sinus. This dissection is usually self-limiting and tends to seal off in a few weeks without producing clinical complications; rarely, it may progress to a type A retrograde aortic dissection with involvement of supraaortic vessels. Careful selective cannulation of both ostia and a very soft first injection to document the catheter position is the best way to prevent such severe complications that may result in the death of a patient with previously normal coronary arteries.

Embolism of thrombotic material during catheterization procedures has three potential origins: the catheters (thrombi generated during the procedure), the left ventricle (intramural thrombus after a myocardial infarction), and atherosclerotic aortofemoral plaques. Appropriate heparinization and frequent flushing of the catheters can prevent the first mechanism. Left ventricular embolism can be prevented by avoiding left ventriculography in patients with left ventricular thrombi that can be easily recognized by echocardiography. Preventing the third mechanism is much more difficult, since protruding aortic plaques (which are quite common in older patients undergoing diagnostic or therapeutic procedures), may be ruptured and mobilized by catheters. Embolization and resulting ischemia can occur in any territory (femoropopliteal, renal, mesenteric, cerebral, or coronary territories), although more frequently in the cerebral circulation. Transient ischemic events are rare (0.1–0.2%) and permanent disability occurs in only 0.05–0.1% of large series of patients undergoing intravascular procedures.

Air embolism, although easily preventable with appropriate catheter filling and flushing techniques, is in fact quite frequent during intravascular procedures. Since air bubbles are not soluble in contrast media, large bubbles

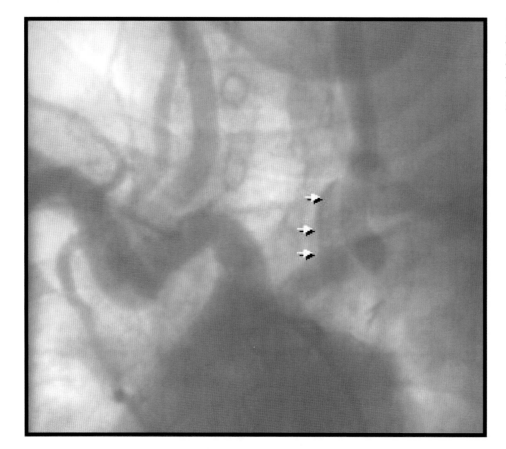

Figure 4.3
Aortography at the ascending aorta level with visualization of the supraortic vessels. A dissection can be seen at the origin of the left subclavian artery (arrows).

located in catheters will enter right, left, or both coronary arteries, producing a sudden and almost complete distal coronary occlusion associated with severe bradycardia, hypotension and ischemic ECG changes. Temporal relationship with a catheter change and/or manipulation of manifold connections may help to establish the diagnosis of air embolism, although ostial coronary dissection should always be excluded by a contrast injection. Air bubbles running down the distal coronary bed can be documented by angiography. The clinical picture may be quite dramatic, but tends to be short-lasting, with spontaneous resolution within a few minutes – although it might be very serious in patients with severe coronary disease or left ventricular dysfunction. During this time frame, until spontaneous resolution, oxygen administration, fluid infusion, and vagolytic agents (atropine) may help to speed up symptom resolution. Early recognition of this characteristic picture may avoid aggressive resuscitation maneuvers such as endotracheal intubation or pacemaker insertion.

Complications arising from contrast use

All contrast media used contain iodine, which absorbs X-rays and gives these agents the radio opacity required for examination of the vessel lumen. All of them are derivatives of triiodobenzoic acid, differing in ionic characteristics (ionic or nonionic), osmolarity (high or low), and viscosity. Hyperosmolarity is responsible for most of the side-effects, including general (nausea, vomiting, and flushing), hemodynamic (hypotension, increase in left ventricular diastolic pressure, and left ventricular dysfunction), electrophysiological (extreme sinus bradycardia, asystole, AV block, and ventricular fibrillation), and renal (renal failure) side-effects. The older agents are ionic and hyperosmolar (five times plasma osmolarity), while contemporary agents are either ionic (dimers of triiodobenzoic acid) or nonionic and have a lower osmolarity (twice the plasma osmolarity) and fewer side-effects. Nonionic agents (although more expensive) are progressively replacing ionic contrast.[6–8]

Mild allergic reactions (nausea, hives, and mild bronchospasm) are infrequent with modern contrast media, and severe reactions (laryngospasm and anaphylactic shock) are very rare (0.001%), although they may be life-threatening. Appropriate treatment for anaphylactic shock (adrenaline, fast-acting steroids, and endotracheal intubation) should always be ready for use in all catheterization laboratories. Recurrence after a previous allergic reaction is frequent, but can be prevented in over 90% of cases by pretreatment with steroids (starting the day before) and H_1 histamine receptor blockers.

Renal failure is a well-known complication after contrast administration. Hypovolemia, contrast-induced

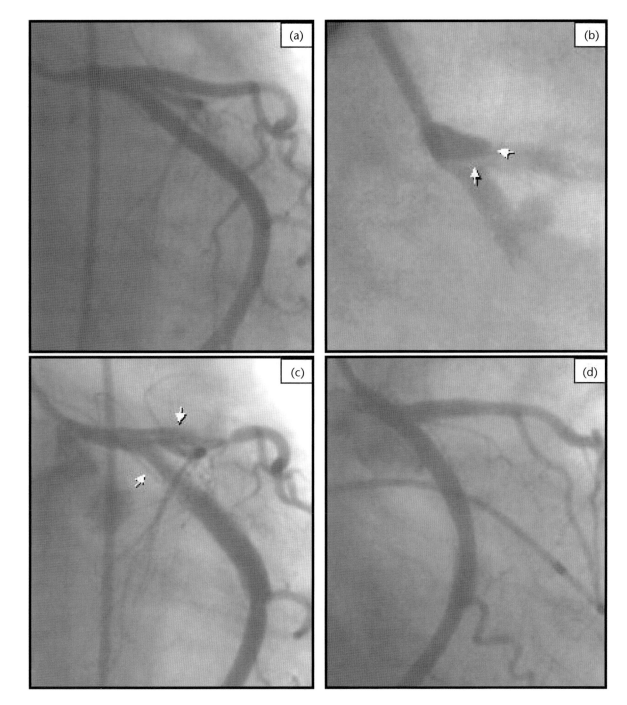

Figure 4.4
Dissection of the left main coronary artery in a patient with previously normal coronary arteries. (a) Angiography of the left main coronary artery before dissection. (b) Catheter-induced dissection of the left main with compromise of distal flow to the left anterior descending (LAD) and circumflex (LCx) arteries. (c) Extension of the dissection to the mid portion of LAD and LCx arteries. (d) Angiographic result after stenting of the left main, LAD, and LCx arteries with restoration of TIMI III flow.

renal vasoconstriction, and a direct toxic effect are all mechanisms that play a role. Older, diabetic, hypovolemic patients with previous cardiac failure and/or mild to moderate renal insufficiency who have received a large volume of contrast are at a high risk for renal failure. Fluid administration (saline infusion 1000 ml in 6 hours before and 1000 ml after the procedure) can prevent the devel-opment of renal failure.[9,10] In old patients or those with left ventricular dysfunction, a slower infusion (along 12 hours) of hyposaline solution will minimize the risk of pulmonary edema upon hydration. Although some authors have advocated the use of calcium antagonists, theophylline, dopamine, atrial natriuretic peptide, or acetylcysteine to prevent contrast medium-related renal

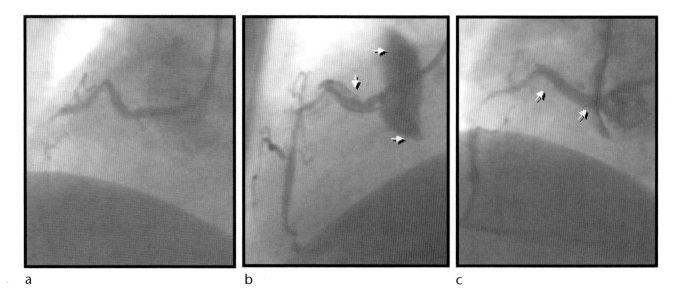

a   b   c

Figure 4.5
Guiding-catheter induced dissection of the right coronary artery at the ostial level (a). The dissection progressed retrogradely to the right Valsalva sinus and aortic wall (b). It persisted after stent implantation (arrows) in the proximal right coronary artery (c).

impairment, this has been questioned by others. The administration of mannitol or diuretics after contrast medium use may also help to prevent renal failure provided that volume administration completely compensates urine loses. Renal failure is usually polyuric and occurs within the first 24 hours after contrast administration, although it may also be oliguric in patients with previous renal failure. It usually lasts for 2–4 days; then creatinine levels tend to decrease to previous levels. Renal function should be monitored after the procedure in all high-risk patients and in those who have received a high volume of contrast medium. Should renal impairment occur, renal function and serum electrolytes should be monitored daily, because a few patients will require hemodialysis until recovery is achieved.

Arrhythmia and conduction defects

With contemporary contrast media, severe cardiac arrhythmia (ventricular tachycardia or fibrillation) is infrequent in stable patients, and whenever it happens it is related to excessive volume injection in a small right coronary artery. In these patients, defibrillation will be performed once the patient has lost consciousness. No other life support measures or antiarrhythmic therapy are required, and most patients will be discharged from the hospital as expected. In unstable patients (those with acute myocardial infarction, acute vessel closure, severe pulmonary edema, or cardiogenic shock), ventricular tachycardia–fibrillation is secondary to ischemia, hypoxia, or poor hemodynamics; this may be

recurrent, and the patient will require additional life support measures and antiarrhythmic drug therapy.

Other tachyarrhythmias (atrial flutter or fibrillation) are relatively rare, and in most cases are associated with heart failure and valvular or pulmonary disease and require similar treatment to other circumstances.

Transitory conduction disturbances are not rare during percutaneous interventions. Extreme sinus bradycardia, asystole, and first-, second-, and third-degree AV block can occur during vessel puncture (vasovagal reaction), right coronary artery contrast injection, intracoronary nitroglycerin, adenosine or verapamil administration, deep intubation of the right coronary artery, distal embolization, or vessel closure. They are usually self-limiting and usually respond adequately to cough and atropine, except in the cases of severe inferior ischemia, where a transient intravenous pacemaker may be required.

New conduction defects (new bundle branch block) are rare and occur more frequently during right ventricle or left ventricle catheterization. Progression towards complete heart block is rare, but may persist for several hours. When this appears under ischemic conditions (acute myocardial infarction or acute vessel closure), it has the same meaning as when it occurs spontaneously (ischemia involving a large myocardial segment) and may not revert even after successful angioplasty of the occluded vessel.

Prolonged hypotension

Hypotension during intravascular procedures may be due to contrast effect, vasovagal reaction, anaphylactic reaction, or myocardial ischemia.

Transient hypotension, even severe, is relatively frequent during invasive procedures, and is mostly related to vasovagal reaction during vascular punctures. It is usually due to vasovagal reflex and is associated with severe bradycardia; it usually responds to volume administration and vagolytic drugs. When it is severe, persists for more than 5 minutes, does not respond to volume administration and atropine, or is associated with ECG changes, one should consider an ischemic etiology due to air embolism, thrombotic embolization, acute vessel closure, or dissection. Any of these circumstances may require a different treatment approach.

In patients with severe cardiac failure, the procedure may worsen heart failure and progress to cardiogenic shock. In such instances, progression is usually slow, and treatment should be that of cardiogenic shock with inotropic agents, vasodilators, and mechanical support, in addition to a percutaneous procedure whenever this is suitable and indicated.

Coronary spasm

Severe coronary spasm may occur during diagnostic or therapeutic procedures.[11] Spasm is more frequent at the right coronary ostium during diagnostic cardiac catheterization and is sometimes associated with progressive diffuse spasm of the right coronary artery and acute ischemic ECG changes. Coronary spasm may also occur in the left coronary ostium, particularly when left main disease is present. Diagnosis of spasm versus severe lesion in a coronary ostium may be difficult. Administration of intracoronary nitroglycerin, the use of a smaller catheter, and a careful analysis of pressure waveform may all be required to clarify whether a coronary obstruction is due to an atherosclerotic obstructive lesion or to a mild lesion with associated spasm. Occasionally, spasm may be generalized, simulating very small coronary arteries.

Cardiac perforation and tamponade

With careful manipulation of contemporary catheters, cardiac perforation during diagnostic procedures is extremely rare either in the right or in the left side of the heart. The most frequent cause of right ventricular perforation (excluding ablative electrophysiological procedures) is the performance of an endomyocardial biopsy, although it can also occur after pacemaker insertion. On the left side, the use of straight wires to cross stenotic aortic valves is the most frequent cause of perforation. In both cases and depending on the size of the perforation, tamponade may occur in a few minutes (which is easy to recognize) or in a

matter of hours (giving an insidious clinical picture that is difficult to recognize). Aortic rupture and cardiac tamponade may also occur in patients with type I aortic dissection undergoing aortic root aortography. Transeptal catheterization (almost always performed during mitral valvuloplasty procedures) may be complicated by atrial perforation (right or left) and cardiac tamponade, particularly during the learning curve of the technique. Experienced operators may keep this risk below 0.5%.

Cardiac tamponade, either acute or subacute, is a rare but life-threatening complication that should be confirmed or ruled out by physical examination and echocardiography in any patient with unexplained prolonged hypotension after a diagnostic or therapeutic procedure. A pericardiocentesis kit should be always ready to use in any catheterization laboratory.

Death

Diagnostic cardiac catheterization is a safe procedure and mortality is very low (0.1%), particularly in stable patients. Old (>80 years) patients and patients with cardiogenic shock, renal failure, acute infarction, or severe left main or three-vessel disease are at increased risk of death in the 24 hours following catheterization – but this is not necessarily related to the procedure. Mortality on the table is very rare in diagnostic procedures and is usually related to ischemia associated with incessant ventricular arrhythmias or cardiogenic shock in already very sick patients or in patients with major complications (left main dissection or cardiac tamponade). Delayed mortality attributable to cardiac catheterization is due to acute renal failure, pulmonary infections, left ventricular failure, or ischemic events.

Other complications

Catheter kinking and rupture

Cannulation of the right coronary artery requires clockwise catheter rotation. Sometimes, particularly in cases with severe aortic tortuosity, rotation is not transmitted to the tip of the catheter, resulting in the catheter kinking at the level of the femoral artery. If unrecognized, persistence in rotation may produce complete catheter rupture and loss of part of the catheter into the vascular system. Careful observation of the distal catheter pressure waveform is the best way to detect kinking early and prevent catheter rupture. Once the catheter has ruptured, retrieval should be performed at the iliac level using either conventional catheters and wires or specially designed retrieval catheters (snares). Success is achieved in most cases; otherwise surgical removal of the foreign body will be required.

Catheter entrapment

Entrapment in a metallic cardiac valve can occur if the catheter is positioned through the valve. To prevent this risk, mechanical valves should never be crossed. If an aortic gradient is considered to be necessary, a transeptal approach to the left ventricle is safer.

Infections

These are very rare in catheterization laboratories in a standard surgical setting. Endocarditis attributable to cardiac catheterization is exceptional, and at present no prophylactic antibiotic therapy is recommended even in patients with mechanical prostheses. Secondary infection of large hematomas may occasionally occur, and surgical drainage is then required.

Cholesterol embolization

This is a very rare complication associated with intravascular procedures and contrast use. Clinical pictures are of progressive (over several weeks) renal failure, usually irreversible, and distal limb ischemia. Cholesterol crystals can be documented in renal and limb capillaries.

Complications specific to therapeutic procedures

Coronary dissections

Coronary dissections may be located at any coronary ostium (due to damage by the guiding catheter) or at the treated lesion site (pressure-related or wire-related damage). Dissections[12] are a very common finding after interventional procedures, as documented by angiography (intraluminal defects, extraluminal opacification, or a flap at a dilatation site), intravascular ultrasound (endocardial flaps), or at autopsy. Highly calcified/fibrotic lesions and a large mass of plaque that require a high pressure to remove balloon waste are the circumstances more frequently associated with dissections, along with subintimal penetration by the wire in chronic total occlusions.[13–15] The NHLBI classified dissections from A to F, although a simpler classification of mild, moderate, or severe (with associated flow impairment) may also be useful. Large, severe dissections with significant residual stenosis, flow impairment, or associated ischemic changes have a poor prognosis (acute vessel closure) and are in fact the most frequent cause of acute vessel closure during percutaneous interventions. In the stent era, most lesions in vessels larger than 2.5 mm are treated with a stent. Small dissections proximal or distal to the stent have a good prognosis and may not need to be treated with additional stents.[16] When dissections are very long (>30 mm) and cannot be treated with a single stent, prolonged long-balloon inflation with or without spot stenting of the proximal or distal part of the dissection or complete coverage of the dissection with several stents are reasonable strategies to seal off the dissection, maintain coronary distal flow, and minimize the amount of metal. Dissections in small vessels can be treated with glycoprotein IIb/IIIa platelet receptor inhibitors and prolonged, low-pressure balloon inflation.

Acute vessel closure

This is the most frequent complication during coronary angioplasty and in the first few hours afterwards. The rate of acute vessel closure was 2–7% after balloon angioplasty, while in the stent era it occurs in about 1–2% of cases.[17–20] Classical angina pain and ECG changes are usually present, and hemodynamic impairment will depend on the amount of ischemic myocardium. Acute vessel closure is usually due to coronary dissection, thrombosis, spasm, significant residual stenosis, stent subexpansion, or a combination of these. It occurs more frequently in cases of total occlusion, acute myocardial infarction, and thrombus-containing lesions, and in small vessels.[21,22] Activated clotting time (ACT) should be checked and additional heparin administered (to ACT > 200 ms); intracoronary nitroglycerin should be administered and a coronary angiography performed. Upon angiographic confirmation of acute vessel closure, a floppy wire should be gently positioned in the distal vessel, and frequently some distal flow is restored with this. Special care must be taken to avoid going subintimal with the wire or crossing the struts of the stent. Angiography is not always helpful in defining the exact cause of vessel occlusion, and in some cases intravascular ultrasound may help to clarify this. After balloon inflation, residual dissections should be treated with implantation of an additional stent, with the aim of permanent vessel patency restoration. In the case of stent subexpansion, high-pressure expansion of the stent should be performed. If a large thrombus burden is present a glycoprotein IIb/IIIa inhibitor should be administered.

Upon flow restoration, immediate improvement of chest pain and ECG changes is obtained, but even transitory (<15 minutes) coronary occlusion is usually associated with at least a mild elevation of troponin and CK-MB values, with increasing values as ischemia time prolongs.

Subacute stent thrombosis

Subacute thrombosis is defined as angiographically documented stent occlusion occurring more than 24 hours but less than 30 days after the procedure (Figure 4.6) and is associated with acute ischemia, infarction, hemodynamic instability, and even death. Nowadays, its rate (with the general use of aspirin and a thienopyridine antiplatelet agent and high-pressure stent implantation) is around 1%; it used to be 3–5 times higher in the early 1990s. Small stent size, long or multiple stents, discontinuation of antiplatelet therapy (due to drug intolerance/allergy, bleeding complication, or noncompliance), residual dissection or thrombus, suboptimal results, stent subexpansion, and the presence of significant nontreated lesions in the same vessel are all risk factors for subacute thrombosis.[23–25] The most important preventive measure is to achieve an optimal final result using appropriately sized stents deployed at high pressure under aggressive antiplatelet therapy including glycoprotein IIb/IIIa inhibitor administration in high-risk lesions.[26–28] If clinical ischemia occurs, cardiac catheterization and immediate angioplasty should be performed. Extra care should be taken with the wire, which should be very soft and floppy to ensure a free pass through the stent lumen and not across stent struts. Subacute thrombosis is almost always associated with acute myocardial infarction, and the rise in cardiac markers will depend on the ischemic territory and the delay to successful reperfusion. If mechanical reperfusion cannot be performed immediately, thrombolysis should be performed as soon as possible if the ischemic territory is big enough to fulfil current indications for fibrinolysis.[29]

Side-branch compromise

Side branches originating in segments treated with balloon angioplasty or stent implantation may be adversely affected (Figure 4.7) by the procedure.[30–33] Side-branch impairment will depend on severity of the pre-angioplasty lesion, the vessel size, and the amount of plaque in the parent vessel that may protrude into it. As a general rule, side branches without ostial involvement will remain patent while severely diseased vessels will develop flow impairment or occlusion after dilatation of the main vessel.

The clinical picture will depend on the distribution territory of the side branch, and may vary from mild chest pain without ECG changes and minimal increase in troponin or CK-MB levels to large transmural myocardial infarction with development of new Q-waves and large increases in biological markers of myocardial necrosis.

In general, dilatation (or stenting) side branches with a high risk of closure prior to parent vessel stenting is recommended, followed by new dilation (or stent implantation) of the side branch if required after parent vessel dilatation.

Distal embolization

During angioplasty, particles of different sizes and materials (thrombus, debris of atherosclerotic plaque including cholesterol, collagen, foam cells, and fibrin, and platelet-rich thrombus) might cause distal obstruction of the coronary arteries (distal embolization; Figure 4.8) or obstruction of the microvasculature (no-reflow phenomenon). Several factors related to the patient (unstable angina or acute/recent myocardial infarction), the lesion (ulcerated or thrombotic lesions, total occlusion, or saphenous vein graft lesions), or the procedure (high-pressure dilation or rotational atherectomy) are associated with a higher risk of both distal embolization and the no-reflow phenomenon.[34,35] Pretreatment with glycoprotein IIb/IIIa inhibitors may decrease this complication, as may the use of several distal protection devices.[36,37] These devices have an aspiration system, a collecting emboli system (filters, baskets, etc.), or a combination of both.[38,39] Clinical application of these devices (at least five of which have been marketed already) is being tested, and at present their cost-effectiveness is still to be determined.

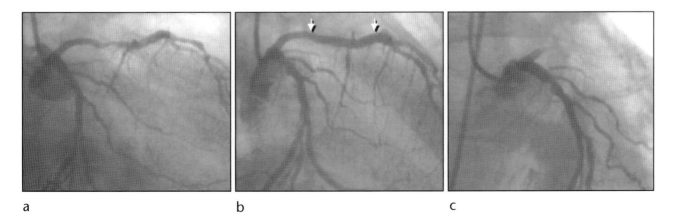

a   b   c

Figure 4.6
Subacute occlusion. (a) Pre-angioplasty LAD lesion. (b) After stent deployment. (c) LAD occlusion 5 days after stent implantation.

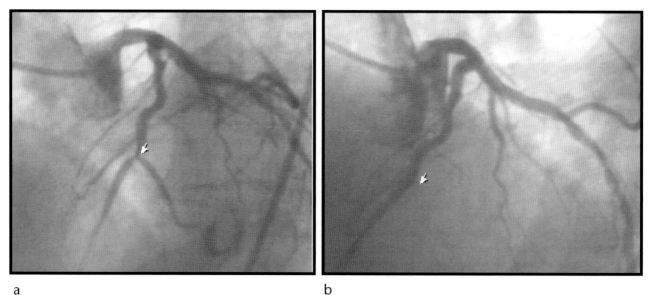

a   b

Figure 4.7
Side-branch occlusion. (a) Severe LAD lesion involving the origin of a diagonal branch. (b) Occlusion of the diagonal branch after stent implantation in the LAD artery.

Distal embolization can be defined as an image, not previously present, of hyperclarity or haziness located downstream from the dilated segment that becomes evident after an interventional procedure. It is usually associated with acute ischemic pain, ECG changes, and subsequent elevation of cardiac markers. Once this complication has occurred, several maneuvers of uncertain efficacy have been proposed to mechanically fracture the thrombus (vigorous movements at the embolization site with a deinflated balloon or small size balloon inflation), glycoprotein IIb/IIIa inhibitors, and intracoronary thrombolysis. In a matter of minutes, most cases tend to show an improvement in distal coronary flow, angina pain, and ischemic ECG changes.

No-reflow phenomenon

The no-reflow phenomenon can be described as an acute reduction in anterograde coronary flow not explained by abrupt closure, dissection, high-grade stenosis, spasm, or distal embolization. The mechanisms responsible for this phenomenon are multifactorial and characterized by an increase in microvascular resistance, due to spasm (thromboxane-induced capillary vasospasm), microemboli (atheroma debris or platelet or neutrophilic plugs), or endothelial damage (due to oxygen free-radical-mediated injury during ischemia–reperfusion, cytokines and other vasoactive substances that induce inflammation, edema, and necrosis).

The incidence of no-reflow varies from 0.5% in elective angioplasties, 2–10% after rotablation, 2–10% in total occlusions, 5–12% in acute myocardial infarction, and 3–18% in degenerated saphenous vein graft angioplas-

ty.[40,41] No-reflow is associated with an onset or increase in chest pain and ischemic ECG changes that frequently persist for more than 1 hour. A significant increase in cardiac markers will occur, and in the case of myocardial infarction mortality increases 2–8 times compared with that of patients with normal distal flow (TIMI III flow).[42]

Treatment strategies include repeated boluses of intracoronary nitroglycerin (200 μg each), verapamil (50–100 μg up to 1 mg), adenosine (40 μg each), or nitroprusside, and appropriate treatment of hemodynamic and rhythm disturbances with fluids, intraaortic balloon pump, vagolytic drugs, electric stimulatation, etc.

Coronary spasm

Coronary spasm is quite frequent during therapeutic procedures, but can be easily treated with intracoronary nitroglycerin and cannot be considered a complication unless it is associated with clinical consequences. It may appear at the ostium, at the lesion site, or anywhere in the vessel; it may be limited to a short segment or extend over a very long one and be associated with partial or total vessel occlusion. The main problem is that spasm may mimic other conditions such as ostial coronary disease, coronary dissections, acute vessel closure, distal embolization, or the presence of a lesion in a nondiseased segment, and may thus result in a misleading diagnosis. Coronary spasm almost always responds properly to intracoronary nitroglycerin, which should therefore always be administered before therapeutic decisions are made regarding new, unexplained or bizarre angiographic images. This simple maneuver may prevent the implantation of stents in non-existent lesions. In the case of

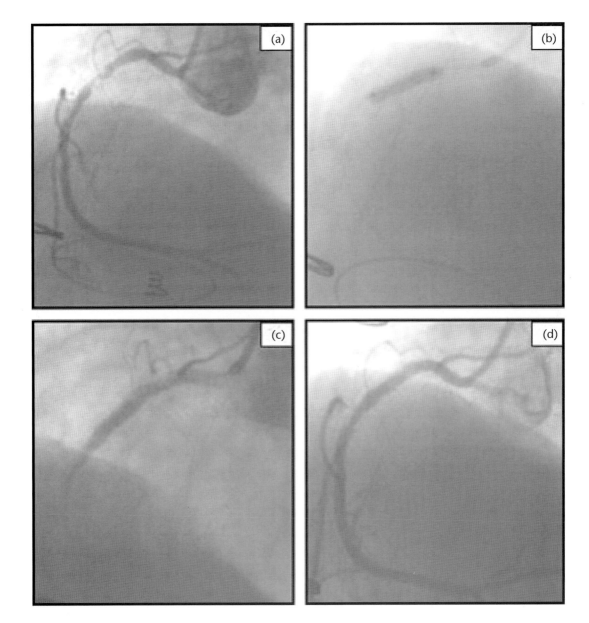

Figure 4.8
Distal embolization. (a) Pre-angioplasty right coronary artery lesion. (b) Stent deployment. (c) No residual stenosis, but severe flow impairment. (d) After nitroglycerin adenosine and abciximab administration, distal flow is TIMI III.

ostial left or right coronary spasm, sublingual or even intravenous nitroglycerin perfusion for several minutes may be required to completely relieve coronary spasm.

Vessel perforation/cardiac tamponade

Coronary perforation is a life-threatening complication that can be recognized by the presence of contrast extravasation beyond the arterial wall. Clinical consequences (hemodynamic instability and associated ischemia) will depend on the

amount and destination of extravascular flow and the ischemia produced by distal vessel occlusion. Perforation may be caused by guidewire, balloon, or more aggressive atherectomy and laser techniques. In large series, rupture occurred in less than 0.3% of cases during balloon angioplasty, in up to 1% during high-pressure stenting, and in 1–2% after rotablation or excimer laser angioplasty.[43–45] Wire-related perforation is more frequent in total chronic occlusion angioplasty due to subintimal dissections that may progress to the adventitia, particularly in the case of stiff wires, which may also perforate distal coronary segments. Balloon- or stent-related perforation is usually due to balloon rupture or oversized or high-pressure inflation. Perforation during atherectomy is related to distal curves in the case of rotational atherectomy and to excessively deep cutting in the case of directional atherectomy. Extra care with technical aspects will minimize this complication.

Clinical and angiographic features may be very variable:

1. Small, even initially inadvertent leakage into the pericardial space may present as a delayed and frequently difficult-to-recognize cardiac tamponade.
2. Mild to moderate perivascular staining (Figure 4.9) without hemodynamic compromise usually presents as chest discomfort of variable degree. Resolution may occur within a few minutes, either spontaneously or after prolonged balloon inflation.
3. Severe and widespread perivascular contrast medium staining with or without pulsated leakage may be associated with vessel occlusion. In such cases, the main symptoms are due to severe myocardial ischaemia.
4. Severe perivascular staining with washout of contrast and leaking into the pericardial space is associated with the clinical picture of acute cardiac tamponade (Figure 4.10) and eventually circulatory shock in a matter of minutes.

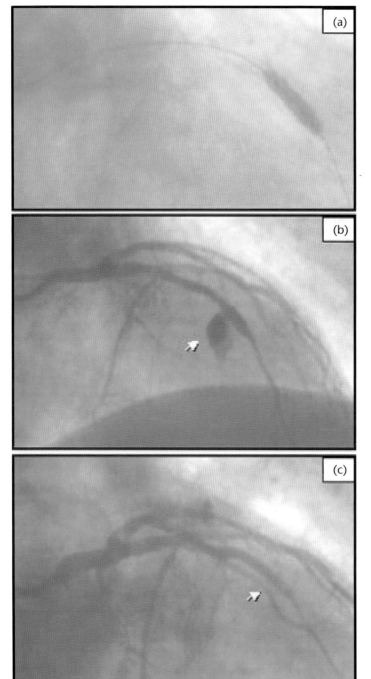

(a)

(b)

(c)

Figure 4.9
Vessel rupture during overdimensioned balloon inflation. (a) Balloon inflation. (b) Large contrast extravasation after balloon deflation. (c) After prolonged balloon inflation, no extravasation is observed.

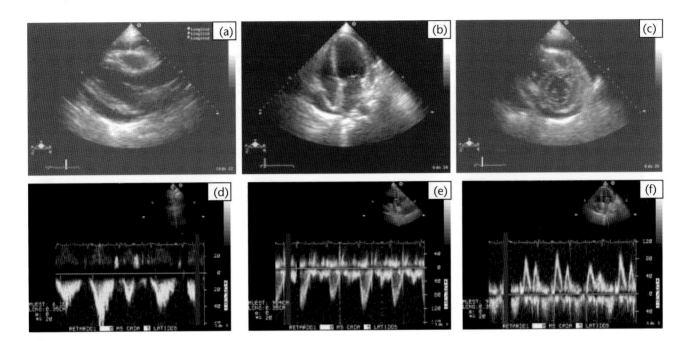

Figure 4.10
Large pericardial effusion with signs of cardiac tamponade after coronary angioplasty: two-dimensional echocardiography. (a) Subcostal view. (b) Apical view. (c) Four-chamber view of a large pericardial effusion. (d) Pulsed Doppler examination of suprahepatic veins with a predominant systolic wave, small diastolic wave, and increment of reversed component. (e) Continuous Doppler of aortic flow with significant variations during respiratory cycle. (f) Pulsed Doppler of transmitral flow with inspiratory variation of E-wave velocity. All three Doppler signs are typical of cardiac tamponade.

The treatment strategy will include sealing the leak, hemodynamic stabilization, and pericardiocentesis if required. Immediate sealing of the leak can be obtained with low-pressure prolonged balloon inflation at the perforation site. This measure may stabilize the patient for several minutes, but is usually associated with ischemia (a perfusion balloon will decrease distal ischemia). After a few minutes, the balloon can be deflated and an angiographic and clinical assessment performed. If the rupture is sealed off and the hemodynamic situation is stable, no further measures other than careful watching will be required. If perforation is still present, the balloon should be inflated again and a polytetrafluoroethylene (PTFE)-covered stent[46–48] deployed at the perforation site. Cardiac tamponade is an emergency situation that is diagnosed and treated based on clinical and angiographic grounds, and echocardiographic confirmation, although helpful, is not mandatory before proceeding to urgent pericardiocentesis. In a few patients, surgery will be still required if there is persistent bleeding after pericardial drainage.

Stent dislodgement

Stents may slip off the balloon. This complication was more frequent (1–2%) with rigid, non-premounted, first-generation stents, and has decreased (<0.5%) with low-profile, flexible, premounted third-generation devices.

Severe proximal tortuosity, calcification, poor guiding catheter backup, and a combination of the above are all risk factors for stent dislodgement. Prevention of stent dislodgement includes appropriate material selection, good guiding catheter support and alignment, appropriate predilatation or debulking if required, and good selection of patients for direct stenting.

A stent may be dislodged from the delivering balloon either outside or inside the coronary circulation. In the first case (usually when guiding wire and balloon slip off the coronary artery or when a dislodged stent is being retrieved into the guiding catheter), it may embolize anywhere into the systemic circulation, usually in the femoro-popliteal territory. Ischemic symptoms in the affected territory are rare, since stents tend to migrate towards small distal vessels whose occlusion will be asymptomatic from a clinical point of view. Frequently, the place of embolization will remain unknown even after X-ray examination. In this case, careful watching for cerebral, mesenteric, or renal ischemic symptoms should be undertaken without specific prophylactic or therapeutic measures.

Stents dislodged from the balloon into the coronary circulation proximal to the target lesion should be either retrieved or expanded in situ. Before any decision is made, several aspects should be taken into consideration, such as the position of the stent (in the left main coronary artery or elsewhere), the integrity of the stent, persistence of the wire inside the stent, persistence of the balloon distal to the stent, and the vessel size. The priority is avoidance of ischemic complications. After this, the stent should be retrieved, bearing in mind that the deployment of a stent in a proximal coronary segment is not a major issue.[49–51] Possible scenarios are as follows:

1. The wire is still inside the stent, the balloon is distal, the stent is intact or mildly distorted, and the balloon can be withdrawn into the stent. The stent can be delivered in place, unless it is in the distal left main overriding left anterior descending or left circumflex arteries, or retrieved as detailed below.
2. The wire is still inside the stent, the balloon is distal, the stent is intact or mildly distorted, and the balloon cannot be withdrawn into the stent. The balloon should be kept distal to the stent inflated a half-atmosphere, and the balloon and stent gently retrieved (after good alignment has been obtained) into the guiding catheter at the descending aortic level (to avoid missing the stent in the cerebrovascular territory).
3. The stent has been dislodged from the balloon but the wire is still there. One should attempt to recross the stent with a new 1.5 mm balloon, inflate it, and then redilate with a larger balloon, matched to vessel size.
4. The stent is severely distorted, the wire is off, and it is impossible to recross with a wire. In the case of a large vessel, another wire can be positioned distal in the coronary artery; the stent can be pushed against the vessel by means of another stent placed parallel to the dislodged one, which can be excluded from the coronary circulation.
5. When the stent is the left main artery and it is a large vessel, it can be retrieved by means of a retrieval snare. If the left main artery is small then one should consider deployment of an additional stent or send the patient for surgical revascularization before clinical signs of left main ischemia develops.

Other complications

Wire rupture

This is exceptional with careful manipulation of PTCA material. It is almost always due to distal entrapment of the wire and subsequent rupture. If the piece is small and distal, it may be left in place, although occlusion of a distal branch will probably occur. If a large piece of wire remains in the coronary artery, retrieval of as much wire as possible should be performed using tools such as a retrieval catheter or a parallel wire.

Longitudinal or pinhole balloon rupture

This is infrequent and may result in vessel dissection/ rupture, although most of the time it does not result in clinical problems.

Transverse balloon rupture

This can also occur. It usually occurs at the proximal segment of coronary arteries and may have severe ischemic consequences.

References

1. Johnson LW, Lozner EC, Johnson S, et al. Coronary arteriography 1984–1987: a report of the Registry of the Society for Cardiac Angiography and Interventions. Results and complications. Cathet Cardiovasc Diagn 1989;17:5.
2. Laskey W, Boyle J, Johson LW, and the Registry Commitee of the Society for Cardiovascular Angiography and Interventions. Multivariate model for prediction of risk of significant complication during diagnostic cardiac catheterization. Cathet Cardiovasc Diagn 1993;30:185.
3. Tan KH, Sulke N, Taub N, Sowton E. Clinical and lesion morphologic determinants of coronary angioplasty success and complications. J Am Coll Cardiol 1995;25:855–65.
4. Scanlon PJ, Faxon DP, Audet AM, et al. ACC/AHA guidelines for coronary angiography: a report of the American College of Cardiology/American Heart Association Task Force on Practice Guidelines (Committee on Coronary Angiography). J Am Coll Cardiol 1999;33:1756–824.
5. McCann RL, Schwartz LB, Pieper KS, et al. Vascular complications of cardiac catheterization. J Vasc Surg 1991;14:375.
6. Schaub F, Theiss W, Busch R, et al. Management of 219 consecutive cases of postcatheterization pseudoaneurysm. J Am Coll Cardiol 1997;30:670–5.
7. Hill JA, Winniford M, Cohen MB, et al. Multicenter trial of ionic versus nonionic contrast media for cardiac angiography. The Iohexol Cooperative Study. Am J Cardiol 1993;72:770–5.
8. Bertrand ME, Esplugas E, Piessens J, et al. Influence of nonionic, isosmolar contrast medium (ioxaglate) on major adverse cardiac events in patients undergoing percutaneous transluminal coronary angioplasty: a multicenter, randomized, double-blinded study. Circulation 2000; 101:131–6.
9. Solomon R, Werner C, Mann D, et al. Effects of saline, mannitol and furosemide on acute decrease in renal function induced by radiocontrast agents. N Engl J Med 1994;331:1416.
10. Stevens MA, McCullough PA, Tobin KJ, et al. A prospective randomized trial of prevention measures in patients at high risk for contrast nephropathy. J Am Coll Cardiol 2000;33:403–11.
11. Bertrand ME, Le Blanche JM, Tilmant PY, et al. Frequency of provoked coronary arterial spasm in 1089 consecutive patients undergoing coronary arteriography. Circulation 1982:65:1299–306.
12. Huber MS, Mooney JF, Madison J, et al. Use of a morphologic classification to predict clinical outcome after dissection from coronary angioplasty. Am J Cardiol 1991; 68:467–71.
13. Capaletti A, Margonato A, Rosano G, et al. Short- and long-term evolution of unstented nonocclusive coronary dissection after coronary angioplasty. J Am Coll Cardiol 1999; 34:1484–8.

14. Cripps TR, Morgan JM, Rickards AF, et al. Outcome of extensive coronary artery dissection during coronary angioplasty. Br Heart J 1991;66:3–6.

15. Black AJ, Namay DL, Niederman AL, et al. Tear or dissection after coronary angioplasty. Morphologic correlates of an ischemic complication. Circulation 1989;79:1035–42.

16. Alfonso F, Hernandez R, Goicolea J, et al. Coronary stenting for acute coronary dissection after coronary angioplasty: implications of residual dissection. J Am Coll Cardiol 1994;24:989–95.

17. Lincoff AM, Popma JJ, Ellis SG, et al. Abrupt vessel closure complicating coronary angioplasty: clinical, angiographic and therapeutic profile. J Am Coll Cardiol 1992;19:926–35.

18. Resnic FS, Ohno-Machado L, Selwyn A, et al. Simplified risk score models accurately predict the risk of major in-hospital complications following percutaneous coronary intervention. Am J Cardiol 2001;88:15–19.

19. Cutlip DE, Baim DS, Ho KK, et al. Stent thrombosis in the modern era: a pooled analysis of multicenter coronary stent clinical trials. Circulation 2001;103:1967–71.

20. Holmes DR Jr, Garratt KN, Popma J, et al. Stent complications. J Invasive Cardiol 1998;10:385–395.

21. Leopold J, Jackobs A. Treatment of closure and threatened closure. In: Strategic Approaches in Coronary Intervention, 2nd edn. Ellis SG and Holmes DR, eds. Philadelphia: Lippincott Williams & Wilkins, 2000.

22. Piana RN, Paik GY, Moscucci M, et al. Incidence and treatment of 'no-reflow' after percutaneous intervention. Circulation 1994;89:2514–18.

23. Leon MB, Baim D, Popma J, et al. Clinical trial comparing three antithrombotic drug regiments after coronary stenting. N Engl J Med 1998;339;1665–71.

24. Moussa I, Di Mario C, Reimers B, et al. Subacute stent thrombosis in the era of intravascular ultrasound-guided coronary stenting without anticoagularion: frequency, predictors and clinical outcome. J Am Coll Cardiol 1997;29:6–12.

25. Moussa I, Oetgen M, Roubin G, et al. Effectiveness of clopidogrel and aspirin versus ticlopidine and aspirin in preventing stent thrombosis after coronary stent implantation. Circulation 1999;99:2364–6.

26. Casserly IR, Hasdai D, Berger P, et al. Usefulness of abciximab for treatment of early coronary artery stent thrombosis. Am J Cardiol 1998:82:981–5.

27. Ellis SG, Lincoff AM, Miller D, et al. Reduction in complications of angioplasty with abciximab occurs largely independently of baseline lesion morphology. J Am Coll Cardiol 1998;32:1619–23.

28. Garot P, Himbert D, Juliard JM, et al. Incidence, consequences, and risk factors of early reocclusion after primary or rescue percutaneous transluminal coronary angioplasty for acute myocardial infarction. Am J Cardiol 1998;82:554–8.

29. Hasdai D, Garratt KN, Holmes DR, et al. Coronary angioplasty and intracoronary thrombolysis are of limited efficacy in resolving early intracoronary stent thrombosis. J Am Coll Cardiol 1996:28:361–7.

30. Mathias DW, Niooney JF, Lange HW, et al. Frequency of success and complications of coronary angioplasty of a stenosis at the ostium of a branch vessel. Am J Cardiol 1991;67:491–8.

31. Fishman DL, Savage MP, Leon MB, et al. Fate of lesion-related side branches after coronary artery stenting. J Am Coll Cardiol 1993;22:1641–6.

32. Arora RR, Raymond RE, Dimas AP, et al. Side branch occlusion during coronary angioplasty: incidence, angiographic characteristics and outcome. Cathet Cardiovasc Diagn 1989;18:210–12.

33. Weinstein JS, Baim DS, Sipperly ME, et al. Salvage of brach vessel during bifurcation lesion angioplasty: acute and long-term follow-up. Cathet Cardiovasc Diagn 1991;22:1–6.

34. Lefkovits J, Holmes DR, Califf RM, et al, for the CAVEAT III Investigators. Predictors and sequelae of distal embolizaiton from the CAVEAT II trial. Circulation 1995;92:734–40.

35. Bhargava B, Kornowski R, Mehran R, et al. Procedural results and intermediate clinical outcomes after multiple saphenous vein graft stenting. J Am Coll Cardiol 2000;35:389–97.

36. Mark KH, Challapalli R, Eisenberg MJ, et al, for the EPIC Investigators. Effect of platelet glycoprotein IIb/IIIa receptor inhibition on distal embolization during percutaneous revascularization of aorcocoronary saphenous vein graft. Am J Cardiol 1997;80:985–8.

37. Matthew V, Grill DE, Scott CG, et al. Clinical studies: the influence of abciximab use on clinical outcome after coronary vein graft interventions. J Am Coll Cardiol 1999;34:1163–9.

38. Baim DS, Wahr D, George B, et al. Randomized trial of a distal embolic protection device during percutaneous intervention of saphenous vein aortocoronary bypass graft. Circulation 2002;105:1285–90.

39. Baldus S, Koster R, Elsner M, et al. Treatment of aorto-coronary vein graft lesions with membrane convered stents. A multicenter surveillance trial. Circulation 2000;102:2024–7.

40. Abbo KM, Dooris M, Glazier S, et al. Features and outcomes of no-reflow after percutaneous coronary interventions. Am J Cardiol 1995;75:778–82.

41. Ito H, Okamura A, Iwakura K, et al. Myocardial perfusion patterns related to thrombolysis in myocardial infarction perfusion grades after coronary angioplasty in patients with acute anterior wall myocardial infarction. Circulation 1996: 93;1993–9.

42. Ito H, Marayuma A, Iwakwa A et al. Clinical implications of the 'no reflow' phenomenon: a predictor of complications and left ventricular remodelling in reperfused anterior wall myocardial infarction. Circulation 1996;93:223–8.

43. Liu F, Erbel R, Hande M, Ge J. Coronary arterial perforation: predictors, diagnosis, management and prevention. In: Strategic Approaches in Coronary Intervention, 2nd edn. Ellis SG and Holmes DR, eds. Philadelphia: Lippincott Williams & Wilkins 2000:501–4.

44. Ellis SG, Ajluni S, Arnold AZ, et al. Increased coronary perforation in the new device era. Incidence, classification management and outcome. Circulation 1994;90:2725–30.

45. Ajluni SC, Glazier S, Blankenship L, et al. Perforations after percutaneous coronary interventions: clinical, angiographic, and therapeutic observations. Cathet Cardiovasc Diagn 1994;32:206–12.

46. Gercken U, Lansky AJ, Buellesfeld L, et al. Results of the Jostent coronary stent graft implantation in various clinical settings: procedural and follow-up results. Catheter Cardiovasc Interv 2002;3:353–60.

47. Elsner M, Auch-Schwelk W, Britten M, et al. Coronary stent grafts covered by a polytetrafluoroethylene membrane. Am J Cardiol 1999;84:335–8.

48. Lopez A, Heuser RR, Stoerger H, et al. Coronary artery application of an endoluminal polytetrafluorethylene stent graft: two center experience with the Jomed JOSTENT. Circulation 1998;17 (Suppl I):I–1016.

49. Garrat K. Coronary stent retrieval: devices and techniques. In: Strategic Approaches in Coronary Intervention, 2nd edn. Ellis SG and Holmes DR, eds. Philadelphia: Lippincott Williams & Wilkins, 2000.

50. Chevalier B, Glatt B, Guyon P, et al. Current indications and results of stent retrieval techniques. J Am Coll Cardiol 2000;35:64A(abst).

51. Eggebrecht H, Haude M, von Birgelen C, et al. Nonsurgical retrieval of embolized coronary stents. Catheter Cardiovasc Interv 2000;4:432–40.

5

Vascular access

I Patrick Kay

The femoral approach

Femoral artery localization

Femoral artery puncture is the standard approach in gaining access to the left heart. The common femoral artery should be punctured in preference to the superficial or profunda (see Figure 5.1). The technique used to cannulate this vessel is germane to arterial puncture elsewhere in the body. The Seldinger technique is used. First the vessel is located by palpating below the inguinal ligament in the region of the inguinal skin crease. The ideal position for puncture is approximately 2 inches below the inguinal lig-

ament and slightly lateral to the position of the vessel. This approach increases the chances of cannulating the common femoral artery and not the superficial femoral or profunda. This minimizes the frequency of local vascular complications. Puncture of the artery at or above the inguinal ligament makes catheter advancement difficult and predisposes to inadequate compression, haematoma formation and retroperitoneal bleeding following sheath removal. Puncture of the artery more than 3 cm below the inguinal ligament increases the chance that the superficial femoral or profunda is punctured, increasing the risk of false aneurysm formation or thrombotic occlusion due to small vessel calibre. Because the superficial

Figure 5.1
Schematic diagram showing the right femoral artery and vein coursing underneath the inguinal ligament. The arterial incision should be placed 3 cm below the ligament and directly over the pulsation of the femoral artery. The venous incision should be placed at the same level but approximately 1–2 cm more medial.

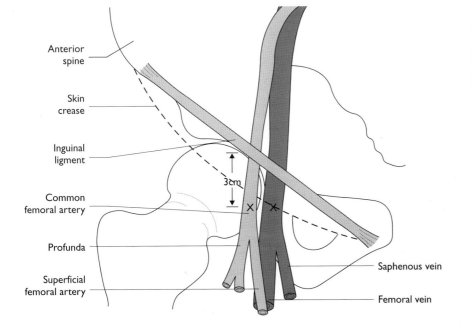

Anterior spine

Skin crease

Inguinal ligament

3cm

Common femoral artery

Profunda

Superficial femoral artery

Saphenous vein

Femoral vein

femoral artery frequently overlies the femoral vein, low venous punctures may pass inadvertently through the superficial femoral artery, leading to excessive bleeding and possibly arteriovenous fistula formation.

Femoral artery puncture

First the femoral artery is localized with middle and index fingers of the left hand. With the fingers stable the area distal is anaesthetized using 10–20 ml of lignocaine. A discrete cut (3–5 mm) is made in the skin using a scalpel blade over the femoral artery. The tissue deep to this cut may be dilated further using various tools, the commonest being the curved 'mosquito' forceps. This approach decreases the resistance that is encountered by the advancement of the needle and sheath. The likelihood that vascular bleeding will become manifest as oozing through the puncture site rather than hidden in a deep haematoma is increased.

Then the vessel is punctured with the needle. The needle may be attached to a syringe or it may be open ended. The experienced operator may sense the artery at the tip of the needle through the transmitted palpation. Once pulsatile flow is confirmed a 0.035 inch wire can be advanced into the vessel toward the heart. Occasionally the wire will turn distally and remanipulation will be required. Hence, fluoroscopic confirmation of the position of the wire is mandatory, especially early in the operator's learning curve. Resistance should not be overcome by force, rather screening and gentle manipulation is recommended. Similarly caution should be exercised in routinely puncturing both walls of the artery as this may translate to an increased risk of hematoma and groin complications, particularly in the age of glycoprotein IIb/IIIa receptor blockers. The needle is then withdrawn. Over the wire a sheath is advanced. The sheath is commonly between 5 French and 8 French in diameter. Through the sheath various diagnostic catheters and interventional guiding catheters may be introduced.

Troubleshooting

Previous catheterization through the femoral artery may lead to scarring. This can make insertion of the sheath difficult on subsequent occasions. Predilation may be necessary using either the dilator of the sheath or specifically designed commercially available stiffer dilators. If the artery can be cannulated, but the 0.035 inch J wire is unable to be advanced beyond the tip of the needle, then the angle of the needle to the vessel should be gently adjusted, by tilting the needle or by lateral/medial movement. If the wire is still unable to be advanced then the wire should be withdrawn to ensure that there is good

flow. Once flow has been assured then a Terumo Glidewire (Terumo Corporation, Tokyo, Japan) or ACS 0.018 inch extra support wire (Guidant, Temecula, CA, USA) can be considered. If flow is poor or absent then the needle should be removed. After a period of compression, a further puncture may be attempted.

If the artery can be cannulated, but the 0.035 inch J wire is unable to be advanced due to excessive calcification, tortuosity or other anatomical factors, an 0.018 inch angioplasty wire such as the ACS extra support may be inserted through the needle and passed through the iliac vessels to the descending aorta. Predilation can then be performed using the introducer of the sheath or other predilators. If this passage is difficult then a 10 cc syringe filled with contrast may be taken and a cine run of the iliac vessels made. This will ensure that any likely anatomical difficulties are well defined.

If there is excessive calcification or tortuosity in the iliac vessels, rapid passage can be made using a Terumo Glidewire or similar, and the insertion of a long sheath. A long sheath should always be inserted if the operator is contemplating angioplasty under such circumstances.

If dissection occurs in the passage of the guiding catheter wire or sheath then left heart catheterization should be relocated to the other groin or a radial approach considered. Fortunately, true arterial compromise from the femoral approach is rare.

If insertion of the sheath is difficult due to an iliac stenosis, then the operator may wish to stent this vessel to facilitate expeditious placement of the sheath.

On occasions the operator will be faced with the prospect of prosthetic graft puncture. This is not an absolute contraindication, however the operator should be aware that passage through the synthetic tissue may be difficult when inserting the sheath. Thromboembolism and graft infection are recognized complications of this approach. The use of Terumo Glidewires and steerable guiding catheter wires may be useful in this context.

Certain systemic diseases are associated with a greater frequency of groin complication. These include the aged, severe aortic stenosis, systemic hypertension, gross obesity and systemic anticoagulation. Fortunately the vascular complications of catheterization via the femoral artery are not great. Generally speaking there are few patients who have an absolute contraindication to femoral artery catheterization.

Femoral vein puncture

Femoral vein puncture is commonly performed prior to arterial puncture. The artery is used as a landmark to facilitate venous puncture. After the instillation of local anesthetic and a short nick created in the skin, the needle is advanced at 45° cephalad with a 10 ml syringe attached to the distal end. Gentle suction is maintained at all times.

Once dark red blood suggestive of venous puncture is withdrawn, the needle is stabilized with the left hand and the syringe removed. Blood-flow will be non-pulsatile. The 0.035 inch J wire can then be advanced into the vein. The vein is commonly compressed on deep movement of the needle meaning that flow of blood into the syringe is only seen on *withdrawal* of the needle. The sheath can then be passed over the 0.035 inch J wire.

Note that the vein can be left temporarily with the J wire in situ, whilst attention is drawn to the arterial puncture. This approach may be advantageous as there will be minimal distortion of the arterial puncture site, which may be caused by the placement of the venous sheath.

Femoral sheath removal

Sheath removal generally is performed by a dedicated group of staff in most departments. These individuals may be nursing staff whose task is to ensure safe sheath removal, or invasive/interventional fellows in training. Very simply good initial training is the key to reproducible successful results, followed by an adequate volume of cases to maintain clinical skill.

Sheath removal from the femoral vein is simple and only requires pressure for a matter of minutes before haemostasis is obtained. After routine coronary angiography, during which no or only a small dose of heparin is used, the sheath may be removed immediately. Removal of smaller sheaths (5 and 6 French) will only require brief periods of compression. Certain centers advocate brief periods of manual compression, followed by the use of a compression device. Others insist on more prolonged periods of manual compression followed by the use of pressure bandages.

After an angioplasty has been performed there will normally be a wait of between 4 and 6 h before the sheath is removed. This is to allow clearance of the heparin administered during the procedure. Recent data suggests that the use of bivalrudin at the time of percutaneous intervention, allows for immediate sheath removal after the intervention, earlier times to ambulation and may facilitate same-day discharge in 26% of patients.[1] Clearly, the potential for complications associated with arterial sheath removal increase with larger sheaths and the concurrent use of glycoprotein IIb/IIIa receptor blockers.

The brachial artery approach

The brachial artery is well approached by cutdown or direct puncture. The techniques are described in other texts. Critics of this approach describe complications due to bleeding, arterial compromise and to brachial nerve damage. It is this author's opinion that the radial approach offers an efficacious and safer option.

The radial artery approach

The radial approach offers certain advantages over femoral catheterization and angioplasty; these include a decreased risk of serious bleeding and early mobilization. The radial technique was initially pioneered by Lucien Campeau for diagnostic coronary studies. Kiemeneij and colleagues[2] adapted the transradial approach for coronary angioplasty and stenting, by combining miniaturized angioplasty equipment compatible with the small size of the radial artery. In August 1992 the first patients were treated via this route at the Amsterdam Department of Interventional Cardiology (ADIC) of the Onze Lieve Vrouwe Gasthuis (OLVG) in Amsterdam. Since catheterization and percutaneous intervention have become commonplace using the right radial approach (Figure 5.2). The technique is now sufficiently robust that positive safety and feasibility trials on outpatient angioplasty have been described. A few caveats will aid the reader in facilitating the process.

Patient selection

First assess the patient for suitability for the radial approach. Broadly speaking the following are contraindications to the radial approach:

Absence of a radial artery pulsation.

Radial dominant circulation as evidenced by the Allen test or saturation in combination with plethysmography.

The novice would be wise to avoid this approach in acute myocardial infarction or haemodynamic instability and in those with considerable tortuosity to the aortic root and great vessels. With experience, the radial approach is ideal for the performance of primary or rescue angioplasty. Under these circumstances the patient is frequently heavily anticoagulated, implying that the risk of significant bleeding will be reduced by the radial approach.

Patient preparation

1. The patient is counseled on the advantages and disadvantages of this approach. Patients are informed that they will be aware of sheath/guiding catheter movement. Equally the instillation of 'the cocktail' (heparin, verapamil and/or nitroglycerin and lignocaine) may be noted.

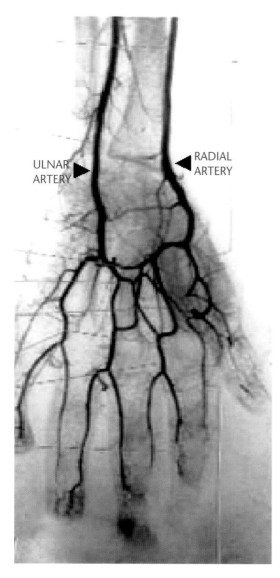

Figure 5.2
Arteriogram demonstrating the position of the radial and ulnar arteries.

2. The Allen's test is favorable suggesting a significant/ dominant ulnar circulation.
3. Administer a sedative as per catheter laboratory protocol.
4. Remove all jewellery from the area and shave and disinfect the arm.
5. Ensure that venous access has been obtained on the opposing upper limb.

The Allen's test

The relative significance of the radial and ulnar circulation can be established by performing the Allen's test (Figures 5.3a and 5.3b):

1. Firmly compress the radial and ulna arteries simultaneously. Then ask the patient to open and close their fingers, making a fist on each occasion. By performing this action the hand will blanch. Ulnar artery compression is then released. The Allen's test is positive if the colour of the hand returns to normal in 10 s. This indicates that the ulnar circulation is intact and that it is safe to perform the procedure via the radial approach. If the hand remains pale the test is negative, suggesting suboptimal circulation through the ulnar system. An alternative route for catheterization should then be selected.
2. Plethysmography may also be used to assess the presence of functioning collaterals. The sensor is clipped onto the thumb and the ulnar and radial arteries compressed. The curve will duly flatten. If at the release of pressure over the ulnar artery the plethysmography curve returns, collaterals are present. If the curve does not return immediately wait an extra minute. Collateral recruitment may result in a slow return of flow and pressure. If you then repeat the test and the curve comes back more rapidly, there are functioning collaterals. A persistent absence of a curve means that there are no collaterals. Under these circumstances the radial artery should not be punctured.

Local anaesthesia

Most operators instill 3–5 ml of lignocaine 1–2% prior to puncture. Generally speaking this volume is sufficient to guarantee adequate anaesthesia, but also importantly it minimizes the risk of distortion of the local anatomy due to administration of an excessive volume. Consequently radial artery puncture can be accurately and safely performed. Some operators will choose to perform a skin incision prior to arterial puncture, whereas others will widen the puncture site once the wire is in situ. The width of the incision should be sufficient to permit the smooth passage of the introducer sheath. Care should be taken not to create a deep incision as this may damage the radial artery. Equally the incision should be longitudinal to the artery and not transverse, as the latter risks complete transsection of the radial artery. A rounded blade is preferable.

Arterial puncture

Palpate the radial artery with the pulp of index and middle fingers. Lift the index finger and puncture at an angle of 45 degrees from lateral to medial.

Aim to puncture the artery as distal as possible (at least 1 cm proximal to the styloid process). This prevents perforation of the retinaculum flexorum and inadvertent

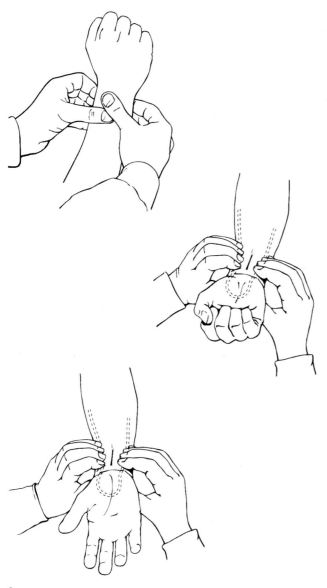

a

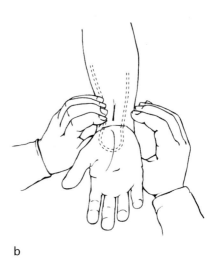

b

Figure 5.3

(a) Occlude both the radial and ulnar arteries with manual compression. With the patient's hand held up, have them clench their fist tightly closed. Next have the patient lower their arm and open their hand in a relaxed position. Avoid hyperextension of the wrist. Maintain compression of both arteries. (b) Release pressure over the ulnar artery. Observe the hand for return of colour. If the ulnar artery is patent and there is an intact palmar arch, colour will return to the hand within 10 s. If the delay is greater than 10 s then there is slow filling in the ulnar artery or incomplete palmar collateral circulation. Finally release pressure over the radial artery and make sure that there is no reactive hyperemia of the land. (Reproduced from A Physicians Guide: The Radial Approach to Angiography and Intervention by CJ Cooper, MD for Cordis, A Johnson & Johnson Company, with permission.)

puncture of a superficial branch of the radial artery. Additionally this permits more proximal attempts at puncture should the first attempt fail. Typically once pulsatile backflow of blood is noted the wire can be passed as for other access routes. The sheath can then be rotated (sometimes a screwing motion is appropriate) into the vessel. Frequently operators will instill the cocktail of medication at this stage, so as to minimize spasm, prior to proximal advancement of the sheath and passage of the guiding catheter.

Various prepackaged needle/wires/sheaths are available from competing companies, which facilitate the passage of the wire through the needle in a stable and controlled manner (Figure 5.4). The following are an example:

1. Arrow puncture set (Arrow International Corporation, USA)

2. Terumo introducer sheath (Terumo Corporation, Japan)

3. Side hole sheath (Medkit Corporation and Terumo Corporation, Japan)
   This side hole sheath can deliver vasodilator directly to the endothelium of the radial artery.

4. Emcee coated sheath (Boston Scientific Scimed, USA).

5. Cordis Transradial Kit (Cordis, a Johnson and Johnson Company, USA)

Sheath insertion

A long sheath will minimize trauma to the radial artery and permit smooth movement of the guiding catheter to the proximal vessel without spasm. Similarly the necessary

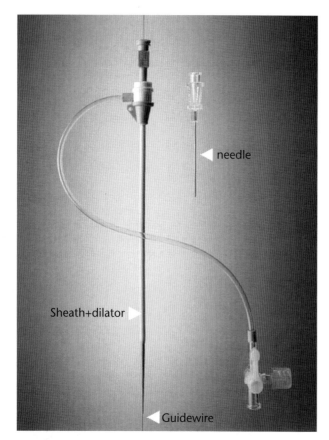

needle

Sheath+dilator

Guidewire

Figure 5.4
Avanti + Transradial kit (Cordis, a Johnson & Johnson Company). This comprises a sheath introducer with vessel dilator, a guidewire and a needle. This is a typical example of a short-sheath kit.

torque may be applied to locate the ostia of the coronary vessels without causing undue spasm. Should significant spasm occur at the time of removal of the sheath, then the administration of spasmolytics should be performed via the side-port of the sheath.

Short sheaths are used by many experienced operators as they permit ready removal of the sheath at the termination of the procedure.

Guiding catheter selection and advancement

Once the sheath is in position, the 0.035 inch wire can be advanced to the ascending aorta. To minimize spasm, especially with highly tortuous or dilated proximal vessels a Terumo Glidewire can be used. If the exchange of guiding catheters is necessary the operator should consider the use of a 0.035 inch exchange wire. This again minimizes trauma to the vessel, especially where there are anatomical difficulties or there has been spasm in the vessel.

Guiding catheter selection

Below we have selected a series of guiding catheters that the operator may find useful. The operator will rapidly create a 'favourites' list:

- Kimny wiseguide (Boston Scientific Scimed)
- MUTA wiseguide (L&R) (Boston Scientific Scimed)
- Radial Curve (Boston Scientific Scimed)
- The Mann IM Guiding catheter (Boston Scientific Scimed)
- Fajadet L & R (Cordis, a Johnson & Johnson Company)

Haemostasis

Recently compression devices have become available which facilitate sheath removal at the termination of the case. These include:

- Radistop (Radi Medical Systems)
- Radstat (Wake Heart Associates)
- Hemoband (TZ Medical)

Complications
Prevention and management of radial artery spasm

Radial artery spasm is commonly associated with transradial cannulation. Usually the problem is mild and only noticeable on withdrawal of the radial sheath. Rarely spasm may be so severe that the sheath can only be removed by using profound physical force. This has been associated with radial artery rupture. Spasm in the artery may be caused by puncture, sheath introduction, guidewire or guiding catheter manipulations or patient anxiety.

Prevention

1. **Patient selection:** avoid small radial arteries. Also do not choose individuals who have extensive peripheral vascular disease for your first cases, as femoral stenoses and tortuosity may well be reflected in the anatomy of the great vessels.
2. **Patient sedation:** first inform the patient about the likely sensations experienced during the procedure. Secondly provide adequate sedation as part of the premed. Some individuals may well require prophylactic analgesia. Consider also the application of topical lidocaine-prilocaine cream (EMLA®) 2 h prior to puncture.

3. **Intrarterial administration of a spasmolytic cocktail**

This cocktail may be introduced at the time of puncture, prior to sheath introduction. This increases the probability that the injected drug will reach the arterial wall. Alternatively a sheath with side-holes may be used to maximize infiltration of medication. A further alternative is the introduction of the sheath about 1–2 cm into the vessel before medication is injected. Typical components of the cocktail are:

    Glyceryl trinitrate 200 mcg
    Verapamil 5 mg
    Lignocaine 50 mg
    Heparin 5000–10 000 IU

Note that the latter two drugs are both acidic and may induce local irritation and spasm. Some operators prefer to inject heparin into the ascending aorta or intravenously for this reason.

4. **Sheath selection**

There are pros and cons to the selection of long and short sheaths in association with the radial route. Short sheaths are believed to cause less spasm at the time of introduction. If the operator is forced to manipulate the catheter frequently or with force then the short sheath will not protect the artery from local irritation and potentially spasm caused by this manoeuvre. The counter argument may be made for long sheaths. Generally speaking the novice is encouraged to start off using the 20–25 cm long sheath until the stage in which their handling skills of the catheter in the aorta is proficient. A trial of the short sheath may then be undertaken depending on the operator's preference.

5. **Guidewire selection**

Guidewires between 0.025 and 0.035 inch are commonly used. Hydrophilic wires may be useful in preventing spasm. Similarly the use of exchange length wires may be useful in minimizing vessel trauma. Avoid the use of guidewires with a sharp 'J' tip as these may be prone to select side branches excessively or to go retrograde on insertion.

6. **Guiding catheter selection**

No one guiding catheter will suit all operators hence it is important to become familiar with a single or group of catheters. The fewer the manipulations and exchanges, the quicker and less complicated the procedure will be.

Management of spasm

If despite the above precautions radial spasm occurs or persists such that the sheath is difficult to withdraw, then consider the following approach:

    Minimize all pain
    Give nifedipine 10 mg sublingually

Nitroglycerin 200 mcg IA (repeated)
Verapamil 5 mg IA
Warm compress over the forearm

If the above does not permit easy sheath withdrawal then wait 1 h. At the end of this time ensure adequate analgesia and try again.

If none of the above appear to work then an axillary block may be helpful.

Clinical trials

A randomized comparison between transradial, transbrachial and transfemoral PTCA with 6F guiding catheters was performed by Kiemeneij and colleagues in 900 patients.[3] Primary end points were entry site and angioplasty related. Secondary end points were quantitative coronary analysis after PTCA, procedural and fluoroscopy times, consumption of angioplasty equipment and length of hospital stay. Successful coronary cannulation was achieved in 279 (93.0%), 287 (95.7%) and 299 (99.7%) patients randomized to undergo PTCA by the radial, brachial and femoral approaches, respectively. PTCA success was achieved in 91.7%, 90.7% and 90.7% of patients, with 88.0%, 87.7% and 90.0% event free at 1-month follow-up, respectively (p = non significant). Major entry site complications were encountered in seven patients (2.3%) in the transbrachial group, six (2.0%) in the transfemoral group and none in the transradial group (p = 0.035). Transradial PTCA led to asymptomatic loss of radial pulsations in nine patients (3%). Procedural and fluoroscopy times were similar, as were consumption of guiding and balloon catheters and length of hospital stay ([mean $\pm$ SD] 1.5 $\pm$ 2.5, 1.8 $\pm$ 3.8 and 1.8 $\pm$ 4.2 days, respectively). The authors concluded that with experience, procedural and clinical outcomes of PTCA were similar for the three subgroups, but access failure is more common during transradial PTCA. Major access site complications were more frequently encountered after transbrachial and transfemoral PTCA.

The OUTCLAS study assessed the safety and feasibility of transradial angioplasty (TRA) on an outpatient basis.[4] Analysis included cost-effectiveness and an assessment of patient comfort. Included were 159 patients treated with balloon angioplasty or intracoronary stent placement, all performed via the radial artery with 6 French guiding catheters. Patients were selected for same-day discharge based on the absence of any adverse predictor for subacute occlusion or unfavorable clinical outcome during the first 24 h after successful PTCA. One hundred and six (66%) patients were discharged 4–6 h after PTCA. Stents were used in 40% of patients. There were no cardiac or vascular complications. The authors concluded that outpatient PTCA, performed via the radial artery, is both safe and feasible in a large part of a routine PTCA population.

The same group analysed the feasibility, safety and predictive factors of success of stent implantation without balloon predilatation (direct stenting) in 250 patients undergoing elective stent implantation via the TRA approach.[5] Coronary interventions were undertaken predominantly via the transradial route using 6 French guiding catheters. Direct stent implantation was attempted using AVE GFX II coronary stent delivery systems. Two hundred and sixty-six direct stent implantations were attempted in 250 patients. Direct stenting was successful in 226 (85%) cases. Out of 40 (15%) cases where direct stenting failed, balloon predilatation facilitated stent implantation in 39. Predictive factors for failure of direct stenting on multivariate analysis were circumflex lesions ($P < 0.01$), complex lesions ($P < 0.01$), and longer stents ($P < 0.001$). The authors concluded that direct stent implantation was safe and feasible in the majority of cases with a low rate of complications.

Subsequent studies have looked at the efficacy of transradial angioplasty in the context of acute myocardial infarction (primary angioplasty).[6] Not only are the angioplasty results as good as the femoral approach, but also the risk of severe bleeding, transfusion and pseudoaneurysm was reduced. The procedure time was not increased in experienced hands. Such studies suggest an economic advantage based on a briefer in-hospital period both among elective admissions and those with acute coronary syndromes and myocardial infarction.

Kiemeneij and colleagues reported the incidence and outcome of radial artery occlusion following transradial angioplasty.[7] They evaluated 563 patients with a normal Allen's test. Patients were evaluated at the time of discharge and at 30 days. At discharge 5.3% demonstrated radial artery occlusion. At 30 days 2.8% of arteries were occluded. All were asymptomatic, with no further therapy required. These figures have been corroborated by other studies.

References

1. Ormiston JA, Shaw BL, Panther MJ et al. Percutaneous coronary intervention with bivalirudin anticoagulation, immediate sheath removal and early ambulation: a feasibility study with implications for day-stay procedures. Catheter Cardiovasc Interv 2002;55:289–93.
2. Kiemeneij F, Laarman GJ. Percutaneous transradial artery approach for coronary stent implantation. Cathet Cardiovasc Diagn 1993;30:173–8.
3. Kiemeneij F, Laarman GJ, Odekerken D et al. A randomized comparison of percutaneous transluminal coronary angioplasty by the radial, brachial and femoral approaches: The Access Study. J Am Coll Cardiol 1997;19:1269–75.
4. Slagboom T, Kiemeneij F, Laarman GJ, van der Wieken R, Odekerken D. Actual outpatient PTCA: results of the OUTCLAS pilot study. Catheter Cardiovasc Interv 2001;53:204–8.
5. Laarman G, Muthusamy TS, Swart H, et al. Direct coronary stent implantation: safety, feasibility, and predictors of success of the strategy of direct coronary stent implantation. Catheter Cardiovasc Interv 2001;52:443–8.
6. Mathias DW, Bigler L. Transradial coronary angioplasty and stent implantation in acute myocardial infarction. J Inv Cardiol 2000;12:547–9.
7. Stella PR, Kiemeneij F, Laarman GJ, et al. Incidence and outcome of radial artery occlusion following transradial artery coronary angioplasty. Cathet Cardiovasc Diagn 1997;40:156–8.

6

Basic coronary angiography: techniques, tools and troubleshooting

John Ormiston, Mark Webster, Barbara O'Shaughnessy

The objective of coronary angiography is to record details of coronary anatomy, including the pattern of arterial distribution and anatomical or functional pathology.

Arterial access

Most procedures are undertaken using a percutaneous approach from the femoral artery. Radial or brachial access is sometimes employed.

Coronary angiographic catheter shapes

Angiographic catheters are preshaped (Figure 6.1) for specific tasks. The most commonly used catheter shapes are JL4 and JR4 for study of the left and right coronary arteries, respectively, and a pigtail for left ventriculography. A JL5 is an appropriate first-choice left coronary catheter in older males, particularly if they are tall or hypertensive.

The most common diameters employed are 5 French (5 Fr) and 6 Fr, but diameters from 4 Fr to 8 Fr are used. Optimal opacification of coronary arteries with 4 Fr catheters requires power-assisted contrast injection.

Catheter advancement to the ascending aorta

Once arterial access has been attained, the catheter is advanced over a guidewire (usually 0.035 or 0.038 inch diameter with a J-shaped tip) into the ascending aorta immediately above the aortic valve.

Problem: inability to advance the guidewire to the ascending aorta

Causes

1. The guidewire has passed into a branch vessel.
2. The guidewire is folding back on itself (e.g. in an abdominal aortic aneurysm).
3. The guidewire has passed subintimally and is dissecting the arterial wall.
4. The guidewire is having difficulty negotiating tortuosity, especially in the iliac arteries.
5. The guidewire is having difficulty traversing an arterial stenosis.

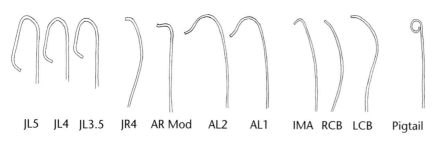

JL5   JL4   JL3.5   JR4   AR Mod   AL2   AL1   IMA RCB LCB   Pigtail

Figure 6.1
Common coronary angiographic catheter shapes. JL, Judkins left; JR, Judkins right; AR, Amplatz right; AL, Amplatz left; IMA, internal mammary artery; RCB, right coronary bypass; LCB, left coronary bypass.

Solutions

Fluoroscopy may show the cause, such as coiling in an abdominal aortic aneurysm. If not, carefully advance the diagnostic catheter to near the wire tip. Remove the wire and inject a very small volume (e.g. 0.5 ml) of radiographic contrast medium to determine whether there is arterial dissection (catheter in the arterial wall). If the contrast disappears rapidly, there is no dissection, and a 5–10 ml forceful hand injection can safely be made. This injection will usually define an anatomical problem such as tortuosity or stenosis and provide a road map for advancement of a steerable wire (e.g. Wholey J wire, Mallinckrodt, St Louis, MO) or of a hydrophilic coated wire such as a Glidewire (Terumo, Japan).

A long sheath may straighten arterial bends, especially in the iliac arteries, allowing easier subsequent catheter manipulation. If it has been difficult to pass a wire, it is wise to make subsequent catheter changes over a wire rather than removing the catheter and wire and starting afresh.

Connection to manifold

When the guidewire and catheter are in the ascending aorta, the guidewire is removed. To ensure that there is no air or clot within the catheter, a syringe is connected to the catheter to aspirate and discard approximately 5 ml of blood. Alternatively, the catheter is allowed to 'bleed back'. The catheter is then connected to the three-port manifold (Figure 6.2), which is a closed system allowing pressure monitoring, catheter flushing with saline, and radiographic contrast administration. Connection to the manifold is performed with saline flushing and with fluid 'bleeding back' from the catheter to exclude air.

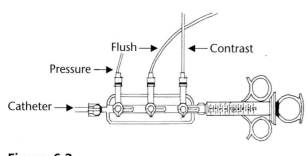

Flush →   ← Contrast
Pressure →
Catheter →

Figure 6.2
Manifold connections.

Observe the hemodynamic pressure waveform and note systolic and diastolic pressures so that you will better understand subsequent pressure changes.

Contrast injection technique

The injection syringe, full of contrast, is held with the handle elevated so that any bubbles rise to the plunger and are less likely to be injected into the patient. Contrast must be injected at a sufficient rate to briefly replace the blood in the coronary artery with continuous reflux into the aortic root. If there is insufficient reflux into the root, there may be failure to reveal an ostial lesion. Before injecting contrast, check that there is no arterial pressure damping (see below).

Problem: poor-quality angiographic pictures

Causes

1. Poor catheter engagement so that there is non-selective contrast injection.
2. Inadequate contrast volume or injection rate.
3. Failure to move the angiography table to bring regions of interest to the center of the angiographic field, where spatial and contrast resolution are best.

Nitroglycerin administration

Nitroglycerin should be administered routinely (either sublingually or by coronary injection) before coronary angiography. If there is suspicion of coronary arterial spasm, especially catheter-tip-induced spasm, intracoronary nitroglycerin 200–400 μg is administered. Nitroglycerin may abolish apparent stenoses due to spasm or unmask true stenoses by dilating the vessel adjacent to a stenosis.

Catheter engagement of the left main coronary artery

Obliquity for coronary artery engagement

The 50° left anterior oblique (LAO) view (image intensifier angled 50° from vertical towards patient's left; see Figure 6.11 below) profiles best the origin of the left (and right) coronary arteries. It is the best obliquity (Figure 6.3) in which to attempt engagement of these arteries.

Choice of catheter shape

The left Judkins-shape catheter with a 4 cm curve (JL4) will usually find the left coronary ostium (Figure 6.4). If the aortic root is larger or smaller than average, a larger (JL5) or smaller (JL 3.5) curve, respectively, may be needed.

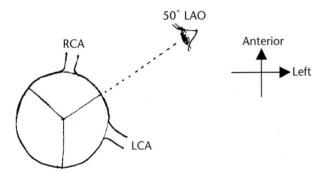

Figure 6.3
The origins of the left and right coronary arteries are best profiled in a 50° LAO projection.

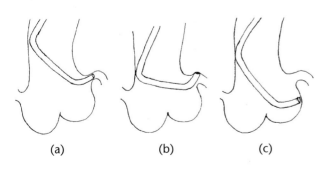

Figure 6.4
In (a), the Judkins shape is correctly aligned in the left coronary artery. In (b), the shape is too small, predisposing to pressure damping and increasing the risk of subintimal contrast injection (dissection). In (c), the shape is too large to engage the coronary artery.

> ## Problem: failure to engage the left main coronary artery
>
> ### Causes
>
> 1. Judkins curve too long or too short.
> 2. Ostium site displaced somewhat from the most common site.
> 3. Very rarely, the left main coronary artery will arise from the right sinus of Valsalva close to or in conjunction with the right coronary artery.

Solutions

An injection of 5–10 ml of contrast close to the expected site of the artery may show the ostium and provide a roadmap for engagement or selection of a more appropriately sized Judkins curve. If the Judkins curve is marginally too long, then the tip of the curve can be altered by pushing the catheter down onto the aortic valve for 5–10 seconds, to bend the tip upwards, followed by catheter withdrawal to engage the left coronary ostium.

Sometimes, deep inspiration or expiration will enable engagement.

Rarely, an Amplatz shape (e.g. AL1, AL2, or AL3) may be required.

> ## Problem: selective engagement of either the left anterior descending or left circumflex artery
>
> ### Cause
>
> Short left main coronary artery or separate orifices for left anterior descending and circumflex arteries.

Solution

With the catheter selectively in one artery, carry out angiography in projections appropriate for that vessel. If the left anterior descending is engaged with a JL4 shape, the circumflex can be selectively engaged with a larger curve such as JL5. Conversely, if the circumflex has been selectively engaged with a JL4 shape, the left anterior descending can be engaged with a smaller curve (JL3.5). Selective injection of each artery sequentially provides good opacification. Withdrawing the catheter close to the ostium and allowing regurgitant contrast to opacify the non-engaged artery usually provides suboptimal opacification.

Problem: failure to find the circumflex or left anterior descending coronary artery

Causes

1. Anomalous origin of the artery (especially the circumflex) from the right sinus close to or in conjunction with the right coronary artery (Figure 6.5).
2. Short left main coronary artery or double orifice (see above).
3. Occluded circumflex.

Solutions

1. An anomalous left circumflex arising from the right sinus can be selectively engaged with a catheter, such as an RCB catheter, that is straighter than a JR4. Sometimes, an Amplatz right shape is useful.
2. If there is a short left main coronary artery, contrast injection after partial withdrawal of the catheter may reveal this.
3. If the circumflex is occluded, it will opacify by collateral filling (except if the artery has occluded in the previous few days before collaterals have had the opportunity to develop).

Problem: pressure damping (reduction of systolic pressure, diastolic pressure or both) upon engagement of a coronary artery

This may cause arrhythmia or myocardial depression, especially when contrast is injected.

Causes

1. Coronary artery stenosis (e.g. left main stenosis).
2. 'Roofing' of catheter tip. The end hole of the catheter is directed against the wall of the coronary artery, preventing transmission of arterial pressure.
3. Catheter-tip-induced spasm (most common in the right coronary artery, but occasionally in the left).
4. Engagement of the catheter in a small branch (e.g. the conus branch of the right coronary artery).
5. Air or thrombus in the catheter, manifold, tubing, or pressure transducer.

Solutions

1. If the problem is due to 1–4 above, withdrawal of the catheter from the coronary artery will restore pressure to normal. If the pressure does not return to normal, there is a strong possibility of air or thrombus in the system, and the catheter should be removed from the body and the system checked.
2. A small (<1 ml) contrast injection will often demonstrate the problem such as 3–6 below.
3. Engagement of a small conus branch. Withdraw the catheter.
4. If the cause is a severe proximal stenosis, such as left main coronary stenosis, limit the number of views to those necessary to display coronary anatomy sufficiently for planning subsequent revascularization. If pressure damping is severe, disengagement of the catheter between contrast injections is wise.
5. 'Roofing' (see Figure 6.4b above) may be limited by withdrawing the catheter a little or changing to a different shape such as a larger Judkins curve for the left coronary artery.
6. Spasm may be abolished by intracoronary administration of 200–400 μg of nitroglycerin. Catheter-induced spasm is more common in the right coronary artery than the left.

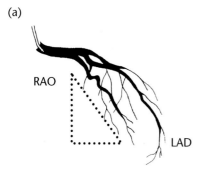

(a)

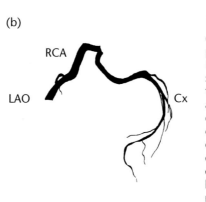

(b)

Figure 6.5
(a) Right anterior oblique (RAO) projection of the left coronary artery. No branches of the left coronary artery supply the circumflex territory (dotted triangle), raising the possibility of anomalous circumflex, occluded circumflex, or double orifice left coronary system with selective injection of the left anterior descending (LAD) coronary artery. (b) Left anterior oblique (LAO) projection showing the left circumflex (Cx) arising from the right coronary artery (RCA).

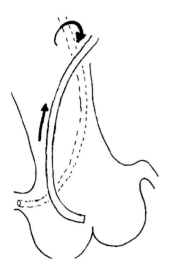

Figure 6.6
To engage the right coronary artery, advance the JR4 catheter to the aortic valve then simultaneously withdraw and rotate in a clockwise direction.

Catheter engagement of the right coronary artery

The origin of the right coronary artery is best profiled in the 50° LAO projection (see figure 6.3 above).

Advance the JR4 catheter so that it lies 1–2 cm above the aortic valve (Figure 6.6). Apply traction to the catheter as you rotate it in a clockwise direction (Figure 6.6). As the catheter rotates, reduce the torque so that the tip does not 'overshoot' the ostium and to reduce the chance of deep engagement.

Problem: failure to find the right coronary artery

'Flush' occlusions of coronary arteries 'do not' occur. There is always some 'stump', and an occluded artery will opacify by collateral flow.

Causes

The most common cause is that the origin of the right coronary artery arises more superiorly and leftwards than normal (Figure 6.7). It may arise from the left sinus close to the left main coronary artery.

Solutions

1. A 5–10 ml rapid injection of contrast and cine acquisition may display the origin and provide a roadmap for engagement.

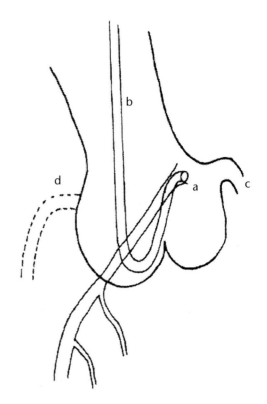

Figure 6.7
Anomalous origin of the RCA more leftward and more superiorly than usual, as shown in this 50° LAO projection. a, anomalous right coronary artery; b, AL1 (Amplatz left 1 angiographic catheter), c, left coronary artery; d, usual site of origin of right coronary artery.

2. The leftward origin of the right coronary artery can most readily be engaged with an Amplatz (e.g. AL1 or AL2) catheter shape. This catheter should be advanced to lie close to the left main coronary artery, then rotated clockwise with test injections to seek the origin which may lie anywhere between the left main coronary origin and the usual site for a right coronary ostium.

Angiographic study of grafts

Grafts arising from the ascending aorta

Read the surgical report to find out how many grafts there are, and whether or not these are sequential grafts. The report may provide clues to where the grafts arise from the aorta and the course that they may take.

The relative positions of the origins of vein grafts or nonpediculated ('free') arterial grafts are best delineated in the 40° RAO view of the ascending aorta (Figure 6.8). This is the best view in which to engage the graft ostia.

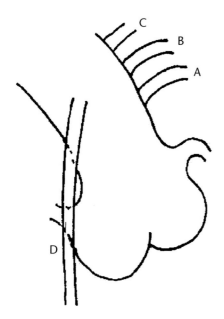

Figure 6.8
Sites of origin of grafts from the ascending aorta displayed in the 40° RAO projection. A is the left anterior descending graft, B the diagonal graft, C the obtuse marginal graft, and D the right coronary artery graft.

Engagement of the leftward-arising grafts (Figure 6.8: A, B, or C).

Advance a left coronary bypass graft catheter (LCB) to the ascending aorta immediately above the aortic valve. Rotate the tip so that in the 40° RAO obliquity it is directed forward, then withdraw the catheter slowly, making small test injections.

Engagement of a right graft (Figure 6.8: D)

Select a catheter straighter than a JR4 shape (e.g. a right coronary bypass (RCB) shape) to engage a right coronary graft if it arises on the right side of the aorta as projected in the RAO 40° obliquity. Advance the RCB catheter to a position high in the ascending aorta immediately upstream from the arch. Remove the wire, flush onto the manifold, rotate the catheter tip to point rightward in this projection, then advance it down the ascending aorta, making test injections if engagement is suspected. Some surgeons place the right coronary graft so that it arises leftward from the aorta in the RAO 40° obliquity, and this often can be determined from the operation report.

If grafts cannot be engaged with LCB or RCB catheters, Amplatz shapes can be tried. It is tempting to try to engage grafts with the JR4 catheter following right coronary angiography, but opacification with this catheter

is frequently suboptimal because of poor engagement. If your objective is to obtain high-quality graft angiograms, it is better to select the appropriate catheter from the outset.

If a graft 'stump' is found, it should be filmed in orthogonal views so that it can be recognized and distinguished from a second 'stump'. If there have been multiple surgical revascularization procedures, there may be multiple graft 'stumps' from previous operations.

If a graft cannot be located, this does not necessarily mean it is occluded. Proof of occlusion is finding the appropriate graft 'stump' and demonstrating target vessel opacification from the native circulation by collateral flow and/or antegrade native vessel flow. Occasionally, an aortogram may help determine whether a graft is patent, and aid subsequent selective cannulation of its ostium.

Internal mammary grafts

Left internal mammary graft

Using an internal mammary artery (IMA) catheter, the left subclavian artery is engaged in the 50° LAO projection (Figure 6.9). This best separates the origins of the great vessels arising from the arch. The left subclavian artery (LSA) arises immediately posterior to the projection of the trachea across the arch (stippled area in Figure 6.9). Pass a 0.035 or 0.038 inch J-shaped wire (b) into the subclavian, beyond the IMA, distally into the axillary artery. Pass the IMA catheter (a) over the wire beyond the origin of the left internal mammary artery (position c). Then, after changing to the 40° RAO projection, which best profiles the origin of the this IMA, slowly withdraw the catheter, rotating counterclockwise to turn the catheter tip anteriorly towards the IMA. Make small test injections of contrast to locate the IMA origin.

Right internal mammary graft

Engage the brahciocephalic artery, which in the 50° LAO projection arises from the aortic arch immediately anterior to projection of the trachea across the arch (BC in Figure 6.9). Record on cine a contrast injection into this artery to provide a roadmap for the passage of a 0.035 inch J-shaped wire beyond the origin of the RIMA and into the right axillary artery (e in figure 6.9). Advance the catheter (d) to a few centimeters beyond the origin of the RIMA and remove the wire (f in Figure 6.9). In the same 50° LAO projection, withdraw the catheter slowly, while rotating clockwise to turn the catheter tip anteriorly. Make contrast test injections to locate the RIMA origin.

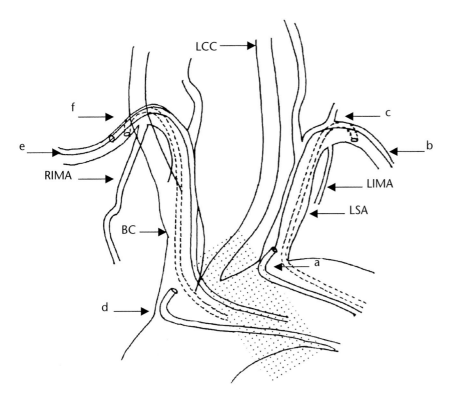

Figure 6.9
Engagement of the internal mammary arteries in the 50° LAO. The stippled region is the projection of the trachea across the aorta. The left subclavian artery (LSA) arises distally to the trachea and the brachiocephalic (BC) anteriorly. BC, brachiocephalic artery; LCC, left common carotid; LIMA, left internal mammary artery; LSA, left subclavian artery; RIMA, right internal mammary artery; RSA, right subclavian artery.

> *Problem: failure to pass the 0.035 inch J-shaped guidewire distal to the internal mammary origin*

Solution

A Glidewire (Terumo) may pass distally and provide sufficient support for advancement of a 5F or 6F IMA catheter. Alternatively, a Wholey wire may be steered into position.

> *Problem: failure to engage the internal mammary artery*

Solution

After a small test injection, record on cine a 5–10 ml rapid contrast injection. If the catheter is close to the origin but not engaged, sometimes inspiration or changing arm position may facilitate engagement. Alternatively, a 0.014 inch angioplasty wire advanced into the internal mammary may facilitate engagement.

Left ventriculography

Advance the pigtail catheter over a 0.035 inch J-shaped guidewire to the aortic root, then withdraw the wire 5–10 cm into the catheter. Rotate the catheter so that the tail lies anteriorly, then gently probe the aortic valve with the wire. When the wire crosses the valve, advance the catheter to a stable position in the mid left ventricular cavity (Figure 6.10). Connect to the manifold to record left ventricular pressure. The pigtail is connected to the power injector, and less than 1 ml of blood is withdrawn into the syringe of the injector to ensure that the system is free of air. Left ventriculography is usually performed with a power injection of 35–40 ml of contrast at approximately 15 ml/s, with cine being recorded in the 30° RAO. Transaortic pressure is recorded on catheter withdrawal across the aortic valve.

> *Problem: inability to cross the aortic valve with the J-shaped guidewire*

Solution

Use a conventional guidewire or Glidewire with a straight tip through an AL1-shaped angiography catheter.

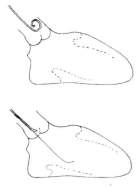

1. Advance pigtail catheter proximal to aortic root then withdraw the wire 5-10 cms into catheter Rotate the catheter so that the tail lies anteriorly.

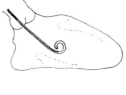

3. Advance the pigtail catheter over the 0.035î wire.

2. Cross the aortic valve with the 0.035î wire

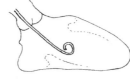

4. Withdraw the wire, flush the catheter, connect to the pressure manifold and obtain a stable catheter position within the mid LV cavity

Figure 6.10
Crossing the aortic valve and positioning the pigtail angiographic catheter within the left ventricular cavity in the 30° RAO projection.

Gently probe the aortic valve with wire while rotating the AL1 catheter so that each probing is to a somewhat different aspect of the aortic valve. Once the valve is crossed with the wire, advance the AL1 catheter into the ventricle, remove the wire, and pass an exchange length wire so that the AL1 catheter can be exchanged for a pigtail shape.

Nomenclature for angiographic projections

X-rays pass from the X-ray tube beneath the table, through the patient to an image intensifier, which is above the patient. The standard nomenclature for left and right

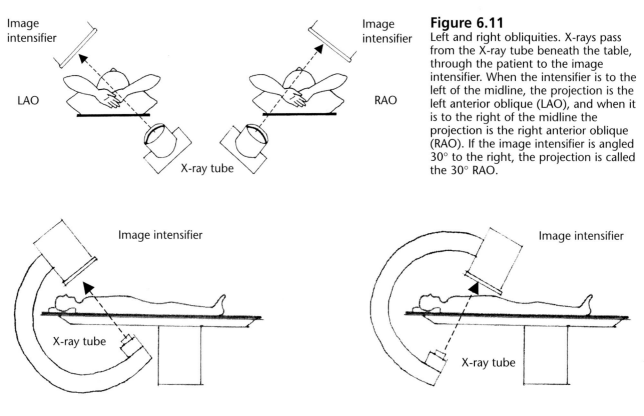

Figure 6.11
Left and right obliquities. X-rays pass from the X-ray tube beneath the table, through the patient to the image intensifier. When the intensifier is to the left of the midline, the projection is the left anterior oblique (LAO), and when it is to the right of the midline the projection is the right anterior oblique (RAO). If the image intensifier is angled 30° to the right, the projection is called the 30° RAO.

Figure 6.12
Cranial and caudal angulation. When the image intensifier is angled toward the head, the projection is called cranial angulation, while when it is angled toward the feet, the projection is called caudal angulation.

obliquities (Figure 6.11) and cranial and caudal angulation (Figure 6.12) is demonstrated here.

Standard Green Lane/Mercy angiographic projections

Left coronary artery projections (vessel segments best demonstrated by this obliquity)

See Figure 6.13.

Right coronary artery projections

See Figure 6.14.

Concluding advice

Always review your angiographic recordings before finishing the procedure. The standard projections may not reveal anatomy adequately and additional projections may be needed. Never end a procedure until you are certain that all vessels, including branch points, have been adequately demonstrated. Think about what the therapeutic strategy is likely to be. If it is percutaneous, has the anatomy, such as of a chronic complete occlusion, been adequately shown for the interventionalist to assess suitability for intervention? If it is surgical, have the target vessels for grafts been demonstrated to best advantage, especially if they are opacifying by collateral flow?

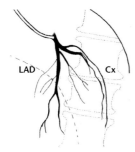

50° LAO with 30° cranial
(Left main, LAD, diagonal, proximal Cx, distal RCA by collaterals)

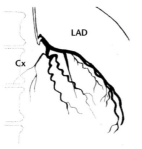

40° RAO
(LAD, Circumflex)

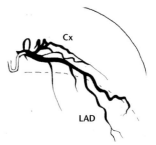

30° RAO with 35° cranial
(Left main, LAD, diagonals)

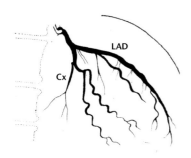

30° RAO with 25° caudal
(LAD, circumflex, intermediate, distal left main)

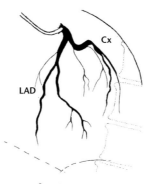

60° LAO
(circumflex, distal RCA by collaterals)

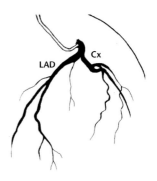

Left Lateral
(LAD, circumflex)

Figure 6.13
Left coronary artery projections.

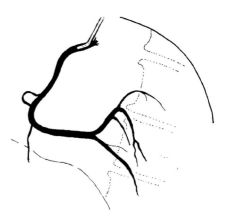

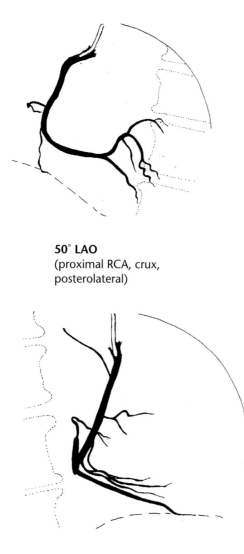

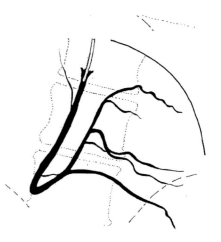

50° LAO
(proximal RCA, crux,
posterolateral)

30° LAO, 20° cranial
(proximal RCA, crux,
posterolateral)

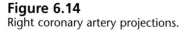

RAO 40°
(proximal RCA, posterior
descending)

PA, 30° cranial
(posterior descending, crux,
posterolateral)

Figure 6.14
Right coronary artery projections.

7

Right heart catheterization and hemodynamic profiles

Arthur W Crossman, Brett M Sasseen

Indications

Right heart catheterization involves the measurement of right heart pressures, assessment of oxygen content from the right heart chambers, and calculation of valve areas when appropriate. Indications for right heart catheterization include the evaluation of intracardiac shunts, valvular heart disease, and dyspnea not explained by noninvasive evaluation (e.g. by history, physical examination, chest X-ray, or echocardiography).[1]

The American College of Cardiology (ACC) recommends right heart catheterization in the management of heart failure patients in whom the diagnosis is uncertain, such as in differentiating cardiogenic from noncardiogenic shock or in patients with coexisting pulmonary disease, in heart failure patients requiring intensive pharmacologic management, in patients who are heart transplant candidates, in patients with suspected pericardial tamponade, or in decompensated heart failure patients undergoing noncardiac surgery.[2]

In the setting of acute myocardial infarction, the use of right heart catheterization is suggested in the diagnosis and management of specific complications, including low cardiac output and cardiogenic shock as a consequence of left ventricular (LV) failure, acute mechanical complications (mitral regurgitation from papillary muscle rupture or ischemia, ventricular septal rupture or free wall rupture), or complicated right ventricular infarction.[2]

In patients undergoing cardiac surgery, right heart catheterization is recommended for patients with low cardiac output or in the management of pulmonary hypertension in hypotensive patients.[2]

In patients with primary pulmonary hypertension, right heart catheterization is indicated in the exclusion of post-capillary causes (left heart failure) of pulmonary hypertension, in the management of primary pulmonary hypertension with vasodilator therapy, and in patients who are candidates for lung transplantation.[2]

Equipment
Catheters, tubing, connectors, and stopcocks

After appropriate venous access has been obtained, accurate hemodynamic monitoring can be accomplished with meticulous attention to forming and flushing the connections to the sheath, proper manifold and pressure transducer setup, as well as careful equipment selection. In general, shorter, stiffer, and wider-bore catheters, tubing with a low-density liquid devoid of air bubbles, and a limited number of stopcocks and connections are preferred due to the resulting higher natural frequency.[3]

Improper damping, excessively compliant tubing, or small air bubbles within the tubing may decrease the natural frequency of the system substantially, which may lead to damping and overshoot of the waveforms. Micromanometers have natural frequencies significantly higher than optimal fluid-filled systems, and are used for accurate measurement of high-frequency events such as ventricular pressure rise (dP/dt) and other parameters of ventricular performance during the first 40–50 ms of ventricular systole.[4]

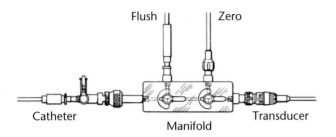

Figure 7.1
Typical pressure measurement system. A manifold with stopcocks is connected to the fluid filled catheter and transducer with two sidearms for flush and zero-line connections. (Adapted from Baim DS and Grossman W. Grossman's Cardiac Catheterization, Angiography, and Intervention. Philadelphia: Lippincott Williams and Wilkins, 2000.[2])

Manifold, transducer, and zero line

Manifolds with three to four side ports are now available in most cardiac catheterization laboratories. Stopcocks attach lines to the side ports and allow pressure recordings, flushing, injections, and waste disposal at various times during the procedure. The pressure and zero-lines are usually connected to the first side port. Saline flush is connected to the second. Contrast is connected to the third port, and waste is connected to the fourth (Figure 7.1).

Transducers are electrical strain gauges that function under the principle of the Wheatstone bridge. If the transducer is placed above mid-chest level, pressure measurements may be falsely lowered. If the transducer is placed below the mid-chest level, readings may be spuriously elevated. One end of the zero-line is connected to the pressure transducer manifold, and the other end is connected to a manifold at mid chest level. Calibration of the transducer is achieved by filling the zero-line, manifold, and pressure transducer with saline. This step also requires connecting a mercury manometer to the free port of the mid-chest manifold with 100 mmHg transmitted to all pressure transducers.

Recording paper

Time lines are vertical lines placed on recording paper at constant time intervals ranging from 0.01 to 5 s. Shorter time intervals should be used for faster paper speeds and longer time intervals for slower paper speeds. One-second time lines are used in routine cases. The paper speed can also be varied over a range of 5–500 mm/s. Most laboratories use 25 mm/s paper speed for many of the measurements.

Oxygen consumption measuring devices

Most laboratories now use devices employing the polarographic or paramagnetic technique to measure oxygen consumption. The metabolic rate meter uses a polarographic oxygen sensor cell, a hood, and a variable-speed blower with a servo feedback loop connected to the oxygen sensor that controls blower speed (blower ventilation) based on oxygen sensing. With the Douglas bag method, the patient breathes into an airtight bag, inspires room air, and expires air into the bag. After a specified time, room air oxygen and Douglas bag gas volumes are then determined. Oxygen consumption is then calculated based on O_2 consumption and CO_2 production from the gas volumes. With either method, these measurements should be made at a steady state when the patient is hemodynamically stable to ensure accurate readings. Oxygen consumption may also be estimated as 3 ml O_2/kg or 125 ml/min/m² × body surface area. Arteriovenous oxygen (AVO_2) difference is calculated from the arterial − mixed venous (pulmonary artery) O_2 content difference. The O_2 content is calculated as O_2 saturation × 1.36 × Hg (g/dl) × 10.

Oximeter

The use of oxygen saturation, rather than oxygen content, is a more accurate way of calculating the shunt fraction in patients. The oxygen content may vary considerably, depending on the level of the patient's hemoglobin, any presence of carboxyhemoglobin, and hemoglobinopathies such as sickle cell disease. Oximeters such as the AVOXimeter use multiple wavelengths of light transmitted through a small sample of heparinized blood to record the optical density of the transmitted wavelength. This technique enables determination of the concentrations of hemoglobin, oxyhemoglobin, methemoglobin, and carboxyhemoglobin, thus eliminating sources of error in the measurement of oxygen content.

Access and catheter advancement

Venous access is usually obtained using a single wall puncture technique. With femoral access, the anterior iliac crest and pubic tubercle determine the plane of the inguinal ligament (Figure 7.2). The arterial pulse is then palpated 2 cm below the plane of the inguinal ligament. This corresponds to the junction of the middle and lower third of the femoral head. The femoral vein is located 0.5–1.0 cm medial to the arterial pulse After local anesthesia has been administered, a small nick is placed over

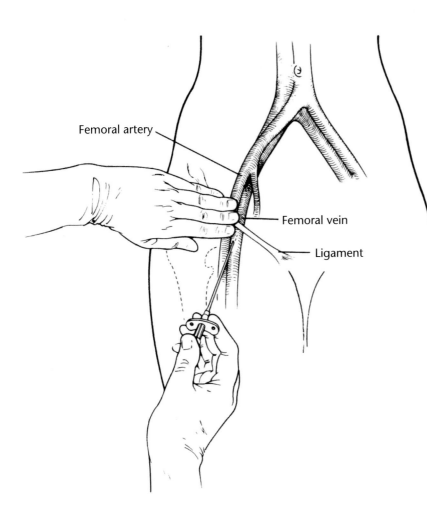

Femoral artery

Femoral vein

Ligament

Figure 7.2
Schematic of the right femoral access site. The arterial pulse is palpated 2 cm below the inguinal ligament. The femoral vein is located approximately one fingerbreadth medial to the arterial pulse. (Adapted from Tilkian AG, Daily AK. Cardiovascular Procedures: Diagnostic Techniques and Therapeutic Procedures. St Louis MO: Mosby, 1986[38] with permission from Elsevier.)

the venous entry site. An 18-gauge needle with a fluid-filled syringe is then placed at a 45° angle cephalad while applying gentle suction. Venous blood (nonpulsatile and dark) will then fill the syringe. If the vein has not been entered, the needle should be flushed and repeat efforts, either more medial or lateral, should be made. The needle then enters the subcutaneous tissue and is withdrawn a few millimeters at a time. If the artery is entered, the needle is removed and pressure held for 5 minutes. A vein that has been entered during a femoral arterial puncture should be used only if the needle did not puncture both the artery and the vein on the same pass. Placement of a sheath through both the artery and vein would create an arteriovenous fistula, possibly causing significant bleeding. When blood is aspirated, the syringe is removed and a 0.035 or 0.038 inch guidewire is advanced 30 cm into the vessel unless resistance is met. The sheath and dilator are inserted over the wire while rotating them gently as they are advanced. The sheath is aspirated to withdraw blood and then flushed with heparinized saline. At the end of the case, the sheath is removed and manual pressure is applied over the vein for 5–10 minutes to obtain adequate hemostasis.

Venous access can also be obtained via the internal jugular, brachial, or subclavian veins. With internal jugular

access, the neck, lateral to the trachea on either side, is prepared in a sterile fashion. The internal jugular vein is lateral to the carotid artery, medial to the external jugular vein, and usually just lateral to the outer edge of the medial head of the sternocleidomastoid muscle. With the patient supine without a pillow under the head, the sternal and clavicular heads of the sternocleidomastoid muscle are palpated after the patient turns the head 30° to the left side. The position of the carotid artery is also palpated. A small wheal of lidocaine is injected near the top of the triangle, where the two muscle heads meet, lateral to the carotid artery. A 23-gauge needle attached to the lidocaine syringe is placed in a position perpendicular to the skin level, just lateral to the carotid and gently advanced, with negative pressure on the syringe, until venous blood is withdrawn. Then, this needle may be left in place, or removed. An 18-gauge needle attached to a syringe is placed in the same spot as the 'finder' needle and advanced until venous blood is returned. The 'finder' needle is then removed, if this has not already been accomplished. The 18-gauge needle is then angled toward the head until 45° from the skin, and the guide wire is advanced approximately 12–15 cm. If premature ventricular contractions are seen, the wire should be slowly withdrawn 2–3 cm. The sheath should be placed over the wire

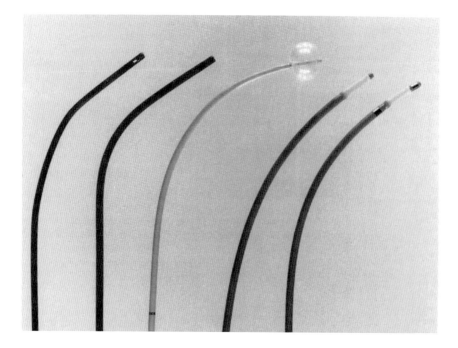

Figure 7.3
Right heart catheters. From left to right: Goodale–Lubin, Cournand, Swan–Ganz (two types), and Baim–Turi catheter with bipolar electrodes (USCI). (Adapted from Baim DS and Grossman W. Grossman's Cardiac Catheterization, Angiography, and Intervention. Philadelphia: Lippincott Williams and Wilkins, 2000.[2])

using the standard Seldinger technique. Some physicians have used intravascular ultrasound to guide access to the internal jugular vein.

Some of the conditions of patients in whom an internal jugular approach might be preferable include:

- pulmonary hypertension;
- tricuspid regurgitation or stenosis;
- right atrial or ventricular dilatation;
- anomalous inferior vena cava;
- suspected femoral or iliac vein thrombosis;
- renal vein thrombosis

Catheter selection is based on the frequency response of the catheter, torquability, and safety. Stiffer, larger-bore catheters, such as the Goodale–Lubin catheter, have better frequency response, are more torquable, steerable, and able to accommodate larger wires. Consequently, they have a greater potential for perforation due to their stiffness. Smaller, less stiff catheters are much less likely to cause pulmonary artery perforation (Figure 7.3). Most balloon-tipped catheters, such as the Swan–Ganz catheter, are appropriate for right heart pressure measurements (Figure 7.4).

As the initial step, the pulmonary artery catheter is flushed and attached to the venous manifold. Then it is inserted into the sheath and advanced up the inferior vena cava. The catheter should not deviate from a paraspinous

position, which may indicate entry into a renal or hepatic vein if this is the case. The catheter should then be withdrawn slightly and rotated, and then advanced above the diaphragm and into the right atrium. Advancement of the catheter should always occur with the balloon inflated, while withdrawal of the catheter should occur with the balloon deflated. Waveform analysis and oximetry will help locate the position of the catheter. A deviation of the catheter from the expected course may indicate anomalous anatomy. Once the catheter is positioned into the right atrium, gentle clockwise rotation and advancement of the entire catheter – not just of the catheter at the sheath entry site – will allow the catheter to track along the anterior and anteromedial wall of the right atrium, the location of the tricuspid valve. A larger right atrium may require a larger bend in the catheter to cross the tricuspid valve with this maneuver. In a dilated right atrium, the catheter may need to be positioned against the lateral wall of the atrium, so that a reverse loop in the catheter will form, allowing it to cross the tricuspid valve (Figure 7.5). If excessive counterclockwise rotation and advancement occurs as the catheter is pointed against the lateral wall of the right atrium, the catheter tip will be positioned into the superior vena cava. Care should be taken, as clockwise rotation of the catheter tip may result in entrapment in the right atrial appendage, while a posteromedial advancement of the catheter tip may lead to crossing of a patent

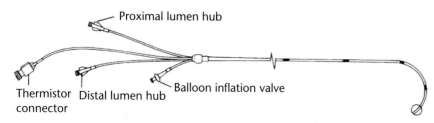

Proximal lumen hub

Thermistor connector   Distal lumen hub   Balloon inflation valve

Figure 7.4
Triple-lumen Swan–Ganz catheter equipped for thermodilution assessment of cardiac output. (Adapted from Tilkian AG, Daily AK. Cardiovascular Procedures: Diagnostic Techniques and Therapeutic Procedures. St Louis MO: Mosby, 1986[38] with permission from Elsevier.)

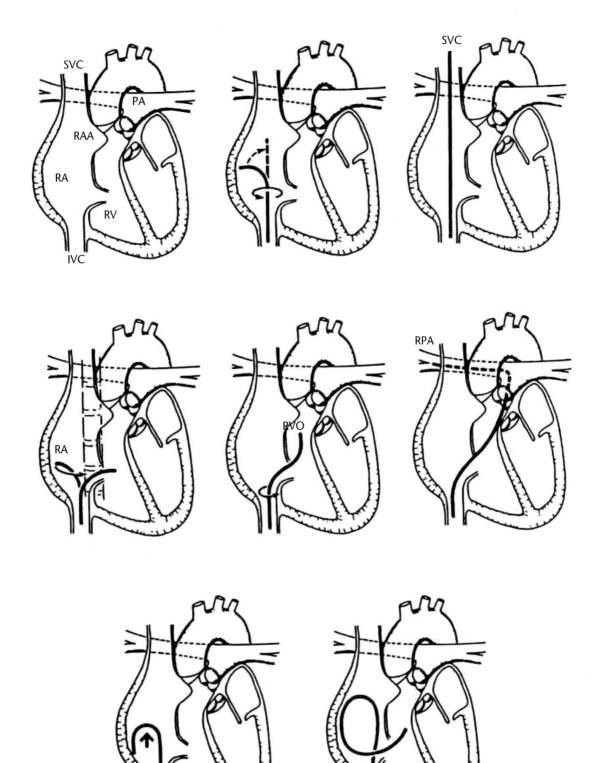

Figure 7.5
Illustration of pulmonary artery catheter manipulations from right femoral access. See text for details. SVC, superior vena cava; PA, pulmonary artery; RAA, right atrial appendage; RA, right atrium; RV, right ventricle; IVC, inferior vena cava; RVO, right ventricular outflow; RPA, right pulmonary artery; HV, hepatic vein.

foramen ovale. An inferior–posterior advancement of the catheter may result in coronary sinus entry (Figure 7.5).

Once inside the right ventricle, the pressure is again recorded. The catheter tip should then be positioned to lie horizontally and just to the right of the patient's spine. Clockwise rotation of the catheter in this position causes the tip to point upward and slightly posteriorly in the direction of the right ventricular outflow tract. If the catheter is not in this position, advancement may lead to injury or arrhythmias. An inspiration by the patient may ease catheter advancement into the pulmonary artery and to the pulmonary capillary wedge position. If there is significant ventricular enlargement, a reverse loop (as indicated above) may enable the catheter tip to cross the tricuspid valve in a more superior position. A curved J wire may be used to guide placement of the catheter into the pulmonary artery, but should only be used with the catheter tip pointing superiorly into the right ventricular outflow tract. Advancement of the catheter into the pulmonary capillary wedge position should be performed with care, as patients with significantly elevated pulmonary pressures are at higher risk of pulmonary arterial rupture. The pulmonary capillary wedge pressure is then recorded. Subsequently, the balloon is deflated and the catheter is withdrawn slightly into to the pulmonary artery. Pulmonary artery pressure is then measured and another blood sample is taken for oximetry.

Placement of the Swan–Ganz catheter into the pulmonary artery when using an internal jugular approach should be performed in a similar manner. The catheter should be advanced when the balloon is inflated. Swift but careful advancement of the catheter will allow easy positioning of the catheter into the pulmonary capillary wedge or pulmonary artery position without excessive manipulation. If no pressure waveforms are encountered after advancing the catheter 15–20 cm, the catheter may be located in the inferior vena cava, which will require repositioning. When utilized to stiffen the catheter, the guidewire should remain within the catheter, unless excess coiling occurs in the right atrium or ventricle. In that situation, the wire may be advanced, but, again, only when the catheter is pointed in a superior direction in the right ventricular outflow tract.

Pressure waveforms and measurement

A cardiovascular pressure wave occurs as blood within the heart or vessels exert pressure. The pressure wave is created by cardiac muscular contraction and is transmitted along a closed, fluid-filled column to a pressure transducer, which converts the mechanical pressure to an electrical signal. The pressure wave may be considered a complex periodic fluctuation in force per unit area, with 1 cycle being defined as the time interval from the onset of one systole to the onset of the subsequent systole. The fundamental frequency of cardiac pressure generation is defined as the number of cycles per second. Fourier defined complex waves as the summation of sine waves of various frequencies and amplitudes. A Fourier series represents complex waveforms by expressing various sine wave frequencies as multiples of the fundamental frequency, also known as harmonics. At a heart rate of 60, the fundamental frequency is 1 cycle per second, or 1 Hz. The first 10 harmonics are 1–10 Hz. A system should be able to respond with equal output over this range of input frequencies to achieve accurate recordings. The natural frequency of a system is that frequency with which a system will oscillate in the absence of friction after being shock-excited. Damping refers to dissipation of the energy of oscillation of the system.

Pressure waveform characteristics are determined by reflected waves, presence of artifacts, and errors in zeroing, balancing, or calibration. The measured pressure wave is the summation of the forward pressure and the reflected or backward pressure wave.[5,6] Pressure reflections occur throughout the arterial tree, with the major point of reflection being the distal abdominal aorta.[6] Hypovolemia, hypotension, vasodilator drugs, and the strain phase of the Valsalva maneuver decrease the influence of reflected waves. Vasoconstriction, hypertension, and aorto-iliac obstruction augment pressure wave reflections. Pressure peaks occur earlier as the catheter tip approaches the distal source of reflection. This can be demonstrated by comparing the timing of peak pressure between the central aorta and the distal aorta.[5–7] Systolic pressure amplification also occurs in the periphery and may be the result of reflected waves. As the pressure wave travels down the arterial tree, systolic pressures in the radial, brachial or femoral arteries are augmented by 20–50 mmHg (Figure 7.6). Adjustments for peripheral augmentation are necessary in valve area measurements.

Various artifacts may also lead to inaccurate pressure waveform recordings. These include catheter whip artifact, end-pressure artifact, catheter impact artifact, and deterioration in frequency response. Catheter whip artifacts are the result of acceleration of fluid within the catheter as the catheter moves within the heart and great vessels. This artifact is particularly common when measuring pressure in the pulmonary arteries. End-pressure artifact occurs when an end-hole catheter tip faces upstream into the direction of blood flow. The kinetic energy of the flowing blood is converted partly into pressure as it suddenly stops moving upon colliding with fluid in the catheter tip. Catheter impact artifact occurs when the catheter impacts upon structures within the heart or great vessels. These structures may impart a pressure transient within the range of the natural frequency of the catheter transducer system. This occurs commonly with pigtail catheters as they are impacted with the opening of mitral valve leaflets.

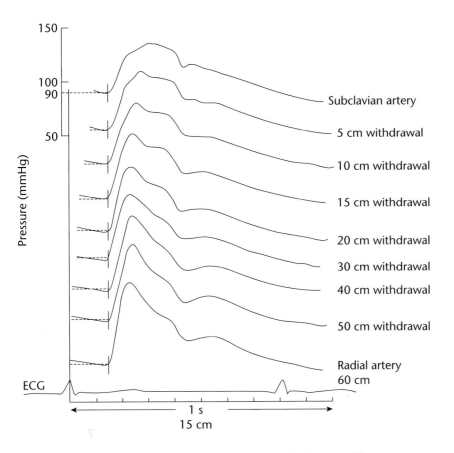

Figure 7.6
Relationship of timing and amplitude of peak pressure recordings with catheter distance from the aortic valve. As the catheter tip is moved further away from the aortic valve, the onset of the pressure waveform is delayed, while the peak pressure occurs earlier and the amplitude of the recorded pressure is greater. (Adapted from Baim DS and Grossman W. Grossman's Cardiac Catheterization, Angiography, and Intervention. Philadelphia: Lippincott Williams and Wilkins, 2000.[2])

Inaccurate pressure recordings are commonly the result of errors in zeroing. All manometers must be zeroed at the mid-chest level. The zero-level will change as the patient's body position moves, and should be altered accordingly. Transducers should be calibrated before each case. This can be done manually with a mercury manometer or electronically with electrical calibration signals. Simultaneous calibration of all pressure transducers should be done to eliminate any pressure differentials caused by unequal amplification of the same pressure signal. This may be the result of small air bubbles present in one or more of the transducer systems. Therefore, adequate flushing of the zero-line and all pressure lines is very important.

Right heart catheterization protocol

Appropriate zeroing of the transducer should occur first. Calibration of all pressure transducers should be performed simultaneously. The catheter should then be advanced into the right atrium and flushed. Then a phasic pressure should be recorded with 40 mmHg scale and at 25 mm/s paper speed. Mean pressure is recorded at 10 mm/s paper speed. The catheter is then advanced into the right ventricle, and the phasic pressure is recorded at

25 mm/s paper speed. The catheter is then advanced to the pulmonary capillary wedge position, and the phasic pressure is recorded with 25 mm/s paper speed. The mean pressure is recorded at 10 mm/s paper speed. The balloon is deflated and the catheter is pulled back into the pulmonary artery. Phasic pressures are recorded at 25 mm/s paper speed and mean pressures at 10 mm/s. (See the specifics of the protocol below.)

Notes on pulmonary capillary wedge pressure

Wedge pressures are obtained when an end-hole catheter tip is wedged into a blood vessel facing a capillary bed. Damping can occur in the presence of a small, constricted capillary bed, constricted precapillary arterioles or venules, or other sources of obstruction such as microthrombi. A catheter wedged in the distal pulmonary artery measures pulmonary venous pressure, which in turn approximates the left atrial pressure in the absence of cor triatriatum or pulmonary venous obstruction. The time delay, diminished y descent and damping of the wedge pressure can lead to inaccurate transmitral gradients[8,9] (Figure 7.7).

When measuring the pulmonary capillary wedge pressure, proper positioning can be confirmed by obtaining an

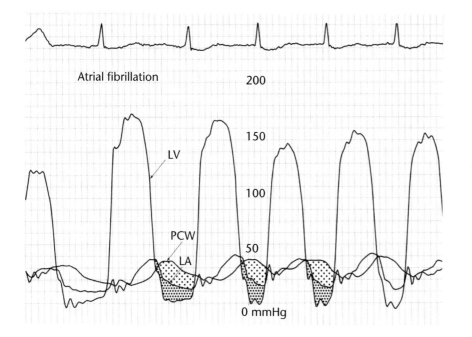

Atrial fibrillation

LV

PCW
LA

200

150

100

50

0 mmHg

Figure 7.7
Simultaneous recording of the left ventricular (LV), pulmonary capillary wedge (PCW), and left atrial (LA) pressures in mitral stenosis. Due to the time delay and blunted *y* descent of the PCW pressure waveform, use of PCW pressure tracing may overestimate the mitral valve gradient in mitral stenosis. Phase-shifting the PCW pressure tracing will eliminate much of this spurious increase in gradient. (Adapted from Murphy JG. Mayo Clinic Cardiology Review, 2nd Edn. Philadelphia: Lippincott Williams and Wilkins, 2000.[9])

oxygen saturation sample greater than 95% and comparing the timing of the *a* and *v* waves with the timing of the ECG and left ventricular pressure. Although not routinely done, a small injection of 2 ml of contrast, demonstrating a lack of contrast washout after 15 s, confirms proper positioning.

Pulmonary capillary wedge pressure overestimates left atrial pressure in patients with acute respiratory failure, chronic obstructive lung disease with pulmonary hypertension, pulmonary venoconstriction, or heart failure with volume overload. Significant errors may be introduced in patients with mitral valve disease or mitral valve prostheses when using pulmonary capillary wedge pressures to estimate left atrial pressure. A transseptal technique should be considered in these cases.

Right and left heart catheterization protocol

For mitral and aortic valve assessment and evaluation of restrictive or constrictive physiology, a left heart catheterization should be performed in addition to the right heart catheterization. After arterial access is obtained, but prior to placing the pigtail catheter in the left ventricle, simultaneous femoral artery (from the sheath) and central aortic phasic and mean pressure tracings should be recorded, with 25 mm/s and 10 mm/s paper speed, respectively. Then the pigtail catheter is advanced across the aortic valve into the left ventricle. No more than 3 minutes should pass without withdrawal, wiping, and flushing of the catheter. In aortic stenosis patients, the pigtail catheter should be one French size smaller than the sheath to pre-

vent damping of the femoral arterial tracing. Gentle manipulation of the guidewire is necessary to avoid damaging or perforation of the aortic valve. Once the pigtail is in the left ventricle, the zero-pressure line is checked. Left ventricular and femoral artery pressures are recorded with 200 mmHg scale, 25 mm/s for phasic and 10 mm/s for mean pressure tracings.

Normal hemodynamics

The collection of hemodynamic data is an essential part of the cardiac catheterization. A routine protocol ensures accurate and complete collection of all information in an efficient manner. Below is one example of the methods used. Such a protocol allows simultaneous pressure measurements across the heart. Most hemodynamic questions may be answered by following such a protocol. However, some hemodynamic measurements are necessary for specific clinical situations. Figure 7.8 demonstrates normal hemodynamic tracings, including simultaneous LV, aortic, LA, and RV pressure tracings.

The routine collection of right and left heart hemodynamic data with blood oxygen saturations and cardiac output measurements may be accomplished safely in just a few minutes. Cardiac output by thermodilution or by the Fick method (oxygen consumption method) is routine. The Fick method is often used in the assessment of valvular lesions. Arterial or left ventricular, right atrial, and pulmonary artery oxygen saturations are collected routinely. Multiple oxygen saturation samples are obtained throughout the right and left heart for intracardiac shunt detection.

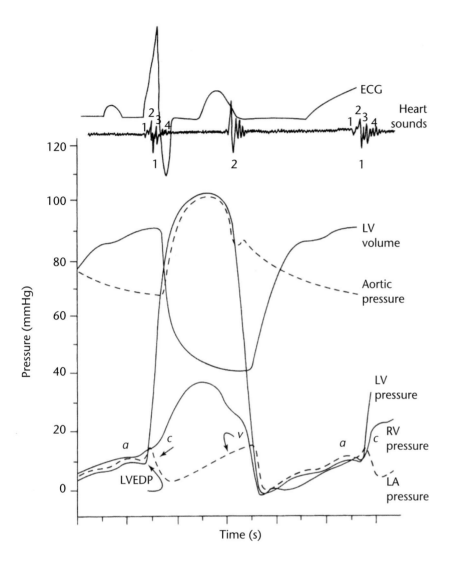

Figure 7.8
Normal morphology and timing of left ventricular (LV), right ventricular (RV), left atrial (LA), and aortic pressure waveforms in relationship to each other, ECG intervals, and heart sounds. Isovolumetric contraction begins at the initiation of the LV upstroke (see LVEDP arrow) and ends with the aortic valve opening. Isovolumetric relaxation begins at the dicrotic notch with aortic valve closure and ends at the final portion of the LV downslope. (Adapted from Kern MJ. The Cardiac Catheterization Handbook, 3rd Edn. St Louis, MO: Mosby, 1999[1] with permission from Elsevier.)

Right heart catheterization protocol[1]

1. Properly zero the catheter and transducer. Ensure that the catheter is flushed.
2. Advance the catheter into the inferior vena cava (IVC) and obtain oxygen saturation.
3. Advance the catheter into the right atrium (RA). Zero-check the pressure. Record the pressure on a 40 mmHg scale: phasic, mean, and phasic pressures. (Phasic pressures are recorded on 25 mm/s paper speed and mean pressures on 10 mm/s paper speed for all recordings.)
4. Turn the recorder off.
5. Advance the catheter to the right ventricle (RV).
6. Record the phasic pressure.
7. Turn the recorder off.
8. Advance the catheter to the pulmonary capillary wedge (PCW) position.

9. Record phasic/mean/phasic pressures with the catheter in the wedge position.
10. Turn the recorder off.
11. From the PCW position, deflate the balloon and withdraw the catheter slightly for pulmonary artery (PA) pressure.
12. Record phasic/mean/phasic pressures.
13. Turn the recorder off.
14. Obtain blood oxygen saturation samples.

Left heart catheterization protocol[1]

Right heart studies are often measured prior to left heart hemodynamic assessment. Simultaneous left and right heart pressures will provide the most accurate information for many clinical situations.

Simultaneous aortic and femoral artery pressure

1. Insert a pigtail catheter through an arterial sheath.
2. Advance the catheter to the aortic valve.
3. Flush the catheter. Zero the pigtail pressure (200 mmHg scale).
4. Flush the sheath. Zero the sheath pressure (200 mmHg scale).
5. Record simultaneous central aortic and femoral artery (FA) (sheath) pressures (phasic/mean/phasic: 25 mm/s paper speed for phasic pressures and 10 mm/s paper speed for mean pressures).
6. Zero-check both pressures again.

Aortic valve assessment

1. Advance a pigtail catheter into the left ventricle.
2. Check the zero-pressures of both sheath and pigtail catheters after flushing.
3. Record LV and FA pressures (25 mm/s paper speed, 200 mmHg scale): phasic/mean FA/phasic pressure (100 mm/s paper speed if an aortic valve gradient is present).

Combined left and right heart catheterization protocols[1]

Start with a PA catheter in the wedge position and with a pigtail catheter in the LV before pullback.

Aortic valve assessment

This is performed as above.

Mitral valve assessment

1. Check the zero-pressures of the PCW, FA, and LV after catheters and sheath have been flushed.

2. Record simultaneous LV and PCW pressures on 40 mmHg scales at 50 mm/s paper speed: phasic/mean PCW/phasic pressures.
3. Let the balloon down, withdraw the catheter to the PA position (25 mm/s paper speed, 40 mmHg scale), and record phasic/mean/phasic PA pressures.
4. Use 100 mm/s paper speed if a mitral valve gradient is present.

Cardiac output

1. Perform Fick oxygen collection (Waters oximetry hood).
2. Measure thermodilution outputs × 3.
3. Obtain LV and PA oxygen saturation samples.

Right heart pullback (Figure 7.9)

1. Check zero-pressures in PA catheter and pigtail catheter.
2. Turn recorder on (25 mm/s paper speed, 40 mmHg scale).
3. Record PCW-to-PA pullback, recording phasic/mean/phasic pressures.
4. Record PA-to-RV pullback.
5. Continue recording RV and add LV pressure to establish presence of constrictive/restrictive physiology (100 mm/s paper speed, 40 mmHg scale).
6. Zero-check LV pressure.
7. Record RV-to-RA pullback: phasic/mean/phasic (25/20/25 mm/s paper speed, 40 mmHg scale).

Ventricular hemodynamics (may be performed after ventriculography)

1. Zero-check LV and FA pressures.
2. Record postventriculography LV end-diastolic pressure (100 mm/s paper speed, 40 mmHg scale).
3. Perform LV pullback to aorta along with simultaneous FA pressure (25 mm/s paper speed, 200 mmHg scale).

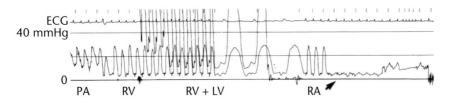

Figure 7.9
Example of normal pressure waveforms recorded during a pullback from the pulmonary artery to the right atrium. Note simultaneous recording of the right and left ventricular waveforms at slow and fast paper speeds. (Adapted from Kern MJ. The Cardiac Catheterization Handbook, 3rd Edn. St Louis, MO: Mosby, 1999[1] with permission from Elsevier.)

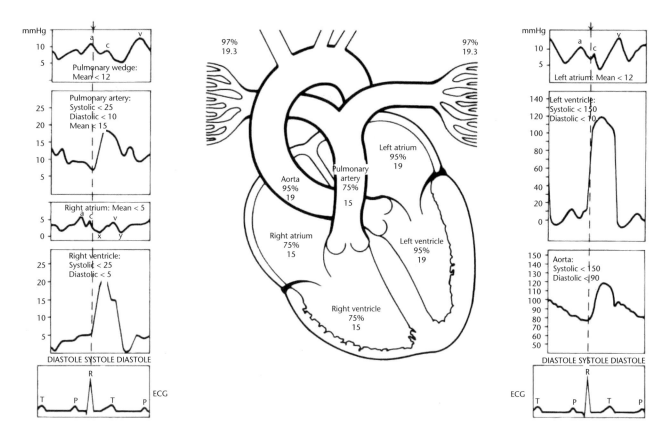

Figure 7.10
Illustrations of normal right and left heart pressure waveforms. The dashed lines indicate the onset of systole. On the left, are the pulmonary wedge, pulmonary arterial, right atrial, and right ventricular waveforms. On the right are the left atrial, left ventricular, and aortic waveforms. The values are the upper limits of normal mean and phasic blood pressures for each chamber. Also listed in the center panel are the normal oxygen saturations and volume percentages for each chamber. (Adapted from Kern MJ. The Cardiac Catheterization Handbook, 3rd Edn. St Louis, MO: Mosby, 1999[1] with permission from Elsevier.)

4. Obtain mean aortic pressures.
5. Zero-check pressures.

The normal mean RA pressure is less than 5 mmHg, while the normal mean LA pressure is less than 12 mmHg. The RA pressure waveform is demonstrated in Figures 7.10–7.12. The a wave represents the increase in RA pressure during atrial contraction. The c wave represents pressure imparted on the right atrium with closure of the tricuspid valve. The v wave represents RA pressure increase as a result of forward venous flow, or passive filling after ventricular systole. The x descent represents the fall in RA pressure during relaxation after closure of the tricuspid valve, while the y descent represents the fall in RA pressure after opening of the tricuspid valve in early diastole. Inspiration decreases phasic and mean RA pressures and may lead to an exaggerated y descent. The LA pressure wave morphologies and sequences are similar to those of the RA, but unlike the RA waves, the v waves in the left atrium tend to be larger than the a waves. As seen in figure 7.11, the LA waveform appears earlier in time than either the RA or PCW wave forms.

A typical RV pressure waveform is demonstrated in Figures 7.9 and 7.10. The normal RV systolic pressure is less than 25 mmHg and the diastolic pressure is less than 5 mmHg. During systole, the RV wave tracing demonstrates a decreased dP/dt compared with the LV waveform, and the peak pressure occurs slightly earlier.

A normal pulmonary pressure waveform is seen in Figure 7.10. A normal PA systolic pressure is less than 25 mmHg, while the diastolic pressure is less than 10 mmHg. The mean PA pressure is less than 15 mmHg.

The PCW pressure tracing is seen in Figures 7.10 and 7.11. A normal mean PCW pressure is less than 12 mmHg. The waveform morphology with a properly wedged catheter is similar to the LA pressure waveform, and also contains a, c, and v waves. The LA pressure waveforms precede those of the PCW pressure by 100–150 ms. This delay must be compensated for in calculating transmitral gradients.

Normal LV systolic pressure is less than 140 mmHg, and the LV end-diastolic pressure is less than 10 mmHg. Isovolumetric contraction occurs at the peak of the R wave of the QRS complex and results in a rapid increase in dP/dt. This takes place with the onset of the upstroke of the LV waveform and ends with the opening of the aortic

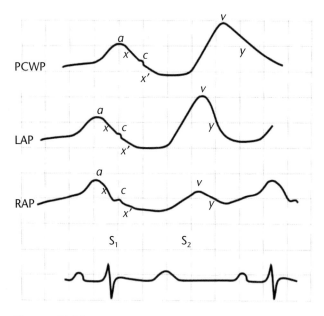

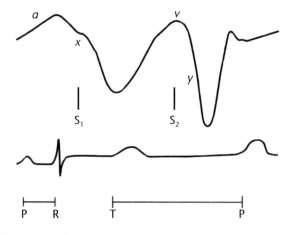

Figure 7.12
Sharp *x* and *y* descents of the right atrial pressure tracing in constrictive pericarditis. (Adapted from Murphy JG. Mayo Clinic Cardiology Review, 2nd Edn. Philadelphia: Lippincott Williams and Wilkins, 2000.[9])

Figure 7.11
Simultaneous pulmonary capillary wedge pressure (PCWP), left atrial pressure (LAP), and right atrial pressure (RAP) in relationship to the ECG. Note the delay as well as the blunted *y* descent in the PCWP waveform. This may lead to overestimation of the mitral valve gradient in patients with mitral stenosis. (Adapted from Murphy JG. Mayo Clinic Cardiology Review, 2nd Edn. Philadelphia: Lippincott Williams and Wilkins, 2000.[9])

valve (Figures 7.8 and 7.10). In the absence of LV outflow tract obstruction, peak LV systolic pressure is equal to the peak proximal aortic systolic pressure. Normal diastolic pressure tracings demonstrate a gradual increase in pressure during diastole. End-diastole is marked by a slight abrupt increase in pressure with the atrial contraction, which corresponds to the LV *a* wave (Figures 7.8, 7.11, and 7.12). Commencement of isovolumetric relaxation corresponds to the end of the T wave on the ECG. This period begins with closure of the aortic valve, represented by the dicrotic notch, and ends with the final portion of the LV waveform downstroke. Normal aortic systolic pressure is less than 140 mmHg and normal diastolic pressure is less than 80 mmHg. The rate of pressure rise *dP/dt* is less than that of the LV pressure rise, and the onset of pressure rise is delayed the further away from the aortic valve the pressure is measured. The terminal portion of the peak systolic pressure waveform occurs earlier when measured by a catheter positioned more distal to the aortic valve (Figure 7.6). The dicrotic notch represents a slight increase in aortic pressure after closure of the aortic valve. An improperly prepared transducer catheter system may result in significant artifact at the dicrotic notch.

Abnormal hemodynamics

Increased atrial pressure is the result of atrioventricular (AV) valvular stenosis or regurgitation, left-to-right shunts,

hypervolemia, congestive heart failure, cardiac tamponade, and constrictive and restrictive disease processes.

Elevated *a* waves are due to hypertrophy or decreased ventricular compliance, mitral or tricuspid valve stenosis or insufficiency, atrial ventricular dissociation when the atrium contracts against a closed AV valve, and decreased atrial compliance.

Absence of *a* waves is due to atrial arrest, atrial fibrillation, or atrial flutter. A falsely lowered *a* wave may be seen in patients with a large *c*–*v* wave.

Large *v* waves occur in the presence of increased flow such as in an atrial septal defect (ASD) or ventricular septal defect (VSD), AV valvular insufficiency, or atrial fibrillation. Large *v* waves on a PCW tracing may result from significant mitral regurgitation (MR), but are not specific or sensitive for MR. They can be seen in any condition associated with increased LA pressure such as reduced compliance in rheumatic heart disease, infiltrative heart disease or post cardiac surgery. In addition, large *v* waves can also be seen with increased LA volume such as in cases of VSD, congestive heart failure, or mitral stenosis.

An exaggerated *x* and *y* descent occur with constrictive pericarditis or with restrictive cardiomyopathy. In addition, an exaggerated *x* descent occurs with cardiac tamponade. LA and RA pressures equilibrate with a large ASD, constrictive pericarditis, or tamponade. In constrictive pericarditis, RA pressure increases with inspiration. Sawtooth deformities of the atrial pressure waveform occur during atrial flutter. Pacemakers and multifocal atrial tachycardia may lead to multiple pressure waveform morphologies. Dissociation of atrial and ventricular pressure waves may occur with Ebstein's abnormality (atrialization of the right ventricle) or in the setting of ventricular tachycardia.

The 'dip and plateau' configuration of the RA pressure waveform, or 'M' configuration, as seen in constrictive pericarditis, is the result of the effect of attenuation of diastolic filling on atrial pressure and flow (Figures 7.12 and 7.13).

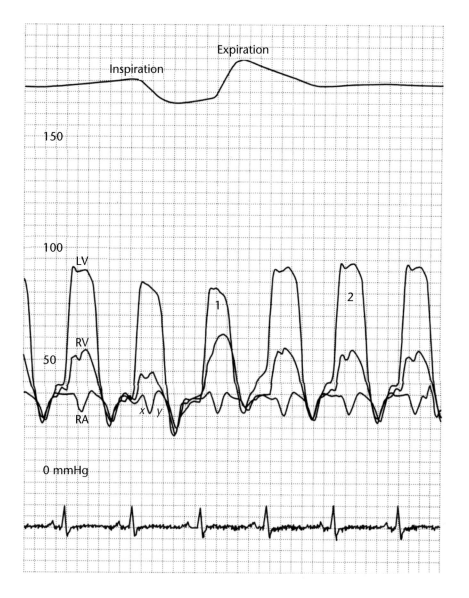

Figure 7.13
Simultaneous right atrial (RA), right ventricular (RV), and left ventricular (LV) pressure tracings in constrictive pericarditis. Note the prominent *x* and *y* descents in the right atrial pressure waveform and discordance of the left and right ventricular waveforms with inspiration and expiration, demonstrating ventricular interdependence; during inspiration, the RV pressure increases, while the LV pressure decreases. (Adapted from Murphy JG. Mayo Clinic Cardiology Review, 2nd Edn. Philadelphia: Lippincott Williams and Wilkins, 2000.[9])

Systolic ventricular pressures are increased with pulmonary or systemic hypertension and with pulmonary stenosis, aortic stenosis, or aortic insufficiency. Systolic pressures are decreased with hypovolemia, congestive heart failure (CHF), an extensive myocardial infarction, and tamponade.

LV end-diastolic pressure elevations are due to hypervolemia, hypertrophy, decreased compliance, CHF, tamponade, and aortic regurgitation. Low diastolic pressures are due to tricuspid or mitral stenosis and hypovolemia. The *a* wave on the LV pressure tracing may be absent or missing with tricuspid or mitral stenosis, tricuspid or mitral insufficiency (if RV or LV compliance is increased), severe aortic insufficiency, atrial fibrillation, flutter, or arrest.

Elevated pulmonary artery pressures are due to primary or secondary pulmonary hypertension, large left-to-right shunts, peripheral pulmonary stenosis, and increased pulmonary venous pressures, such as from mitral stenosis, mitral regurgitation, or CHF. Decreased pulmonary pres-

sures are due to hypovolemia, pulmonic stenosis (valvular or subvalvular), Ebstein's anomaly, hypoplastic right heart syndrome, and tricuspid stenosis and atresia.

Aortic pressure is increased in systemic hypertension and coarctation of the aorta if the pressure is measured above the obstruction. Aortic pressure is decreased with hypovolemia, aortic stenosis, and decreased LV systolic function, such as in shock.

Aortic stenosis may also cause *pulsus parvus et tardus*, or a weak and delayed pulse, such as in the carotid or radial pulses.

A wide aortic pulse pressure is secondary to aortic insufficiency, systemic hypertension, or a large left-to-right shunt (open ductus, aortopulmonary window, truncus arteriosus communis, or perforated sinus of Valsalva aneurysm). A narrow aortic pulse pressure is caused by aortic stenosis, heart failure, cardiac tamponade, and shock.

A pulsus paradoxus (>10 mmHg arterial systolic pressure decrease with inspiration) is caused by cardiac tamponade. Pulsus alternans (alternating strong and weak arterial pulses) may occur with severe heart failure.

A pulsus bisferiens occurs in combined aortic stenosis and regurgitation, aortic regurgitation alone, and in hypertrophic cardiomyopathy. The pressure waveform morphology demonstrates two peaks during ventricular systole. The first peak is the percussion wave and the second, lower-amplitude, peak is the tidal wave.

A dicrotic pressure wave pattern, in which the second peak of the waveform is in diastole immediately after the second heart sound, is seen in significant LV dysfunction, cardiac tamponade, or hypovolemic shock. A systolic pressure wave is followed by a large diastolic pressure wave of lower amplitude after aortic valve closure and occurring at the dicrotic notch.

Hypertrophic cardiomyopathy

The Brockenbrough sign may be used to characterize hypertrophic cardiomyopathy with an outflow gradient (Figure 7.14). A post premature ventricular contraction (PVC) beat in a patient with a dynamic LV outflow tract obstruction, such as in hypertrophic cardiomyopathy, will result in an increased gradient between the aortic and LV pressures, a decrease in aortic pressure, and a diminished aortic pulse pressure.

Constrictive pericarditis and restrictive cardiomyopathy

Restrictive and constrictive waveforms appear similar, and are difficult to distinguish without respiratory maneuvers.

Typically, constrictive pericarditis is associated with equalization of diastolic pressures with LV end-diastolic pressure (LVEDP) – RV end-diastolic pressure (RVEDP) less than 5 mmHg, PA systolic pressure less than 60 mmHg, and the RVEDP greater than one-third of the RV systolic pressure (RVSP)[10,11] (Figure 7.13). Typically, the RA pressure does not fall with inspiration (Kussmaul's sign) (Figure 7.13). An inspiratory increase by greater than 5 mmHg in the gradient between PCW and LV diastolic pressures is associated with constrictive physiology. In addition, interdependence of RV and LV pressures may be seen with respiratory maneuvers; inspiration causes an initial increase in RV systolic pressure along with a decrease in LV systolic pressure, and the opposite occurs with expiration (Figure 7.13).

Restrictive cardiomyopathy is usually associated with some separation of RV and LV end-diastolic pressures (usually >5 mmHg difference), severe pulmonary hypertension with the PA systolic pressure greater than 60 mmHg, and the RVEDP/RVSP ratio less than one-third. Volume loading has been used to separate the RV and LV end-diastolic pressures in patients with restrictive cardiomyopathy, but this has only been studied in a few patients.[11] Respiration causes concordant changes in both RV and LV systolic pressures, with both RV and LV systolic pressures slightly decreasing with inspiration and both increasing with expiration.

Hemodynamic calculations

Once the hemodynamic data are collected, computations enhance quantitation of cardiac function. We provide formulae here for the more common calculations needed. The reader is referred to other sources for specific derivations and applications.[1]

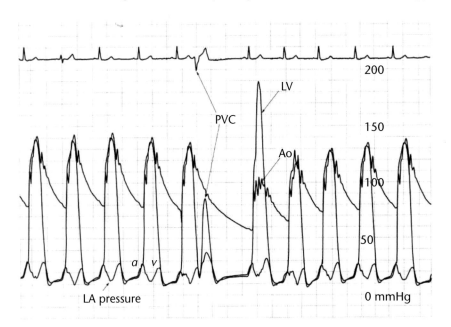

Figure 7.14
Brockenbrough–Braunwald–Morrow sign. In hypertrophic obstructive cardiomyopathy after a premature ventricular contraction occurs, the left ventricular (LV) outflow tract gradient increases, the aortic (Ao) systolic blood pressure decreases, and the aortic pulse pressure decreases. (Adapted from Murphy JG. Mayo Clinic Cardiology Review, 2nd Edn. Philadelphia: Lippincott Williams and Wilkins, 2000.[9])

Cardiac output (CO) by the Fick method (oxygen consumption)

$$CO = \frac{O_2 \text{ consumption (ml / min)}}{AV\ O_2 \text{ difference (ml } O_2 \text{ /100 ml blood} \times 10}.$$

Oxygen consumption is measured from a metabolic 'hood' or Douglas bag. It may also be estimated as 3 ml O_2/kg or 125 ml/min/m^2 × body surface area. AV O_2 (arteriovenous oxygen) difference is calculated from arterial – mixed venous (pulmonary artery) O_2 content. O_2 content = oxygen saturation × 1.36 × hemoglobin (g/dl) × 10.

Cardiac index (CI, l/min/m^2)

$$CI = \frac{CO \text{ (l / min)}}{BSA \text{ (m}^2)}.$$

Stroke volume (SV, ml/beat)

$$SV = \frac{CO \text{ (l / min)}}{HR \text{ (bpm)}}.$$

Stroke index (SI, ml/beat/m^2)

$$SI = \frac{SV \text{ (ml / beat)}}{BSA \text{ (m}^2)}.$$

Stroke work (SW, g · m)

SW = (mean LV systolic pressure – mean LV diastolic pressure) × stroke volume × 0.0144.

Flow

Cardiac output in the catheterization laboratory can be determined by the Fick method or the indicator dilution method. As oxygenated blood circulates across the arteriovenous vascular bed, oxygen is extracted by the tissues, and the blood becomes relatively deoxygenated. It then returns to the pulmonary circulation to become oxygenated. For a given amount of oxygen supply (oxygen consumption) and oxygen demand (tissue oxygen extraction or arteriovenous oxygen difference), enough blood flow must be present in enough volume per unit time for the supply to equal the demand:[12]

$$flow = \frac{supply \text{ (ml / min)}}{demand \text{ (ml / l)}}.$$

In other words, the oxygen content that is extracted from tissues must be supplied in adequate amounts by blood flow across the tissue bed. Adolph Fick described this principle in 1870.

In humans, the cardiac output is given by

$$CO = \frac{O_2 \text{ consumption (ml / min)}}{(AV\ O_2 \text{ saturation difference)} \times \text{hemoglobin (g / dl)} \times 1.36 \times 10}.$$

Oxygen extraction (demand) is the difference between oxygen content in oxygen-saturated arterial blood and that in oxygen-desaturated mixed venous blood (pulmonary arterial blood). Oxygen content is calculated by multiplying hemoglobin × 1.36 × 10 × arterial or venous oxygen saturation.[13,14] The most reliable site for obtaining mixed venous oxygen saturation is the pulmonary artery.[15,16] A small right-to-left shunt occurs in the systemic arterial circulation due to bronchial and Thebesian venous drainage. Because this shunt is small, systemic arterial oxygen saturation can be used as a substitute for pulmonary venous oxygen saturation.

Cardiac output assessment by the Fick technique is the most accurate method of determining cardiac output, particularly in patients with low cardiac output or with irregular rhythms. Oxygen consumption can be indirectly measured by a metabolic rate meter or Douglas bag as previously described, or it may be assumed to be 125 ml/min/m^2 and multiplied by body surface area. Simultaneous reliable measurements of the arteriovenous oxygen content difference and oxygen consumption are essential for accurate cardiac output determination. Air bubbles in the blood sample, oxygen-saturated blood obtained from a pulmonary artery catheter in the wedge position, and blood overly diluted with heparin may contribute to errors in oxygen saturation measurement. The Fick method assumes a steady state for measurement of oxygen consumption and extraction. Prior to collection of blood for oxygen saturation determination, it is very important that measurements be made when the patient is hemodynamically stable and is in a stable respiratory pattern. Supplemental oxygen should be discontinued at least 10–15 minutes before determination of the cardiac output by the Fick method. If a steady state is not achieved due to anxiety or dyspnea, during which a measurement of oxygen is falsely elevated, then the cardiac output will be spuriously high. If shallow breathing (alveolar hypoventilation) occurs, as with oversedation, the oxygen consumption is falsely low, and therefore the cardiac output determination will also be falsely low.

The indicator dilution method is based on the principle that a known amount of an indicator injected into the central circulation mixes completely with blood and changes concentration as it flows into a distal location.[17] Single injection and continuous infusions are the two general types of method used. An indicator such as indocyanine green dye or room-temperature saline of a known amount is injected proximally to a central chamber, with adequate mixing of blood, followed by continuous measurement of indicator concentration as a function of time. The change in the indicator concentration (or temperature) is plotted over time, and the area under the curve is then utilized to calculate the cardiac output[17,18] (Figure 7.15).

The indicator dilution method is the most accurate technique in patients with higher cardiac output states.[19] It is inaccurate in the presence of irregular heart rhythms and in the presence of significant regurgitation of a valve between the injection and sampling sites. The thermodilution method with cold saline is the most commonly used version of this analysis. Advantages of the thermodilution technique include the following:

- It does not require blood withdrawal.
- It does not require an arterial puncture.
- The indicator is inexpensive and inert.
- There is almost no recirculation of saline.

The thermodilution technique requires a pulmonary artery balloon flotation catheter (Swan–Ganz) with a thermistor at the end. The method uses ice water or water at room temperature. The proximal port, the right atrium, is the site for rapid infusion, while the distal site is used for pressure measurements. With the thermodilution technique, approximately 10 ml of saline (iced or at room temperature) is injected through the proximal port of the Swan–Ganz catheter. An external thermistor measures the

temperature of the injectate. When the injectate completely mixes with blood, a decrease in temperature is detected by the distal thermistor. Temperature change as a function of time is plotted on y and x coordinates, respectively, and the area under the curve becomes the integral of the temperature change over the time of measurement (Figure 7.15).[18] In both methods, the area under the curve is inversely related to cardiac output. The variability in the thermodilution method is as high as 15–20%.

Notes on thermodilution technique[1]

1. If the catheter is coiled excessively in the right atrium or ventricle, poor positioning of the distal thermistor in relation to the proximal port may occur. The catheter may need to be straightened out with a guidewire.
2. Thermodilution systems require a computation constant of 0.825 in the cardiac output determination.[20] The computer should be set with the proper computation constant.
3. Inject the proper amount of injectate. In adults, 10 ml of saline is the proper volume, while 5 ml may be used in pediatric patients.
4. Avoid warming the injectate with the palm of the hand. This will introduce an error into the calculation.
5. Coordinate the injection with the start button by the technician.
6. The bolus of saline should be rapidly delivered at a constant rate.

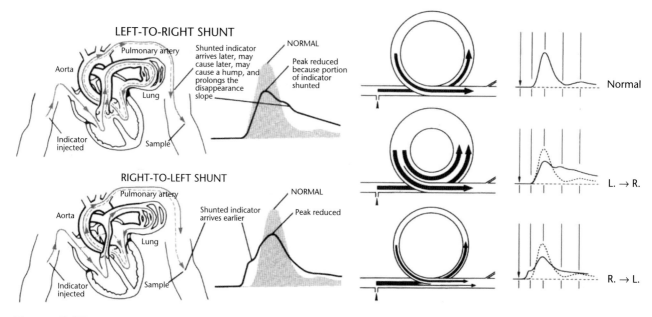

Figure 7.15
Illustration of the indicator dilution method for determining left-to-right and right-to-left shunts. (Adapted from Kern MJ. The Cardiac Catheterization Handbook, 3rd Edn. St Louis, MO: Mosby, 1999[1] with permission from Elsevier.)

7. Multiple outputs (three or four) should be obtained and averaged.
8. The thermodilution technique is inaccurate with significant tricuspid regurgitation or in patients with low cardiac output. The Fick method should be used in these situations.

Resistance

Determination of vascular resistance is based on Poiseuille's law:

$$Q = \frac{\pi(P_{in} - P_{out})r^4}{8\eta l},$$

where Q is the volume flow, P_{in} and P_{out} are the incoming and outgoing pressures, η is the viscosity of the fluid, l is the length of the tube, r is the radius of tube. Poiseuille's law is based on steady-state laminar flow of a homogenous fluid through a rigid tube. Therefore, the application to humans is only approximate. By rearranging Poiseuille's law, $\Delta P/Q = 8\eta l/\pi r^4$ = resistance. Because blood flow is pulsatile and is a nonhomogeneous fluid in a nonlinear, elastic vascular bed, resistance as described by the above law has limited use in human studies. Therefore, it is used primarily in an empiric manner to aid in clinical decision making.

The following formulae are used to describe resistance in various vascular beds.

Pulmonary vascular resistance (PVR, Wood Units)

$$PVR = \frac{\text{mean PAP} - \text{mean LAP (or PCWP)}}{CO},$$

where PAP, LAP, and PCWP are the pulmonary artery, left atrial, and pulmonary capillary wedge pressures, respectively.

Total pulmonary resistance (TPR, Wood Units)

$$TPR = \frac{\text{mean pulmonary artery pressure}}{CO}.$$

Systemic vascular resistance (SVR, Wood Units)

$$SVR = \frac{\text{mean aortic pressure} - \text{mean right atrial pressure}}{CO}.$$

Converting to resistance in metric units (dyn · s · cm^{-5})

SVR, PVR, TPR units × 80.

Mean pulmonary capillary wedge pressure can be substituted for mean left atrial pressure.[8,21,22] The units are empiric, and called Wood Units after Dr Paul Wood. These units are mmHg/l/min = Hybrid Resistance Unit (HRU) = Wood Unit. As indicated above, a Wood Unit can be converted to dyn·s·cm^{-5} (metric resistance units) by multiplying with a factor of 80. As predicted by Poiseuille's law, resistance is altered with hematocrit changes (increased viscosity), during growth (change in length and radius of blood vessels) and with changes in vascular radius.

Shunts

An intracardiac shunt is an abnormal connection between a left and right heart chamber. The blood flow may be directed left to right or right to left, or may be bidirectional. These shunts are often detected by clinical findings. Unexplained arterial desaturation, or an unexpectedly high pulmonary artery oxygen saturation should prompt assessment for the presence of a shunt. Table 7.1 lists locations of intracardiac shunts based on 'step-ups' of oxygen saturation. Effective blood flow is the theoretical flow in the circuit that would exist without any shunting. A left-to-right shunt increases the amount of blood to the right heart. Therefore, the effective blood flow is equal to the pulmonary blood flow plus the shunt flow. With a right-to-left shunt, the systemic blood flow is increased by the amount of the shunt. Therefore, the effective blood flow is equal to the systemic flow plus the shunt flow. (Figure 7.16).

Shunt calculations

$$\text{Pulmonary blood flow } (Q_p) = \frac{O_2 \text{ consumption}}{PVO_2 - PAO_2},$$

where PVO_2 is the pulmonary venous oxygen content and PAO_2 is the pulmonary arterial oxygen content.

$$\text{Systemic blood flow } (Q_s) = \frac{O_2 \text{ consumption}}{SAO_2 - MVO_2},$$

where SAO_2 is the systemic arterial oxygen content and MVO_2 is the mixed venous oxygen content.

$$\text{Shunt radio} = \frac{Q_p}{Q_s}.$$

Table 7.1 Cardiac shunt locations

Locations	Earliest step-up location (for left-to-right shunts)
Atrial septal defects:	
Primum (low)	Right atrium, right ventricle
Secundum (mid)	Right atrium
Sinus venosus (high)	Right atrium
Partial anomalous pulmanory venous return (pulmonary veins entering right atrium)	Right atrium
Ventricular septal defects:	
Membranous (high)	Right ventricle
Muscular (mid)	Right ventricle
Apical (low)	Right ventricle
Aorticopulmonary window (connection of aorta to pulmonary artery)	Pulmonary artery
Patent ductus arteriosus (normally closed aorta – pulmonary artery connection at birth)	Pulmonary artery

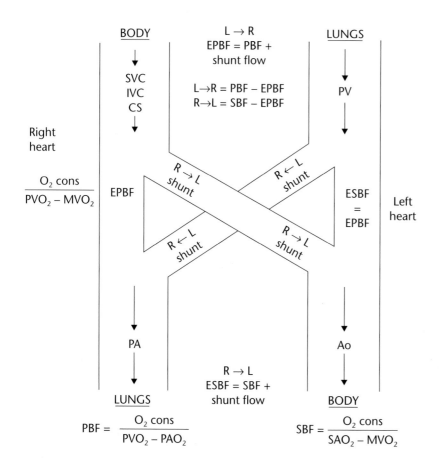

Figure 7.16
Illustration of left-to-right and right-to-left intracardiac shunting The ratio of pulmonary to systemic blood flow can be used to quantify the magnitude of a left-to-right or right-to-left shunt. A bidirectional shunt quantification involves a more complex equation. PBF, pulmonary blood flow; EPBF, effective pulmonary blood flow; SBF, systemic blood flow; ESBF, effective systemic blood flow; O_2 cons, oxygen consumption; PAO_2, pulmonary arterial oxygen saturation or content; PVO_2, pulmonary venous oxygen saturation or content; MVO_2, mixed venous oxygen saturation or content, SAO_2, systemic arterial oxygen saturation or content; SVC, superior vena cava; IVC, inferior vena cava; CS, coronary sinus; Ao, aorta; PA, pulmonary artery. (Adapted from Kern MJ. The Cardiac Catheterization Handbook, 3rd Edn. St Louis, MO: Mosby, 1999[1] with permission from Elsevier.)

Formula for Q_p/Q_s (shortened formula):

$$\frac{Q_p = (SAO_2 - MVO_2) = Art - MV}{Q_s = (PVO_2 - PAO_2) = PV - PA},$$

where Art is the arterial O_2 saturation, MV is the mixed venous O_2 saturation, PV is the pulmonary venous O_2 saturation, and PA is the pulmonary arterial O_2 saturation.

Formulae for bidirectional shunts:

$$\text{left-to-right shunt} = \frac{Q_p(MVO_2 - PAO_2)}{MVO_2 - PV * O_2},$$

$$\text{right-to-left shunt} = \frac{Q_p(PV * O_2 - SAO_2)(PAO_2 - PV * O_2)}{(SAO_2 - MVO_2)(MVO_2 - PV * O_2)}.$$

*If the pulmonary vein is not entered, use 98% $\times$ O_2 capacity.

A simpler formula for a quick approximation in bidirectional shunting may be used. The effective blood flow is the hypothetical amount that would exist in the absence of any left-to-right or right-to-left shunting:

$$Q_{eff} = \frac{O_2 \text{ consumption (ml / min)}}{PVO_2 \text{ content (ml / l)} - MVO_2 \text{ content (ml / l)}},$$

$$\text{left-to-right shunt} = Q_p - Q_{eff},$$

$$\text{right-to-left shunt} = Q_s - Q_{eff}.$$

Oximetry procedure

If a shunt is suspected, an oximetry run should be performed. After pressures and cardiac output have been determined, the oximetry run can commence with the catheter tip in the right or left pulmonary artery. The catheter must be flushed and waste blood aspirated. Approximately 2 ml samples of blood are obtained from the pulmonary artery, regions of the right ventricle, mid and low right atrium, superior vena cava, and inferior vena cava above and below the hepatic vein. In addition, an arterial sample or left ventricular sample should also be obtained. If it is possible to cross an atrial septal defect easily, a pulmonary venous sample may also be obtained. Saturation syringes should be heparinized with less than 0.5 ml. Saturations are determined sequentially with an end-hole catheter or a pulmonary artery catheter. Localization of the catheter tip can be determined fluoroscopically or by identification of pressure waveform.

Oxygen step-up

A left-to-right shunt is demonstrated when a significant increase of oxygen content in that chamber or vessel exceeds that of a proximal chamber beyond normal variation in oxygen content between the right heart chambers [23–26] (Table 7.2). A step-up in oxygen saturation at the pulmonary artery by more than 7% above the right atrial saturation demonstrates a left-to-right shunt. Similarly, the desaturation of arterial blood samples to a similar degree indicates a significant right-to-left shunt. This type of shunt should be distinguished from oxygen desaturation due to lung disease or atelectasis, and may be accomplished with administration of 100% O_2. Intracardiac shunts do not improve with oxygen supplementation. In determining the site of a right-to-left shunt, sequential sampling can be made from the left atrium (pulmonary vein), left ventricle, and aorta. Echocardiography with a bubble study is helpful in localizing an intracardiac shunt.

Mixed venous blood is usually assumed to be the blood from the pulmonary artery. In a left-to-right shunt, mixed venous blood oxygen content must be measured in the chamber just proximal to the site of step-up. With an atrial septal defect, the mixed venous blood is 3 (SVC) + IVC/4.[27] If pulmonary venous blood is not sampled, and the patient does not exhibit bidirectional shunting (i.e. arterial desaturation), the pulmonary venous oxygen saturation is assumed to be 95%. If the systemic oxygen saturation is less than 95%, one must determine whether a right-to-left shunt exists (administer 100% O_2). If there is an intracardiac right-to-left shunt, then an assumed value for pulmonary venous oxygen of 98% oxygen capacity should be used to calculate the pulmonary blood flow. If arterial desaturation is present and is not due to a right-to-left shunt, then the observed systemic arterial oxygen saturation should be used in the pulmonary blood flow calculation.

A Q_p/Q_s less than 1.5 is usually associated with a small left-to-right shunt, and often may be followed carefully. A Q_p/Q_s greater than 2.0 is consistent with a large left-to-right shunt, and may be an indication for surgery.

Limitations of the oximetry method

- Oximetry may not detect small (<20%) shunts.
- The blood flow calculations assume a steady state during the run and during measurements of oxygen consumption.
- The oximetry method also assumes complete mixing instantly and that blood samples obtained are representative of blood in the particular compartment.
- A high systemic flow tends to equalize the arteriovenous oxygen difference across a given vascular bed.[25] Therefore, with a high systemic blood flow, the mixed venous oxygen saturation is higher than normal, and intrachamber variability is blunted. In contrast, when the systemic blood flow is reduced, a larger step-up is required before a significant left-to-right shunt may be detected.

Indicator dye curves are more sensitive for detecting small right-to-left shunts, but cannot localize the shunt. A shunt is determined to be present when early recirculation of dye occurs. Shunts less than 25% can be detected easily

Table 7.2   Oximetric criteria for detection of left-to-right shunts

Level of shunt	Criteria for significant step-up				Approximate minimal Q_p/Q_s required for detection (assuming SBFI = 3 (min/m²)	Possible causes of step-up
	Mean of distal chamber samples	Mean of proximal chamber samples	Highest value in distal chamber	Highest value in proximal chamber		
	O_2% sat	O_2 vol%	O_2% sat	O_2 vol%		
Atrial (SVC/IVC to RA)	≥7	≥1.3	≥11	≥2.0	1.5–1.9	Atrial septal defect; partial anomalous pulmonary venous drainage; ruptured sinus of Valsalva; VSD with TR; coronary fistula to RA
Ventricular (RA to RV)	≥5	≥1.0	≥10	≥1.7	1.3–1.5	VSD; PDA with PR; primum ASD; coronary fistula to RV
Great vessel (RV to PA)	≥5	≥1.0	≥5	≥1.0	≥1.3	PDA; aorto-pulmonary window; aberrant coronary artery origin
Any level (SVC to PA)	≥7	≥1.3	≥8	≥1.5	≥1.5	All of the above

with this technique.[28] A single sampling technique is used in which dye is injected proximal to a shunt (antecubital vein), with sampling distal to the shunt (brachial artery) (Figure 7.15). Left-to-right shunting shows additional flow through the pulmonary circulation (larger upward circle), with the dye dilution curve showing reduced maximal deflection with a later recirculation hump as dye recirculates through the lungs, and a prolonged slow clearance (Figure 7.15, middle panel). With a right-to-left shunt and addition of flow to the systemic circulation, a relatively reduced pulmonary flow (smaller upward circle) is seen (Figure 7.15, lower panel). Dye curves show an early shoulder due to a portion of the indicator passing directly to the arterial circulation, a flattened peak, and attenuated late downstroke. The areas beneath the curves are used for quantitation of the shunts.

Alternatively, a double sampling technique can be used where dye is injected into the pulmonary artery and sam-ples are obtained in the right ventricle and ascending aorta.[29] Early appearance of dye in the right ventricle concomitant with the appearance of dye in the ascending aorta would indicate a left-to-right shunt.

Valve area calculations

Valve area calculations are based on two hydraulic formulae developed by Dr Richard Gorlin and his father in 1951.[30] The general formula is

$$\text{area} = \frac{\text{flow}}{44.3C\,\Delta(\text{pressure})},$$

where C is an empiric constant. Since flow occurs across the atrioventricular and semilunar valves at different times during the cardiac cycle, flow is modified to reflect these differences. Thus, for the aortic valve, the cardiac output is divided by the heart rate × the systolic ejection period, while for the mitral valve, cardiac output is divided by the heart rate × the diastolic filling period.

The formula for any valve area calculation is

$$\text{area (cm}^2) = \frac{\text{valve flow (ml/s)}}{44.3C\sqrt{\text{MVG}}},$$

where MVG is the mean valvular gradient. For the semilunar valves and tricuspid valve, $C = 1$, while for the mitral valve, $C = 0.85$.[31] Valve flow is measured in milliliters per second during the diastolic or systolic flow period.

Mitral valve flow

$$\frac{\text{CO (ml/min)}}{\text{diastolic filling period (s/min)}}.$$

The diastolic filling period (s/min) is the diastolic period (s/beat) × heart rate and is measured as the time between mitral valve opening and mitral valve closing at end-diastole (Figure 7.17).

Aortic valve flow

$$\frac{\text{CO (ml/min)}}{\text{systolic ejection period (s/min)}}.$$

The systolic ejection period (s/min) is equal to the systolic period (s/beat) × heart rate and is measured as the time between aortic valve opening and the aortic valve closing (Figure 7.17).

By rearranging the Gorlin equation as Δ (pressure) = [flow/(valve area)(44.3)]² for a given valve area, the pressure increase is proportional to the square of the increase in flow. Therefore, a doubling of the flow rate will quadruple the pressure gradient.

To calculate the mitral valve area, simultaneous recordings of the left ventricular (LV) and pulmonary capillary wedge (PCW) pressure or left atrial (LA) pressure tracings are made.[8] The PCW pressure occurs later in time than the LV pressure, and therefore, phase shifting of the PCW pressure tracing is necessary. When measured directly, the true LA v-wave peak occurs within the downslope of the LV tracing. Therefore, the peak of the PCW v wave should be moved so that most of the v wave is within the LV tracing (Figure 7.17). In a patient with mitral stenosis, Figure 7.7 above demonstrates how the lack of phase shifting of the PCW pressure can significantly overestimate the mitral valve gradient. The diastolic filling period (DFP) is the time from mitral valve opening to mitral valve closing. Multiple DFPs should be measured (5 if the patient is in sinus rhythm, and 10 if the patient is in atrial fibrillation). This distance in centimeters is converted to seconds, depending on the paper speed (usually 1 s is 10 cm). After phase-

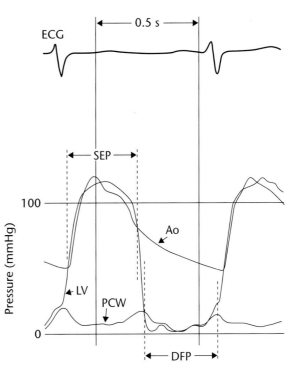

Figure 7.17
Simultaneous left ventricular (LV), aortic (Ao), and pulmonary capillary wedge (PCW) pressure tracings. The systolic ejection period (SEP) and diastolic filling period (DFP) are also marked. (Adapted from Baim DS and Grossman W. Grossman's Cardiac Catheterization, Angiography, and Intervention. Philadelphia: Lippincott Williams and Wilkins, 2000.[2])

shifting the PCW pressure waveform, the area between the PCW and LV pressure tracings during the diastolic filling period is planimetered and the average of 5 tracings is utilized (10 in the presence of atrial fibrillation) to yield the mean transvalvular gradient. This area in cm² is converted to mmHg, depending on the conversion factor (based on the number of cm/mmHg from the scale used). The calculated cardiac output, mean DFP, and mean valve gradient are inserted in the mitral valve Gorlin equation to yield the mitral valve area in cm².

Example of mitral valve area calculation[1] (Figure 7.18)

1. Cardiac output = 3500 ml/min.
2. Heart rate = 80 bpm.
3. Scale factor = 1 cm = 3.9 mmHg (40 mmHg full scale).
4. Planimeter 5 LV–PCW areas (10 in the presence of atrial fibrillation).
5. Calculate the mean valve gradient:

$$MVG = \frac{\text{area} \times \text{scale factor}}{\text{DFP}} = \frac{9.46 \text{ cm}^2 \times 3.9 \text{ mmHg}/1 \text{ cm}}{3.4 \text{ cm}}$$

$$= \frac{36.9}{3.4} = 10.85 \text{ mmHg}.$$

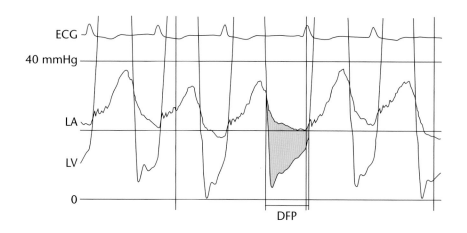

Figure 7.18
Calculation of the mean mitral valve gradient. After appropriate phase-shifting of the PCW pressure, the area between the LV and PCW pressure tracings is planimetered. This area represents the mean valve gradient across the mitral valve.

6. Determine the mitral valve flow:

$$\frac{CO\ (ml/min)}{DFP \times HR} = \frac{3500\ ml/min}{3.4\ cm \times (1\ s/10\ cm) \times 80\ bpm}$$

$$= \frac{3500}{0.34 \times 80} = 128.7.$$

7. Determine the mitral valve area:

$$\frac{mitral\ valve\ flow}{0.85 \times 44.3 \times \sqrt{10.85}} = \frac{128.7}{0.85 \times 44.3 \times 3.3} = \frac{128.7}{124.3} = 1.0\ cm^2.$$

An improperly wedged catheter tip may result in a damped mean pulmonary artery wedge pressure and thus a falsely high transmitral gradient. In patients with prosthetic mitral valves, the PCW pressure overestimates the LA pressure. Overestimation is in part by large v waves increasing the phase delay, making correction and alignment of pressure tracings difficult. Direct LA pressure measurement is the most accurate method. Transseptal

catheterization should be performed to confirm large pressure gradients in patients with suspected prosthetic mitral stenosis. Cardiac output determinations calculate net forward flow and do not account for forward flow plus regurgitant flow when significant mitral regurgitation occurs with mitral stenosis. Therefore, the mitral valve area may be underestimated in these patients with mixed mitral stenosis and regurgitation.

Aortic valve area determination is similar to that of the mitral valve, except that the systolic ejection period (SEP) is used in place of the DFP, and the constant $C = 1.0$ is used instead of 0.85. The LV and central aortic or peripheral arterial pressure tracings are displayed simultaneously and the area between the curves is planimetered 5 times (10 times if atrial fibrillation is present) to give an average mean aortic valve gradient. If femoral artery (FA) and LV pressures are used, the FA pressure tracing will need to be phase-shifted in time (to the left) and in gradient (downward, depending on the pressure gradient between central aortic and FA pressure tracings) (Figures 7.19 and

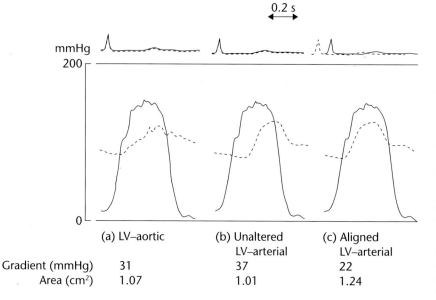

	(a) LV–aortic	(b) Unaltered LV–arterial	(c) Aligned LV–arterial
Gradient (mmHg)	31	37	22
Area (cm²)	1.07	1.01	1.24

Figure 7.19
Effects of unchanged and phase-shifted arterial waveforms in aortic stenosis. Prior to phase-shifting, simultaneous femoral and central aortic pressures are recorded to determine if any peripheral augmentation is present. (a) shows LV and central aortic pressure tracings. (b) shows how a delay in the femoral artery waveform increases the pressure gradient. In (c), phase-shifting has been performed, but the mean valve gradient is now underestimated by 9 mmHg due to femoral artery pressure augmentation. This is corrected by adjusting the peripheral arterial waveform downward by the amount of augmentation over the central aortic pressure. (Adapted from Baim DS and Grossman W. Grossman's Cardiac Catheterization, Angiography, and Intervention. Philadelphia: Lippincott Williams and Wilkins, 2000.[2])

7.20). This value also needs to be converted from cm² to mmHg by a conversion factor based on the scale used. The systolic ejection period is converted from cm to s by using the factor 1 s/10 cm if a 100 mm/s paper speed is used. Once the mean aortic gradient and the SEP have been calculated, the valve area can be determined from the formula.

The mean aortic pressure gradient is measured by planimetry of the superimposed aortic and LV pressure tracings. The peak-to-peak gradient is not equivalent to the mean gradient for mild and moderate stenosis; however, this may be close in value to the mean gradient for severe stenosis. The delay in pressure transmission of a peripheral waveform will spuriously increase the gradient, while peripheral augmentation will falsely reduce the gradient across the aortic valve. Consequently, phase-shifting the femoral arterial wave form as indicated above is necessary (Figures 7.19 and 7.20). A catheter tip in the LV outflow tract can also underestimate the gradient across the aortic valve, since a pressure gradient usually exists between the LV and the LV outflow tract.[33] Optimally, a second catheter may be positioned directly above the aortic valve to reduce transmission delay and femoral pressure amplification.

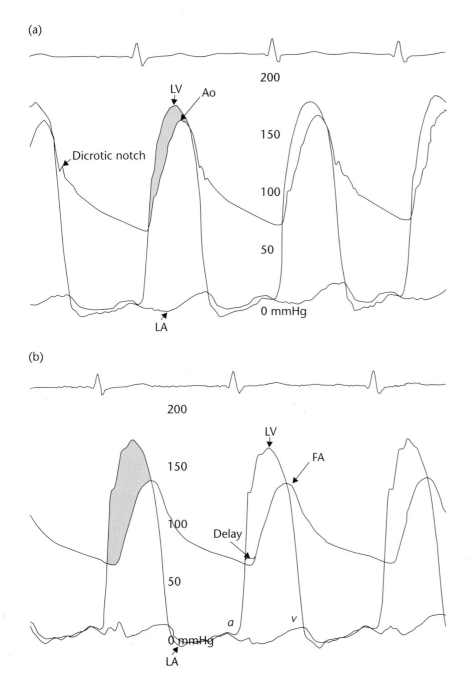

(a)

(b)

Figure 7.20
Simultaneous left ventricular and aortic (a) or peripheral arterial (b) waveforms. In (a) one catheter is placed in the left ventricle (LV), and the other catheter is placed in the proximal ascending aorta (Ao). Accurate measurements of the true pressure gradients are obtained in this manner. In (b), one catheter is placed in the LV, and the femoral sheath is used to measure peripheral arterial pressure (FA). This peripheral waveform needs to be adjusted as in Figure 7.18 to account for time delay and peripheral augmentation. (Adapted from Baim DS and Grossman W. Grossman's Cardiac Catheterization, Angiography, and Intervention. Philadelphia: Lippincott Williams and Wilkins, 2000.[2])

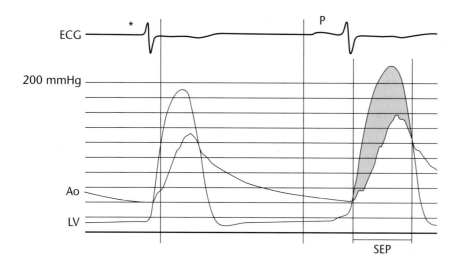

Figure 7.21
Calculation of aortic valve area. After appropriate phase-shifting of the femoral artery tracing, the area between the femoral arterial and left ventricular waves is planimetered. This area represents the mean aortic valve gradient.

Example of aortic valve area calculation[1] (Figure 7.21)

1. Heart rate (HR) = 60 bpm.
2. Cardiac output (CO) = 5000 ml/min.
3. Determine scale factor to convert recording deflection from cm to pressure by directly measuring paper calibration lines of 200 mmHg. 1 cm = 19.4 mmHg.
4. Record 5 aortic–LV gradients if the patient is in sinus rhythm and 10 aortic–LV gradients if the patient is in atrial fibrillation. Recordings should be on 100 mm/s paper speed.
5. Phase-shift the upstroke of the femoral artery tracing to match the upstroke of the LV pressure tracing. Planimeter each recording and then average. Area = 12.20 cm².
6. Determine the systolic ejection period:

$$SEP = 4.1 \text{ cm} \times 1 \text{ s}/10 \text{ cm} = 0.41 \text{ s}.$$

7. Determine the mean valve gradient:

$$MVG = area \times scale\ factor\ /\ SEP$$
$$= \frac{12.2 \text{ cm}^2 \times 19.4 \text{ mmHg} / 1 \text{ cm}}{4.1 \text{ cm}}$$
$$= \frac{236.68}{4.1} = 57.7 \text{ mmHg}.$$

8. Determine the aortic valve flow:

$$\frac{CO}{SEP \times HR} = \frac{5000}{0.41 \text{ s}/\text{beat} \times 60 \text{ bpm}} = \frac{5000}{24.6} = 203.2.$$

9. Determine the aortic valve area:

$$\frac{\text{aortic valve flow}}{1.0 \times 44.3 \times \sqrt{\text{gradient}}} = \frac{203.2}{44.3 \times \sqrt{57.7}} = \frac{203.2}{44.3 \times 7.5} = 0.61 \text{ cm}^2.$$

In low-flow states, the Gorlin formula overestimates the aortic valve area. Consequently, a modified Gorlin formula has been used.[34] In the setting of low cardiac output, low transaortic valve gradient, and significant aortic stenosis, an infusion of dobutamine or nitroprusside may distinguish between a small calculated aortic valve area due to low cardiac output and true aortic stenosis.[35]

Valve resistance is equal to the mean valve gradient divided by cardiac output per second of systolic (aortic valve) or diastolic (mitral valve) flow. Since resistance is less flow-dependent, it may be used to distinguish patients with true severe aortic stenosis from those with low-cardiac-output aortic stenosis. A simplified formula for calculating aortic valve resistance is[32]

aortic valve resistance =

$$\frac{(\text{mean gradient}) (\text{systolic ejection period}) (\text{heart rate}) \times 1.33}{\text{cardiac output } (1/\text{min})}$$

Aortic regurgitation

A characteristic hemodynamic feature in aortic regurgitation is the widened pulse pressure. In addition, the femoral arterial waveform demonstrates a brisk pressure upstroke. Figure 7.22 shows severe aortic regurgitation with rapidly increasing LV diastolic pressure, a wide aortic pressure, and near-equalization of aortic and LV pressure at end-diastole.

Mitral regurgitation

Large *v* waves in the PCW or LA pressure waveforms may represent LV pressure transmitted from a regurgitant mitral valve. The PCW *v* wave occurs on the downslope of the LV pressure waveform (Figure 7.23). Large *v* waves reflect changes in the pressure–volume filling curve of the

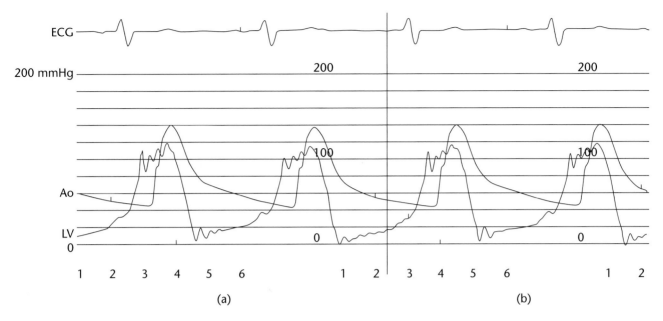

Figure 7.22
Severe aortic regurgitation. Notice the wide pulse pressure of the aortic pressure tracing (Ao), the brisk upstroke of the aortic waveform, and the near-equalization of pressures between the left ventricle (LV) and aorta at end-diastole.

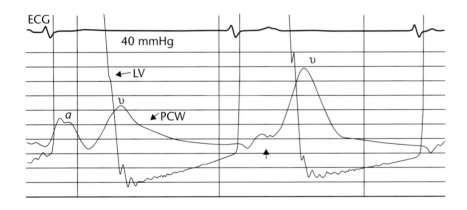

Figure 7.23
Severe mitral regurgitation. A large *v* wave is present on the PCW tracing.

atrium, and therefore may be due to valvular mitral regurgitation or stenosis, or other conditions in which the pressure–volume relationship is altered (high atrial volume due to ventricular septal defect or stiffening of chamber elasticity due to ischemia or hypertrophy).

Tricuspid valve gradients

Small gradients (5 mmHg) across the tricuspid valve may lead to important symptoms. Two large-lumen catheters to measure simultaneous RA and RV pressures are required. Pressures through these catheters should be matched before placement in the RA and RV to avoid technical error. The formula for the mitral valve area should be used; however, the Gorlin constant for this valve has not been determined.[1]

Pulmonary valve gradients

A pulmonary valve gradient may be determined by catheter 'pullback', continuously measuring pressure during catheter withdrawal from the pulmonary artery to the RV. However, two catheters or double-lumen Cournand catheters are more precise and can record simultaneous PA and RV pressures. No formula exists for pulmonary valve area, and prognostic data are based on RV pressure.[1]

Complications (Table 7.3)

The most common problem is encountered with the catheter in the right ventricle, or right ventricular outflow tract, which may lead to transient advanced atrioventricular heart block, right bundle branch block, or ventricular

Table 7.3   Complications of right heart catheterization

	Major	*Minor*
Access	Pneumothorax Hemothorax Tracheal perforation (subclavian route)	Hematoma Thrombosis
Intracardiac	Right ventricular perforation Heart block (right bundle branch block) Pulmonary rupture Pulmonary infarction	Cellulitis Ventricular arrhythmias

arrhythmias. Most arrhythmias are self-limiting and do not require treatment. Repositioning of the catheter is usually sufficient to terminate the arrhythmia. Sustained ventricular arrhythmias have been reported in patients with electrolyte abnormalities, severe acidosis, or myocardial ischemia. In patients with left bundle branch block, a temporary pacemaker may be needed if right bundle branch block occurs. Rarely, in patients with severe pulmonary hypertension, aggressive placement of the catheter in the pulmonary capillary wedge position, particularly without the balloon tip inflated, may result in pulmonary artery rupture, which may be devastating. This may be confirmed with dye injection through the pulmonary artery catheter. Tamponade of the bleeding with the catheter balloon tip inflated at the site of injury may halt bleeding. Emergency surgery may also be required in this life-threatening condition.

References

1. Kern MJ. The Cardiac Catheterization Handbook, 3rd edn. St Louis, MO: Mosby, 1999.
2. Baim DS, Grossman W. Grossman's Cardiac Catheterization, Angiography, and Intervention, 6th edn. Philadelphia: Lippincott Williams & Wilkins, 2000.
3. Mueller HS, Chatterjee K, Weintraub WS. Bedside right heart catheterization. J Am Coll Cardiol 1998;32:840–64.
4. Faisetti HL, Mates RE, Green DG, et al. Vmax as an index of contractile state in man. Circulation 1971;43:467.
5. Murgo JP, Westerhof N, Giolma JP, et al. Manipulation of ascending aortic pressure and flow wave reflections with Valsalva manuever: relationship to input impedance. Circulation 1981;63:122–32.
6. Murgo JP, Westerhof N, Giolma JP, et al. Aortic input impedance in normal man: Relationship to pressure wave forms. Circulation 1980;62:105.
7. McDonald DA. Blood Flow in Arteries, 2nd edn. Baltimore: Williams & Wilkins, 1974.
8. Lange RA, Moore DM Jr, Ciggaroa RG, et al. Use of pulmonary capillary wedge pressure to assess severity of mitral stenosis: Is true left atrial pressure needed in this condition? J Am Coll Cardiol 1989;13:825–31.
9. Murphy JG. Mayo Clinic Cardiology Review, 2nd edn. Philadelphia: Lippincott Williams & Wilkins, 2000.
10. Higano ST, Elie A, Tahirkheli NK, Kern MJ. Hemodynamics rounds series II: Hemodynamics of constrictive physiology: influence of respiratory dynamics on ventricular pressures. Cathet Cardiovasc Intervent 1999;46:473–86.
11. Vaitkus PT, Kussmaul WG. Constrictive pericarditis versus restrictive cardiomyopathy: a reappraisal and update of diagnostic criteria. Am Heart J 1991;1431–41.
12. Fick A. Uber die messung des Blutquantums in den Herzentrikeln. Sitz der physic-Med geswurtzbert 1870;16.
13. Bernhart FW, Skeggs L. The iron content of crystalline human hemoglobin. J Biol Chem 1943;147:19.
14. Diem K (ed). Documenta Geigy — Scientific Tables, 6th edn. Ardsley, NY: Geigy Pharmaceuticals, 1962:578.
15. Dexter L, et al. Studies of congenital heart disease II. The pressure and oxygen content of the blood in the right auricle, right ventricle and pulmonary artery in control patients. J Clin Invest 1947;26:554.
16. Barratt-Boyes BG, Wood EH. The oxygen saturation of blood in the venae cavae, right heart chambers and pulmonary vessels of healthy subjects. J Lab Clin Med 1957;50:93.
17. Stewart GN. Researches on the circulation time and on the influences which affect it: IV. The output of the heart. J Physiol 1997;22:159.
18. Weisel RD, Berger RL, Hechtman HB. Current concepts measurement of cardiac output by thermodilution. N Engl J Med 1975;292:682.
19. Grandetie, AV, et al. Thermodilution method overestimates low cardiac output in humans. Am J Physiol 1983;245(Heart Circ Physiol 14):H690.
20. Forrester JS, et al. Thermodilution cardiac output determination with a single flow directed catheter. Am Heart J 1972;83:306.
21. Rappaport E, Dexter L. Pulmonary 'capillary' pressure. Meth Med Res 1958;7:85.
22. Connolly DC, Kirklin JW, Wood CH. The relationship between pulmonary artery pressure and left atrial pressure in man. Circul Res 1954;2:434.
23. Lange RA, Moore DM Jr, Cigarroa RG, Hillis LD. Use of pulmonary capillary wedge pressure to assess severity of mitral stenosis: Is true left atrial pressure needed in this condition? J Am Coll Cardiol 1989;13:825.
24. Dexter L, et al. Studies of congenital heart disease. II. The pressure and oxygen content of blood in the right auricle, right ventricle and pulmonary artery in control patients with observations on the oxygen saturation and source of pulmonary capillary blood. J Clin Invest 1947;26:554.

25. Antman EM, Marsh JD, Green LH, Grossman W. Blood oxygen measurements in the assessment of intracardiac left to right stunts: a critical appraisal of methodology. Am J Cardiol 1980;46:265.

26. Barratt-Boyes BF, Wood EH. The oxygen saturation of blood in the venae cavae, right heart chambers and pulmonary vessels of healthy subjects. J Lab Med 1957;50:93.

27. Freed MD, Miettinen OS, Nadas AS. Oximetric determination of intracardial left to right shunts. Br Heart J 1979;42:690.

28. Flamm MD, Cohnke, Hancock EW. Measurement of systemic cardiac output at rest and exercise in patients with atrial septal defect. Am J Cardiol 1969;23:258.

29. Castillo CA, Kyle JC, Gilson WE, Rowe GG. Simulated shunt curves. Am J Cardiol 1966;17:691.

30. Swan HJC, Wood EH. Localization of cardiac defects by dye-dilution curves recorded after injections of T-1824 at multiple sties in the heart and great vessels during cardiac catheterization. Proc staff meet Mayo Clin 1953;28:95.

31. Gorlin R, Gorlin G. Hydraulic formula for calculation of area of stenotic mitral valve, other cardiac valves and central circulatory shunts. Am Heart J 1951;41:1.

32. Cohen MV, Gorlin R. Modified orifice equation for the calculation of mitral valve area. Am Heart J 1972;84:839.

33. Cannon JD, Jr., Zile MR, Crawford FA, Jr., Carabello BA. Aortic Valve resistance as an adjunct to the Gorlin formula in assessing the severity of aortic stenosis in symptomatic patients. J Am Coll Cardiol 1992;20:1517

34. Lange RA, Moore DM, Cigarroa RG, Hillis LD. Use of pulmonary capillary wedge pressure to assess severity of mitral stenosis: Is true left atrial pressure needed in this condition? J AM Coll Cardiol 1989;13:825.

35. Pasipoularides A. Clinical assessment of ventricular ejection dynamics with and without outflow obstruction. J Am Coll Cardiol 1990;15:859.

36. Cannon SR, Richards KL, Crawford M. Hydraulic estimation of stenotic orifice area: a correction of the Gorlin formula, Circulation 71:1170–1178, 1985.

37. Keelan ET, McBane RD, Higan ST, et al. Does dobutamine infusion during cardiac catheterization help in assessment of the patient with low output/low gradient aortic stenosis. Circulation 1994;90(Suppl): I–52 (abst).

38. Tilkian AG, Daily EK. Cardiovascular Procedures: Diagnostic Techniques and Therapeutic Procedures. St Louis, MO: Mosby, 1986.

39. Kern MJ. Hemodynamic Rounds: Interpretation of Cardiac Pathophysiology from Pressure Waveform Analysis. New York: Wiley-Liss Inc, 1993.

8

Balloon angioplasty

Ken Kozuma

Plain 'old' balloon angioplasty

Percutaneous coronary balloon angioplasty was initiated in 1977 by Andreas Gruentzig and his colleagues. In those days, balloon angioplasty had a high risk (>3%) of myocardial infarction due to acute closure of the dilated vessels.[1] Coronary stenting has solved such acute complications, and has become the standard percutaneous interventional procedure. Currently, stenting is performed in more than 80% of percutaneous coronary interventions (PCI) for the treatment of de novo stenosis.[2] However, balloon angioplasty remains essential in daily interventional practice, and is undoubtedly necessary for the pre-dilatation and post-dilatation of stents, treatment of in-stent restenosis, and for small or large vessels. In these situations, stents have not added any benefit over balloon angioplasty.

New anti-restenosis strategies such as brachytherapy and drug-eluting stents have gained the spotlight in the interventional cardiology field. After the introduction of intracoronary brachytherapy, plain balloon angioplasty regained interest among interventional cardiologists, because the combination of stenting and brachytherapy was found to be inappropriate and unsafe.[3,4] Higher stent thrombosis rates and increased restenosis have been observed in this setting, while brachytherapy after balloon angioplasty better results than balloon angioplasty without radiation (R Kuntz, ACCIS presentation, 2001). Appropriate balloon angioplasty technique becomes even more relevant in the era of drug-eluting stents, as balloon injury in the adjacent segments outside the stent may be the sole mechanism responsible for restenosis. Finally, one should realize that a balloon catheter is the main component of the stent

delivery system and has a major impact on flexibility. In this chapter, we will describe the indications for and technique of balloon angioplasty.

Historical perspective

In 1977, Gruentzig and his colleagues performed the first coronary angioplasty in a living human in an operating room. This intraoperative angiogram showed obvious improvement of the lumen at the time of subsequent restudy.[5] Gruentzig[6] performed percutaneous transluminal coronary angioplasty (PTCA) for the first time outside the operating room in September 1977. The National Heart, Lung, and Blood Institute (NHLBI) initiated a registry for PTCA among 73 sites worldwide. Knowledge from this registry and live demonstration courses directed by Gruentzig greatly helped the dissemination of PTCA up to 1980. However, in those days, the equipment for PTCA was quite primitive and bulky. Guiding catheters were 9 or 10 French (Fr) made of solid polytetrafluoroethylene (PTFE). In the early 1980s, guiding catheters and introducer sheaths were improved for PTCA. First-generation balloon catheters were fixed to the guidewire, which made it difficult to cross tight or tortuous lesions. The next step in percutaneous intervention was the development of steerable guidewires[7] to allow good control for the operator and advancement to distal sites in the treated coronary arteries. This system was developed by Simpson in 1981 and the success rates of PTCA increased tremendously. Guiding catheters and balloon catheters have been improved remarkably over the past decade. Currently, 6 Fr is the most common catheters size, while 5 Fr guiding catheters are also available. Initially, balloon catheters used over-the-wire systems, but new monorail systems have become popular as they allow the use of short guidewires, which facilitates the performance of PTCA by a single operator. With the progression in balloon technology, such as the use of different types of balloons, better materials, better coatings, and lower-profile systems,[8] the balloon catheter now permits improved delivery, increased comformability, higher burst pressure, and lower compliance for more accurate balloon sizing. All of these advancements have enabled higher success rates in the setting of balloon angioplasty (nearly 90%) as well as in all other coronary interventions (>90%).

Balloon technology

Construction of balloon catheters

The balloon catheter consists of three parts: the shaft, the lumen, and the balloon (Figure 8.1). The shaft refers to the area between the hub and the balloon. The shaft size influences the performance of the catheter. A larger shaft gives greater pushability and faster inflation/deflation times. A smaller shaft design may be better in flexibility, visualization, and crossability, but may compromise pushability and wire moveability. There are mainly two types of shafts available: hypotube and corewire types. The hypotube is superior in terms of the balance between small profile and pushability (Maverick 2, Viva, Arashi, Gemini, Stormer, Maestro, among others). The corewire shaft is superior in terms of flexibility (Sierra, Bonnie, Hayate Pro, CrossSail, among others).

Lumen technology has been developed to give superior pushability and trackability. Bilumen and triple-lumen designs were used initially (Figure 8.2). Currently, the coaxial shaft, which is a tube within a tube, is the most popular type. The innermost space is the lumen for the guidewire. The outer space is the inflation/deflation lumen. This low-profile shaft enables the kissing balloon technique using 6 Fr guiding catheters. Since the wire is in the center, the catheter push and also the amount of forward columnar force are uniformly distributed along the length and circumference of the shaft.

Balloons are constructed of different types of material and are bonded onto the shaft. The distal tip is an important element of the balloon technology. The distal tip is usually tapered, which allows it to cross the lesion less traumatically in order to get the balloon in position. The profile of the distal tip will determine how much push is needed to get across the lesion. Coating is also one of the most important determinants for the ability to cross the lesion. The inner lumen of the catheter is also coated to allow for better wire movement. A hydrophilic coating is superior in crossabilty. A slippery characteristic is not suitable for in-stent restenosis, since the balloon will easily slip out of the lesion when it is inflated. Balloon materials will be discussed later.

Types of balloon catheters

There are several different types of balloons: over-the-wire; monorail (sliding rail or rapid exchange); on-the-wire; and perfusion (Figures 8.1 and 8.3).

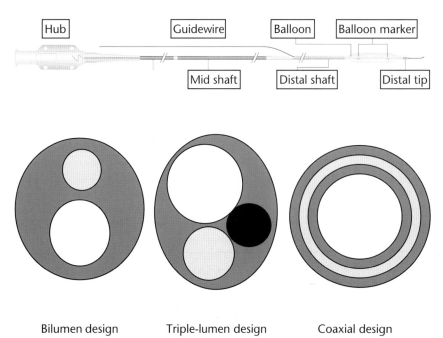

Figure 8.1
Construction of the balloon catheter (monorail type).

Hub | Guidewire | Balloon | Balloon marker
Mid shaft | Distal shaft | Distal tip

Figure 8.2
Construction of balloon shafts. The bilumen and triple-lumen designs have higher profiles. The coaxial type is the current standard.

Bilumen design   Triple-lumen design   Coaxial design

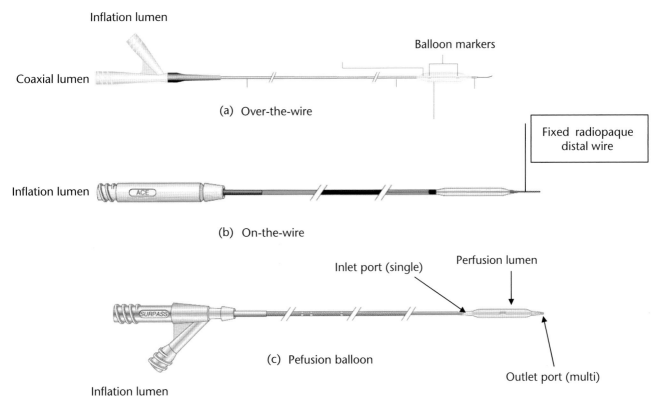

Inflation lumen

Coaxial lumen

Balloon markers

(a) Over-the-wire

Fixed radiopaque
distal wire

Inflation lumen

(b) On-the-wire

Inlet port (single)

Perfusion lumen

(c) Pefusion balloon

Outlet port (multi)

Inflation lumen

Figure 8.3
Construction of balloon catheters (other than monorail – see Figure 8.1). (a) Over-the-wire system. (b) On-the-wire system. (c) Perfusion balloon.

Over-the-wire system (Figure 8.3a)

The over-the-wire system requires two operators to manipulate the catheter. In this type of system, the guidewire and balloon catheter move independently of each other. The catheter has a lumen through its entire length that tracks over a guidewire. The operator can exchange balloon catheters only with a 300 cm exchange length wire or specific products (Trapper or Magnet) in order to maintain the wire position across the lesion. A major disadvantage is increased exposure to radiation because the fluoroscopy needs to be on during the placement of the balloon.

Monorail system (sliding rail or rapid exchange system; Figure 8.1)

The monorail catheter is a catheter where only the distal 15–25 cm of the balloon catheter tracks over the guidewire. The advantage of this system are less procedural time, a single operator, reduced fluoroscopy time, and no additional devices for the exchange.[9] The monorail system is therefore most popular system currently.

On-the-wire system (Figure 8.3b)

The on-the-wire balloon is a system often referred to as a fixed system. The guidewire and balloon are on the system. The guidewire cannot be advanced independently over the balloon. This system does not allow for guidewire exchange. The advantage of this system is that it has the lowest profile. Its disadvantages are the inability to exchange for another balloon catheter without having to recross the lesion and the need to remove the whole system if the wire tip becomes damaged.

Perfusion balloon (Figure 8.3c)

This catheter may be either an over-the-wire or a monorail design. It is a balloon catheter that has perfusion side holes proximal and distal to the actual balloon. As the balloon is inflated, the perfusion side holes allow blood to enter the catheter through the proximal holes, flow within the inflated balloon, and exit the catheter's distal side holes. The advantage of this system is that the balloon can be inflated for longer periods of time without causing chest pain due to the distal blood flow provided. This type

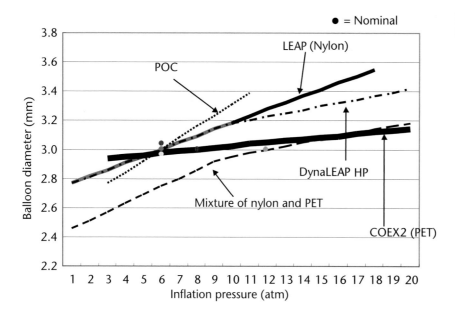

Figure 8.4
Comparison of balloon compliance.

of balloon is exclusively used for specific situations, such as coronary perforation and abrupt closure, that cannot be recovered by a stent. The disadvantage of this system is the decreased trackability due to its larger diameter.

Balloon materials

Most balloons are composed of one or a combination of the following materials. The differences are mainly in terms of elasticity, which influences balloon compliance (Figure 8.4).

Polyolefin copolymer (POC)

This is the most compliant of all balloon materials. POC has the greatest elasticity or ability to stretch. Balloon sizing is important when using this material, because over-sizing can easily occur. In addition, compliant balloons tend not only to stretch in diameter but also to overexpand into the areas of least resistance, i.e. proximal and distal to the lesion (known as 'dog-boning'). Therefore, angiographic dissection has been observed more commonly and to a significantly greater extent among patients undergoing POBA with compliant balloons. Crossability may be superior in this type.

Polyethylene (PE)

This is less compliant than POC, and has moderate elasticity characteristics.

Nylon

This is a thick material, which is compliant at higher pressures. Nylon tends to have higher mean burst pressures.

Polyethylene terephthalate (PET)

This is a noncompliant strong balloon material. PET creates a thicker-walled balloon. These factors allow physicians to work at higher pressures. Therefore, a hard calcified lesion or post-stent dilatation would be suitable for a balloon using this material.

POBA indications

In the beginning, PTCA was limited to patients who were symptomatic, clinically stable, and had good left ventricular function and were good candidates for coronary artery bypass surgery. Lesion indication was also limited. The patients had to have single-vessel disease with proximal, discrete, concentric, noncalcified, non-occluded, non-angulated stenoses that did not involve major side branches. In the early 1990s, indications for PTCA have been remarkably expanded. Because of the enthusiasm with new interventional devices, plain balloon angioplasty was nicknamed plain 'old' balloon angioplasty (POBA). However, this procedure still remains an important component of the interventional arena, whereas most of the so-called 'new devices', except for stents, have proven to be ineffective.

Nowadays, elderly patients and those with acute myocardial infarction, unstable angina, or poor left ventricular function are treated with coronary interventions. Patients with multivessel disease, left main and bypass grafts, calcified, angulated, bifurcated, or totally occluded lesions can be candidates in the proper conditions. Contraindications may be limited to very high-risk patients with some acute disease such as cerebral hemorrhage, gastrointestinal bleeding, acute severe infection (i.e. sepsis), and allergy to heparin and antiplatelet agents.

Table 8.1   Indications for POBA

Clinical indications
- Patients with evident ischemia with significant obstructive lesions
  - Acute myocardial infarction
  - Unstable angina
  - Stable angina
  - Depressed left ventricular function
  - Elderly
  - Post coronary artery bypass surgery

Morphologic indications
- Sites
  - Single and multivessel
  - Left main (protected or unprotected[†])
  - Saphenous vein[†]
  - Arterial grafts
- Lesions
  - Discrete, concentric*
  - Tandem, long, eccentric, diffuse
  - Angulated
  - Bifurcation (for side branch[†])
  - Total and subtotal occlusions
  - Ostial, proximal[†]
  - Mid and distal
  - Calcified
  - In-stent restenosis*
  - Small and large vessels*

* Good indications for POBA.
[†] Relative contraindications for POBA.

Lesion morphology may not be an absolute contraindication in the current era of coronary interventions. However, it is nevertheless important to note that we always have to estimate the benefit from the intervention for the patient in each case. If the risk of the intervention exceeds the benefit, we cannot intervene.

General indications for POBA are listed in Table 8.1. Among these indications, a few may be considered to favor POBA over other new approaches. First, POBA gives equivalent effects to stenting in treating small vessels.[10–12] In particular, so-called 'stent-like results' may be obtained in this setting. It has been demonstrated that stents give greater and more certain neointimal growth than POBA, despite the latter providing higher initial lumen gain. In a small vessel, it is rather difficult to gain enough lumen to compensate for the later loss even when using coronary stents. Second, as already described, POBA has a better outcome than stenting in the setting of intracoronary brachytherapy. Other contraindications such as metal allergy and contraindications for ticlopidine or clopidogrel should also be considered.

Successful angioplasty begins with an understanding of the lesion. Balloon type and material selection are very dependent on the type, location, severity, and morphology of the lesion.

1. *Long lesions.* These are defined as lesions greater than 20 mm in length. These lesions may be treated with a long balloon catheter in order to avoid causing dissection at the edges of the atheroma.[13] Long balloon catheters are available in 30 and 40 mm lengths.

2. *Soft lesions.* These may be of recent development and have a high concentration of lipid. To dilate soft lesions, low inflation pressure will be sufficient.

3. *Bifurcated lesions.* A bifurcation lesion is a complex lesion associated with increased complications and decreased success rate after angioplasty. Contributing factors are extensive disease, elastic recoil, increased chance of dissection, and increased chance of side-branch occlusion. Two or three guidewires and multiple balloon catheters may be necessary to treat bifurcation lesions (kissing balloon technique, KBT). Low-profile balloon catheters (VIVA, Marverick 2, Maestro, Stormer, among others) using a hypotube shaft are appropriate for KBT if the operator wants to dilate after stenting and is using 6 Fr guiding catheters.

4. *Calcified lesions.* These contain cholesterol, connective tissue, and arterial muscle cells. They have a greater chance of dissection and perforation. The preferred choice of balloon catheter is a noncompliant balloon that allows higher inflation pressures in an attempt to crack the lesion. A Rotablator may be required to allow dilatation of heavily calcified lesions.

5. *Bend (angle) lesions.* These are described as lesions on an angulated segment of the coronary artery. They have a higher complication and restenosis rate when angioplastied.[13] The complication rate contributes to the vessel trauma as the vessel is straightened when the balloon is inflated. POBA may not be enough to treat bend lesions, in which case stenting would be preferred.

6. *Total occlusions.* These are lesions that are completely occluded. A 1.5 mm high-crossability balloon would be the first choice of balloon size for a first pass through a total occlusion if it is very hard. Outcome predictability is strongly influenced by the length and duration of the occlusion (success rates are lower for lesions over 3 months old).[14] Chronic occlusions have been shown to involve higher equipment costs, greater amounts of contrast use, longer periods of fluoroscopy,[15] a lower recanalization rate, and higher incidences of reocclusion and restenosis.[16,17] Stenting has improved the outcome of patients undergoing PCI especially in this type of lesion.[18]

7. *Ostial lesions.* The success rates in treating lesions at the opening of the coronary vessel are decreased because of elastic recoil, abrupt closure, and dissection caused by the guiding catheter. The rate of restenosis is also high. Other strategies may be significantly better for treatment of these lesions.

8. *Saphenous vein graft (SVG).* SVG lesions are extremely high-risk lesions for POBA because of the high incidence of distal embolization. Stenting with distal

protection devices may produce a more successful outcome.[19]

9. *Thrombus.* Lesions containing thrombus are also at high risk of embolization. It is strongly recommended that heparinization and potent antiplatelet therapies be employed for reducing the clot prior to angioplasty unless it is in the setting of acute ST-elevation myocardial infarction (ASTMI). Regardless of the higher risk of distal embolization and microvascular damage, stenting has a better outcome for AMI patients than POBA.[20–22] Furthermore, distal protection devices may improve the risk of these types of lesions.

10. *In-stent restenosis.* This is a major problem for current PCI because of the very high incidence of restenosis. Until the advent of brachytherapy, no new devices have had a better outcome than POBA for the treatment of in-stent restenosis.[23–25] It is important to note that POBA is the most appropriate procedure in the setting of intracoronary radiotherapy, as already described. Although the 'Cutting balloon' failed to show its efficacy in preventing restenosis in the treatment of in-stent restenosis[26] (the Reduce II trial), it is technically useful for the dilatation of in-stent restenosis, since its blades prevent slip from the lesion during balloon inflation.

11. *Others.* As already mentioned, a small vessel (<2.5 mm) is one of the good indications for POBA. A large vessel (>4.0 mm) may also be a good indication for POBA because of the lower incidence of restenosis[27] and the lower availability of coronary stents. The proximal left anterior descending (LAD) artery is also known to be a higher risk lesion for restenosis,[28,29] and requires stenting. For an ostial LAD, atherectomy may be useful to avoid compromising the major side branch (circumflex).

Mechanisms of dilatation and restenosis

Balloon angioplasty is a mechanical dilatation of the lesion that results in tearing of the media and compression of the atherosclerotic plaque. The dilating force is a function of the pressure (hydrostatic force) put in the balloon, the tension being determined by the balloon diameter (according to Laplace's Law) inside the balloon wall, the balloon material/compliancy, and the vector force (the amount of constriction; Figure 8.5). Therefore, balloon size and balloon compliance are the major determinants for successful mechanical dilatation. A larger balloon will have more severe constriction of the balloon and greater dilating force at a lower pressure. A noncompliant balloon will maximize dilating force and concentrate it at the harder segment of the lesion (Figure 8.6).

In intravascular ultrasound investigations, dissection is observed in up to 60–70% of dilated segments.[30,31] Dissection may be necessary for optimal results after balloon angioplasty. Angiographic restenosis is currently recognized as 50% diameter stenosis by quantitative coronary angiography in any study. Clinical restenosis is different. Patients who have recurrent symptoms or objective signs of ischemia are considered to have clinical restenosis. Since ischemia is determined by the relative supply and demand of the coronary circulation, clinical restenosis can be less objectively defined. Restenosis is the biggest issue after PCI. In particular, balloon angioplasty has a higher restenosis rate (30–50%) compared with stenting. The differences are due to the scaffolding effect of stenting on vessel shrinkage (elastic recoil and constrictive remodeling) and gaining a larger lumen. In other words, vessel remodeling is a major cause for restenosis after balloon angioplasty, and the degree may be larger

Figure 8.5
Mechanisms of balloon dilatation. The components of the dilating force are the vector force, the tension, and the pressure of the balloon.

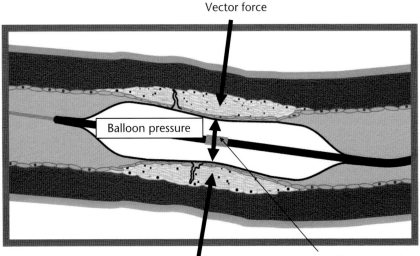

Vector force

Balloon pressure

Tension (hoop stress)

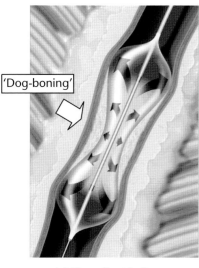

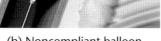

(a) Compliant balloon　　　(b) Noncompliant balloon

Figure 8.6
Difference between compliant and noncompliant balloons. (a) A compliant balloon tends to be oversized at the edges, with less dilatation at the obstructive segment of the lesion ('dog-boning'). (b) A noncompliant balloon gives a predictable amount of pressure at the lesion without uncontrolled radial and longitudinal growth.

than that of restenosis due to neointimal proliferation. Pathophysiological mechanisms for restenosis may additionally be more complex. Once the balloon injures the vessel, platelets, endothelial cells, and inflammatory cells are recruited to the vessel wall from the adventitia, and growth factors such as platelet-derived growth factor (PDGF), epidermal growth factor (EGF), fibroblast growth factor (FGF), transforming growth factor (TGF), and insulin-like growth factor (IGF) are released from these cells. Thrombin may also be involved in stimulating smooth muscle cell proliferation. The phenotypes of myofibroblasts and smooth muscle cells are switched to synthetic types from contractile types, and they begin to migrate from the adventitia to the lumen (neointima) through the fracture or tear in the media and internal elastic membrane. Extracellular matrix composed of proteoglycans and collagen subtypes is also produced by these cells and increases the volume of neointima. After this phase of proliferation, vascular shrinkage, namely remodeling, occurs, producing collagen, and this phenomenon may be similar to tissue contraction as seen in wound healing.

Complications

Death, myocardial infarction, and abrupt closure are considered as major complications of balloon angioplasty.

Death can be due to myocardial infarction, bleeding, embolization, and serious vascular complications requiring emergency surgery.

Abrupt closure is usually associated with flow-limiting intimal flaps, suboptimal dilatation, or medial dissections. Stents have almost solved this complication due to their scaffolding property.[32,33] However, in limited settings, such as small vessels that cannot be treated with coronary stents, only balloon angioplasty can be applicable. Careful attention should be paid to the presence of intimal flaps or

medial dissections. In addition, coronary brachytherapy combines poorly with coronary stents. Therefore, the technique of POBA alone is more important than before.

Coronary perforation may be less frequent during a POBA procedure than during other procedures such as atherectomy and stenting. This complication in the setting of balloon dilatation is usually associated with an oversized balloon, calcification, angulated eccentric lesions, and guidewire perforation. The operator should be very cautious when advancing a stiff and hydrophilic-coated guidewire. Recently developed guidewires, which are more completely covered with hydrophilic coating, can cross lesions very easily, but may easily penetrate the coronary artery.

Arterial injury, either coronary or aortic, may be caused by the tips of guiding catheters. Guiding catheters that tend to jump into the coronary ostium should be avoided. Careful attention should be made when using large (8 Fr or more) guiding catheters during insertion into a coronary ostium with atherosclerosis, in order to avoid serious injury. Dissection of the left main coronary artery, the ostium of the right coronary artery, and the ascending aorta often leads to a fatal complication.

The incidence of these major complications depends on the operator's skill and on patient selection.

Procedure of POBA

Puncture of the vascular access site

Currently, femoral, brachial, and radial arteries are used for access sites for coronary intervention. Although each site has its own advantages and disadvantages, any approach can be applicable for balloon angioplasty through 6 Fr guiding catheters, and even through 5 Fr guidings. The transradial approach may have a limitation when using bulky devices such as atherectomy devices (7–8 Fr guiding catheters are required). Considering that 80% of current interventions involve stenting, a routine transradial approach may be advantageous in terms of reducing the effects of hemostasis and bleeding complications. Recently, suture-mediated closure devices and sealing devices have been developed, which may save physicians' efforts in the removal of the sheath. It is important to note that complications related to vascular access depend on the operator's skill as well as other complications.

Guiding catheters

A guiding catheter should be placed in a coaxial position in the coronary ostium in order to obtain adequate backup and to avoid coronary injury. Selection of a guiding catheter can be the same as for other interventional devices. In brief, the Judkins catheter is selected for the usual lesions. An experienced operator may also use these standard types of catheters for complex lesions by inserting them deeply into the coronary artery. Amplatz and other catheters with additional backup (Voda, EBU, XB, CLS, Muta, and Ikari) may be useful for the treatment of complex lesions such as chronic total occlusions and calcified and tortuous lesions. Balloon angioplasty does not usually need strong backup catheters. However, bailout stenting is often required in cases of dissection, abrupt closure, and suboptimal results. On such occasions, stronger backup guiding may be helpful.

Advancing the guidewire

The development of the steerable guidewire is one of the revolutions in interventional cardiology. The over-the-wire system was a major advance in equipment technology, allowing manipulation of the guidewire independently from the balloon catheter. One can get support from the balloon catheter, when using an over-the-wire system. Nowadays, however, the rapid exchange (monorail) system is becoming more popular than the over-the-wire system. This system allows catheters to be charged by one operator, as already described. With progression in guidewire technology, the ability to reach more difficult coronary destinations has become easier, even without balloon catheter support.

Guidewires should be advanced while being rotated slowly and following a guiding map on the screen. For bifurcated lesions, it is sometimes necessary to insert two guidewires for each branch (KBT; see the discussion above on POBA indications – point 3). In cases of difficult coronary stent placement or balloon introduction, two guidewires may be necessary in the same coronary artery (buddy wire technique).

Selection of balloon catheters

The functional properties of a balloon catheter may be determined by the following: (i) crossability; (ii) rated burst pressure; (iii) steerability of the guidewire; (iv) the degree of compliance; (v) the length and size of the balloon; (vi) the capability of rewrapping; (vii) the speed of deflation; (viii) equality of the dilatation pressure on the balloon surface; (ix) the capability of coronary perfusion. For example, lesions with chronic total occlusions are usually hard and require lower profile balloons with superior crossability. Crossability consists of trackability (the ability to reach the lesion) and pushability (the ability to pass the lesion). Nylon elastomer may be a suitable material for higher-crossability balloons. For calcified lesions and post stent dilatation, high-rated burst pressure and shorter balloons may be better. PET may be used for high-pressure balloon inflations. The size of the balloon should be based on the reference vessel diameter, in accordance with online quantitative coronary angiography (QCA) or visual estimation. A balloon/artery ratio of around 1.1 is currently recommended. Perfusion balloons are useful for hemostasis at the site of coronary perforation. It is important to keep in mind that the balloon increases its diameter in relation to balloon pressure.

Advancement of the balloon catheter

It is usually easy to advance the balloon catheter over the guidewire. However, very cumbersome lesions such as those that are tortuous, diffusely calcified, or chronically occluded need additional techniques. In order to succeed in crossing difficult lesions, the following techniques can be applied: the use of stronger back-up catheters, deep insertion of the guiding catheter, adding vibration, pushing the balloon while pulling the guidewire, the use of a stiff guidewire (so-called 'extra-support type'), and the buddy wire technique.

Positioning of the balloon catheter and dilatation of the lesion

The balloon should be inflated in the proper position, since balloon injury often causes a restenotic reaction. The most severe segment of the stenosis should be covered by the central part of the balloon, especially in cases of hard calcified lesions. Sometimes, however, the balloon should be placed across the entire atheromatous segment in order to avoid causing a dissection. Long balloons may be useful for this purpose. The balloon inflation duration at the appropriate site should be 30–120 s for POBA. Repetitive dilatation and slowly increasing pressure may be effective in preventing acute recoil and abrupt closure. For bailout of dissections, long inflations with a perfusion balloon used to be performed, but stenting may be better for this purpose in the current clinical era.

Assessment of the results of the procedure

After finishing the balloon angioplasty, the result is determined angiographically and clinically. Successful balloon angioplasty used to be defined by visual assessment as follows: (i) more than 20% dilatation compared with pre procedure; (ii) residual diameter stenosis less than 50%; (iii) good flow (TIMI grade 3). In the era of stenting in interventional cardiology, the standard of success has become stricter than before. Usually, the percentage diameter stenosis post stent implantation should be less than 20% in the current standard of PCI. Quantitative assessment has become more popular for the prediction of patient outcome. The gold standard measurement for assessment of the objective severity of stenosis is quantitative coronary angioplasty (QCA). QCA has demonstrated important ideas, such as minimal lumen diameter (MLD), late loss, and late loss index. MLD and reference diameter are the most significant predictors for restenosis.[32,34] Trans-stenotic gradients used to be a major tool for the assessment of the result in the early days before the development of QCA.[35] In the 1990s, pressure guidewires and flow wires have shown considerable ability to assess procedural success.[36,37] Intravascular ultrasound (IVUS) is the best tool to estimate procedural results and to understand the mechanism of dilatation and restenotic reactions. However, many trials have failed to demonstrate the efficacy of IVUS guidance in reducing restenosis rates.

Conclusions

Although many new devices have been developed for PCI, balloon angioplasty still retains an important role in the main arena of interventional cardiology. Understanding the technique of balloon angioplasty is fundamental for all interventional cardiologists.

References

1. Gruentzig AR, King SB 3rd, Schlumpf M, Siegenthaler W. Long-term follow-up after percutaneous transluminal coro-nary angioplasty. The early Zurich experience. N Engl J Med 1987;316:1127–32.
2. Holmes DR Jr, Savage M, LaBlanche JM, et al. Results of Prevention of REStenosis with Tranilast and its Outcomes (PRESTO) trial. Circulation 2002;106:1243–50.
3. Leon MB, Teirstein PS, Moses JW, et al. Localized intracoro-nary gamma-radiation therapy to inhibit the recurrence of restenosis after stenting. N Engl J Med 2001;344:250–6.
4. Morino Y, Limpijankit T, Honda Y, et al. Late vascular response to repeat stenting for in-stent restenosis with and without radiation: an intravascular ultrasound volumetric analysis. Circulation 2002;105:2465–8.
5. Gruentzig AR, Myler RK, Hanna EH, Turina MI. Coronary transluminal angioplasty. Circulation. 1977;55/56:84 (abst).
6. Gruentzig AR. Translumination dilatation of coronary artery stenosis (letter to editor). Lancet 1978;i:263.
7. Simpson JB, Baim DS, Robert EW, Harrison DC. A new catheter system for coronary angioplasty. Am J Cardiol 1982;49:1216–22.
8. Finci L, Meier B, Roy P, et al. Clinical experience with the Monorail balloon catheter for coronary angioplasty. Cathet Cardiovasc Diagn 1988;14:206–12.
9. Linnemeier TJ, McCallister SH, Lips DL, et al. Radiation exposure: comparison of rapid exchange and conventional over-the-wire coronary angioplasty systems. Cathet Cardiovasc Diagn 1993;30:11–14.
10. Briguori C, Nishida T, Adamian M, et al. Coronary stenting versus balloon angioplasty in small coronary artery with complex lesions. Cathet Cardiovasc Interv 2000;50:390–7.
11. Kastrati A, Schomig A, Dirschinger J, et al. A randomized trial comparing stenting with balloon angioplasty in small vessels in patients with symptomatic coronary artery disease. ISAR–SMART Study Investigators. Intracoronary stenting or angioplasty for restenosis reduction in small arteries. Circulation 2000;102:2593–8.
12. Park SW, Lee CW, Hong MK, et al. Randomized comparison of coronary stenting with optimal balloon angioplasty for treatment of lesions in small coronary arteries. Eur Heart J 2000;21:1785–9.
13. Ellis SG. Coronary lesions at increased risk. Am Heart J 1995;130:643–6.
14. Meier B. Total coronary occlusion: a different animal? J Am Coll Cardiol 1991;17:50B–7B.
15. Bell MR, Berger PB, Menke KK, Holmes DR Jr. Balloon angioplasty of chronic total coronary artery occlusions: What does it cost in radiation exposure, time, and materi-als? Cathet Cardiovasc Diagn 1992;25:10–15.
16. Stewart JT, Denne L, Bowker TJ, et al. Percutaneous trans-luminal coronary angioplasty in chronic coronary artery occlusion. J Am Coll Cardiol. 1993;21:1371–6.
17. Puma JA, Sketch MH Jr, Tcheng JE, et al. Percutaneous revascularization of chronic coronary occlusions: an overview. J Am Coll Cardiol 1995;26:1–11.
18. Buller CE, Dzavik V, Carere RG, et al. Primary stenting versus balloon angioplasty in occluded coronary arteries: the Total Occlusion Study of Canada (TOSCA). Circulation 1999;100:236–42.
19. Baim DS, Wahr D, George B, et al. Randomized trial of a distal embolic protection device during percutaneous inter-vention of saphenous vein aorto-coronary bypass grafts. Circulation 2002;105:1285–90.
20. Stone GW, Brodie BR, Griffin JJ, et al. Clinical and angio-graphic follow-up after primary stenting in acute myocardial

infarction: the Primary Angioplasty in Myocardial Infarction (PAMI) stent pilot trial. Circulation 1999;99:1548–54.

21. Brodie BR, Stuckey TD. Mechanical reperfusion therapy for acute myocardial infarction: Stent PAMI, ADMIRAL, CADILLAC and beyond. Heart 2002;87:191–2.

22. SoRelle R. Stents are the CADILLAC of care. Controlled Abciximab and Device Investigation to Lower Late Angioplasty Complications. Circulation 2002;105:e9094–5.

23. Di Mario C, Marsico F, Adamian M, et al. New recipes for in-stent restenosis: cut, grate, roast, or sandwich the neointima? Heart 2000;84:471–5.

24. Moustapha A, Assali AR, Sdringola S, et al. Percutaneous and surgical interventions for in-stent restenosis: long-term outcomes and effect of diabetes mellitus. J Am Coll Cardiol 2001;37:1877–82.

25. Dietz U, Rupprecht HJ, de Belder MA, et al. Angiographic analysis of the angioplasty versus rotational atherectomy for the treatment of diffuse in-stent restenosis trial (ARTIST). Am J Cardiol 2002;90:843–7.

26. Mauri L, Bonan R, Weiner BH, et al. Cutting balloon angioplasty for the prevention of restenosis: results of the Cutting Balloon Global Randomized Trial. Am J Cardiol 2002; 90:1079–83.

27. de Feyter PJ, Kay P, Disco C, Serruys PW. Reference chart derived from post-stent-implantation intravascular ultrasound predictors of 6-month expected restenosis on quantitative coronary angiography. Circulation 1999;100:1777–83.

28. Ashby DT, Dangas G, Mehran R, et al. Comparison of clinical outcomes using stents versus no stents after percutaneous coronary intervention for proximal left anterior descending versus proximal right and left circumflex coronary arteries. Am J Cardiol 2002;89:1162–6.

29. Ellis SG, Shaw RE, Gershony G, et al. Risk factors, time course and treatment effect for restenosis after successful percutaneous transluminal coronary angioplasty of chronic total occlusion. Am J Cardiol 1989;63:897–901.

30. Peters RJ, Kok WE, Di Mario C, et al. Prediction of restenosis after coronary balloon angioplasty. Results of PICTURE (Post-IntraCoronary Treatment Ultrasound Result Evaluation), a prospective multicenter intracoronary ultrasound imaging study. Circulation 1997;95:2254–61.

31. Schroeder S, Baumbach A, Mahrholdt H, et al. The impact of untreated coronary dissections on acute and long-term outcome after intravascular ultrasound guided PTCA. Eur Heart J 2000;21:137–45.

32. Kuntz RE, Gibson CM, Nobuyoshi M, Baim DS. Generalized model of restenosis after conventional balloon angioplasty, stenting and directional atherectomy. J Am Coll Cardiol 1993;21:15–25.

33. Lincoff AM, Topol EJ, Chapekis AT, et al. Intracoronary stenting compared with conventional therapy for abrupt vessel closure complicating coronary angioplasty: a matched case-control study. J Am Coll Cardiol 1993;21:866–75.

34. Mintz GS, Popma JJ, Pichard AD, et al. Intravascular ultrasound predictors of restenosis after percutaneous transcatheter coronary revascularization. J Am Coll Cardiol 1996;27:1678–87.

35. De Bruyne B, Pijls NH, Paulus WJ, et al. Transstenotic coronary pressure gradient measurement in humans: in vitro and in vivo evaluation of a new pressure monitoring angioplasty guide wire. J Am Coll Cardiol 1993;22:119–26.

36. Serruys PW, di Mario C, Piek J, et al. Prognostic value of intracoronary flow velocity and diameter stenosis in assessing the short- and long-term outcomes of coronary balloon angioplasty: the DEBATE Study (Doppler Endpoints Balloon Angioplasty Trial Europe). Circulation 1997;96:3369–77.

37. Pijls NH, Bech GJ, et Gamal MI, et al. Quantification of recruitable coronary collateral blood flow in conscious humans and its potential to predict future ischemic events. J Am Coll Cardiol 1995;25:1522–8.

9

Coronary stenting

Marco A Costa

Introduction

Charles Dotter[1] first proposed the use of prosthetic devices to improve vessel patency after percutaneous balloon angioplasty in 1964. More than two decades had passed before Jacques Puel and colleagues[2] implanted the first stent in a human coronary artery in Toulouse, France. With the refinement of technology, landmark studies such as the Belgian Netherlands STENT (BE-NESTENT)[3] and the Stent Restenosis (STRESS) study[4] trials were able to demonstrate the better long-term coronary patency after stenting compared with balloon angioplasty. Currently, stents represent over 80% of all percutaneous coronary revascularization procedures performed worldwide. The success of these devices is primarily due to their mechanical ability to promote large acute gains in lumen dimensions and prevent negative vascular remodeling. The aim of this chapter is to summarize the current stent designs, techniques, and clinical indications.

Stent design

Since the early days, stent design has been altered to afford more flexibility, greater radial strength, and minimal metallic coverage[5] (Figure 9.1). The ultimate goal has been to reconcile these paradoxical features and produce a flexible device that can be deployed safely without compromising its primary scaffold function. Other important features of coronary stents are strut thickness, radiopacity, crossing profile, degree of foreshortening, and recoil. Stents can be made of stainless steel, cobalt-based alloy,

tantalum, nitinol, or polymer. The growing use of stents has stimulated the introduction of a number of different stent designs (Table 9.1).[5,6] There are five basic design types: tubular, coil, ring, multi-design, and mesh. Stents can be further categorized according to their mechanism of expansion (self-expanding or balloon-expandable). Some stent designs are similar, whereas others differ significantly, but none have incorporated all of the characteristics of an ideal stent. In principle, thin-coil stents are very flexible, but provide uneven expansion and tend to recoil, whereas thick, tubular stents provide superior coverage of the lesion and greater radial support, but lack flexibility, maneuverability and conformability.

Stainless steel, balloon-expandable stents are the most common type of stents currently used in clinical practice. Thus, the balloon delivery system has a major impact on device performance, with a direct influence on flexibility[7,8] and crossing capability. The ability of a stent to span an obstruction depends on the profile of the crimped stent (Table 9.2), the amount of friction of the delivery system against the vessel wall, the flexibility[7] of the stent and of the delivery system, and the pushability of the delivery catheter. Attempts have been made to decrease the amount of balloon protrusion outside the stent in order to minimize vessel trauma in adjacent coronary segments during deployment (Figure 9.2). However, a perfect match between stent and balloon length has not yet been achieved by any manufacturer.

Experimental and clinical studies have provided contradictory results regarding the significance of stent design in predicting long-term outcomes and restenosis.[9–14] The mechanical behavior of coronary stents may differ between in vivo and in vitro situations. This is due to the elastic properties of the arterial wall, which may be significantly altered by the presence of disease. With

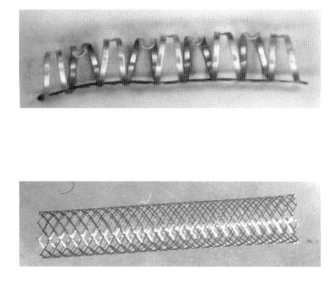

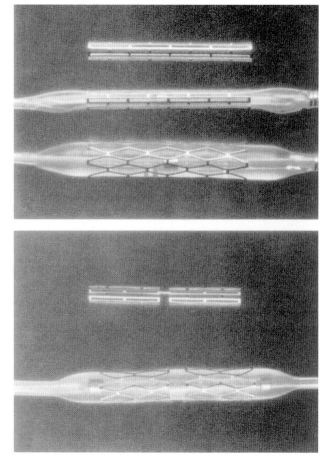

Figure 9.1
First-generation coronary stents. Expanded Palmaz–Schatz stent (original design, left upper panel; modified design with articulation, left bottom panel), Gianturco–Roubin-II (GRII) Stent (right upper panel) and Wallstent (right bottom panel). (Right hand panel reproduced from Kutryk MJ, Serrys PW. Coronary Stenting; Current Perspectives. A Companion to the Handbook of Coronary Stenting. London: Martin Dunitz, 1999.[15])

the exception of the GR-II versus Palmaz–Schatz stent study, which demonstrated the superiority of the tubular stent, early clinical trials reported similar outcomes of different stent designs.[12–14] In the experimental laboratory, Rogers and collaborators[10] have shown that increasing the number of struts per cross-section from 8 to 12 was associated with a twofold reduction in neointimal thickening after 28 days. In contrast, increasing only strut thickness from 125 to 200 μm had no significant impact on early luminal thrombus or late intimal thickening. Others have shown that thicker struts induce greater neointimal proliferation in the clinical setting, particularly in small vessels.[11,15–17] In practice, how-

ever, it seems that the impact of stent design on neointimal proliferation has not been a major determinant of stent selection. Rather, clinicians have selected stents based on their deliverability and acute success predictability. Recently, cobalt-based alloy stents became clinically available. Cobalt-chromium is stronger and more radiopaque than stainless steel, which allow the production of a stent with thinner struts, lower profiles (<0.40″), better flexibility and similar radial strength as compared to similar stent designs made of stainless steel. As these features are directly related to procedural success, cobalt-chromium stents may soon become the first choice to many operators.

Table 9.1 Different stent designs

Stent design	Stent	Composition	Manufacturer	Strut thickness (mm)	Recoil (%)	Shortening (%)	Radiopacity	Marker
Coil	GRII	Stainless steel	Cook	0.076	9–11	0	Low	On stent
	Wiktor	Tantalum	Medtronic	0.13	9	4	High	None
	Angiostent	Platinum/iridium	Angiodynamics	0.127	7	12	High	No
	Freedom	Stainless steel	Global	0.175	5–9	0	Low	No
Slotted tube	MAC Carbon Stent	Stainless steel	AMG	0.085	3	1	Low	None
	Biodivysio SV	PC-coated	Biocompatibles/Abbot	0.05	1	4	Low	None
	Biodivysio AS	Stainless steel		0.091	2	4	Low	None
	Biodivysio OC	Stainless steel		0.091	4	4	Low	None
	Teneo Tenax-XR	a-SiC:H/tantalum	Biotronik	0.08	5	3	Low	On stent
	LP Stent	Stainless steel	Boston Scientific	0.1	2	3–5	Low	None
	Carbostent Sirius, 4 cells	Stainless steel	Sorin	0.075	3–5	0	Low	Yes
	Cook V-Flex	Stainless steel	Cook	0.07	1	0	Low	None
	Palmaz–Schatz	Stainless steel	Cordis, J&J	0.07	6	8	Low	None
	BxVelocity	Stainless steel	Cordis, J&J	0.14	2.5	1.7	Medium	None
	BxSonic	Stainless steel	Cordis, J&J	0.14	2.4	1.7	Medium	None
	P-S 153	Stainless steel	Cordis, J&J	0.062	5	8	Medium	None
	PURA-A	Stainless steel	Devon	0.12	2	1–5	Low	None
	PURA Vario AL/AS	Stainless steel	Devon	0.07	3	5	Low	None
	Megaflex Genius	Stainless steel	Eurocor	0.12	1	1	High	None
	ACS Multilink	Stainless steel	Guidant	0.06	6	5	Low	None
	JoStent Flex/Plus	Stainless steel	Jomed	0.09	4	5	Low	None
	beStent 2	Stainless steel	Medtronic	0.085–0.095	2	0	Low	On stent
	R Stent	Stainless steel	ORBUS	0.13	3	0	Medium	None
	Diamond Flex AS	Stainless steel	Phytis	0.075	3–5	1	Low	None
	Radius	Nitinol	Scimed	0.11	0	3	Medium	None
	Carbostent Sirius	Stainless steel	Sorin	0.075	3–5	0	Low	On stent
	Carbostent Syncro	Carbon-coated	Sorin	0.075	3–5	0	Low	On stent
	Tsunami	Stainless steel	Terumo	0.08	5	5	Low	None
Mesh	Wallstent	Stainless steel	Schneider	0.1	—	20	Medium	None
Multiple ring	Multilink Pixel	Stainless steel		0.099	4	11	Medium	None
	Multilink Tetra	Stainless steel		0.091–0.124	2–3	3–4	Medium	None
	Multilink Penta	Stainless steel		0.091–0.124	2–3	3–4	Medium	None
	Multilink Ultra	Stainless steel		0.127–0.101	2	5	Medium	None

Table 9.1 Different stent designs (continued)

Stent design	Stent	Composition	Manufacturer	Strut thickness (mm)	Recoil (%)	Shortening (%)	Radiopacity	Marker
Multicell	Express	Stainless steel	Boston Scientific	0.132	5	5	High	None
	NIR, 7 cells and 9 cells	Stainless steel	MediNonel, BSC	0.1	3	3	Low	None
	NIR Royal	Gold		0.1	5	3	High	None
Sinusoidal ring	AVE S660	Stainless steel	Medtronic	0.127	2	1.5	Medium	None
	beStent (4 crowns)	Stainless steel		0.085–0.095	1.6–2.2	0	Low	Yes
	AVE S670	Stainless steel		0.127	3	3	Medium	None
	AVE S7	Stainless steel		0.102	2	3	Medium	None

	Profile (mm)		
Table 9.2 Crossing profile and conformability of coronary stents			
Stent	Mounted on 2.5 mm balloon:	Mounted on 3.0 mm balloon:	Conformability[a]
Biodivysio SV	0.84		+++
Multilink Pixel	0.93		+++
AVE S660	0.99		++++
JoStent		1.0	+++
Carbostent	1.02	1.04	+++
Multilink Penta	1.04	1.07	+++
Biodivysio AS		1.07	+++
Express	1.02	1.09	+++
AVE S670		1.09	++++
R stent		1.1	+++
Multilink Tetra	1.04	1.12	+++
NIR-Sox	1.09	1.12	+
BxSonic	1.07	1.14	++
beStent 2	1.07	1.17	+++
BxVelocity	1.07	1.17	++

[a] +, poor; ++, acceptable; +++, good; ++++, excellent.

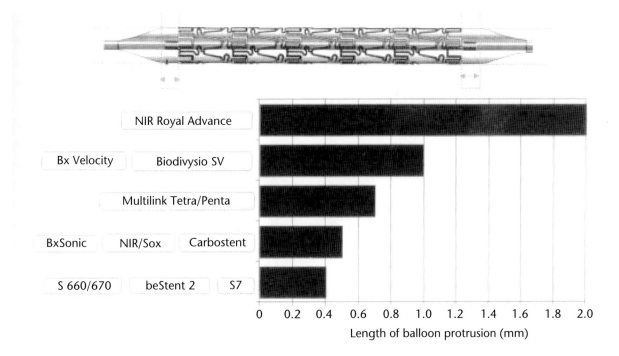

Figure 9.2
Length of balloon protrusion outside the stent.

Stent technique

Stent technique has changed considerably since Sousa (São Paulo, Brazil) and colleagues implanted the first Palmaz–Schatz stent, the prototype of current balloon-expandable tubular stents, in a human coronary artery in 1987 (Figure 9.3). The use of aggressive anticoagulation regimens was standard in the early days of coronary

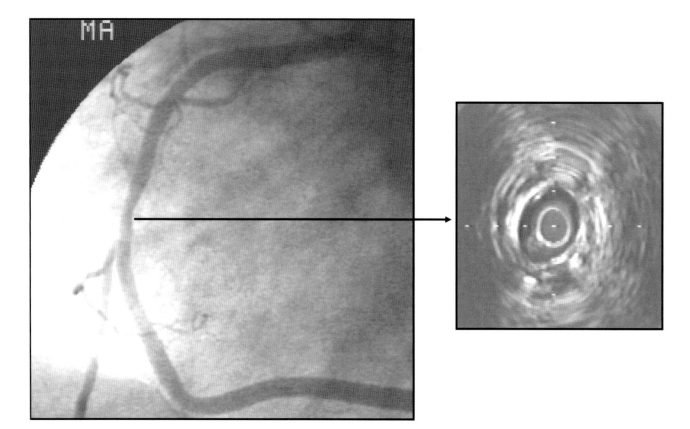

Figure 9.3
Human right coronary artery 13 years after the implantation of the first Palmaz–Schatz Stent. Intravascular ultrasound cross-section at the minimal lumen area, showing minimal intimal proliferation. (Courtesy of Professor J Eduardo Sousa, MD, PhD, São Paulo, Brazil.)

stents due to the catastrophic consequences of stent thrombosis. The anticoagulation protocol in the BENES-TENT[3] included 250–500 mg of aspirin daily and 75 mg of dipyridamole three times a day continued for 6 months. During the procedure, a continuous infusion of dextran (1000 ml) and a bolus dose of 10 000 U of heparin were used, followed by a combination of heparin and oral warfarin for the next 36 hours. Warfarin therapy was continued for 3 months. Despite this very aggressive anticoagulation regimen, stents were still facing skepticism due to the high incidence of thrombotic complications.[18]

Colombo and his group[19] demonstrated that normalization of the rheology inside the stent, as well as its inflow and outflow, was more important than anticoagulation therapy to minimize the intrinsic thrombogenic nature of stents. They demonstrated that most of the angiographically satisfactory stent deployments still showed incomplete apposition or inadequate expansion on intravascular ultrasound. The use of larger noncompliant balloons and/or higher inflation pressures to optimize stent expansion and apposition, combined with ticlopidine and aspirin antiplatelet therapy alone, produced very low thrombosis rates and similarly a low incidence of vascular complica-

tions. Other trials confirmed the efficacy of dual therapy with aspirine–ticlopidine over anticoagulation with warfarin.[20] These revolutionary concepts became routine clinical practice and paved the way for a widespread acceptance of coronary stents.

Stent sizing and inflation pressure

Selection of appropriate stent size is a critical step for both acute and long-term success. There should be a balance between stent size and inflation pressure so that deployment is optimized without compromising procedure safety. The balloon–artery ratio should remain between 1.0 and 1.1. As improvements in current stent designs evolve, less adjunctive balloon dilatation may be needed. Noncompliant balloons should be used when postprocedure dilatation is performed.

Intravascular ultrasound (IVUS) studies have shown that, even when high inflation pressures are applied, approximately one-third of the angiographically satisfactorily deployed stents are still underexpanded.[21] However, the systematic use of very high-pressure (>18 atm) balloon inflations or oversizing stents, or both, based on the assumption that the vessel would be bigger than observed on angiography, is not recommended and may be hazardous. The risk of oversizing stents involves edge dissection and vessel perforation,[22] while undersizing may increase the chance of stent thrombosis due to incomplete apposition and restenosis due to unsatisfactory lumen gain.[23] Currently, IVUS is the only guide to optimally size the stent, but the results of randomized studies have not demonstrated the long-term benefit of IVUS-guided stent deployment as compared with angiographically guided procedures.[24]

Provisional stenting

The strategy of balloon angioplasty with a stand-by stent to be implanted whenever needed (so-called provisional stenting) may represent a reduction in costs and good long-term outcome when a 'stent-like' result is obtained with balloon angioplasty alone.[25] Before unconditionally applying the strategy of provisional stenting in daily practice, one should consider that routine stent implantation was cost-effective in the BENESTENT II trial,[26] and that the subgroup of patients with 'stent-like' results after angioplasty had a clinical outcome that was still 6% inferior to that of the stented patients.

It is unlikely that 'stent-like' results will be achieved by angioplasty without adjunctive IVUS or physiological assessment, which may ultimately increase the cost of the procedure. Indeed, preliminary data from the DEBATE II trial,[27] in which optimal results were guided by quantitative coronary angiography (QCA) (residual diameter stenosis < 35%) and Doppler flow wire (CFR > 2.5) measurements, showed that both unconditional and provisional stenting strategies had similar 1-year clinical outcome and that unconditional stenting was more cost-effective. An interesting and somewhat puzzling finding was that an improvement in event-free survival at 1 year was further achieved by stent implantation after an initial 'stent-like' balloon angioplasty. In view of these considerations, a strategy of provisional stenting will not improve clinical outcome or reduce costs of percutaneous procedures,[25,28] but it may postpone stenting in up to 50% of patients, which may have some benefit, considering the insidious and 'malignant' problem of in-stent restenosis, particularly in patients with small coronary arteries.

Direct stenting

The standard stent implantation technique involves predilation with a balloon to open the vessel and to facilitate passage and positioning of the stent. Reduction in both cost and restenosis rate may be further obtained by applying a strategy of direct stenting (without balloon predilatation),[28] although the benefit of direct stenting on angiographic outcome needs to be confirmed in randomized clinical trials. With improvements in stent flexibility and a decrease in the crossing profiles of new-generation stents, particularly the new cobalt-chromium stents, direct stent placement without balloon predilatation has become more widespread.[28] This technique is theoretically less traumatic to the vessel wall, and may be particularly beneficial in the presence of thrombus[29] or when treating degenerated vein grafts. Direct stenting is associated with shorter procedure times and decreased utilization of contrast agents and equipment without compromising clinical outcome.[30,31] However, tight or heavily calcified lesions, particularly those located in tortuous vessels, may lead to a greater risk of stent dislodgement from the delivery balloon and potential embolization of the stent. Predilatation would also be preferred when precise positioning of the distal end of the stent is mandatory. Potentially poor visualization of the vessel distal to the stent may occur, particularly in critical stenoses. The use of a proximal anatomical landmark, such as a side branch or calcium spot, to guide stent positioning is usually helpful during direct stenting. The use of extra support guidewires and optimal catheter guide support are recommended.

Spot stenting

The concept of using the shortest possible stent only in the particular segments of a lesion where the luminal result does not meet IVUS criteria for an optimal result after balloon angioplasty – so-called 'spot stenting' – has been proposed by Colombo and colleagues.[32] This is an attractive strategy, given the poor outcomes of long lesions treated with very long (>32 mm) stents. In a nonrandomized study, clinical events and target lesion revascularization rates were lower in the spot stenting group than in the conventional stenting group (22% versus 38% and 19% versus 34%, respectively).[32] The cost-effectiveness of such a strategy has yet to be determined. When considering the spot stenting strategy, one should also realize that IVUS guidance is required. The strategy of a non-IVUS-guided provisional stent placement may lead to bailout stenting in one-third of patients, with a threefold increased risk of periprocedural infarction, as reported in a recent randomized study.[33]

The relationship between lesion length and vessel size[34] should always be considered when choosing one strategy (unconditional long stenting) or another (spot stenting). The use of long stents to treat vessels larger than 3.5 mm in diameter provides acceptable restenosis rates, whereas minimizing stent length is important in small vessels.[34] Finally, one should consider the fact that one stent not only provides better outcome but is also cheaper than multiple stents.[35]

Clinical indications and stent selection

Initially, stents were only approved for abrupt or threatened vessel closure during balloon angioplasty.[36] Excepting the lack of randomized clinical trials comparing coronary stenting versus medical therapy, acceptable clinical indications supported by reasonable levels of scientific evidence are listed below:

1. Primary reduction of restenosis in de novo, focal lesions in vessels larger than 3.0 mm.[3,4,26]
2. Primary reduction of clinical events in focal lesions in located saphenous vein grafts.[37]
3. Chronic total coronary occlusions.[38]
4. Primary treatment of myocardial infarction.[39]
5. Primary reduction of restenosis in long coronary lesions.[32,33]
6. Multivessel coronary disease in a nondiabetic patient with good ventricular function.[40,41]
7. Treatment of restenosis after balloon angioplasty.[42]

It is nevertheless important to note that the landmark BENESTENT and STRESS trials were accepted by clinicians as being positive overall, despite a subacute thrombosis rate of 3.7%, longer hospital stay, and more vascular and bleeding complications with stents. Moreover, the long-term clinical outcomes of patients treated with balloon angioplasty or stent in the STRESS trial were not significantly different.

The most appropriate percutaneous treatment for small vessels remains debatable. A number of clinical trials have been designed to demonstrate the superiority of stenting over balloon angioplasty to treat small (<2.8 mm) coronary vessels, but only a few have attained this goal.[43–45] The lack of customized small vessel stents and an insufficient number of patients may explain the negative results.

The predictable acute success of coronary stents may tempt clinicians worldwide to use stents in a variety of clinical and anatomical situations outside the scientific indications mentioned above. Nevertheless, unprotected left main stenosis remains a contraindication for stenting, unless the patient is not a candidate for bypass surgery.

Finally, coronary revascularization should be indicated only for significant coronary stenosis (>50% diameter stenosis). Borderline obstructions, between 50% and 60% diameter stenosis in locations other than the left main, should be treated only if ischemia is demonstrated. These recommendations should be applied for all revascularization procedures, including coronary stenting.

Stent selection

The overall performance of new-generation stent designs is excellent, with few exceptions. Some stents are more flexible than others or have a smaller crossing profile (Table 9.2) and therefore are more deliverable. However, only a minority of cases will require a specific stent design. Further, restenosis rates among different stent designs are similar. Generally, all stents are suitable for implantation in native coronary arteries. Few stents, however, have been designed for specific situations. The Multilink Ultra Stent (Guidant, Temecula, CA), as well as the polytetrafluoroethylene (PTFE)-covered JoStent Graft (JoMed, Rangendingen, Germany), are specifically made for vein graft implantation. Covered stents or stent grafts have also been used to treat coronary ruptures and aneurysms, but their routine application in native coronary arteries is limited due to the risk of side-branch occlusion. Table 9.3 illustrates some of the situations that may benefit from a particular stent characteristic.

Table 9.3 Selection of stent for specific conditions.	
Clinical and anatomical situation	*Desirable stent features*
Calcified lesions	Good radial support, low friction
Calcified vessels	Low friction, high flexibility, low crossing profile, good radial support
Lesion located on a curve (>90°)	High conformability and flexibility
Proximal vessel tortuosity	High flexibility, low friction, low crossing profile
Bifurcation involving large side branch	Open cell design
Ostial lesions	Good radial support, good radiopacity
Vein grafts, thrombus-containing lesion, total occlusions	Good lesion coverage and radial support
Small vessels	Thin stent strut, high flexibility
Diffuse disease	Minimal balloon overhand
Significant vessel tapering	Minimal balloon overhand
Direct stenting	Low crossing profile, low friction, high flexibility
Vessel perforation	Covered stents

References

1. Dotter CT, Judkins MP. Transluminal treatment of arteriosclerotic obstruction. Description of a new technique and a preliminary report of its application. Radiology 1989;172:904–20.

2. Puel J, Juilliere Y, Bertrand ME, et al. Early and late assessment of stenosis geometry after coronary arterial stenting. Am J Cardiol 1988;61:546–53.

3. Serruys PW, de Jaegere P, Kiemeneij F, et al. A comparison of balloon-expandable-stent implantation with balloon angioplasty in patients with coronary artery disease. Benestent Study Group. N Engl J Med 1994;331:489–95.

4. Fischman DL, Leon MB, Baim DS, et al. A randomized comparison of coronary-stent placement and balloon angioplasty in the treatment of coronary artery disease. Stent Restenosis Study Investigators. N Engl J Med 1994;331:496–501.

5. Kutryk MJB, Serruys PW. Coronary Stenting. Curent Perspectives. A Companion to the Handbook of Coronary Stents. London: Martin Dunitz, 1999.

6. Colombo A, Stankovic G, Moses JW. Selection of coronary stents. J Am Coll Cardiol 2002;40:1021–33.

7. Ormiston JA, Dixon SR, Webster MW, et al. Stent longitudinal flexibility: a comparison of 13 stent designs before and after balloon expansion. Cathet Cardiovasc Interv 2000;50:120–4.

8. Holmes DR Jr, Lansky A, Kuntz R, et al. The PARAGON stent study: a randomized trial of a new martensitic nitinol stent versus the Palmaz–Schatz stent for treatment of complex native coronary arterial lesions. Am J Cardiol 2000;86:1073–9.

9. Edelman ER, Rogers C. Stent-versus-stent equivalency trials: Are some stents more equal than others? Circulation 1999;100:896–8.

10. Garasic JM, Edelman ER, Squire JC, et al. Stent and artery geometry determine intimal thickening independent of arterial injury. Circulation 2000;101:812–18.

11. Escaned J, Goicolea J, Alfonso F, et al. Propensity and mechanisms of restenosis in different coronary stent designs: complementary value of the analysis of the luminal gain-loss relationship. J Am Coll Cardiol 1999;34:1490–7.

12. Baim DS, Cutlip DE, O'Shaughnessy CD, et al. Final results of a randomized trial comparing the NIR stent to the Palmaz–Schatz stent for narrowings in native coronary arteries. Am J Cardiol 2001;87:152–6.

13. Baim DS, Cutlip DE, Midei M, et al. Final results of a randomized trial comparing the MULTI-LINK stent with the Palmaz–Schatz stent for narrowings in native coronary arteries. Am J Cardiol 2001;87:157–62.

14. Heuser R, Lopez A, Kuntz R, et al. SMART: the microstent's ability to limit restenosis trial. Cathet Cardiovasc Interv 2001;52:269–77; discussion 278.

15. Kastrati A, Dirschinger J, Boekstegers P, et al. Influence of stent design on 1-year outcome after coronary stent placement: a randomized comparison of five stent types in 1,147 unselected patients. Cathet Cardiovasc Interv 2000;50:290–7.

16. Briguori C, Sarais C, Pagnotta P, et al. In-stent restenosis in small coronary arteries: impact of strut thickness. J Am Coll Cardiol 2002;40:403–9.

17. Kastrati A, Mehilli J, Dirschinger J, et al. Intracoronary stenting and angiographic results: strut thickness effect on restenosis outcome (ISAR–STEREO) trial. Circulation 2001;103:2816–21.

18. Serruys PW, Strauss BH, van Beusekom HM, et al. Stenting of coronary arteries: Has a modern Pandora's box been opened? J Am Coll Cardiol 1991;17:143B–54B.

19. Colombo A, Hall P, Nakamura S, et al. Intracoronary stenting without anticoagulation accomplished with intravascular ultrasound guidance. Circulation 1995;91:1676–88.

20. Leon MB, Baim DS, Popma JJ, et al. A clinical trial comparing three antithrombotic-drug regimens after coronary-artery stenting. Stent Anticoagulation Restenosis Study Investigators. N Engl J Med 1998;339:1665–71.

21. Fitzgerald PJ, Oshima A, Hayase M, et al. Final results of the Can Routine Ultrasound Influence Stent Expansion (CRUISE) study. Circulation 2000;102:523–30.

22. Hoffmann R, Haager P, Mintz GS, et al. The impact of high pressure vs low pressure stent implantation on intimal hyperplasia and follow-up lumen dimensions; results of a randomized trial. Eur Heart J 2001;22:2015–24.

23. Kuntz RE, Safian RD, Carrozza JP, et al. The importance of acute luminal diameter in determining restenosis after coronary atherectomy or stenting. Circulation 1992;86:1827–35.

24. Schiele F, Meneveau N, Vuillemenot A, et al. Impact of intravascular ultrasound guidance in stent deployment on 6-month restenosis rate: a multicenter, randomized study comparing two strategies – with and without intravascular ultrasound guidance. RESIST Study Group. REStenosis after Ivus guided STenting. J Am Coll Cardiol 1998;32:320–8.

25. Al Suwaidi J, Berger PB, Holmes DR Jr. Coronary artery stents. JAMA 2000;284:1828–36.

26. Serruys PW, van Hout B, Bonnier H, et al. Randomised comparison of implantation of heparin-coated stents with balloon angioplasty in selected patients with coronary artery disease (Benestent II). Lancet 1998;352:673–81.

27. Serruys PW, de Bruyne B, Carlier S, et al. Randomized comparison of primary stenting and provisional balloon angioplasty guided by flow velocity measurement. Doppler Endpoints Balloon Angioplasty Trial Europe (DEBATE) II Study Group. Circulation 2000;102:2930–7.

28. Brito FS Jr, Caixeta AM, Perin MA, et al. Comparison of direct stenting versus stenting with predilation for the treatment of selected coronary narrowings. Am J Cardiol 2002;89:115–20.

29. Loubeyre C, Morice MC, Lefevre T, et al. A randomized comparison of direct stenting with conventional stent implantation in selected patients with acute myocardial infarction. J Am Coll Cardiol 2002;39:15–21.

30. Carrie D, Khalife K, Citron B, et al. Comparison of direct coronary stenting with and without balloon predilatation in patients with stable angina pectoris. BET (Benefit Evaluation of Direct Coronary Stenting) Study Group. Am J Cardiol 2001;87:693–8.

31. Wilson SH, Berger PB, Mathew V, et al. Immediate and late outcomes after direct stent implantation without balloon predilation. J Am Coll Cardiol 2000;35:937–43.

32. Colombo A, De Gregorio J, Moussa I, et al. Intravascular ultrasound-guided percutaneous transluminal coronary angioplasty with provisional spot stenting for treatment of long coronary lesions. J Am Coll Cardiol 2001;38:1427–33.

33. Serruys PW, Foley DP, Suttorp MJ, et al. A randomized comparison of the value of additional stenting after optimal balloon angioplasty for long coronary lesions: final results of the additional value of NIR stents for treatment of long coronary lesions (ADVANCE) study. J Am Coll Cardiol 2002;39:393–9.

34. Serruys PW, Kay IP, Disco C, et al. Periprocedural quantitative coronary angiography after Palmaz–Schatz stent implantation predicts the restenosis rate at six months: results of a meta-analysis of the BElgian NEtherlands Stent study (BENESTENT) I, BENESTENT II Pilot, BENESTENT II and MUSIC trials. Multicenter Ultrasound Stent In Coronaries. J Am Coll Cardiol 1999;34:1067–74.

35. Hoffmann R, Herrmann G, Silber S, et al. Randomized comparison of success and adverse event rates and cost effectiveness of one long versus two short stents for treatment of long coronary narrowings. Am J Cardiol 2002;90:460–4.

36. Roubin GS, Cannon AD, Agrawal SK, et al. Intracoronary stenting for acute and threatened closure complicating percutaneous transluminal coronary angioplasty. Circulation 1992;85:916–27.

37. Savage MP, Douglas JS, Jr., Fischman DL, et al. Stent placement compared with balloon angioplasty for obstructed coronary bypass grafts. Saphenous Vein De Novo Trial Investigators. N Engl J Med 1997;337:740–7.

38. Sirnes PA, Golf S, Myreng Y, et al. Sustained benefit of stenting chronic coronary occlusion: long-term clinical follow-up of the Stenting in Chronic Coronary Occlusion (SICCO) study. J Am Coll Cardiol 1998;32:305–10.

39. Stone GW, Grines CL, Cox DA, et al. Comparison of angioplasty with stenting, with or without abciximab, in acute myocardial infarction. N Engl J Med 2002;346:957–66.

40. Serruys PW, Unger F, Sousa JE, et al. Comparison of coronary-artery bypass surgery and stenting for the treatment of multivessel disease. N Engl J Med 2001;344:1117–24.

41. Abizaid A, Costa MA, Centemero M, et al. Clinical and economic impact of diabetes mellitus on percutaneous and surgical treatment of multivessel coronary disease patients: insights from the Arterial Revascularization Therapy Study (ARTS) trial. Circulation 2001;104:533–8.

42. Erbel R, Haude M, Hopp HW, et al. Coronary-artery stenting compared with balloon angioplasty for restenosis after initial balloon angioplasty. Restenosis Stent Study Group. N Engl J Med 1998;339:1672–8.

43. Kastrati A, Schomig A, Dirschinger J, et al. A randomized trial comparing stenting with balloon angioplasty in small vessels in patients with symptomatic coronary artery disease. ISAR–SMART Study Investigators. Intracoronary stenting or angioplasty for restenosis reduction in small arteries. Circulation 2000;102:2593–8.

44. Koning R, Eltchaninoff H, Commeau P, et al. Stent placement compared with balloon angioplasty for small coronary arteries: in-hospital and 6-month clinical and angiographic results. Circulation 2001;104:1604–8.

45. Doucet S, Schalij MJ, Vrolix MC, et al. Stent placement to prevent restenosis after angioplasty in small coronary arteries. Circulation 2001;104:2029–33.

10

Ablative techniques in coronary intervention

Paul S Gilmore

Directional coronary atherectomy

Directional coronary atherectomy (DCA) ablates plaque by cutting and physically removing the plaque material from the coronary artery. A rotating cutting blade (approximately 2000 rpm) within the distal cutting window section of the catheter is advanced across the window and cuts or shears the plaque by rotating the cutting edge. A chamber to house the resected material is contained within the catheter distal to the window (Figure 10.1). To ablate and retrieve an atherosclerotic obstruction, the device is advanced over the wire to the lesion and multiple passes are made, cutting the material and storing it in the catheter housing. A low-pressure balloon is inflated at the lesion location to press the open cutting area towards the wall of the vessel where the plaque is being ablated. Balloon deflation allows circumferential rotation of the entire catheter to orient the cutting window towards the remaining obstruction. The catheter must be removed from the body to retrieve the plaque debris. Reinsertion of the catheter and repetitive atherectomy are performed until the angiographic or intravascular ultrasound (IVUS) appearance is acceptable. The net impact on the lesion of the catheter is a combination of dottering, cutting, and balloon angioplasty (Figures 10.2–10.4).

Early multicenter studies and trials with the DCA device revealed many interesting concepts and strategies. The first studies were comparisons with balloon angioplasty in the pre-stent era. The initial atherectomy devices were bulky and the learning curves, even at high-volume cathlabs, were not mature when the first multicenter trials started. The anticipated advantage of high enrolment by using a multicenter approach may have been negated by embracing many of these immature learning curves. The initial CAVEAT (Coronary Angioplasty Versus Excisional Atherectomy Trial) and CCAT results demonstrated higher complication rates and costs with attempted stand-alone DCA compared with balloon angioplasty, with no

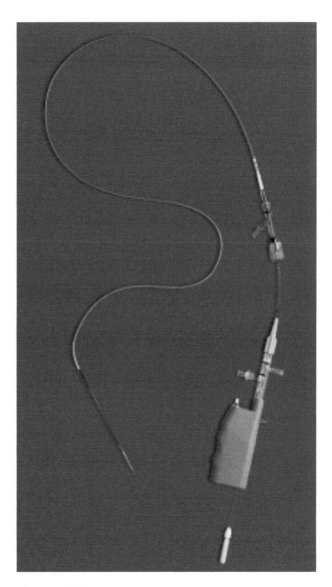

Figure 10.1
Directional coronary atherectomy (DCA) catheter and drive mechanism.

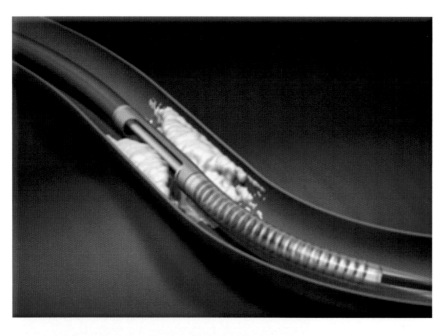

Figure 10.2
Initial DCA placement.

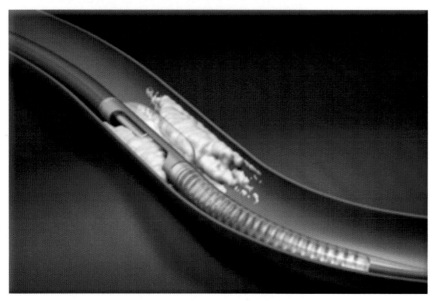

Figure 10.3
DCA: cutting process.

improvement in clinical outcome.[1–3] Issues were raised regarding myocardial enzyme elevation and subclinical infarcts and their impact on mortality and clinical outcomes.[4] Vein grafts were an attractive target due to the relatively sizable volume of obstructive atheroma, but infarcts due to distal embolization and no-reflow remained a problem and results were comparable to these of balloon angioplasty.[4] Still, individual sites with skilled operators continued to have good results, and – even following the negative results of CAVEAT – clinical use of the DCA device increased.[5]

The second series of DCA trials occurred during the development and increasing commercial availability of stents. The atherectomy catheters were improved at about that time by decreasing the size to 7 French (Fr) and softening the nose cone. These trials encouraged adjunctive balloon angioplasty use if the atherectomy results were suboptimal. The OARS (Optimal DCA Restenosis Study) registry determined the effect of high-volume operators in a few centers on the outcome of DCA. The complications were fewer, the success rate was 97.5%, and the 1-year target vessel revascularization rate was 17.8%.[6] The BOAT (Balloon versus Optimal Atherectomy Trial) results (Table 10.1) demonstrated decreased angiographic restenosis rates and no difference in cumulative infarct and death rates. The rate of target vessel revascularization was comparable between groups.[7] By 1998, when the BOAT results were published, the clinical expectations had shift-

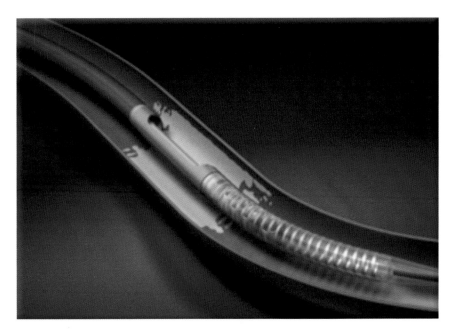

Figure 10.4
Circumferential cutting for maximum debulking.

ed from balloon angioplasty outcomes to stent angioplasty outcomes. The target lesion revascularization rates from DCA studies performed during the late 1990s were in the 15–18% range, comparable to many of the early stent restenosis outcomes.[6,8,9]

One of the seminal contributions of BOAT to interventional cardiology is clarifying the role played by a larger post-procedural lumen size in the restenotic process. 'Bigger is better' became the paradigm for debulking, and 'acute gain', 'late loss', and 'late loss index' joined the lexicon.[7]

Another concept to emerge from the DCA trials was the impact of periprocedural enzyme elevations on subsequent mortality (Table 10.1). This potential has been mitigated by the recent demonstration of reduced infarcts with intravenous platelet inhibitors.[10] The difference in outcomes between different locations and operators

raised the issue of learning curves and the development of expertise when the number of procedures is relatively low.

The SOLD (Stenting after Optimal Lesion Debulking) registry used IVUS imaging in an effort to ablate lesions to a percentage plaque area of less than 60%. The percentage plaque area was defined as vessel cross-sectional area (CSA) minus lumen CSA divided by vessel CSA. With this approach, the restenosis rate in the DCA/stent group was 11%, versus 21% in the stent group. The target lesion revascularization rate was 7% in the DCA/stent group, versus 19% in the stent group.[11]

The AMIGO (Atherectomy before Multilink Improves lumen Gain Outcome) trial results were presented by Dr Antonio Columbo at the American College of Cardiology 2002 Meetings. The intent of the study was to determine the restenosis rates of the ACS MULTILINK stent in patients with and without pre-stent DCA. There were no differences between patients who had DCA prior to stenting and those who did not. The primary outcomes of binary restenosis, major adverse cardiac events (MACE) at 6 and 12 months, and target vessel failure were not significantly different between groups.

Table 10.1   Balloon versus Optimal Atherectomy Trial (BOAT): complications (% of patients)

Complication	DCA	PTCA
Any CK-MB elevation	34	14
CK-MB > 3× normal	16	6
CK-MB > 5× normal	9	4
CK-MB > 8 or	6	2
CK-MB > 3, with missing CK-MB		
In-hospital death rate	0.0	0.4
1-year cumulative death rate	0.06	1.6

DCA, directional coronary atherectomy; PTCA, percutaneous transluminal coronary angioplasty; CK-MB, creatine kinase MB isoenzyme.

Applications of DCA

In the absence of an overarching reason for using DCA in native coronaries or saphenous vein grafts (SVGs), what are the patient- or lesion-specific indications for increasing procedural costs and demanding more operator expertise? Ostial lesions exhibit above-average restenosis rates. The probability of SVG ostial lesion restenosis[12] is unchanged by using DCA prior to stenting versus stenting alone, in that success rates, complication rates and 1-year follow-up are nearly the same. Bramucci et al[13] described low TLR rates with DCA and stenting of ostial left anterior descending (LAD) lesions. Left main ostial stenosis does seem to respond better to DCA/stent compared with stent alone.[14]

Lesion characteristics that favor the application of DCA are ostial location, especially protected left main and LAD segments, and eccentric plaque distribution where plaque shift could compromise side-branch or left main blood flow.

Unfavorable lesion characteristics are heavy calcification, tortuous vessels, vessels less than 3 mm in diameter, and degenerated vein grafts.

The optimal endpoints when performing DCA should be similar to the OARS intent. The final result should be a less than 15% residual following adjunctive balloon inflations, evidence of tissue extraction, TIMI 3 flow and, if a stent is used, no residual stenosis. IVUS guidance may help determine the residual plaque CSA and maximize the effect of atherectomy on the lesion and vessel.[8,9]

Rotational ablation

The Rotablator (Boston Scientific, Natick, MA) uses an over-the-wire, high-speed, rotating burr to ablate plaque (Figures 10.5–10.6). The mechanical characteristics of rotational ablation of plaque with the Rotablator are a fascinating application of physics to coronary artery interventions.

The main tenets of rotational ablation are differential cutting and orthogonal displacement of friction by rotating the burr at very high speeds. Ablation of plaque results in fragmentation of the plaque components into particulate

emboli, 90% of which are smaller than red blood cells. There is little impact of particulate emboli on the distal vascular bed when appropriate techniques are used. The debris is eventually cleared by the reticuloendothelial system in the spleen, liver, and bone marrow.

Differential cutting is the ability to selectively ablate atherosclerotic material while sparing the normal vessel wall. Diseased plaque is inelastic and does not deflect away from the rotating burr. The more elastic undiseased vessel wall stretches when in contact with the burr and little damage is done, though denuded endothelium has been described.[15] While all types of plaque are ablated, the calcific plaque typifies the inflexible rigid material that is pulverized into microscopic fragments by the friction caused by the diamond microchips embedded into the head of the elliptical burr, which is rotating at high speed (up to 200 000 rpm, with a working range of 150 000–170 000 rpm). While it is friction that ablates the plaque, it is important to reduce heat generation by meticulous technique. Some of the theoretical benefits of rotational atherectomy are minimizing vessel wall stretch and elastic recoil, both with the initial technique and with subsequent adjunctive balloon dilatation. There should be less barotrauma with stand-alone rotational ablation, and if balloon use is adjunctive following ablation, then low inflation pressures should be used. A smoother channel resulting from ablation, with less turbulent flow, fewer tears, and less disruption, may translate into fewer complications in the form of subacute thrombosis or eventual restenosis.[16] The technical application of rotational ablation includes a continuous flush through the sheath housing the burr. The patient should be treated with the usual aspirin and heparin anticoagulation, with nitrates and calcium blockers

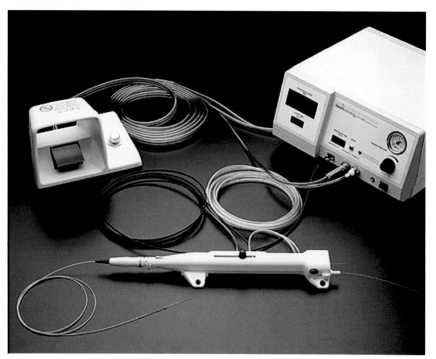

Figure 10.5
Rotablator equipment.

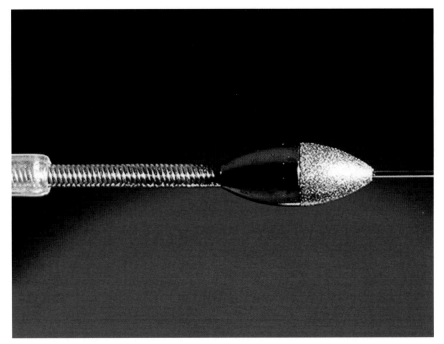

Figure 10.6
Close-up of Rotablator burr.

being useful for avoiding coronary spasm. A decrease in slow and no-reflow phenomena and reduction in creatine kinase (CK) enzyme totals have been noted with the use of intravenous platelet inhibitors.[17] An optional lubricant derived from olive oil and egg whites may be used. Two prominent burr selection strategies have been tested, and currently the most favorable approach is to use the stepped burr method. The target burr-to-artery ratio is 0.6–0.7. The initial burr size selection is based on the amount of obstruction (ablation) anticipated. Long, severely diseased segments may require sequential increases in burr diameter of 0.25 mm to 0.5 mm from a relatively conservative initial burr selection of less than 0.5 burr-to-artery ratio. A short discrete lesion in a large vessel may require a single aggressively sized burr with a burr-to-artery ratio of 0.7–0.8. The maximum drop in rotational speed while ablating the lesion should be less than 5000 rpm. Limiting the engagement of the burr in the lesion to less than 30 s will reduce heat build-up in the artery wall and surrounding tissues and allow antegrade blood flow during the breaks between lesion engagements. If adjunctive balloon angioplasty is used following ablation, low inflation pressures to minimize barotrauma and brief inflation durations to minimize the potential for decreased distal flow are advised.[18,19]

Unfavorable lesion characteristics include local thrombus at the intended site, although 'balloon-undilatable' infarct-related arteries might still require rotational ablation to allow balloon dilatation and stent placement. Severe left ventricular dysfunction suggests a limited capacity to tolerate any decrease in perfusion or function, much less slow or no-reflow. SVGs, due to the large amount of obstruction and thinner walls, limit the application of rotational ablation to lesions in the body of the

grafts. We have on occasion used the Rotablator on aorto-ostial SVG anastamotic locations, which (much like protected or unprotected left main lesions) are usually debulked prior to stenting with or without IVUS guidance. In vessels with spontaneous dissection, it is difficult to insure placement of the wire in the true lumen. Chronic total occlusions may be addressed only with proven guidewire passage into the distal vessel. Favorable lesion attributes are heavily calcified lesions, small vessels, diffuse disease involving long coronary segments, and bifurcation lesions where balloon dilatation or stenting makes side-branch occlusion likely. Side branches smaller than 1.5 mm that have over 70% stenoses occlude significantly less often with rotational ablation and stenting then stenting alone.

Predictors of complications include deceleration over 5000 rpm for longer than 10 s or deceleration over 7000 rpm for more than 5 s. Prophylactic temporary pacing or pretreatment of atropine in right coronary artery (RCA) applications help avoid transient hypotension or bradycardia, which can compromise blood flow in the interventional artery.[19]

Clinical trials with the Rotablator have investigated success rates in various settings as well as generating comparative results amongst treatment strategies. The ERBAC study compared rotational atherectomy versus laser angioplasty versus balloon percutaneous transluminal coronary angioplasty (PTCA) for native de novo coronary lesions. Procedural success was significantly higher in the rotational ablation group, with an 89.2% success rate, compared with 79.9% in the balloon group and 77.2% in the laser group. There were no differences among groups in death, coronary artery bypass grafting (CABG), Q-wave myocardial infarction, or non-Q-wave myocardial infarction. The bailout stenting rate varied from 0.5% (rotational ablation) to 1.7% (laser), with the balloon group requiring bailout stenting in 0.9% of interventions. The restenosis rates were 47% in the balloon group, 59% in the laser group and 57% in the rotational ablation group.[19]

DART compared PTCA with rotational ablation in type A or B1 lesions.[20] De novo or restenotic lesions in vessels of 2.0–2.9 mm in size were eligible for randomization. In this study, 223 patients were randomized to the rotational ablation group, with 221 patients in the PTCA group. Procedural success was excellent, with 99% of the rotational ablation and 100% of the balloon patients having a successful procedure. Bailout stenting was performed in 6% of the rotational ablation and 14% of the PTCA patients ($p = 0.01$). Slow/no-reflow was observed and treated in 8% of the rotational and 0.5% of the balloon patients ($p = 0.01$). Major dissection occurred in 8% of the rotational ablation and 16% of the PTCA patients ($p = 0.05$). Emergency treatment was needed in 10% of the PTCA patients and no rotational ablation patients ($p = 0.05$). The results were not statistically different between groups regarding acute gain, late loss, loss index ratio, or angiographic restenosis (52% rotational ablation and 48% PTCA). The target lesion revascularization rates were 22% and 18% in the rotational ablation and PTCA groups, respectively.

Much like the early DCA experience, when initial results were attributed to inadequate technique and too divergent a population, with BOAT and OARS following CAVEAT, the DART study was followed by STRATAS (Study to determine Rotablator and Transluminal Angioplasty Strategy) to determine the best burr selection strategy for safety, primary success, and angiographic restenosis.[21] The routine strategy used a burr-to-artery ratio of less than 0.7 and a balloon inflation pressure of less than 4 atm. The aggressive strategy used a burr-to-artery ratio of more than 0.7 and an inflation pressure of 1 atm on less.

The STRATAS results and complications typify the results of rotational ablation and balloon trials (Tables 10.2 and 10.3). An aggressive rotational ablation strategy followed by low-pressure inflations or as a stand-alone technique did not lower restenosis rates compared with the conservative rotational ablation strategy. Adverse clinical events were comparable between groups.

SPORT (Stenting Post Rotational atherectomy Trial) compared debulking with high-speed rotablation with balloon dilatation prior to planned stent deployment.[22] Eligible lesions were moderately calcified and/or long lesions (>15 mm diameter) in vessels less than 3.2 mm in diameter. The primary study endpoint was target vessel failure at 6 months. Additional endpoints were MACE and

Table 10.2   Study to determine Rotablator and Transluminal Angioplasty Strategy (STRATAS): results

Procedural results	Routine	Aggressive	p
Adjunctive PTCA	97	83	0
Maximal pressure (atm)	5.8	1.7	0.01
Number of burrs	1.9	2.7	0.02
Maximum burr size	1.8	2.1	0
Burr/artery ratio (QCA)	0.71	0.82	0
Angiographic success rate (%)	95.5	94.7	NS
Final MLD (mm)	1.97	1.95	NS
Residual DS (%)	26	27	NS
Follow-up MLD (mm)	1.26	1.16	NS
Follow-up DS (%)	53	56	NS
Late loss index	0.54	0.62	NS

PTCA, percutaneous transluminal coronary angioplasty; QCA, quantitative coronary angiography; MLD, minimal lumen diameter; DS, degree of stenosis.

Table 10.3   STRATAS: complications (% of patients)

Complication	Routine	Aggressive	p
Death	1.6	0.4	NS
Urgent CABG	2	0	0.03
Q-wave myocardial infarction	1.2	1.2	NS
Slow reflow	7.7	15.7	0
No-reflow	7.7	15.2	0.01
CK-MB > 5 × normal	7	11	NS
Target vessel revascularization	19.5	22.3	NS

CABG, coronary artery bypass grafting; CK-MB, creatine kinase MB isoenzyme.

angiographic restenosis at 6 months. Baseline quantitative coronary angiography (QCA) is compared in Table 10.4. Angiographic, procedural, and clinical success rates are compared in Table 10.5. Follow-up data are compared in Table 10.6. A modest increase in procedural success did not translate into long-term improvement or reduced angiographic restenosis.

Having considered rotational ablation in the pre-stent era and as an adjunctive to stenting, the next step was to investigate it as a primary treatment strategy for in-stent restenosis. The BARASTER trial compared rotational ablation, rotational ablation plus balloon, and balloon for in-stent restenosis. The ARTIST (Angioplasty versus Rotablation for the Treatment of diffuse In-stent Restenosis) trial compared rotational ablation plus low-pressure PTCA (<6 atm) with PTCA (mean inflation pressure 12.7 atm) for in-stent restenosis.[23-25] Binary angiographic restenosis (>50% diameter stenosis) was 51.2% in the PTCA group and 64.8% in the rotational ablation group ($p = 0.039$). MACE-free survival occurred in 91.1% (mean follow-up 7 months) of the PTCA group and 79.6% of the rotational ablation group (mean follow-up 8 months). More than half of the patients with diffuse in-stent restenosis had recurrent restenosis, regardless of which treatment method was used. In the ARTIST outcome data, balloon treatment was preferable to rotational ablation followed by low-pressure balloon inflation. In patients undergoing brachytherapy, there was no clinical benefit to debulking prior to brachytherapy.[26]

The improved procedural success rate in complex and highly calcified lesions justifies the expense and time involved in performing rotational atherectomy in certain situations. Heavily calcified vessels and any vessel that cannot be dilated by a conventional balloon technique are appropriate situations for rotational ablation. In addition, long diffusely diseased vessels and bifurcation lesions respond well to debulking. SVG ostia and native coronary ostia may require debulking prior to stent implantation due to the 'aortic' nature of the stenosis as opposed to native coronary arteriosclerosis. There is no benefit to using rotational ablation for debulking in-stent restenosis, although the same side-branch protection may be afforded as in native bifurcation lesions if balloon dilatation would compress plaque into a side branch.

Table 10.4   Comparison of baseline QCA

	PTCA + Stent	Rota + Stent	P value
	N=364	N=349	
Lesion length (mm)	16.0	17.0	NS
RVD (mm)	2.83 ± 0.48	2.87 ± 0.49	NS
Pre proc MLD (mm)	0.88 ± 0.42	0.87 ± 0.38	NS
% DS Pre procedure	86.0 ± 9.3	85.8 ± 10.4	NS
Post proc MLD (mm)	2.74	2.81	P=0.032
Acute gain	1.86	1.94	P=0.041

Table 10.5   Comparison of angiographic, procedural, and clinical success rates

	PTCA + Stent	Rota + Stent	P value
	N=375	N=360	
Angiographic success (%)	100	100	NS
Procedural success (%)	88.1	93.6	0.0114
Clinical success (%) (procedural success with no MACE)	87.3	91.6	NS

Table 10.6   Comparison of follow-up data

	PTCA + Stent	Rota + Stent	P Value
	N=375	N=360	
6 month follow-up (%)	94.4 (354)	94.4 (340)	NS
clinical angiographic	70	74.7	
TVR (%)	11.5	14.4	NS
Angiographic restenosis (%)	27.6	30.4	NS

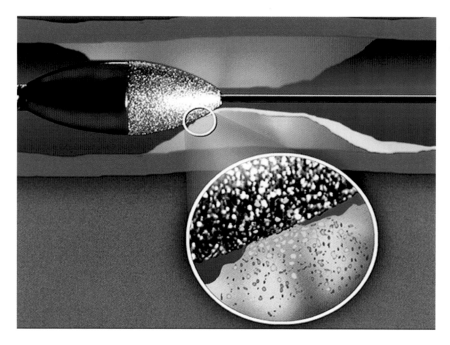

Figure 10.7
Schematic of Rotablator lesion engagement.

Applications of excimer laser coronary angioplasty

None of the ablative or debulking techniques has been demonstrated to be superior to stenting following balloon angioplasty for the treatment of uncomplicated de novo coronary lesions. In complex lesions, eximer laser coronary angioplasty (ELCA) may be superior to PTCA. Preisack[27] compared these techniques in lesions with similar baseline characteristics. Most of the ELCA lesions required final balloon inflations. The success rates were 78% and 80% for ELCA and PTCA, respectively. Favorable lesions for ELCA were bifurcation and ostial lesions and total occlusions.

The use of laser angioplasty in specific lesion situations has developed over the years, including SVGs, complex native lesions, bifurcation settings, in-stent restenosis, and as adjunctive to debulking prior to brachytherapy. The desiccation of acute and thrombotic lesions has been described.[28,29] Chronic total occlusions, including aorto-ostial SVG anastamoses, may be ablated after conventional wire passage or approached by use of a combined wire/0.9 mm laser fiber technique.

Favorable lesions for laser consideration include in-stent restenosis, total occlusions with guidewire passage, and occasionally (if time and resources allow and clinical indications exist) total occlusions with alternating laser fiber and wire probing of occlusions to attempt crossing the occlusion. Long lesions, bifurcation lesions, and small-vessel stenosis can be approached with success rates equal to balloon success. Certain SVG lesions may be safer than conventional balloon angioplasty. Undilatable lesions may be laser-able and allow completion with conventional techniques, although rotation ablation may be preferable for calcified undilatable lesions.

Unfavorable lesions include those located in very tortuous, small, or very distal vessel locations, and tortuous or dissected segments.

Laser angioplasty for in-stent restenosis

Large concentric laser fibers were shown to be safe and effective in debulking in-stent restenoses (ISR) with a 92% success rates.[30] Dahm and Kuon[31] demonstrated 100% efficacy of eccentric fibers using slow ablation rates. Most operators use interrupted lesion engagement and ablation similar to rotational ablation. ISR can be safely ablated with high procedural success rates and relatively low restenosis and target vessel revascularization rates compared with alternative modalities

The LARS (Laser Angioplasty for Restenotic Stents)[32] trial compared excimer laser angioplasty with balloon angioplasty for ISR. Most ISR dilatations involve eventual high-pressure balloon inflations whether or not debulking is utilized. Much of the effect of balloon dilatation is to improve stent expansion from inadequate initial stent placement. IVUS evaluation demonstrates suboptimal initial stent expansion as a frequent component of repeat presentation for ISR. Much of the benefit of balloon dilatation is stent expansion in addition to extrusion of neo-intimal tissue outward through the stent struts.[33]

Large concentric laser fibers were shown to be safe and effective in debulking ISR lesions, with a 92% success rate. Nearly 100% procedural success can be achieved using eccentric fibers and slow ablation rates. Most operators use interrupted lesion engagement and intermittent lesion ablation similar to rotational ablation. ISR can be safely ablated with high procedural success rates and relatively low restenosis rates. Clinical target vessel revascularization rates in the 12.8% region may make this technique preferable to alternative modalities.[34]

Bifurcation lesions

Occlusion of significant side branches occurs with balloon and stent techniques due to shifting of plaque. This shifting may be obviated by the use of debulking, and laser angioplasty may be preferable to alternative techniques in this setting. The use of two wires to protect the side branches is possible, unlike rotational ablation. There are multiple possible constellations of plaque proximal and distal to the side branch as well as within the proximal side branch. Eccentric fiber selection allows direct address of the plaque that is most likely to occlude the side branch subsequent to balloon or stent dilatation.

Thrombus-containing lesions

While safety and effectiveness are demonstrable in acute syndromes and infarct settings, with and without visible thrombus, much of the data were obtained prior to the general availability of the Angiojet (Possis). Small thrombi, in the context of significant atheromatous lesion bulk, may favor the use of laser angioplasty, whereas larger thrombi associated with less obstruction suggest the use of rheolytic thrombectomy.

Total occlusions

Total occlusions, once crossed, may be ablated, although negative remodeling increases the perforation risk in long segments. Occluded aorto-ostial graft lesions can be dilated.

Technical considerations

As with all rigid devices, guiding catheter selection is an integral component of procedural success. The guide diameter must be appropriate for the fiber diameter. Vessel size and lesion severity determine fiber selection. Lesion shape and reference diameter dictate concentric versus eccentric fiber selection. Laser ablation must proceed slowly, since it is dependent on virtual contact with the tissue to actually ablate the plaque rather than dotter the lesion. Advancing fibers must move at less than 0.5 mm/s. Fluence adjustments can be made for more calcified or fibrotic lesions that do not allow initial advancement with the default fluence settings (45 mJ/mm^2 and 25 Hz).

Contrast must be completely cleared from the coronary artery or vein graft prior to lasing. The photoacoustic shock accompanying the delivery of laser energy in a coronary artery with even dilute contrast generates fluoroscopically visible bubbles and leads to a risk of dissection, slow flow, and infarct from occlusion or perforation (author's personal experience and as reported by Van Leeuwen et al[35]). The necessity for contrast clearance and provision of a less obstructed field for lasing resulted in the use of a saline flush via the guide during the laser application and lessened the complication rate.[36]

Technical considerations include the use of eccentric laser fibers in eccentric lesions, especially in the proximal vessels or vein grafts. Concentric fibers generate the maximum debulking effect with the initial pass. With eccentric fibers, the operator can use the wire to pivot the eccentric laser fiber around the central axis of the vessel and ablate a cross-sectional area larger than the catheter area and a larger diameter than the laser fiber. In long lesions such as diffuse ISR or SVGs, and by stopping the advance of the fiber prior to breaking through the distal end of the lesion, multiple circumferential cuts into the plaque can be made, much like DCA, with the wire acting as a pivot, instead of the DCA balloon offsetting the atherectomy window. Rotating the fiber around the central wire position without finishing the distal end of the lesion supports the wire in a relatively fixed position until most of the lesion has been ablated.

References

1. Topol E, Leya F, Pinkerton C, et al. A comparison of directional atherectomy with coronary angioplasty in patients with coronary artery disease. N Engl J Med 1993; 329:221–7.
2. Elliot J, Berdan L, Holmes D, et al. One-year follow-up in the Coronary Angioplasty Versus Excisional Atherectomy Trial (CAVEAT I). Circulation 1995;91:2158–66.
3. Adelman A, Cohen E, Kimball B, et al. A comparison of directional atherectomy with balloon angioplasty for lesions of the left anterior descending coronary artery. N Engl J Med 1993;329:228–33.
4. Holmes D, Topol, E, Califf R, et al. A multi-center, randomized trial of coronary angioplasty versus directional atherectomy for patients with saphenous vein bypass graft lesions Circulation 1995;91:1966–74.
5. Omoigui N, Califf R, Pieper K, et al. Peripheral vascular complications in the Coronary Angioplasty Versus Excisional Atherectomy Trial (CAVEAT-I). Circulation 1995;26:922–30.
6. Simonton CA, Leon MV, Baim DS, et al. 'Optimal' directional coronary atherectomy: final results of the Optimal Atherectomy Restenosis Study (OARS). Circulation 1998; 97:332–9.
7. Baim DS, Cutlip DE, Sharma SK, et al. Final results of the Balloon vs. Optimal Atherectomy Trial (BOAT). Circulation 1998;97:322–31.
8. Sumitsuji S, Suzuki T, Katoh L, et al. Restenosis mechanism after aggressive directional coronary atherectomy assessed by intravascular ultrasound in Adjunctive Balloon Angioplasty following coronary atherectomy study (ABACAS). J Am Coll Cardiol 1997;29:457A.

9. Tsuchikane E, Sumitsuji S, Awata N, et al. Final results of the stent versus directional coronary atherectomy randomized trial (START). J Am Coll Cardiol 1999;34:1050–7.

10. Lefkovits J, Blankenship JC, Anderson K, et al. Increased risk of non-Q MI after directional atherectomy is platelet dependent: evidence from the EPIC trial. J Am Coll Cardiol 1996;28:849.

11. Mousa I, Moses J, De Mario C, et al. Stenting after optimal lesion debulking (SOLD) registry: angiographic and clinical outcome. Circulation 1998;98:1604–9.

12. Ahmed JM, Hong MK, Mehran R, et al. Comparison of debulking followed by stenting versus stenting alone for saphenous vein graft aorto-ostial lesions: immediate and one-year clinical outcomes. J Am Coll Cardiol 2000;35:1560–8.

13. Bramucci E, Repeto A, Ferrario M, et al. Effectiveness of adjunctive stent implantation following directional coronary atherectomy for treatment of left anterior descending ostial stenosis. Am J Cardiol 90:1074–8.

14. Park SJ, Park SW, Lee CW, et al. Long-term outcome of unprotected left main coronary stenting in patients with normal left ventricular function: Is debulking atherectomy prior to stenting beneficial? J Am Coll Cardiol 33(Suppl A):15A.

15. Bass TA, Gilmore PS, White CJ, et al. Surface luminal characteristics following coronary rotational atherectomy (PTRA) versus balloon angioplasty (PTCA): angioscopic, ultrasound and angiographic evaluation. J Am Coll Cardiol 1993;21:444A.

16. Mintz GS, Douek P, et al. Target lesion calcification in coronary artery disease: an intra-vascular ultrasound study. J Am Coll Cardiol 1992;20:1149–55.

17. Gilmore PS, Bass TA, et al. Single site experience with high-speed coronary rotational atherectomy. Clin Cardiol 1993; 1:311–16.

18. Safian RD, Feldman T, Muller DWM, et al. Coronary Angioplasty and Rotablator Atherectomy Trial (CARAT): immediate and late results of a prospective multi-center randomized trial. Cathet Cardiovasc Interv 2001;53:213–20.

19. Vandormael M, Reifart N, Preusler W, et al. Six months follow-up results following excimer laser angioplasty, rotational atherectomy and balloon angioplasty for complex lesions: ERBAC study. Circulation 1994;90:I-213A.

20. Reisman M, Buchbinder M, Sharma SK, et al. A multi-center randomized trial of rotational atherectomy vs. PTCA: DART. Circulation 1997;96(Suppl):I-67.

21. Whitlow PL, Bass TA, Kipperman RM, et al. Results of the Study to determine Rotablator and Transluminal Angioplasty Strategy (STRATAS). Am J Cardiol 2001;87:699–705.

22. Buchbinder M, Fortuna R, Sharma SK, et al. Debulking prior to stenting improves acute outcomes: early results from the SPORT trial. J Am Coll Cardiol 2000;35(Suppl A):8A.

23. Haager PK, Horn B, Klues HG, et al. Advantages of rotablation with adjunctive PTCA versus PTCA alone in the treatment of in-stent restenosis: data from the IVUS sub study of the multi-center randomized ARTIST trial. Circulation 2000;102:432 (abst).

24. vom Dahl J, Dietz U, Silber S, et al. Angioplasty versus rotational atherectomy for treatment of diffuse in-stent restenosis: clinical and angiographic results from a randomized multi-center trial (ARTIST study). J Am Coll Cardiol 2000; 35:83.

25. vom Dahl J, Haager PK, Reineke T, et al. Predictors of recurrent in-stent restenosis following mechanical treatment by angioplasty or rotational atherectomy: results from an angiographically controlled prospective trial (ARTIST study). J Am Coll Cardiol 2000;35:83A.

26. Bass TA, Gilmore P, Zenni M, et al. Debulking does not benefit patients undergoing intracoronary beta-radiation

therapy for in-stent restenosis. Insights from the START trial. (In press.)

27. Preisack MB, Liewald C, Athanasiadis A, et al. Success and procedural outcome of excimer laser coronary angioplasty compared to conventional balloon angioplasty. J Invasive Cardiol 1997;9:10–16.

28. Bonn D. Laser thrombolysis: safe and rapid removal of clots? Lancet 2000;355:1976.

29. Topaz O, Bernardo N, McQueen R, et al. Excimer laser angioplasty in acute coronary syndromes. Cathet Cardiovasc Interv 2000;50:154.

30. Koster R, Hamm CW, Seabra-Gomes R, et al. Treatment of in-stent coronary restenosis by excimer laser angioplasty. Am J Cardiol 1998;80:1424–8.

31. Dahm JB, Kuon E. High-energy eccentric excimer laser angioplasty for debulking diffuse in-stent restenosis leads to better acute and 6-month follow-up results. J Invasive Cardiol 2000;12:343–4.

32. Giri S, Ito S, Lansky AJ, et al. Clinical and angiographic outcome in the Laser Angioplasty for Restenotic Stents (LARS) multi-center registry. Cathet Cardiovasc Interv 2001; 52:24–34.

33. Mehran. Am J Cardiol 1996;78:618–22.

34. Mehran R, Dangas G, Mintz GS, et al. Treatment of in-stent restenosis with excimer laser coronary angioplasty versus rotational atherectomy: comparative mechanisms and results. Circulation 2000;101:2484–9.

35. Van Leeuwen TG, et al. Intraluminal vapor bubble induced by excimer laser pulse causes microsecond arterial dilatation and invagination leading to extensive wall damage in the rabbit. Circulation 1993;87:1258–63.

36. Deckelbaum LI, Natarajan MK, Bittl JA, et al. Effect of intracoronary saline infusion on dissection during excimer laser coronary angioplasty: a randomized trial. J Am Coll Cardiol 1995;26:1264–9.

37. Sharma SK, Duvvuri S, Dangas G, et al. Rotational atherectomy for in-stent restenosis: acute and long-term results of the first 100 cases. J Am Coll Cardiol 1998; 32:1358–65.

38. Reith S. The place of Rotablator for treatment of in-stent restenosis. Semin Interv Cardiol 2000;5:199–208.

39. Appelman YE. Evaluation of the long term function outcome assessed by myocardial perfusion scintigraphy following ECLA compared to BA in longer coronary lesions. Int J Card Imaging 1996;78:618–22.

40. Topaz O, Morris C, Minisi AJ, et al. Enhancement of t-PA induced fibrinolysis with laser energy: in-vitro observations. Lasers Med Sci 1999;14:123–8.

41. Estella P, Ryan TJ, Lanberg JS, et al. Excimer laser assisted coronary angioplasty of lesions containing thrombus. J Am Coll Cardiol 1993;21:1550–6.

42. Topaz, O. Effectiveness of excimer laser coronary angioplasty in AMI or USA. Am J Cardiol 2001;87:849–55.

43. Koster R, Hamm CW, Seabra-Gomes R, et al. Laser angioplasty of restenosed coronary stents: results of a multi-center surveillance trial. J Am Coll Cardiol 1999; 34:25–32.

44. Appleman YEA, Pick JJ, Strikwerda S, et al. Randomized trial of excimer laser versus balloon angioplasty for treatment of obstructive coronary artery disease. Lancet 1996;347:79–84.

45. Stone GW, deMarchena E, Dageforde D, et al. A prospective randomized, multi-center comparison of balloon angioplasty in patients with obstructive coronary artery disease. J Am Coll Cardiol 1997;30:1714–21.

46. Madyoon H, Croushore L. Application of excimer laser coronary angioplasty in bifurcation lesions. Lasers Med Sci 2001;16:108–12.

11

Treatment of complex angioplasty subsets

Carlo Di Mario

Introduction

The mechanical scaffold provided by coronary stents has represented a dramatic improvement in our techniques of percutaneous myocardial revascularization, and this improvement has been particularly valuable for the treatment of complex lesions. In the last few years, however, promising data have been accumulating that may lead to a second revolution based on a stent platform, namely the use of drug-eluting stents that inhibit late intimal hyperplasia and restenosis.[1-4] Again, complex lesions will be the most important target for these new devices, because the restenosis rate for small vessels, bifurcational lesions, and total occlusions is often higher than 30%. If stents have allowed treatment of complex lesions with a low immediate risk and a high success rate, the drug elution process can transform this short-term favorable outcome into a long-term patency and persistent benefit. On the verge of this new revolution, it is particularly difficult to write about the treatment of complex lesions, as our techniques will be drastically modified by the use of these prostheses. In this chapter, we will try, however, to summarize what we know about the treatment of complex lesions with metallic stents in the specific subsets of lesions in bifurcations, lesions located in vessels of small reference diameter, and in chronic total occlusions.

Bifurcational lesions

Often, we consider as bifurcational lesions only those that require a kissing stenting strategy. In reality, 15–20% of the lesions that we have to treat in our daily practice will

entail involvement of branches larger than 2.0 mm that require treatment with balloon dilatation before or after stent placement. Bifurcational lesions in the coronary system are even more frequent. As in every other arterial conduit in the body (carotids and iliacs), plaques tend to accumulate due to rheological phenomena at bifurcation points, and the only reason why we do not treat these cases more frequently is a selection bias to send these patients for surgical treatment. In a review of 285 consecutive patients undergoing bypass surgery at the Royal Brompton Hospital, London, 49% of these patients would have required treatment of at least one bifurcational lesion if revascularization had to be performed using percutaneous techniques. These data clearly illustrate that if we want to extend the applicability of percutaneous revascularization to the majority of the present surgical candidates, we need to provide a safe and durable solution to this problem.

A simple definition of a bifurcation lesion can be the involvement of a side branch with a reference diameter greater than 2 mm in the stenosis. Many classifications have been proposed to distinguish these lesions according to the site of the prevalent narrowing, in the main artery proximal to the bifurcation or at the ostia of the two daughter vessels, with all the possible combinations.[5] Often, however, when dealing with a bifurcation, one is faced with the problem that the ostia of the daughter vessels will become impaired during treatment, even if they did not have significant narrowings to start with. Intravascular ultrasound almost invariably shows that the plaque that develops around a bifurcation involves the origin of all the daughter branches and extends into the proximal funnel for a much longer segment than predicted angiographically. If we add the effect of a plaque shift during dilatation consequent to the well-known phenomenon of axial plaque redistribution in straight vessel segments, it will be clear that these different classifications are often futile, while the treatment strategy is mainly dictated by the size of the vessels involved. Stents were created to cover a straight vessel segment and give uniform scaffolding to the vessel wall. Although specially designed stents have been proposed,[6,7] in practice all-purpose conventional stents are used for treatment of the vast majority of bifurcational lesions, with the obvious problem of creating access and maintaining patency of a side branch with closed cell stent designs. While most of the conventional stents allow enlargement of the cells to a diameter of 2.5–2.7 mm,[8] a careful selection must be made when the branch to be covered with a stent has a diameter greater than 3.0 mm, such as, for instance, the circumflex or left anterior descending (LAD) coronary artery in lesions involving the left main stem. Fifteen years of experience with conventional metallic stents have led to the development of various techniques of treatment and have allowed the evaluation of results both immediately and at follow-up. Unlike simpler lesions in straight segments or even lesions in small vessels and after recanalization of chronic total occlusions, properly conducted multicenter or randomized trials are not available for bifurcational lesions. This lack of data reflects our uncertainties regarding the best possible technique and the poor outcome observed in the initial observational trials. The consensus in the era of current eluting metallic stents can be summarized as follows:

1. Unless severe flow impairment or ostial narrowing develop during treatment of bifurcational lesions at the ostium of a side branch, a single-stent technique is preferable to the use of kissing stents. All kissing stenting techniques, despite their better initial angiographic appearance, are more complex, are time- and material-consuming, and, more importantly, do not provide certainty of a better long-term outcome.

2. Among the multiple techniques proposed for the treatment of bifurcational lesions (T-stenting, culotte, V-stenting, and Y-stenting), only T-stenting survives as a frequently applied option in the case of an insufficient result with implantation of a single stent. The other options are used by a minority of operators in very selected cases (Figure 11.1).

3. Dilating with a balloon through stent struts carries a high risk of deformation of the stent distal to the site of dilatation and, especially if balloons larger than 2.0 mm are used, a final kissing balloon is advised to prevent the deformation process.

All of these considerations, however, may become of only historical interest in the era of drug-eluting stents. If we accept that the stent can act as a platform for local drug release, then all the injured segment should be ideally covered with these antirestenotic devices, suggesting that techniques such as V-stenting or culotte could be resurrected and that the use of two stents to treat bifurcational

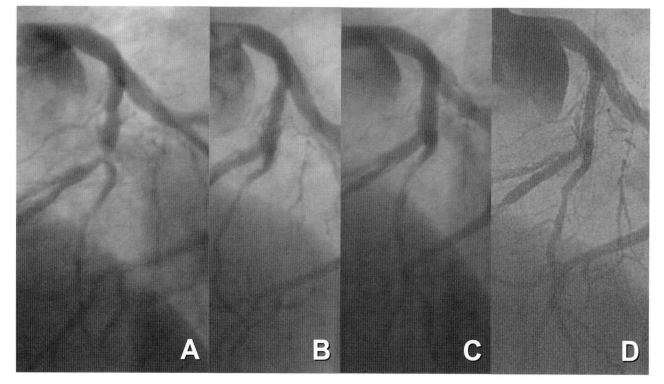

Figure 11.1
Severe stenosis of left anterior descending and first diagonal branch, before treatment (A), immediately after insertion of 2 Duet stents using a culotte technique (B), 6 months after treatment (C), 5 years after treatment (D).

lesions could become routine practice. Conversely, as proper embedding of the stent struts into the vessel wall is essential for timely release of antiproliferative treatment, the possible deformation and change in cell geometry induced by kissing stenting techniques or kissing balloon dilatation are possible causes of late failure in these lesions. Unfortunately, none of the largest trials conducted with drug-eluting stents have given answers to these technical questions, because the presence of major side branches in the stented segment was an exclusion criterion. The only study that specifically addressed the treatment of bifurcational lesions with drug-eluting stents has been recently reported, but is still unpublished (SIRIUS bifurcations).[9] This study was a multicenter randomized trial to assess the feasibility and safety of treatment of patients with true bifurcational lesions (>50% stenosis in both the main vessel and the ostium of side branch) and test two different strategies: the elective use of a kissing stenting technique with the rapamycin-coated drug eluting stent Cypher (Cordis Corporation, Miami, FL) or the implantation of a single rapamycin-coated stent in the main vessel with a simple balloon dilatation across the stent struts for the side branch. The protocol allowed the investigators to switch to double stenting if flow impairment or residual ostial stenosis greater than 50% developed in the side branch, and this option was frequently followed, with 22 out of 43 patients randomized to stent percutaneous coronary angioplasty (PTCA) crossing over to the implantation of two stents. In practice, of the 86 patients randomized, 63 were treated using a double-stenting technique, 22 had a stent for the main vessel and PTCA for the side branch, and 1 patient was excluded because the treatment was not performed on a bifurcational lesion. As expected, as the left main bifurcation was excluded from enrolment, the LAD/diagonal bifurcation was the most frequently treated site (76% in the stent arm and 72% in the stent/PTCA arm). A T-stenting technique was used in the vast majority of cases (95%) in the patients who received two stents. In two-thirds of the cases, the stent in the side branch was deployed before the stent in the main vessel, often with a technique of simultaneous stent insertion, while a stent was implanted initially in the main vessel in the remaining 20 patients. Quantitative angiography showed a small mean reference diameter for the main vessel (2.6 ± 0.4 mm) and, especially, for the side branch (2.1 ± 0.3 mm). The final QCA measurement demonstrated a reduction of the percentage stenosis in the main branch to 11.6 ± 7.7% and in the side branch to 14.4 ± 13.8% if two stents were used and to 23.5 ± 27.2% when only balloon dilatation was performed in the side branch. In practice, in only 72.7% of the patients who received a single stent for the main vessel was angiographic success (TIMI III flow and no stenosis >50%) achieved in the side branch, versus 93.7% of the patients who received two stents. Using a 3-month protocol of combined administration of aspirin and clopidogrel, stent thrombosis was acceptably low (3.5%), with two of these three patients

having this complication 1 and 3 days post procedure showing severe suboptimal results immediately after the procedure. The presence of a single case of late thrombosis (32 days post procedure) seems to confirm also for bifurcational lesions the safety of these rapamycin-coated prostheses in terms of re-endothelialization. Angiographic follow-up was performed in 66 out of 85 patients (78%), and showed an excellent result in terms of restenosis in the main vessel, reduced to 4 out of 66 patients restudied (6.1%), in 3 out of 4 being limited to a focal restenosis at the proximal stent edge. Less satisfactory were the results in the side branch, with a restenosis rate of 22.7% (15 out of 66). The high number of crossovers obviously makes comparison between the two groups difficult, but the use of a second stent, even with drug elution, does not appear to improve the restenosis rate, which was 24.0% in the two-stent groups and 18.7% in the stent/PTCA group. The pattern of restenosis was very typical, with 14 out of the 15 restenoses being very focal at the ostium of the side branch, where in two-thirds of the cases angiography or intravascular ultrasound have confirmed incomplete ostial coverage as the possible cause of the problem.

Registry data from Milan and Rotterdam confirm that bifurcational lesions have revascularization restenosis rates in excess of 10%, even with drug-eluting stents.[10,11] New techniques have been proposed to solve the problem. In the 'crush' technique, the drug-eluting stent implanted in the side branch is deployed very proximal, to cover a few millimeters of the main vessel to ensure complete coverage of the side-branch ostium. The preliminary unpublished data of this technique proposed by Colombo et al suggested that the technique is safe in terms of subacute stent thrombosis, but no data are yet available to confirm that it removes the risk of ostial restenosis in the long term. Other unknown variables are the behavior of different types of drug-eluting stents, such as paxlitaxel-coated stents, and the feasibility of using bifurcated drug-coated stents to ensure optimal lesion coverage. The practical conclusion for the treatment of bifurcational lesions is that a drug-eluting stent in the main vessel can substantially lower the restenosis rate. If an angiographically acceptable result is obtained in the side branch, it might be wise (also for cost containment) to limit the treatment to balloon dilatation or even to avoid recrossing the stent struts and dilating them to prevent strut distortion and uneven drug distribution to the vessel wall (Figure 11.2). If a double-stent technique is used, meticulous attention must be given to ensure full coverage of the ostial lesion, and the ideal technique has yet to be found.

Small vessels

Many randomized studies have addressed the usefulness of routine stent implantation for the treatment of lesions in vessels with a reference diameter smaller or equal to

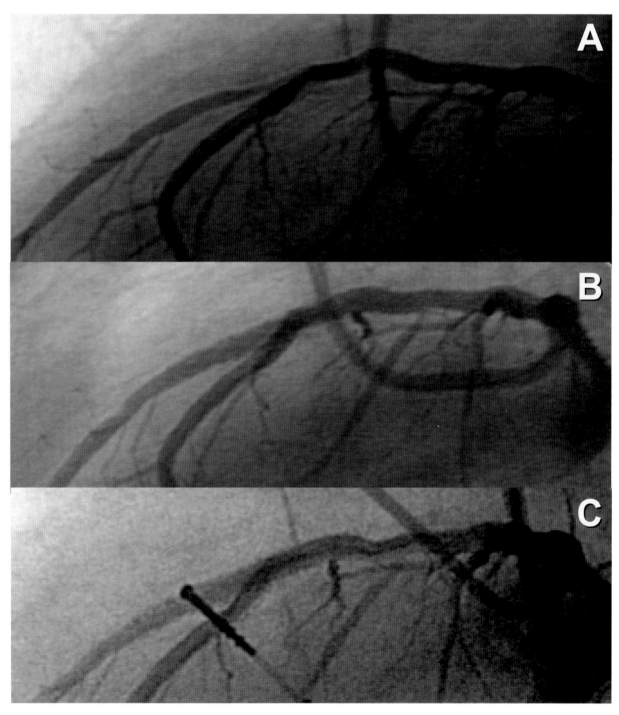

Figure 11.2
Severe stenosis of left anterior descending and first diagonal branch, before treatment (A), immediately after insertion of a Sirolimus eluting Cypher stent on the main vessel and a Driver stent on the diagonal branch using a T-technique (B), 8 months after treatment (C).

2.75–2.50 mm.[12–16] It is interesting to note that the results of these studies were very conflicting, going from a clear positivity in favor of routine use of stents in the BESMART and RAP trials to neutral or negative results in the majority of the other trials (SISA, PARK, ISAR–SMART, MICROSCOPE, and COST). These differences are possibly explained by the different characteristics of the treated lesions (more focal in the first trials) and the more aggressive technique of PTCA used in the latter group of trials. A sort of intermediate position has been proposed by the Milan group and others, recommending that the use of stents for long lesions in small vessels be limited to those segments with sufficient angiographic and ultrasound visualization.[17] In practice, this technique (called spot stenting) has always had limited use, because the decision-making criteria remain subjective and intravascular ultrasound is a demanding and expensive procedure, and it is much easier to completely cover the diseased segment with stents. Still, intravascular ultrasound has certainly played a pivotal role in improving our understanding that these lesions are very heterogeneous and many so-called 'small vessels' actually have a much larger reference diameter and represent the tip of the iceberg of a very diffuse disease process.[18,19] The positive results obtained with techniques of ultrasound-guided or physiology-guided (Doppler or pressure wire measurements) provisional stenting[20–24] can also be applied in this lesion subset. Still, all these proposed techniques will be quickly abandoned if the initial promises of drug-eluting stents also hold in this lesion subset. Although the designs of the initial trials with drug-eluting stents did not include vessels smaller than 2.75 mm, in practice, as the inclusion criteria were only visual, a substantial proportion of patients in all of these trials had vessels of small reference diameter. Table 11.1 reports the results in RAVEL,[25] SIRIUS,[4] and TAXUS II (unpublished data), with vessels divided according to the different reference diameter. As can be seen, the results vary from an outstanding 0% restenosis rate and an absence of late loss in the smaller-vessel cohort of the RAVEL trial to a still-low 18.6% restenosis rate in the longer lesions in small vessels of the SIRIUS trial. Looking at the control group, the absolute difference in terms of restenosis rate is even greater for the smaller-vessel cohort, given the high propensity for restenosis with conventional metallic stents (37% and 42.3% in RAVEL and SIRIUS, respectively). Another important finding of these first trials with drug-eluting stents is that the restenotic

lesions observed were mainly present at the edges of the stented segment, were focal in nature, and therefore were more easily treatable. A consequence of these findings is the trend to use even longer stents to fully cover the diseased segment and avoid injury outside the stent to vessels with severe plaque burden. Unfortunately, the reported trials do not give real information on how the implantation of multiple stents may solve the problem of a truly diffuse disease involving the distal vessels. The initial results from groups able to accumulate large experience with the commercially available rapamycin-coated stents (the RESEARCH study, Rotterdam and Single-Center Experience in Milan) have been reported recently,[26] but are still unpublished. The initial data suggest that subacute stent thrombosis may become an issue when extremely long segments are covered, leading to multiple side branches shut off and distal embolization. Treatment with glycoprotein IIb/IIIa inhibitors and a more prolonged (6–12 months) treatment with combined antiplatelet treatment has been suggested. Also in terms of restenosis, individual cases of in-stent restenosis have been reported and fully characterized, suggesting that segments of incomplete stent expansion and hinge points are the most likely cause of in-stent restenosis, which remains focal in nature in these very long treated segments. Finally, the need for vessel overlapping to ensure optimal delivery does not seem to increase the risk of stent thrombosis or induce untoward side-effects, such as the formation of aneurysms.[27] Another consideration that must be taken into account is how small a vessel can be to receive treatment with these new drug-eluting stents. Although 2.25 mm stents are available (Cypher), it is sometimes difficult to insert these long prostheses into extremely small distal vessels, especially in case of severe proximal tortuosity. The need for more flexible stents and thinner stent struts for these

Table 11.1   Vessel size and in-lesion restenosis rate (%) in randomized drug-eluting stent trials

	Small		Medium		Large	
Trial	CYPHER	Control	CYPHER	Control	CYPHER	Control
RAVEL[a] (N = 238)	0	37	0	26	0	42
US-SIRIUS[b] (N = 702)	18.6	42.3	6.3	36.5	1.3	30.2
TAXUS 2MR[c] (N = 269)	11.4	35.1	2.5	20.6	12.2	16.0
TAXUS SR[c] (N = 267)	13.5	24.4	4.1	20.8	0	14.3

[a] Small <236 mm; medium ≥2.36 and 2.84 mm; large ≥2.84 mm.
[b] Small ~2.3 mm; medium ~2.8 mm; large ~3.3 mm.
[c] Small <2.5 mm; medium ≥2.5 and <3.0 mm; large ≥3.0 mm.

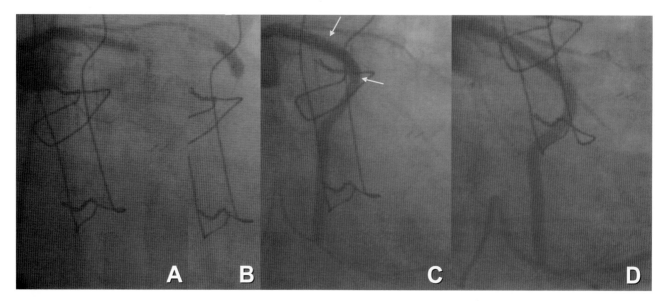

Figure 11.3
Occlusive lesion of a sequential vein graft before treatment (A), with a residual waist in the balloon used for the final stent expansion at 24 Atm (B), immediately after insertion of a 33 mm Sirolimus eluting Cypher stent (C), 7 months after treatment (D).

vessels is probably not cancelled by the availability of antiproliferative drug elution to overcome restenosis.

Chronic total occlusion

Chronic total occlusion is the main cause of the inability to offer percutaneous revascularization in patients with coronary artery disease. The main problem with chronic total occlusion is not the type of stent to use but rather the possibility to cross the occlusion and advance the wire into the true lumen of the distal vessel. Despite reports of increased success rates, treatment of truly old chronic long occlusions has a limited success rate even in experienced hands, and we certainly need a breakthrough in technology to overcome the problem.[28] After having restored a lumen, the chances of restenosis or re-occlusion are prohibitively high, and full coverage of the occluded segment with conventional metallic stents reduces but does not eliminate restenonis, especially in patients with long occlusions and in diabetics, who are also predisposed to re-occlusion.[29–31] Again, for drug-eluting stents in this setting, we only have unpublished registry data, but this experience, still anecdotal, suggests that long-term vessel patency, even in cases of long re-occlusions after previous stent implantation, can be achieved (Figure 11.3).

Conclusions

Drug-eluting stents are likely to completely change our technique of treatment of complex lesions. We are

still in the infancy of this new revolution in interventional cardiology, which could lead to a dramatic increase in the application of this method. The possibility of offering this treatment to the majority of patients with ischemic heart syndromes needs proper handling of the specific issues posed by these challenging lesions.

References

1. Toutouzas K, Di Mario C, Falotico R, et al. Sirolimus-eluting stents: a review of experimental and clinical findings. Z Kardiol 2002;91(Suppl 3):49–57.

2. Sousa JE, Costa MA, Sousa AG, et al. Two-year angiographic and intravascular ultrasound follow-up after implantation of sirolimus-eluting stents in human coronary arteries. Circulation 2003;107:381–3.

3. Morice MC, Serruys PW, Sousa JE, et al., RAVEL Study Group. A randomized comparison of a sirolimus-eluting stent with a standard stent for coronary revascularization. N Engl J Med 2002;346:1773–80.

4. Holmes DR Jr, Leon MB, Moses JW, et al., on behalf of the SIRIUS Trial Investigators. One-year follow-up of the SIRIUS study. A randomized study with the sirolimus-eluting Bx VELOCITY™ in the treatment of patients with de-novo native coronary artery lesions. J Am Coll Cardiol 2003;41:32A.

5. Di Mario C, Airoldi F, Reimers B, et al. Bifurcational stenting. Semin Interv Cardiol 1998;2:65–76.

6. Toutouzas K, Stankovic G, Takagi T, et al. A new dedicated stent and delivery system for the treatment of bifurcation lesions: preliminary experience. Cathet Cardiovasc Interv 2003;58:34–42.

7. Colombo A, Airoldi F, Sheiban I, Di Mario C. Successful treatment of a bifurcation lesion with the Carina Bard stent: a case report. Cathet Cardiovasc Interv 1999;48:89–92.

8. Colombo A, Stankovic G, Moses JW. Selection of coronary stents. J Am Coll Cardiol 2002;40:1021–33.

9. Colombo A, Louvard Y, Raghu C, et al. Sirolimus eluting stents in bifurcation lesions: 6 months angiographic result according to the implantation technique. J Am Coll Cardiol 2003;41;53A.

10. Tanabe K, Lemos PA, Lee CH, et al. The impact of sirolimus-eluting stents on the outcome of patients with bifurcation lesions. J Am Coll Cardiol 2003;41:12A.

11. Airoldi F, Spanos V, Stankovic G, et al. Bifurcational coronary artery lesion treatment with rapamicine-eluting stents: results from a single center experience. J Am Coll Cardiol 2003;41:53A.

12. Kastrati A, Schomig A, Dirschinger J, et al. A randomized trial comparing stenting with balloon angioplasty in small vessels in patients with symptomatic coronary artery disease. ISAR–SMART or angioplasty for restenosis reduction in small arteries. Circulation 2000;102:2593–8.

13. Doucet S, Schalij MJ, Vrolix MC, et al., Stent In Small Arteries (SISA) Trial Investigators. Stent placement to prevent restenosis after angioplasty in small coronary arteries. Circulation 2001;104:2029–33.

14. Park SW, Lee CW, Hong MK, et al. Randomized comparison of coronary stenting with optimal balloon angioplasty for treatment of lesions in small coronary arteries. Eur Heart J 2000;21:1785–9.

15. Koning R, Eltchaninoff H, Commeau P, et al. Stent placement compared with balloon angioplasty for small coronary arteries: in-hospital and 6-month clinical and angiographic results. BESMART (BeStent in Small Arteries Trial) Investigators. Circulation 2001;104:1604–8.

16. Haude M, Konorza TF, Kalnins U, et al. Heparin-coated stent placement for the treatment of stenoses in small coronary arteries of symptomatic patients. Heparin-Coated Stents in Small Coronary Arteries Trial Investigators. Circulation 2003 Mar 11;107:1265–70.

17. Airoldi F, Di Mario C, Presbitero P, et al. Elective stenting in small coronary arteries: results of the Italian prospective multicenter registry MICROSCOPE. Ital Heart J 2002;3:406–11.

18. Colombo A, De Gregorio J, Moussa I, et al. Intravascular ultrasound-guided percutaneous transluminal coronary angioplasty with provisional spot stenting for treatment of long coronary lesions. J Am Coll Cardiol 2001; 38:1427–33.

19. Akiyama T, Moussa I, Reimers B, et al. Angiographic and clinical outcome following coronary stenting of small vessels: a comparison with coronary stenting of large vessels. J Am Coll Cardiol 1998;32:1610–18.

20. Airoldi F, Di Mario C, Takagi T, et al. Provisional stenting in small vessels. Int J Cardiovasc Interv 2001;2:91–8.

21. Schiele F, Meneveau N, Gilard M, et al. Intravascular ultrasound-guided balloon angioplasty compared with stent: immediate and 6-month results of the multicenter, randomized Balloon Equivalent to Stent Study (BEST). Circulation 2003;107:545–51.

22. Serruys PW, de Bruyne B, Carlier S, et al. Randomized comparison of primary stenting and provisional balloon angioplasty guided by flow velocity measurement. Doppler Endpoints Balloon Angioplasty Trial Europe (DEBATE) II Study Group. Circulation 2000;102:2930–7.

23. Di Mario C, Moses JW, Anderson TJ, et al. Randomized comparison of elective stent implantation and coronary balloon angioplasty guided by online quantitative angiography and intracoronary Doppler. DESTINI Study Group (Doppler Endpoint STenting INternational Investigation). Circulation 2000;102:2938–44.

24. Moussa I, Moses J, Di Mario C, et al. Selecting who qualifies for optimal balloon angioplasty versus elective stenting in coronary artery disease (a subanalysis of the DESTINI trial). Am J Cardiol 2002;90:323–5.

25. Regar E, Serruys PW, Bode C, et al. Angiographic findings of the multicenter Randomized Study With the Sirolimus-Eluting Bx Velocity Balloon-Expandable Stent (RAVEL): sirolimus-eluting stents inhibit restenosis irrespective of the vessel size. Circulation 2002;106:1949–56.

26. Saia F, Lemos PA, Degertekin M, et al. Sirolimus-eluting stents for treatment of in-stent restenosis in the real world: preliminary results from the Rapamycin-Eluting Stent Evaluated at Rotterdam Cardiology Hospital (RESEARCH) Registry. J Am Coll Cardiol 2003;41:53A.

27. Abizaid AA, Munoz JS, Seixas AC, et al. Is there any arterial toxic effect after overlapping sirolimus-eluting stents? J Am Coll Cardiol 2003;41:13A.

28. Sheiban I, Dharmadhikari A, Tzifos V, et al. Recanalization of chronic total coronary occlusions: the impact of a new specific guidewire on primary success rate. Int J Cardiovasc Interv 2000;3:105–10.

29. Moussa I, Moses J, Di Mario C, et al. Selecting who qualifies for optimal balloon angioplasty versus elective stenting in coronary artery disease (a subanalysis of the DESTINI trial). Am J Cardiol 2002;90:323–5.

30. Elezi S, Kastrati A, Neumann FJ, et al. Vessel size and long-term outcome after coronary stent placement. Circulation 1998;98:1875–80.

31. Sallam M, Spanos V, Briguori C, et al. Predictors of reocclusion after successful recanalization of chronic total occlusion. J Invasive Cardiol 2001;7:511–15.

12

Primary angioplasty for acute myocardial infarction

Giuseppe De Luca, Harry Suryapranata

Introduction

The management of patients with acute myocardial infarction (AMI) has considerably improved over the past decades, with many factors being involved in the reduction of mortality, including earlier diagnosis and treatment of the acute event, improved management of complications such as recurrent ischemia and heart failure, and general availability of pharmacological therapies such as aspirin, beta-blockers, ACE inhibitors and glycoprotein IIb/IIIa inhibitors.[1] Most attention, however, has been focused on therapies that may restore antegrade coronary blood flow in the culprit artery of the patient with evolving AMI. The two methods to achieve this goal are thrombolytic therapy and immediate coronary angiography followed by primary angioplasty if appropriate.[1]

Angioplasty for AMI was first described as a rescue therapy in the case of failed intracoronary thrombolysis, and was studied extensively as adjunctive therapy, performed immediately (within hours), early (within 1–2 days), late (after 2 days), or electively for inducible ischemia and/or postinfarction angina, after intravenous thrombolytic therapy. Primary angioplasty, without the use of thrombolytic therapy, was described in 1983.[2] It can be applied as an alternative reperfusion therapy in candidates for thrombolytic therapy, and is the only reperfusion option in many patients with AMI inelegible for thrombolytic therapy.

Pathophysiological considerations and concomitant pharmacological treatment

Studies based on autopsy, angiography, and angioscopy have shown that formation of a coronary thrombus on an atherosclerotic plaque, leading to total or subtotal occlusion of the coronary artery, is the key event that causes acute ischemic syndromes. Coronary thrombus formation is usually initiated by disruption or fissuring of the plaque. Typically, this is a lipid-laden plaque with a thin cap, and most of these plaques are not hemodynamically significant before rupture. At the site of rupture, platelets adhere to the arterial wall and release vasoconstrictive and aggregating substances. A platelet thrombus is formed, the coagulation system is activated, and the end-product is a coronary thrombus consisting of aggregated platelets stabilized by fibrin. The result of a mechanical approach to reperfusion is therefore critically dependent on the concomitant use of adjunctive pharmacotherapy to counterbalance the many factors that predispose to further thrombus formation, distal embolization, and reocclusion of the coronary artery.

Several studies have evaluated the value of adding antithrombotic drugs to standard reperfusion therapy in order to find the best treatment for AMI. A randomized study[3] has shown that the administration of a high dose of unfractioned heparin (300 UI/kg), as pretreatment for primary angioplasty, did not result in additional benefits in clinical outcome, but was associated with a higher risk of major bleeding (10% versus 6%) when compared with pretreatment with low-dose heparin (70 UI/kg) or placebo. Recent trials have compared enoxaparin (low-molecular-weight heparin) with unfractioned heparin as adjunctive therapy to thrombolysis,[4,5] showing a significant reduction of ischemic complications in patients receiving enoxaparin in comparison with unfractioned heparin.

Since the introduction of a new powerful class of antiplatelet drug (glycoprotein IIb/IIIa inhibitors), several trials have investigated their role as adjunctive therapy to thrombolysis and primary angioplasty, without reaching conclusive and convincing data. In the GUSTO V trial,[6] 16 588 patients with ST-elevation myocardial infarction were randomly assigned to standard-dose reteplase (8260 patients) or half-dose reteplase and full-dose abciximab (8328 patients). No significant difference was observed in 30-day mortality rate (5.9% versus 5.6%). In the RAPPORT trial,[7] a multicenter, randomized trial of abciximab in patients with AMI undergoing primary angioplasty, a total of 483 patients were assigned to abciximab (bolus plus 12-hour infusion) or placebo. The study did not show a significant reduction of combined endpoint of death and reinfarction in patients treated by abciximab in comparison with placebo at both 30-day follow-up (4.6% versus 5.8%; $p =$ NS) and 6-month follow-up (8.7% versus 11.2%; $p =$ NS), respectively.

In the CADILLAC,[8] a randomized trial involving 2082 patients with AMI assigned (in a 2-by-2 factorial design) to undergo percutaneous transluminal coronary angioplasty (PTCA) or stenting, with or without abciximab administration. In this study, no difference was observed at 6-month follow-up in terms of combined endpoint of death and reinfarction. A significant difference was observed only in target-vessel revascularization (5.7% for stenting plus abciximab versus 16.9% in the PTCA group; $p < 0.001$).

Finally, the PACT trial[9] aimed at the evaluation of benefits of the combined use of thrombolysis and angioplasty. In this trial, 606 patients with ST-elevation AMI were randomly assigned to receive either an intravenous bolus of 50 mg alteplase or placebo, followed by rescue angioplasty/stenting, if TIMI 3 flow was not observed at 90 minutes. The authors found an higher rate of patency in the group that received an early bolus of alteplase (61% versus 34%; $p = 0.001$), but no difference in ejection fraction (58% versus 58%) and in 30-day combined endpoint of mortality and reinfarction was observed (6.6% versus 5.9%, respectively).

Advantages of acute coronary angiography

The safety and diagnostic potential of coronary angiography during the early hours of AMI was reported more than 20 years ago.[10] In addition to being a prelude to angioplasty, acute coronary angiography offers several advantages. Patient management after the acute event is facilitated by knowledge of the coronary anatomy, and allows identification of a large subgroup of patients who can be discharged very early (2–3 days) after the acute event,[11] as well as the 5–10% of patients who have an indication for elective coronary artery bypass grafting on anatomical grounds, such as left main disease and/or severe triple-vessel disease.[12] Some patients presenting with symptoms and signs of AMI should not undergo reperfusion therapy (e.g. some patients with spontaneous reperfusion of the infarct-related coronary artery, or patients with a cardiac event without thrombotic occlusion of a coronary artery, or with a noncardiac condition that may mimic AMI) – and this can only be ascertained by angiography. Finally, patients with aortic dissection extending into the aortic root or with a coronary anatomy unsuitable for angioplasty can be considered for acute surgical intervention. In other words, the major advantage of a primary angioplasty strategy for AMI is the fact that the early therapeutic strategy can be determined according to coronary anatomy and clinical situation, within just a few hours after AMI, as all of these patients will undergo immediate angiography.

Primary angioplasty in patients eligible for thrombolytic therapy

Primary coronary angioplasty, when performed by experienced operators, restores TIMI 3 flow in over 90% of patients, and reocclusion is very low. This compares favorably with the 50–70% of patients who achieve normal flow after thrombolysis (Figure 12.1). These effects on myocardial flow explain the better outcome of patients with AMI treated by primary angioplasty when compared with thrombolysis. An overview of short-term results of 10 comparisons, involving a total of 2606 patients,[13] has shown that, compared with thrombolysis, primary angioplasty results in a lower mortality rate (4.4% versus 6.5%; relative risk 0.66, 95% confidence interval (CI) 0.46–0.94), translating into absolute benefit of 2 lives saved per 100 patients treated with angioplasty rather than thrombolysis. The reduction in the combination of death or nonfatal reinfarction after angioplasty compared with thrombolysis is even more striking (11.9% versus 7.2%; relative risk 0.58, 95% CI 0.44–0.76). With respect to safety, stroke was reduced from 2.0% with thrombolysis to 0.7% with angioplasty (relative risk 0.35, 95% CI 0.14–0.77).

Furthermore, the influence of time delay on clinical outcome has also been investigated in a pooled analysis of all randomized trials comparing primary PTCA and lytic therapy.[14] With increasing time delay to presentation, the

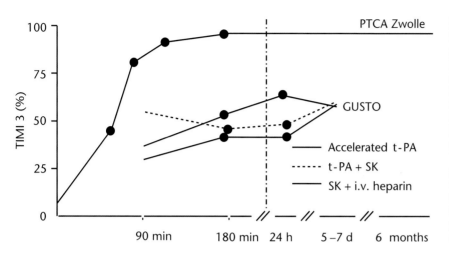

Figure 12.1
Graphical display of TIMI (Thrombolysis in Myocardial Infarction) grade 3 flow immediately after randomization: comparison between the angiographic results from the Zwolle and GUSTO (Global Utilization of Streptokinase and Tissue Plasminogen activator for Occluded coronary artery) trials. The data on TIMI flow in the GUSTO trial were gathered from different patients, who were randomly assigned to angiography at different time intervals after the start of therapy. tPA, tissue plasminogen activator; SK, streptokinase.

mortality rate increases significantly after thrombolysis, while it remains relatively stable after PTCA. Therefore, it seems that prolonged time delay does not affect the benefits of primary angioplasty, when compared with lytic therapy.

Recently, long-term follow-up data of the Zwolle trial have been published on 395 patients randomly assigned to angioplasty or intravenous streptokinase.[15] Clinical information was collected for a mean (± standard deviation) of 5±2 years, and medical charges were compared. A total of 194 patients were assigned to undergo angioplasty and 201 to receive streptokinase. As summarized in Table 12.1, the mortality rate was 13% in the angioplasty group, as compared with 24% in the streptokinase group (relative risk 0.54, 95% CI 0.36–0.87). The cardiac death rate was 6.7% in the angioplasty group and 19.9% in the streptokinase group (p = 0.0001). The Kaplan–Meier curves for overall survival are shown in Figure 12.2. Nonfatal reinfarction occurred in 6% and 22%, respectively (relative risk 0.27, 95% CI 0.15–0.52). The combined incidence of death and nonfatal reinfarction was lower for early events, within the first 30 days, with a relative risk of 0.13 (95% CI

0.05–0.37), as well as for late events, after 30 days, with a relative risk of 0.62 (95% CI 0.43–0.91). The rates of readmission for heart failure and ischemia were lower in the angioplasty group than in the streptokinase group. Total medical charges per patient were similar in the angioplasty group (US$16 090) and the streptokinase group (US$16 813).

That costs are not higher, and in fact even may be lower for primary angioplasty than for thrombolysis, has been shown in several settings.[16] Given the superior safety and efficacy of primary angioplasty, this treatment is now preferred when logistics allow this approach. The results of primary angioplasty are in part dependent on the setting in which it is performed, and therefore the results from various hospitals may differ considerably. This is a consequence of the fundamental difference between a procedure and pharmacotherapy,[17] and has been shown for angioplasty for stable and unstable angina. Quality control, outcome monitoring, and adherence to guidelines and recommendations of task forces of the American College of Cardiology/American Heart Association (ACC/AHA) are therefore of crucial importance.[1]

Table 12.1   Seven-year clinical outcome in patients with AMI randomized to angioplasty (PTCA) or thrombolysis (with streptokinase, SK) in the Zwolle trial

Event	PTCA (n = 194)	SK (n = 201)	p
Mortality	13.4	23.9	0.01
Cardiac death (%)	6.7	19.9	0.001
Cardiac rupture (%)	0.5	1.0	1.0
Heart failure (%)	3.1	10.0	0.01
Sudden death (%)	3.1	9.0	0.02
Reinfarction (%)	6.0	22	0.001
Reintervention (%)	26	52	0.001
Hospital readmission (%)	38	58	0.001
NYHA class I (%)	89	73	0.001
LVEF < 0.40 (%)	14	26	0.006

NYHA, New York Heart Association; LVEF, left ventricular ejection fraction.
Adapted from Zijlstra F et al. N Eng J Med 1999;341:1413–19[15] with permission from the Massachusetts Medical Society.

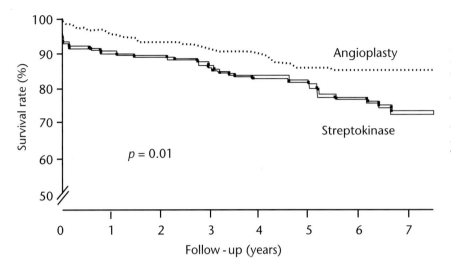

Figure 12.2
Kaplan–Meier survival curves in the Zwolle trial,[15] comparing primary angioplasty with streptokinase, during a follow-up period of 7 years. In patients allocated to angioplasty, the significant reduction in mortality rate, observed before hospital discharge, is even more pronounced at 7-year follow-up, when compared with streptokinase.

Would all patients benefit from primary angioplasty?

Although the benefits of primary angioplasty in comparison with thrombolysis have been demonstrated in randomized trials, the question remains whether primary angioplasty should be performed in all patients with AMI or only in high-risk patients. From 1993 to 1995, a total of 240 patients were involved in a prospective randomized trial: 145 high-risk patients were treated with primary angioplasty and 95 low-risk patients were randomized to undergo primary angioplasty or to receive streptokinase.[18] Patients were considered high-risk when they had a large anterior myocardial infarction, with Killip class 3 or 4 at admission, and/or contraindications for thrombolytic therapy. As shown in Figure 12.3, in the high-risk group,

the mortality rate at 6 months was 11%, the incidence of reinfarction was 3%, and the need for subsequent re-PTCA or coronary artery bypass grafting (CABG) was 14% and 16%, respectively. Among low-risk patients, the incidence of reinfarction and the need for re-PTCA were significantly higher in those patients allocated to streptokinase (16% and 61% versus 3% and 20%, respectively; $p < 0.01$), whereas all other parameters, including mortality rate (2% in each group), were similar between the two groups.

Similar data have also been reported by Ribichini and collegues,[19] who randomized 110 patients with inferior AMI with precordial ST-segment depression to primary angioplasty or thrombolytic therapy. At 1-year follow-up, the incidence of death, reinfarction, or repeat revascularization was 11% in the PTCA group versus 52.7% in the thrombolysis group ($p < 0.0001$).

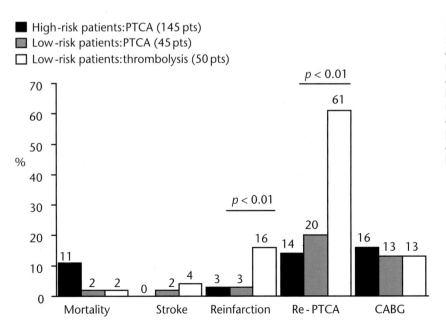

Figure 12.3
Bar graphs show the 6-month clinical outcome of low-risk AMI patients, randomized to thrombolysis or angioplasty. Significantly lower incidences of reinfarction and re-PTCA were observed in the angioplasty group. PTCA, percutaneous transluminal coronary angioplasty; CABG, coronary artery bypass grafting.

Stents and other mechanical devices

In the early years of coronary stenting, the presence of intraluminal thrombus was considered a relative contraindication for stenting. The anticoagulation regimens that were used resulted in a high risk of bleeding and vascular complications. Stenting was therefore restricted to bail-out situations, such as flow-limiting dissections or severe residual stenosis despite balloon dilatations. Despite these two problems, the initial results of stenting were quite favorable. In particular, since the development of safe and effective antiplatelet agents, stenting has had a profound effect on the performance and results of primary angioplasty both in the acute phase and during follow-up. A pooled analysis of data from randomized trials,[20] involving 4120 patients[8,21–26] is depicted in Figure 12.4. The better outcome conferred by stenting is related to a significant reduction in restenosis in comparison with angioplasty.

The impact of stenting is also pertinent to costs – by reducing the rate of restenosis, stent-eligible patients have a reduced need for repeat hospitalization and procedures.[27] As summarized in Table 12.2, 24-month follow-up data from our randomized trial[28] showed the clear benefit of stenting in comparison with balloon angioplasty, with a significant reduction in reinfarction and target vessel revascularization. The cost-effectiveness of primary stenting, compared with balloon angioplasty, for AMI has also been shown (Figure 12.5). Nevertheless, there are important caveats regarding our current knowledge of the role of stenting for AMI. Firstly, the benefit of stenting to reduce the rate of restenosis and the need for repeat revascularization procedures is clear, but the effect of stenting on mortality seems the be absent. Secondly, almost all stent trials have enrolled patients after diagnostic angiography, and thus excluded many patients deemed 'not suitable' for stenting. Results of trials that enroll all patients with acute ST-elevation myocardial infarction and with randomization before vascular access is obtained, are urgently needed. At present, stenting can be advocated for bail-out situations and to reduce restenosis in selected suitable candidates. Further improvements will come from new stent designs and maybe from stents covered with drugs or materials that prevent thrombosis and/or restenosis.

Many new devices have been introduced in the last few years (e.g. directional atherectomy, transcatheter extraction atherectomy (TEC), the Posis Angioget, and the PercuSurge Guardwire System), but so far only few and nonrandomized data are available for patients with AMI.[29–32] Kaplan et al[29] reported their experience in 100 patients with AMI treated with TEC. No reflow was observed in 6% of patients, with an in-hospital mortality rate of 5%, and a total 6-month mortality rate of 10%. The safety and feasibility of TEC in AMI have yet to be proven in the TOPIT (TEC or PTCA in Thrombus) multicenter trial,[30] in which 550 patients with acute coronary syndromes (including AMI) will be randomized to balloon angioplasty or TEC. However, the skills and costs required for these techniques, the loss of time to achieve adequate flow through the infarct-related artery owing to technical preparations, and the risk of not reaching the culprit lesion are major limitations.

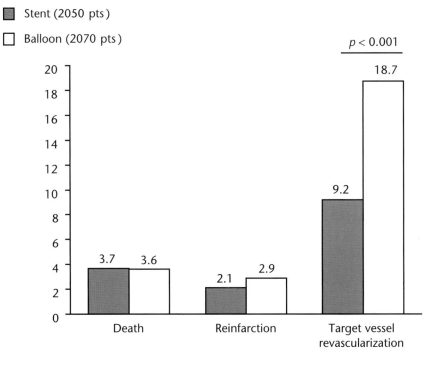

Figure 12.4
Bar graphs showing a pooled data analysis of the 6–12 month clinical outcome of patients with AMI randomized to balloon angioplasty or stenting. Primary stenting has been shown to be superior to balloon angioplasty, and this is mainly due to a significant reduction in restenosis after stenting, when compared with angioplasty.

Table 12.2   Cumulative clinical outcome at 24 months

	Stent (112 pts)	Balloon (115 pts)	p-value
Death	3 (3%)	4 (3%)	1.00
Reinfarction	1 (1%)	10 (9%)	0.01
Death/reinfarction	4 (4%)	13 (11%)	0.04
Target vessel revascularization	15 (13%)	39 (35%)	0.0003
Subsequent bypass surgery	7 (6%)	18 (16%)	0.033
Repeat angioplasty	8 (7%)	21 (18%)	0.016
Cumulative cardiac event-free survival	94 (84%)	71 (62%)	0.0002
Total cost (US$)	15 710	16 466	0.83

Reproduced from Suryapranata H et al. Heart 2001;85:667–71[28] with permission from the BMJ Publishing Group.

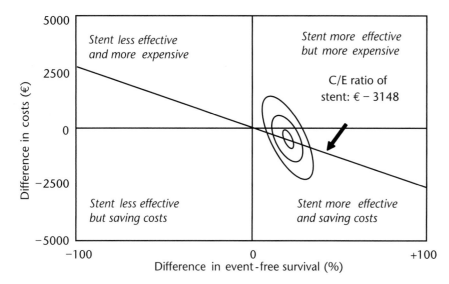

Figure 12.5
Stenting in AMI: Zwolle trial. A bivariate normal distribution of differences in costs and effects in a two-dimensional plane, together with the uncertainties surrounding estimates. A 95% confidence ellipse and a simultaneous confidence region for both costs and effects are depicted. The probability that the inner ellipse includes the true incremental costs and effectiveness is 5%. For the middle ellipse, this is 50%, and for the outer ellipse, 95%. Stenting resulted to be more effective and cost saving, with an incremental cost-effectiveness ratio € − 3148.

Patency of the artery and reperfusion of the myocardium

In experiments with temporary occlusion of a coronary artery in animals, it has been shown that restoration of antegrade flow in an epicardial coronary artery does not always result in effective reperfusion of the affected myocardium, due to damage to distal microvasculature or distal embolization. This has been called the 'no-reflow' phenomenon.

Intracoronary Doppler flow measurements, contrast echocardiography, and magnetic resonance imaging have shown that in a considerable number of patients, flow into the distal myocardium is abnormal or even absent despite a patent epicardial coronary artery.[33] Clinical data show that patients with evidence of adequate myocardial perfusion have an excellent clinical outcome, whereas almost all major adverse clinical events after reperfusion

therapy occur in patients with signs of the 'no-reflow' phenomenon.[33]

A new angiographic parameter to describe the effectiveness of myocardial reperfusion, the myocardial blush grade, has been introduced.[34] As summarized in Table 12.3, we found a direct relationship between myocardial blush grade, ST-segment resolution, enzymatic infarct size, pre-discharge left ventricular function, and mortality.

In day-to-day clinical practice, 12-lead ECG, in particular, resolution of ST-segment elevations after reperfusion therapy, is an excellent and simple method[35,36] that can be applied after all forms of reperfusion therapy. In our previous study,[36] after adjustment for age, sex, infarct location, and previous infarction, the relative risk of death was 6.4 (95% CI 2.7–15.39) among patients with no ST-segment resolution and 3.5 (95% CI 1.5–8) among patients with partial resolution, in comparison with patients with total ST-segment resolution (Figure 12.6).

Several approaches are under investigation to improve myocardial perfusion and to maintain or restore micro-

Table 12.3   Relationship between myocardial blush grade, enzymatic infarct size, left ventricular ejection fraction (LVEF), ST-segment resolution, and mortality

| | Myocardial blush grade | | | |
	3	2	1/0	Trend analysis
LDH_{72}	757 ± 582	1143 ± 879	1623 ± 1147	<0.0001
LVEF (%)	50 ± 10	46 ± 11	39 ± 12	<0.0001
Mortality rate (%)	3	6	23	<0.0001
ST-segment resolution (%)	65	54	27	<0.0001

LDH_{72} indicates enzymatic infarct size from serial lactate dehydrogenase measurements up to 72 h after angioplasty. LVEF was measured by pre-discharge radionucleide ventriculography. Total mortality was assessed after a follow-up of 1.9 ± 1.7 years. ST-segment resolution was evaluated as described elsewhere.[39]
Adapted from van't Hof A. Circulation 1998;97:2302–6.[34]

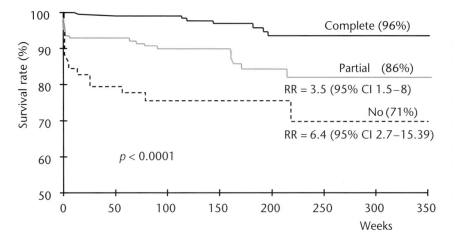

Figure 12.6
Long-term survival after primary angioplasty is related to ST-elevation resolution. At 7-year follow-up, the cumulative survival rate of 96% in patients with complete resolution is significantly higher when compared with that in patients with partial or no ST-segment resolution (86% and 71%, respectively).[36] RR, relative risk; 95% CI, 95% confidence interval. (Reproduced from van't Hof AW et al. Lancet 1997;350:615–19[36] with permission from Elsevier.)

vascular integrity in infarct patients. Adenosine has been studied as an adjunct to fibrinolytic therapy in the AMIS-TAD trial.[37] The use of adenosine did result in smaller anterior infarct size, but there was no reduction in morbidity/mortality. The ESCAMI trial[38] evaluated the efficacy of enopride (a Na^+/H^+ exchange inhibitor) as adjunctive therapy to early reperfusion therapy for AMI, showing no difference in limitation of infarct size or improvement of clinical outcome, in comparison with placebo.

The ECLA group[39] evaluated the impact of additional GIPS (glucose–insulin–potassium solution) infusion on clinical outcome in patients with AMI, showing a 66% reduction in the relative in-hospital mortality risk when GIPS was added to reperfusion (the absolute mortality risk decreased from 15.2% to 5.2%).

The impact of distal embolization after primary angioplasty has been shown in our randomized trial on AMI.[40] The incidence of distal embolization (16% in this series) is surprisingly high during primary angioplasty. It is associated with a significantly lower TIMI 3 flow, a less adequate myocardial blush grade, and a less complete ST-segment resolution, as well as a lower ejection

fraction and a higher enzymatic infarct size, resulting in a poor long-term survival during a follow-up of 6 years (56% versus 91%). Therefore, further clinical research should be aimed towards defining a subgroup of patients at high risk for distal embolization. Furthermore, treatment strategy should also be developed to prevent this event, either by a mechanical approach, such as the use of embolic protective devices, or by a pharmacological approach, using glycoprotein IIb/IIIa inhibitors or adjunctive lytic therapy.

Emergency transfer of AMI patients for primary angioplasty

Only a minority of patients with AMI present to a hospital with the facilities to provide primary angioplasty therapy to all patients with AMI. Most patients present in settings – at home, or in an ambulance, an emergency room, or another hospital facility – that permit the immediate use

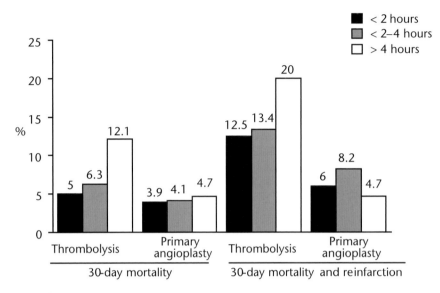

■ < 2 hours
▨ < 2–4 hours
☐ > 4 hours

Figure 12.7
Bar graphs showing a pooled data analysis of clinical outcome of patients with AMI randomized to primary angioplasty or streptokinase.[14] Patients were divided according to the time from onset of ischemia to reperfusion. The mortality rate at 30 days is significantly higher after thrombolytic therapy when compared with angioplasty, particularly in those patients presenting late. But more interestingly, with increasing time delay to treatment, the mortality rate increases considerably after thrombolysis, while it remains relatively stable after angioplasty.

of thrombolytic therapy, but need additional referral and transportation to allow primary angioplasty. This can be organized safely, but the additional time delay would offset some of the benefits, even though the time to therapy is less important for clinical outcome after primary angioplasty compared with thrombolytic therapy (Figure 12.7).[14,41]

In the region surrounding Zwolle (The Netherlands), our hospital is the only center with PTCA facilities, covering an area with up to 1.5 million inhabitants. The surrounding 17 referral hospitals are located at distances as far as 100 km. From 1990 to 1997, a total of 1296 patients have been treated with primary angioplasty at our institution. Of these, 894 were admitted directly to our hospital, while 402 were transferred from other hospitals[42] (Table 12.4). Referral of patients for primary PTCA is not necessarily associated with prolonged time delay, as the time lost during transportation has been caught up by transferring the patients directly into the cathlab. This results in a shorter door-to-balloon time. In fact, the total time delay from symptom onset to the first balloon inflation, of 215 minutes, is quite similar to that observed in nontransferred patients. The clinical outcome at 1 year was comparable between the groups, with respect to the need for re-intervention, reinfarction, and mortality, resulting in event-free

survival rates of 66% and 63%, respectively. These results suggest that transferring patients for primary angioplasty is safe and effective.

These findings have also been confirmed in the PRAGUE multicenter randomized trial,[43] involving a total of 300 patients, presenting at 17 community hospitals, located at less than 75 km from those PTCA centers. Interestingly, this situation is quite similar to our setting. Patients were randomized into three groups: group A (patients treated on site with streptokinase), group B (patients treated with streptokinase and transferred to a PTCA center), and group C (patients transferred immediately for primary PTCA, without streptokinase on board). No significant difference in time delay from symptom onset to reperfusion was observed between transported patients (215 minutes in group C and 220 minutes in group B) and patients treated at the community hospital (192 minutes). Interestingly, the total time delay of 215 minutes in patients tranferred for primary angioplasty is exactly similar to that observed in our trial. As shown in Figure 12.8, the mortality rate and the incidence of reinfarction at 30 days were significantly lower after primary angioplasty, while stroke was only observed in those patients treated with streptokinase. As a result, the combined clinical endpoint of

Table 12.4   Transfer for primary PTCA: clinical outcome at 1 year – the Zwolle experience

Event	Non-transferred (n = 894)	Transferred (n = 402)	p
Primary success (%)	95.7	96.1	
Death (%)	6.7	7.9	0.001
Reinfarction (%)	2.8	5.4	0.02
Re-PTCA (%)	12.1	14.3	1.0
CABG (%)	14.6	17.3	0.01
Event-free	65.9	62.9	0.001

Adapted from Zijlstra et al. Ned Tijdschr Geneeska 1999;143.[42]

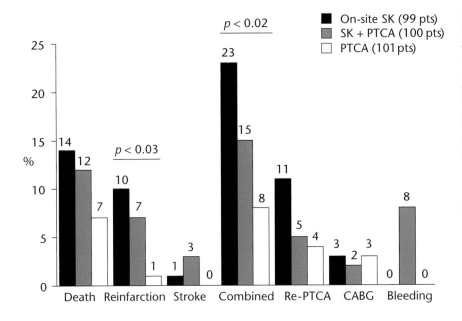

Figure 12.8
Bar graphs showing 30-day clinical outcome of the PRAGUE trial.[42] The mortality rate and the incidence of reinfarction were significantly lower after primary angioplasty, while stroke was only observed in those patients treated with streptokinase (SK). As a result, the combined endpoint of death, reinfarction, or stroke was significantly lower after primary angioplasty, while major bleeding complications occurred only in those patients pretreated with streptokinase.

death, reinfarction, or stroke was significantly lower after primary PTCA (8% in group C, 15% in group B, and 23% in group A), while bleeding complications occurred only in those patients treated with streptokinase. But, more importantly, no deaths or other major complications occurred during transportation in this series. Therefore, the risk of major bleeding complications after thrombolytic therapy is higher than the risk of transportation.

The Danish Trial in Acute Myocardial Infarction-2 (DANAMI-2) (data presented during the 2002 Annual Meeting of the American College of Cardiology) is the first, large randomized trial to compare transfer of patients for PTCA with on-site lytic therapy using 100 mg front-loaded tissue plasminogen activator (tPA). The trial was conducted at 5 PTCA centers and 22 referring hospitals serving almost two-third of the Danish population of 5.4 million. In agreement with the PRAGUE trial, this trial showed that long distance transport for primary angioplasty is safe, with a similar outcome in comparison with on-site primary angioplasty. The cumulative event rate of death, reinfarction, and stroke at 30 days was 8% for patients treated by PTCA and 13.7% for fibrinolysis patients ($p = 0.0003$), with a relative risk reduction of 45%. This was comparable between PTCA centers and referring hospitals.

All of these reports have consistently shown that transferring patients with AMI for primary angioplasty is safe, and improves the outcome in comparison with on-site thrombolysis. In general, it can be stated that the higher the risk of the patient, the greater the potential benefit of primary angioplasty.[44]

Conclusions

The life-saving effect of reperfusion for AMI has been well established. If we define our goal for the future as effective myocardial reperfusion within 2 hours after symptom onset in all patients with AMI, then it is clear that we still have a long way to go.

Earlier diagnosis by 12-lead ECG at home or in the ambulance, rapid transportation, and institution of the best available option should be the first priority. Prehospital diagnosis of AMI allows preparation before patient's arrival and results in an important improvement in the delivery of reperfusion therapy. In patients treated with primary angioplasty, it results in a 30–40 minutes shorter time to first balloon inflation,[45] and where angioplasty is not available, it allows the prehospital and more rapid administration of thrombolytic therapy. Prehospital diagnosis offers as an additional advantage the possibility of considering pharmacological pretreatment on the way to the catheterization laboratory.

Although more research is required into many facets of primary angioplasty, it is clear that this treatment is here to stay. Planning for infarct angioplasty needs to be coordinated and clinical protocols need to be agreed by all involved in the care of patients with AMI. The additional benefits and limitations of new drugs, devices, and combinations of both will be investigated, and may lead to improved patient outcome, but in the years to come, most benefit for our patients will come from dedicated application of the therapeutic possibilities that are available today.

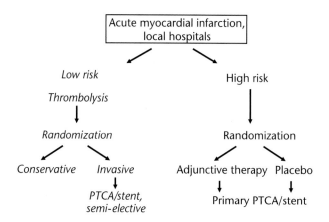

Figure 12.9
Our proposed PTCA strategy for the treatment of AMI. All low-risk patients should be immediately treated at a local hospital with intravenous thrombolysis and subsequently randomized to conservative or invasive strategy (the following day or before hospital discharge), whereas all high-risk patients should be transferred immediately for primary angioplasty, with or without adjunctive pharmacological therapy.

Until more information becomes available, we would like to propose the following PTCA strategy for AMI (Figure 12.9). Patients with AMI admitted at local hospitals should be classified into low-risk and high-risk patients, according to the clinical and ECG findings at admission. Intravenous thrombolysis should be given immediately to low-risk patients, followed by randomization to conservative or invasive strategy, as our previous trial[18] has shown that primary PTCA in these low-risk patients has no additional benefits with regard to mortality. However, to address whether the incidence of reinfarction could be reduced by an adjunctive PTCA procedure, patients allocated to an invasive strategy should be transferred for PTCA or stenting, on a semi-elective basis (the following day or before hospital discharge) whereas all high-risk patients should be transferred immediately for primary PTCA or stenting, with or without pretreatment with adjunctive pharmacological agents.

References

1. Ryan TJ, Antman EM, Brooks NH, et al. 1999 update: ACC/AHA Guidelines for the Management of Patients with Acute Myocardial Infarction: Executive Summary and Recommendations: A report of the American College of Cardiology/American Heart Association Task Force on Practise Guidelines (Committee on Management of Acute Myocardial infarction). Circulation 1999;100:1016–30.

2. Hartzler GO, Rutherford BD, McConahay DR, et al. Percutaneous transluminal coronary angioplasty with and without thrombolytic therapy for treatment of acute myocardial infarction. Am Heart J 1983;106:965–73.

3. Liem AL, Zijsltra F, Ottevanger JP, et al. High-dose heparin as pretreatment for primary angioplasty in acute myocardial infarction: the Heparin in Early Patency (HEAP) randomized trial. J Am Coll Cardiol 2000;35:600–4.

4. Efficacy and safety of tenecteplase in combination with enoxaparin, abciximab, or unfractionated heparin: the ASSENT-3 randomised trial in acute myocardial infarction. Lancet 2001;358:605–13.

5. Antman EM, Louweremburg HW, Baars HF, et al, for the ENTIRE–TIMI 23 Investigators. Enoxaparin as adjunctive antithrombin therapy for ST-elevation myocardial infarction. Results of the ENTIRE–Thrombolysis in Myocardial Infarction (TIMI) 23 trial. Circulation 2002;105:1642–49.

6. Topol EJ; The GUSTO V Investigators. Reperfusion therapy for acute myocardial infarction with fibrinolytic therapy or combination reduced fibrinolytic therapy and platelet glycoprotein IIb–IIIa inhibition: the GUSTO V randomised trial. Lancet 2001;357:1905–14.

7. Brener SJ, Ban LA, Burchenal JEB, et al, on the behalf of the RAPPORT Investigators. Randomized, placebo-controlled trial of platelet glycoprotein IIb/IIIa blockade with primary angioplasty for acute myocardial infarction. Circulation 1998;98:734–41.

8. Stone G, Grined CL, Cox AD, et al, for the Controlled Abciximab and Device Investigation to Lower Late Angioplasty Complications (CADILLAC) Investigators. Comparison of angioplasty with stenting with or without abciximab, in acute myocardial infarction. N Engl J Med 2002;346:957–66.

9. Ross AM, Coyne CS, Reiner JS, et al, for the PACT Investigators. A randomized trial comparing primary angioplasty with a strategy of short-acting thrombolysis and immediate planned rescue angioplasty in acute myocardial infarction; the PACT trial. J Am Coll Cardiol 1999;33:1528–33.

10. DeWood MA, Spores J, Notske R, et al. Prevalence of total coronary occlusion during early hours of transluminal myocardial infarction. N Engl J Med 1980;303:897–902.

11. Grines CL, Marselese DL, Brodie B, et al, for the PAMI-II Investigators. Safety and cost-effectiveness of early discharge after primary angioplasty in low risk patients with acute myocardial infarction. J Am Coll Cardiol 1998;31:967–72.

12. Every NR, Maynard C, Cochran RP, et al, for the Myocardial Infarction Triage and Intervention Investigators. Characteristics, management, and outcome of patients with acute myocardial infarction treated with bypass surgery. Circulation 1996;94(Suppl II);81–6.

13. Weaver WD, Simes RJ, Betriu A, et al, for the Primary Coronary Angioplasty vs Thrombolysis Collaboration Group. Comparison of primary coronary angioplasty and intravenous thrombolyitc therapy for acute myocardial infarction: a quantitative overview. JAMA 1997;278:2093–8.

14. Zijlstra F, Patel A, Jones M, et al. Clinical characteristics and outcome of patients with acute (<2 h), intermediate (2–4 h) and late (>4 h) presentation treated by primary coronary angioplasty or thrombolytic therapy for acute myocardial infarction. Eur Heart J 2002;23:550–7.

15. Zijlstra F, Hoorntje JCA, de Boer MJ, et al. Long-term benefit of primary angioplasty as compared with thrombolytic therapy for acute myocardial infarction. N Engl J Med 1999;341:1413–19.

16. Lieu TA, Gurley RJ, Lundstrom RJ, et al. Projected cost-effectiveness of primary angioplasty for acute myocardial infarction. J Am Coll Cardiol 1997;30:1741–50.

17. Canto JG, Every NR, Magid DJ, et al. The volume of primary PTCA procedures and survival after myocardial infarction. N Engl J Med 2000;342:1573–80.

18. Zijlstra F, Beukema WP, van't Hof A, et al. Randomized comparison of primary coronary angioplasty with thrombolytic therapy in low-risk patients with acute myocardial infarction. J Am Coll Cardiol 1997;29:908–12.

19. Ribichini F, Steffenino G, DellaValle A, et al. Comparison of thrombolytic therapy and primary coronary angioplasty with liberal stenting for inferior myocardial infarction with precordial ST-segment depression. Immediate and long-term results of a randomized study. J Am Coll Cardiol 1998;32:1687–94.

20. Zhu MM, Feit A, Chadow H, et al. Primary stent implantation compared with primary balloon angioplasty for acute myocardial infarction: a meta-analysis of randomized clinical trials. Am J Cardiol 2001;88:297–301.

21. Antoniucci D, Santoro GM, Bolognese L, et al. A clinical trial comparing primary stenting of the infarct-related artery with optimal primary angioplasty for acute myocardial infarction. J Am Coll Cardiol 1998;31:1234–9.

22. Suryapranata H, van't Hof AWJ, Hoorntje JC, et al. Randomized comparison of coronary stenting with balloon angioplasty in patients with acute myocardial infarction. Circulation 1998;97:2502–7.

23. Rodriguez A, Bernardi V, Fernandez M, et al. In-hospital and late results of coronary stents versus conventional balloon angioplasty in acute myocardial infarction (GRAMI Trial) (Gianturco-Roubin in Acute Myocardial Infarction). Am J Cardiol 1998;81:1286–91.

24. Saito S, Hosokawa G, Tanaka S, et al. Primary stent implantation is superior to balloon angioplasty in acute myocardial infarction: final results of the primary angioplasty versus stent implantation in acute myocardial infarction (PASTA) trial. PASTA Trial Investigators. Cathet Cardiovasc Interv 1999;48:262–8.

25. Grines CL, Cox DA, Stone GW, et al. Coronary angioplasty with or without stent implantation for acute myocardial infarction. Stent Primary Angioplasty in Myocardial Infarction Study Group. N Engl J Med 1999;341:1949–56.

26. Millard L, Hamon M, Khalife K, et al. A comparison of systematic stenting and conventional balloon angioplasty during primary percutaneous transluminal coronary angioplasty for acute myocardial infarction. STENTIM-2 Investigators. J Am Coll Cardiol 2000;35:1729–36.

27. van't Hof AWJ, Suryapranata H, de Boer MJ, et al. Costs of stenting for acute myocardial infarction. Lancet 1998;351:1817.

28. Suryapranata H, Ottervanger JP, Nibbering E, et al. Long term outcome and cost-effectiveness of stenting versus balloon angioplasty for acute myocardial infarction. Heart 2001;85:667–71.

29. Kaplan BM, Larkin T, Safian RD, et al. Prospective study of extraction atherectomy in patients with acute myocardial infarction. Am J Cardiol 1996;78:383–8.

30. Kaplan BM, Gregory M, Schreiber TL, et al. A comparison between transcatheter extraction atherectomy and balloon angioplasty in acute coronary syndromes (TOPIT). Circulation 1996;95(Suppl):1846 (abst).

31. Silva JA, Saucido JF, Lanoue AS, et al. For the VeGAS I and VeGas II investigators. Rheolytic thrombectomy using the Posis Angiojet catheter in patients with acute myocardial infarction presenting within 8 hours of symptoms. J Am Coll Cardiol 1998;32(Suppl A):410A (abst).

32. Belli G, Pezzano A, De Biase AM, et al. Adjunctive thrombus aspiration and mechanical protection from distal embolization in primary percutaneous intervention for acute myocardial infarction. Cathet Cardiovasc Interv 2000;50:362–70.

33. Iliceto S, Marangelli V, Marchese A, et al. Myocardial contrast echocardiography in acute myocardial infarction: pathophysiological background and clinical applications. Eur Heart J 1996;17:344–53.

34. van't Hof A, Liem A, Suryapranata H, et al. on the behalf of the Zwolle Myocardial Infarction Study Group. Angiographic assessment of myocardial reperfusion in patients treated with primary angioplasty for acute myocardial infarction. Myocardial Blush Grade. Circulation 1998;97:2302–6.

35. Schroder R, Dissmann R, Bruggermann T, et al. Extent of early ST segment elevation resolution: a simple but strong predictor of outcome in patients with acute myocardial infarction. J Am Coll Cardiol 1994;24:384–91.

36. van't Hof AWJ, Liem A, de Boer MJ, Zijlstra F, on behalf of the Zwolle Myocadial Infarction Study Group. Clinical value of 12-lead electrocardiogram after successful reperfusion therapy for acute myocardial infarction. Lancet 1997;350:615–19.

37. Mahaffey KW, Puma JA, Barbagelata NA, et al. Adenosine as an adjunct to thrombolytic therapy for acute myocardial infarction: results of a multicenter, randomized, placebo-controlled trial: the Acute Myocardial Infarction Study of Adenosine (AMISTAD) trial. J Am Coll Cardiol 1999;34:1711–20.

38. Zeymer U, Suryapranata H, Monassier JP, et al, for the ESCAMI Investigators. The Na$^+$/H$^+$ exchange inhibitor Eniporide as an adjunct to early reperfusion therapy in acute myocardial infarction. Results of the Evaluation of the Safety and Cardioprotective effects of Eniporide in Acute Myocardial Infarction. J Am Coll Cardiol 2001;38:1644–50.

39. Diaz R, Paolasso EC, Piegas LS, et al, on behalf of the ECLA (Estudios Cardiologicos Latinoamerica) Collaborative Group. Metabolic modulation of acute myocardial infarction: the ECLA Glucose–Insulin–Potassium Pilot Trial. Circulation 1998;98:2227–34.

40. Henriques JP, Zijlstra F, Ottervanger JP, et al. Incidence and clinical significance of distal embolization during primary angioplasty for acute myocardial infarction. Eur Heart J 2002;23:1112–17

41. Brodie BR, Stone G, Morice MC, et al. Importance of time to reperfusion on outcomes with primary angioplasty for acute myocardial infarction (results from the Stent Primary Angioplasty in Myocardial Infarction Trial). Am J Cardiol 2001;88:1085–90.

42. Zijlstra F, Suryapranata H, AWJ van't Hof, et al. Gilijke resultaten van primaire percutane transluminale coronaire angioplastiek bij direct en indirect verwezen patienten met acuut myocardinfarct. Ned Tijdschr Geneeskd 1999;143 (10).

43. Widimisky P, Groch L, Zelizko M, et al, on behalf of the PRAGUE Study Group Investigators. Multicenter randomized trial comparing transport primary angioplasty vs immediate

thrombolysis vs combined strategy for patients with acute myocardial infarction presenting to a community hospital without a catheterization laboratory. The PRAGUE study. Eur Heart J 2000;21:823–31.

44. O'Neill WW, de Boer MJ, Gibbons RJ, et al. Lessons from the pooled outcome of the Pami, Zwolle and Mayo Clinic randomized trials of primary angioplasty versus thrombolytic therapy of acute myocardial infarction. J Invasive Cardiol 1998;10:4A–10A.

45. Zijlstra F. Long-term benefit of primary angioplasty compared to thrombolytic therapy for acute myocardial infarction. Eur Heart J 2000;21;1847–9.

13

The role of distal protection devices

Arun Kuchela, Campbell Rogers

Introduction

When discussing the risks and benefits of percutaneous interventions, patients will often ask 'What happens to the stuff? Where does it go?' For many years, the answer was that the material would simply pass into the distal vasculature without any recognized impact. Embolization of thrombus and plaque material was felt to be infrequent. However, evidence to the contrary has slowly been mounting, suggesting that distal embolization is in fact a common occurrence with significant associated adverse effects. The development of devices to prevent distal embolization has further raised the awareness of this event and created a new and expanding aspect of percutaneous intervention. This chapter will briefly describe the currently available devices and the available literature to examine the current role of embolic protection devices.

Distal embolization – evidence and implications

Distal embolization is most commonly recognized angiographically as diminished flow to the distal vascular bed, or 'no reflow'. It is manifested clinically with target organ damage, for example periprocedural myocardial infarction or ischemic neurological event. As outlined by Topol and Yadav,[1] the concept of microvascular embolization was suggested by Willerson and colleagues based on a model of endothelial injury. However, the frequency and impact of distal embolization has been suggested by newer diagnostic modalities. Myocardial contrast echocardiography was used to demonstrate that at least 25% of patients with normal flow on angiography lack perfusion at the tissue level.[2] Nuclear studies have shown that perfusion defects can develop during a procedure without any enzyme evidence[3] and magnetic resonance imaging has demonstrated that microvascular obstruction portends a worse prognosis.[4] Further evidence is provided by the TIMI myocardial perfusion grade, which demonstrated that lower perfusion was related to a higher mortality independent of flow in the epicardial artery.[5]

Evidence regarding the incidence and potential impact of distal embolization can be found in several studies. The CAVEAT trial, which compared directional atherectomy with balloon angioplasty, reported a periprocedural myocardial infarction rate of 7%, which was highly predictive of mortality, bypass, or repeat intervention at 30 days.[6,7] In the CAVEAT-II trial of directional atherectomy in saphenous vein grafts (SVGs), the incidence of distal embolization with percutaneous transluminal coronary angioplasty (PTCA) was 5.1%.[8] However, distal embolization was associated with a statistically significant increase in periprocedural myocardial infarctions and adverse events out to 1 year. The incidence of distal embolization, as suggested by myocardial infarction, in balloon angioplasty of SVGs in a review of published data is approximately 4%.[9] Transluminal extraction atherectomy of SVG lesions had an incidence of distal embolization of 12.8%, which was associated with significantly more in-hospital complications, predominantly myocardial infarction, and lower procedural success.[10] Acute infarct angioplasty for SVG lesions was associated with a postprocedural TIMI grade 3 flow in only 48% of cases and an in-hospital mortality rate of 19%, while 71% of native coronary lesions undergoing angioplasty for acute myocardial infarction had grade 3 flow and a 7.9% in-hospital mortality rate.[11]

The impact of periprocedural myocardial enzyme release has been demonstrated by Hong et al.[12] They determined that major creatine kinase MB isoenzyme (CK-MB) release ($>5 \times$ normal) occurred in 15% of otherwise-successful SVG interventions and that the magnitude of enzyme elevation correlated with 1-year mortality.

Some of the strongest evidence for distal embolization comes from the use of distal protection devices themselves. Webb and colleagues[13] first demonstrated the feasibility and potential implications of distal protection by analyzing the particulate debris from SVG interventions using a balloon occlusion system. The Percusurge GuardWire was employed in 27 SVG interventions and demonstrated an improvement in TIMI grade flow. There also did not appear to be any damage to the vessel associated with the occlusion balloon. The ischemic times were short, approximately 2.5 minutes, and were well tolerated. The retrieved particles were $204 \pm 57\ \mu m$ in major axis and $83 \pm 22\ \mu m$ in minor axis, and consisted of predominantly acellular atheromatous material found under the fibrous cap. Semiquantitative analysis of the plaque material suggested that more debris was released from balloon dilatation than from direct stenting.

Embolic protection devices

Currently, there are several embolic protection devices, falling into three basic categories: distal occlusion balloons, filters, and proximal occlusion balloon/flow reversal (Table 13.1). Distal occlusion balloons are placed distal to the target lesion and used to temporarily occlude flow to the distal vessel, thus trapping all the potentially embolic particles. Filters are also placed distal to the target lesion, but instead maintain flow in the vessel and act to filter out large embolic particles. The proximal occlusion balloon blocks inflow to the vessel and relies upon retrograde flow

Table 13.1　Available embolic protection devices

Occlusion balloon	Distal filter	Proximal occlusion/ flow reversal
Percusurge GuardWire	AngioGuard (Cordis)	Parodi Anti-Emboli System (ArteriA)
	FilterWire EX (Boston Scientific/ Embolic Protection, Inc)	Proxis (Velocimed)
		Kerberos
	CardioShield (MedNova)	
	NetII NG (Guidant)	
	Trap (MicroVena)	
	Interceptor (Medtronic)	

to prevent embolization of particles. Each of these types of devices has its major advantages and disadvantages (Table 13.2). The distal occlusion balloon has a lower crossing profile and more flexibility, and theoretically provides more complete protection. Its major disadvantages include interruption of flow to the target organ, inability to perform an angiogram during balloon inflation, failure to protect proximal side branches, and a requirement for multiple procedural steps. The major advantage of filters is preservation of flow and the ability to perform intraprocedural angiography. Disadvantages include potentially incomplete protection, larger crossing profile, retrieval failure, and potential filter thrombosis/occlusion. Finally, the potential benefits of using a proximal occlusion system include the ability to obtain complete protection prior to

Table 13.2　Advantages and disadvantages of the different types of devices

	Advantages	Disadvantages
Distal occlusion	• Lower crossing profile • Complete distal protection for all particles and humoral mediators	• Interruption of flow • Inability to perform angiogram • Multistep procedure • No protection of side branches
Filters	• Preservation of flow • Ability to perform angiogram during procedure	• Loss of smaller particles and humoral mediators • Larger crossing profile • Potential filter thrombosis
Proximal occlusion/flow reversal	• Complete protection prior to lesion manipulation • Protection of side branches • Ability to use guidewire of choice	• Interruption of flow • Inability to perform angiogram • Larger guide size

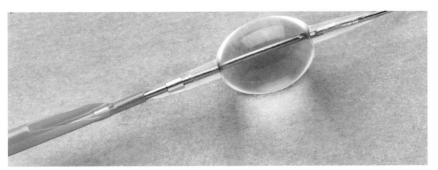

Figure 13.1
PercuSurge GuardWire distal occlusion balloon and aspiration catheter.

lesion manipulation, protection of side branches, and the absence of a requirement to deliver a device distally, allowing the use of any guidewire. The major disadvantages are the interruption of flow and potential poor tolerance of occlusion of large zones of tissue. The following is a brief description of the most common devices in clinical use.

The first device approved by the US Food and Drug Administration (FDA) for distal embolic protection is an occlusion balloon and aspiration system, the Percusurge GuardWire (Medtronic/AVE)[14] (Figure 13.1). The system consists of several coaxial components, the first of which is a 210 cm-long angioplasty wire consisting of a 0.014 inch nitinol hypotube with a 35 mm radiopaque, flexible coil design tip. A 5.5 mm-long elastometric balloon is incorporated into the wire 3.5 cm from the coil tip and can be inflated to between 3.5 and 5.0 mm at low pressures (<2 atm) via a detachable inflation adapter. A 135 cm-long side-hole aspiration catheter (Export) with a 35 cm-long distal monorail wire lumen is used to remove particulate debris before balloon deflation. The GuardWire is used to cross the target lesion and the distal balloon is placed in a region of normal vessel downstream. The balloon is then inflated, preventing antegrade flow down the vessel while the intervention is performed over the GuardWire, all embolic material presumably being trapped proximal to the distal balloon. The Export catheter is then used to aspirate 20–40 ml, which would contain any embolic material. The distal balloon is then deflated and the GuardWire removed. See Figure 13.2.

The AngioGuard (Cordis, J&J) distal protection device consists of a filter integrated into a 0.014 inch stainless steel angioplasty wire. The filter has a nickel–titanium skeleton supporting a polyurethane membrane creating a collection basket (Figure 13.3). The membrane has multiple laser-drilled pores of 100 μm. The basket diameters vary from 4.0 to 8.0 mm and are designed for use in 3.0–7.5 mm vessels. The device is held closed by an outer delivery sheath (2.5 French (Fr)). The AngioGuard requires a 7 Fr guide catheter, and is deployed after crossing the target lesion by pulling back the delivery sheath. A second sheath is used to close the filter and remove it.[15]

The MedNova CardioShield (Neuroshield versions for carotid interventions) (Figure 13.4) is another distal protection filter that functions along the lines of the AngioGuard filter. It consists of a non-nitinol self-expanding system with a porous polymeric membrane and is mounted on a 0.014 inch guidewire. An important feature is that the filter is free to rotate on the guidewire. A delivery catheter is withdrawn to deploy the filter after crossing the target lesion. A second retrieval catheter is used to envelop the filter for removal. Late generations of the MedNova device provide the added functionality of a variety of wire stiffnesses, allowing wire choice based on particulars of a given lesion.

The FilterWire EX (Boston Scientific/Embolic Protection, Inc) (Figure 13.5) is also a filter mounted on a 0.014 inch angioplasty wire. However, it differs from the other filters in that it is mounted off-center. The filter consists of an elliptical, radiopaque, nitinol loop and polyurethane filter with pore holes of approximately 100 μm, and gives a 'fishing net' appearance. The device can be used in vessels between 3.5 and 5.5 mm. The FilterWire has a 3.9 Fr delivery/retrieval sheath and is 6 Fr guide-compatible.

The Net II NG Embolic Protection System (Guidant) is a polyurethane filter on a nitinol frame. It has pore sizes less than or equal to 120 μm. The MicroVena Trap is a braided nitinol filter, with an additional nitinol retrieval basket. It is availablen in various sizes with a 2.9 Fr delivery sheath and a 5 Fr retrieval sheath. Finally, one of the most promising distal protection filters is the Interceptor (Medtronic/AVE). This device is a nitinol basket affixed to a 0.014 inch guidewire. Its first generation required a separate retrieval sheath at the end of the procedure, and clinical experience was reported in the SECURE trial.[16] Subsequent-generation devices have removed the need for complete collapse and retrieval, and allow opening and closing of the device from the proximal end of the wire. This advance greatly simplifies and speeds use.

Three novel proximal occlusion systems have been developed. The first, the Proxis device (Velocimed) consists of a highly flexible 6 Fr balloon-tipped catheter advanced through an 8 Fr guide to a point proximal to the lesion (Figure 13.6). With the balloon inflated and distal flow halted, guidewires and balloons or stents can be introduced. At the conclusion of the procedure, the distal territory is aspirated through the balloon-tipped catheter before flow is restored. This system exploits flow reversal through myocardial capillaries, and allows the implementation of

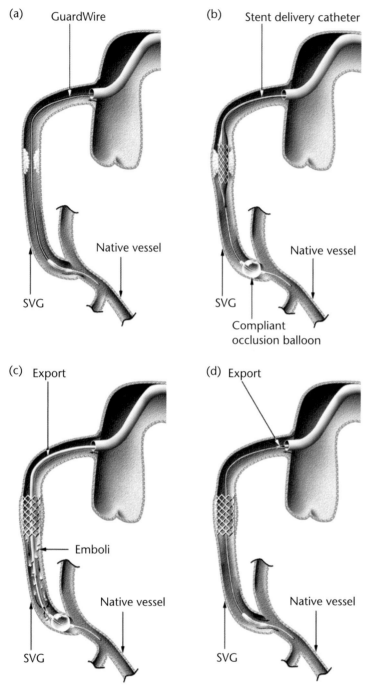

(a) GuardWire

(b) Stent delivery catheter

Native vessel

SVG

Native vessel

SVG

Compliant
occlusion balloon

(c) Export

(d) Export

Emboli

Native vessel

SVG

Native vessel

SVG

Figure 13.2
Schematic representation of the use of the
Percusurge GuardWire system.

protection before any manipulation of the lesion, including
guidewire crossing. It also allows the theoretical protection of all side branches proximal to and distal to the
lesion. Initial clinical experience is underway in Europe,
with early results presented. The second proximal occlusion device (Kerberos, Inc) places a balloon directly on the
tip of the guiding catheter, and has the added feature of
active distal rinsing during aspiration.

Finally, the Parodi Anti-Emboli System (PAESI,
ArteriA Medical Science, Inc.) uses a proximal occlusion
balloon and operates by the theory of flow reversal
(most commonly in the carotid artery). It consists of a
guiding catheter with an occlusion balloon mounted at
the distal end, which occludes the vessel and creates a
negative pressure gradient distally, with resultant retrograde flow.

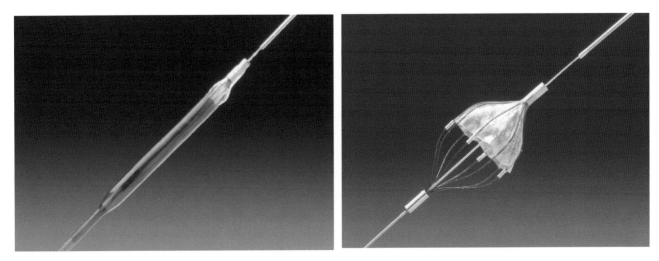

Figure 13.3
AngioGuard filter.

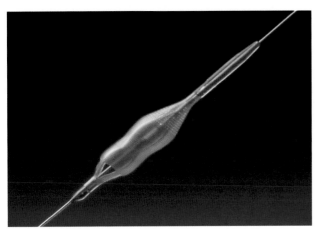

Figure 13.4
MedNova NeuroShield.

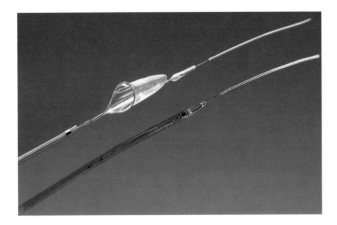

Figure 13.5
The FilterWire EX guidewire filter device and retrieval catheter.

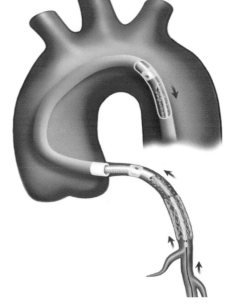

Figure 13.6
Proxis device (Velocimed, Inc.).

Clinical experience

Saphenous vein grafts

With higher rates of distal embolization and increased risk of repeat bypass surgery, SVGs have been a prime target for the development and evaluation of embolic protection devices. Carlino et al[17] reported their initial experience with the Percusurge GuardWire balloon occlusion system in 15 degenerated SVGs from Milan, Italy. The grafts were a mean age of 9.2 ± 4.5 years and the lesions were 27.0 ± 17.0 mm in length. The mean occlusion time for the distal balloon was 4.8 ± 1.2 minutes and a mean of 27.8 ± 10 ml of blood was withdrawn. The TIMI grade flow post intervention was normal in all patients (2.0 ± 0.8 pre procedure) and there was no elevation of CK greater than twice the upper limit of normal, despite a high incidence of lesions with thrombus and ulceration. This study provided further evidence of the feasibility and potential benefit for distal protection in SVG intervention.

The SAFE (Saphenous Vein Graft Angioplasty Free of Emboli) trial was a prospective, controlled, multinational registry to establish the feasibility, safety and efficacy of the Percusurge GuardWire.[18] The study enrolled 103 consecutive patients undergoing 105 SVG lesion-stenting procedures. The lesions had to have a reference diameter of at least 3 mm, and have at least 20 mm of normal vessel distal to the lesion to place the balloon. Major exclusion criteria included recent myocardial infarction, target lesion at the aorto-ostium or after the first anastomosis in a jump graft, ejection fraction (EF) less than 25%, and renal dysfunction. The primary end point was in-hospital MACE, defined as death, myocardial infaction (CK-MB > 3 × normal), emergent bypass surgery, or repeat target vessel revascularization. Major secondary endpoints included no-flow, device success and 30-day adverse event rates. The GuardWire was successfully deployed and aspiration completed in 85% of grafts. The primary reason for failure was inability to steer the GuardWire across tight lesions or tortuous vessels. The GuardWire was felt to be stiffer and transmitted less torque than standard angioplasty wires. The crossing profile of 0.036 inch may have impeded delivery, but this has since been improved to 0.028 inch. There is also a significant learning curve in using the device. TIMI grade 3 flow improved with intervention from 83.5% to 99%. The in-hospital MACE rate was 4.9%, which mostly comprised myocardial infarction. The 30-day event-free survival rate was 94%. The mean balloon inflation time was 5.4 ± 3.7 minutes, and was well tolerat-

ed in all patients. Grossly visible debris was recovered in 91% of patients, and histomorphometric analysis revealed mostly fibrin and plaque elements. Scanning electron microscopy demonstrated most particles to be less than or equal to 96 μm in size (81%). (Figure 13.7) This study was effective in demonstrating the feasibility and safety of the distal occlusion balloon in SVG interventions, as well as providing further evidence regarding embolic particles and the potential benefit to distal protection. SAFE also provided the impetus for a large randomized trial examining the efficacy of distal protection in SVG interventions.

The SAFER (Saphenous Vein Graft Angioplasty Free of Emboli Randomized) trial by Baim et al[19] was the pivotal trial that led to FDA approval of the Percusurge GuardWire for SVG interventions. The study randomized 801 patients with SVG lesions to intervention with either a standard 0.014 inch angioplasty guidewire or a 0.014 inch GuardWire. The lesions had to be greater than 50% diameter stenosis, be located in the mid-portion of the vessel, and have a reference vessel of between 3 and 6 mm. As with the SAFE study, the lesions had to be more than 5 mm from the ostium and have 20 mm of normal vessel distally. The major exclusion criteria were recent myocardial infarction with elevated cardiac enzymes, impaired left ventricular function (LVEF < 25%), baseline creatinine greater than 2.5 mg/dl, and planned use of an atherectomy device. Patients received standard therapy with aspirin and clopidogrel, and were randomized based on operator preselection of glycoprotein IIb/IIIa receptor blocker usage. The primary endpoint was 30-day MACE rate, defined as a composite of death, myocardial infarction (CK-MB > 3 × upper limit of normal), emergent bypass surgery, or target vessel revascularization. Technical success with the GuardWire was achieved in 90.1% of cases, with failures being due to inability to deliver the device, inability to occlude antegrade flow, and inability to aspirate at least 20 ml. There was a 6.9% absolute reduction (42% relative reduction) in the primary endpoint for the GuardWire

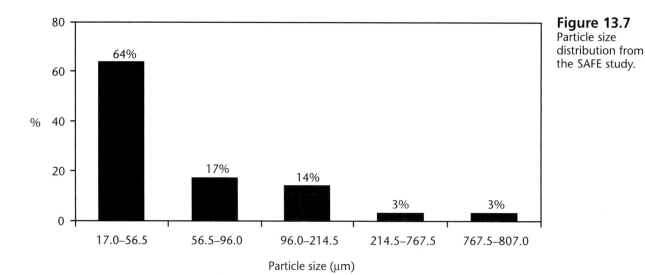

Figure 13.7
Particle size distribution from the SAFE study.

(p = 0.004), which was due primarily to a reduction in myocardial infarctions. This benefit was seen regardless of the use of glycoprotein IIb/IIIa receptor blocker. The GuardWire also achieved higher rates of TIMI grade 3 flow, and a lower incidence of no-reflow. There was also a trend towards mortality reduction with the GuardWire, although the study was not powered to evaluate this. SAFER was the first large-scale trial to show a clear benefit to distal protection, with a reduction in adverse events and no increase in complications. Although only looking at SVG interventions, SAFER does provide an incentive to examine the benefits of distal protection in other interventions where distal embolization causes significant adverse events (e.g. native coronaries and carotid arteries). The FIRE trial was recently completed, comparing the FilterWire (Boston Scientific/EPI) with either no protection or GuardWire protection in SVG stenting. This trial will be the first to allow direct comparison of the relative efficacy and safety of filtering verses distal occlusion approaches for SVG stenting. It is important to acknowledge that, even with protection, adverse events did occur, although the genesis of these events is not clear. Possible contributors include particles released by inflation of the GuardWire itself, incomplete aspiration of particles (particularly those adherent to the occlusion balloon itself), motion of the protection device during the procedure, with transient loss of apposition and escape of particles, or embolic fragments adherent to the stented site, not freely mobile, which embolize in the early postprocedure period.

The phase I and initial cohort from the phase II (FIRE) studies using the FilterWire in SVG interventions have recently been reported.[20] The phase I study described 60 lesions in 48 patients, while the roll-in portion of the phase II study contained 248 lesion in 230 saphenous veins at 65 centers. The phase I study required lesion lengths less than 40 mm, reference vessel diameter of 3.5–5.5 mm, at least TIMI grade 2 flow, and a minimum 2 cm straight segment distal to the lesion. This study identified five technical features that were associated with a higher than expected adverse event rate (21.3% 30-day MACE), and were addressed in the phase II study. These were (i) more than 2.5 cm distance between lesion and distal anastomosis for placement of the filter; (ii) the FilterWire loop placed in the middle of the greater than 2 cm straight landing zone segment; (iii) orthogonal angiographic views to document filter apposition; (iv) avoidance of retracting the entire debris-containing filter into the sheath; and (v) distal protection employed during all SVG dilatations. The phase II study allowed more complex lesions of any length and TIMI 1 flow. The device was successfully delivered in 95.7% of cases in phase I and 96.5% in phase II. The postprocedure TIMI 3 flow was present in 94.7% in phase I, but was similar in phase II. However, there was more glycoprotein IIb/IIIa use in phase II, as well as fewer episodes of no-reflow and distal thromboemboli. There was also a markedly lower 30-day MACE rate of 11.3%, which was largely due to a reduction in periprocedural myocardial

infarction (the MACE rate in the control arm of SAFER was 16.5%[19]). The MACE rate was increased with long lesions, high-grade baseline stenoses, and the presence of thrombus. Nonetheless, the FilterWire was successful in reducing adverse events related to distal embolization, but required a specific set of anatomic and operator-related issues to ensure effectiveness.

Native coronary artery intervention

The frequency and clinical outcome of distal embolization during primary angioplasty for acute myocardial infarction has recently been assessed.[21] Embolization was defined as a distal filling defect with an abrupt 'cutoff' in one of the peripheral coronary artery branches of the infarct-related vessel, distal to the site of angioplasty. In 178 patients undergoing primary angioplasty, distal embolization was observed in 15.2% and was associated with less angiographic success. Myocardial blush scores and ST–T segment resolution were also reduced with distal embolization. These patients also had larger cardiac enzyme leak and lower LVEF at discharge (42% verses 51%; p < 0.01). The long-term mortality rate was higher in patients with distal embolization (44% verses 9%; p = 0.001).

A preliminary report of embolic protection using an occlusion balloon in 39 patients undergoing native coronary intervention with acute, subacute, and chronic disease has demonstrated feasibility in preventing distal embolization.[22] Aggravation of anginal pain occurred in 19 of 36 awake patients, but was well tolerated. Another report described the successful use of the Percusurge GuardWire in 7 of 8 patients with acute myocardial infarction.[23] The immediate angiographic result was excellent and thrombus was aspirated from all successful cases. The EMERALD trial is an ongoing randomized trial of 500 patients presenting with acute myocardial infarction and will randomize patients to primary or rescue percutaneous coronary intervention with or without distal protection using the GuardWire. The primary endpoint of efficacy will be determined by the resolution of ST-segment elevation and myocardial perfusion with technetium-99 sestamibi.

The principal drawback to the occlusion balloon is lack of antegrade flow in the vessel and the resultant ischemia. While this has been well tolerated in SVG interventions, native coronaries are potentially less likely to tolerate prolonged occlusion. Filters, on the other hand, may provide the solution. Grube et al[15] reported their initial experience with the AngioGuard guidewire (Cordis) in 26 patients, 11 SVG lesions, and 15 native coronary lesions. The AngioGuard, as mentioned previously, is a 0.014 inch angioplasty wire with an integrated wire basket and polyurethane filter at the distal end. Eleven of the patients had unstable angina, while two patients were within

48 hours of an acute myocardial infarction. The technical success rate was 96.2%, with inability to deliver the device in one patient. There was no rise in CK or CK-MB levels in either SVG or native coronaries. While the final TIMI grade flow was improved in both types of intervention, the TIMI flow in the SVGs diminished after angioplasty and stent deployment, but returned to normal after removal of the device. This was seen primarily in large grafts with complex lesions, indicating a large embolic load occluding the filter pores. The mean particle size was 0.10 $\pm$ 0.5 mm^2 (range 0.015–20 mm^2) and the mean embolic load per patient was 37 $\pm$ 36 mm^2. Interestingly, the larger particles were found to be aggregates of smaller particles, which could have passed through the 100 μm pores. The particulate was found to be predominantly chronic thrombus and atheromatous material. While this report was not designed to compare the AngioGuard with other forms of distal protection, it does provide evidence for distal embolization in native coronary intervention, as well as the feasibility and safety of a filter for embolic protection in both SVG and native coronaries.

The FilterWire EX was recently evaluated in 35 patients with 36 lesions treated undergoing percutaneous coronary intervention.[24] Twenty-two lesions were located in native coronary arteries and 14 in SVGs. The FilterWire was technically successful in 92% of lesions, 95% of native vessels, and 82% of SVG lesions. Reduced flow was associated with the FilterWire in place (36.1%), and only one patient developed sustained no-reflow after FilterWire removal. Distal branch vessel embolization was found in four (11.1%) cases. The major adverse cardiac event was only 6% and embolic debris was recovered in 82% of these cases.

Carotid artery interventions

The safety and feasibility of carotid artery stenting using distal occlusion balloon protection was reported by Henry et al.[25] They used the Percusurge GuardWire in 48 patients who underwent angioplasty and stenting of 53 internal carotid artery (ICA) stenoses. Immediate technical success was achieved in all patients, and carotid artery occlusion was well tolerated in all but one patient who had multiple, severe carotid lesions, and poor collateralization. Total mean cerebral flow occlusion time was 542 $\pm$ 243 s. One immediate neurologic complication (transient amaurosis) occurred in a patient who had an anastomosis between the external carotid (EC) and ICA territories. While small and nonrandomized, this initial experience does provide evidence of the feasibility and safety of distal protection in carotid artery intervention. Another preliminary study of 46 patients undergoing carotid stenting, with 25 patients having cerebral protection, found a combined event rate of neurologic events or death of 4.34%, with none in the protected group.[26]

A recent report by Schluter et al[27] described a single-center experience with the Percusurge GuardWire for cerebral protection during carotid artery stenting in 96 patients undergoing 102 interventions. The device was deployed in 99 procedures (97%), but was feasible in only 94 (92%) of the interventions. Device failure due to leakage of the valve-sealing mechanism in three patients and balloon intolerance (adverse neurologic response to balloon inflation) in two patients accounted for the cases that were completed without neuroprotection. Three other patients suffered tolerable adverse neurologic responses and completed the procedure. There was one major stroke and two transient ischemic attacks (TIAs) in patients with the device in place, resulting in a procedural success rate of 91% and a periprocedural stroke/TIA rate of 3.4%. Two minor strokes occurred in patients in whom the device could not be deployed, given an intent-to-treat periprocedural neurologic event rate of 5.4%. The stroke rates for symptomatic and asymptomatic patients were 4.6% and 1.9%, respectively. Interestingly, this study did not show a statistically significant benefit to neuroprotection when compared with an event rate of 7.2% from a 5-year prospective analysis by Roubin et al.[28] Although limited by size and lack of randomization, this study does demonstrate that cerebral embolic protection with an occlusion balloon is feasible, with approximately 2% being unable to tolerate the device and a 3.1% intention-to-treat stroke rate. A similar report from a multi-disciplinary group by Whitlow et al[29] in 75 patients found 5% balloon intolerance that did not prohibit stenting, and no major or minor neurologic events, with 100% procedural success.

Subclinical microemboli produce characteristic signals on transcranial Doppler studies (microemboli signals, MES) that have been correlated with increased risk for embolic neurologic events.[30,31] An evaluation of the efficacy of occlusion balloon neuroprotection compared: with unprotected carotid artery stenting revealed three phases of increased MES counts: namely stent deployment, predilation, and postdilation, in order of decreasing counts.[32] Distal balloon protection significantly reduced the frequency of MES, from 164 $\pm$ 108 to 68 $\pm$ 83 (p = 0.002). Most of the MES noted in the protection group occurred during the unprotected phases of sheath placement, wire manipulation, and balloon deflation. The MES observed during the protected phases may have been due to a nonocclusive balloon, embolization via the external carotid artery, or trapped emboli that were inaccessible to the aspiration catheter. While the implications of MES in carotid artery stenting are not yet established, it is evident that occlusion balloon embolic protection can be effective in reducing microemboli.

A prospective registry to evaluate the feasibility and safety of filters for embolic protection has been reported by Reimers and colleagues.[33] They used three different filters (AngioGuard (J&J Cordis), NeuroShield (MedNova), FilterWire EX (Embolic Protection, Inc.)) in 84 patients undergoing elective internal carotid artery stenting. The filter was successful in crossing the lesion in 96.5% of cases (95.8% for AngioGuard, 96.6% for NeuroShield, and 100% for FilterWire EX), with predilatation being required in 6 patients (6.9%). Flow impairment that resolved after the filter was removed was observed in 7.2%, while macroscopically visible debris in the filter occurred in 53% of the cases. The filter was well tolerated by all patients. Only one patient experienced an adverse neurologic event, namely a minor stroke with complete resolution within 1 week. While this study did not utilize transcranial Doppler to evaluate the efficiency of embolic protection, the low neurologic event rate would indicate that cerebral embolic protection with filter devices is feasible and safe. SAPPHIRE (Study of Angioplasty with Protection in Patients at High Risk for Endarterectomy) is a 720-patient randomized, controlled trial that will examine the benefits of the AngioGuard filter in carotid artery stenting.

Macdonald and colleagues[34] have reported on the UK experience with the MedNova NeuroShield filter in 50 patients. The technical success rate was 98% for filter placement/retrieval. There was one minor stroke, with resolution within 48 hours, but no major stokes were associated with the procedure. The 30-day event rate for death or major disability from stroke was 2/50 (4%), of which no cases were atheroembolic. The all-stroke/death rate was 3/50 (6%). The first of two deaths was the result of a fatal hemorrhagic stroke that occurred at 4 days, presumably from reperfusion, and the second was from perforated ventricle caused by a temporary pacing wire. The histology of the particulate retrieved was similar to other studies. Overall, this small study found the NeuroShield to be safe and effective in carotid artery stenting. Another preliminary multicenter study with the NeuroShield in 162 patients undergoing carotid artery stenting demonstrated successful filter deployment in 94% of cases.[35] The overall combined 30-day rate of all-stroke and death on an intention-to-treat basis was 2%, with two minor strokes, two deaths, and no major strokes.

Renal artery interventions

The feasibility of distal protection with the Percusurge GuardWire in renal artery stenting has been reported by Henry et al.[36] Twenty-eight hypertensive patients with 32 renal artery lesions underwent angioplasty and stenting with distal protection. The immediate technical success rate was 100%, with visible debris being aspirated from all patients. The mean renal artery occlusion time was 6.55 ± 2.46 minutes. During a mean follow-up of 6.7 months, both systolic and diastolic blood pressures improved, and no patients experienced a decline in renal function. This preliminary study suggests that renal artery intervention with distal occlusion balloon protection is both feasible and safe.

Particle size

There is a debate regarding the pathogenetic role of large and small embolic particles, and about the relative degrees to which filtering or occlusive devices trap small particles. A recent report indicates that for the Interceptor filter, with nominal pore size of 100 μm, particles far smaller than 100 μm were routinely retrieved during SVG interventions.[37] Furthermore, the aggregate volume of particulate retrieved was identical to that retrieved with the occlusive GuardWire in similar patients.

Conclusions

There is little doubt that distal embolization occurs at the time of vascular intervention, causing target organ damage and associated adverse outcomes. The Percusurge GuardWire is the most studied distal protection device in a variety of vascular territories. It is the only one tested to date in a large randomized controlled trial and proven efficacious in preventing distal embolization and the associated adverse outcomes in SVG interventions. The recently completed FIRE trial will allow direct comparison of filtering and occlusion approaches. The GuardWire and some filters have also been shown to be both feasible and safe for use in native coronary arteries, carotid arteries, and renal arteries. For SVG interventions, the results of the SAFER study may make future device evaluations with an unprotected control arm inappropriate. Nonetheless, new devices and updated versions will continue to be developed in an attempt to further improve the major shortcomings of current devices, including deliverability and completeness of protection. Embolic protection has a clear role in percutaneous interventions that will only continue to expand.

References

1. Topol E, Yadav J. Recognition of the importance of embolization in atherosclerotic vascular disease. Circulation 2000;101:570–80.
2. Ito H, et al. Clinical implications of the 'no reflow' phenomenon. A predictor of complications and left ventricular remodeling in reperfused anterior wall myocardial infarction. Circulation 1996;93:223–8.
3. Koch KC, vom Dahl J, Kleinhans E, et al. Influence of a platelet GPIIb/IIIa receptor antagonist on myocardial hypoperfusion during rotational atherectomy as assessed by myocardial Tc-99m sestamibi scintigraphy. J Am Coll Cardiol 1999;33:998–1004.
4. Wu KC, Zerhouni EA, Judd RM, et al. Prognostic significance of microvascular obstruction by magnetic resonance imaging in patients with acute myocardial infarction. Circulation 1998;97:765–72.

5. Gibson CM, Cannon CP, Murphy SA, et al. Relationship of TIMI myocardial perfusion grade to mortality after administration of thrombolytic drugs. Circulation 2000;101:125–30.

6. Topol EJ, Leya F, Pinkerton CA, et al. A comparison of directional atherectomy with coronary angioplasty in patients with coronary artery disease. The CAVEAT Study Group. N Engl J Med 1993;329:221–7.

7. Harrington RA, Lincoff AM, Califf RM, et al. Characteristics and consequences of myocardial infarction after percutaneous coronary intervention: insights from the Coronary Angioplasty Versus Excisional Atherectomy Trial (CAVEAT). J Am Coll Cardiol 1995;25:1693–9.

8. Lefkovits J, Holmes DR, Califf RM, et al. Predictors and sequelae of distal embolization during saphenous vein graft intervention from the CAVEAT-II trial. Coronary Angioplasty Versus Excisional Atherectomy Trial. Circulation 1995;92:734–40.

9. de Feyter PJ, van Suylen RJ, de Jaegere PP, Topol EJ, Serruys PW. Balloon angioplasty for the treatment of lesions in saphenous vein bypass grafts. J Am Coll Cardiol 1993;21:1539–49.

10. Hong MK, Popma JJ, Pichard AD, et al. Clinical significance of distal embolization after transluminal extraction atherectomy in diffusely diseased saphenous vein grafts. Am Heart J 1994;127:1496–503.

11. Watson PS, Hadjipetrou P, Cox SV, et al. Angiographic and clinical outcomes following acute infarct angioplasty on saphenous vein grafts. Am J Cardiol 1999;83:1018–21.

12. Hong MK, Mehran R, Dangas G, et al. Creatine kinase-MB enzyme elevation following successful saphenous vein graft intervention is associated with late mortality. Circulation 1999;100:2400–5.

13. Webb JG, Carere RG, Virmani R, et al. Retrieval and analysis of particulate debris after saphenous vein graft intervention. J Am Coll Cardiol 1999;34:468–75.

14. Oesterle S, Hayaze M, Baim DS, et al. An embolization containment device. Cathet Cardiovasc Interv 1999;47:243–50.

15. Grube E, Gerckens U, Yeung AC, et al. Prevention of distal embolization during coronary angioplasty in saphenous vein grafts and native vessels using porous filter protection. Circulation 2001;104:2436–41.

16. Schofer J, Chevalier B, Seth A, et al. Stenting of saphenous vein grafts: initial experience with a distal filter protection system in a multicenter trial. Circulation 2001;104(17 Suppl II):II-622–3.

17. Carlino M, De Gregorio J, Di Mario C, et al. Prevention of distal embolization during saphenous vein graft lesion angioplasty. Experience with a new temporary occlusion and aspiration system. Circulation 1999;99:3221–3.

18. Grube E, Schoffer JJ, Webb J, et al. Evaluation of a balloon occlusion and aspiration system for protection from distal embolization during stenting in saphenous vein grafts. Am J Cardiol 2002;89:941–5.

19. Baim DS, Wahr D, George B, et al. Saphenous vein graft Angioplasty Free of Emboli Randomized (SAFER) Trial Investigators. Randomized trial of a distal embolic protection device during percutaneous intervention of saphenous vein aorto-coronary bypass grafts. Circulation 2002;105:1285–90.

20. Stone G, Rogers C, Ramee S, et al. Distal filter protection during saphenous vein graft stenting: technical and clinical correlates of efficacy. J Am Coll Cardiol 2002;40:1882–8.

21. Henriques JP, Zijlstra F, Ottervanger JP, et al. Incidence and clinical significance of distal embolization during primary angioplasty for acute myocardial infarction. Eur Heart J 2002;23:1112–17.

22. Sutsch G, Kiowski W, Bossard A, et al. Use of an emboli containment and retrieval system during percutaneous coronary angioplasty in native coronary arteries. Schweiz Med Wochenschr 2000;130:1135–45.

23. Belli G, Pezzano A, De Biase AM, et al. Adjunctive thrombus aspiration and mechanical protection from distal embolization in primary percutaneous intervention for acute myocardial infarction. Cathet Cardiovasc Interv 2000;50:362–70.

24. Popma JJ, Cox N, Hauptmann KE, et al. Initial clinical experience with distal protection using the FilterWire in patients undergoing coronary artery and saphenous vein graft percutaneous intervention. Cathet Cardiovasc Interv 2002;57:125–34.

25. Henry M, Amor M, Henry I, et al. Carotid stenting with cerebral protection: first clinical experience using the PercuSurge GuardWire system. J Endovasc Surg 1999;6:321–31.

26. Parodi JC, La Mura R, Ferreira LM, et al. Initial evaluation of carotid angioplasty and stenting with three different cerebral protection devices. J Vasc Surg 2000;32:1127–36.

27. Schluter M, Tubler T, Mathey DG, Schofer J. Feasibility and efficacy of balloon-based neuroprotection during carotid artery stenting in a single-center setting. J Am Coll Cardiol 2002;40:890–5.

28. Roubin GS, New G, Iyer SS, et al. Immediate and late clinical outcomes of carotid artery stenting in patients with symptomatic and asymptomatic carotid artery stenosis: a 5-year prospective analysis. Circulation 2001;103:532–7.

29. Whitlow PL, Lylyk P, Londero H, et al. Carotid artery stenting protected with an emboli containment system. Stroke 2002;33:1308–14.

30. Gaunt ME, Martin PJ, Smith JL, et al. Clinical relevance of intraoperative embolization detected by transcranial Doppler ultrasonography during carotid endarterectomy: a prospective study of 100 patients. Br J Surg 1994;81:1435–9.

31. Ackerstaff RG, Moons KG, van de Vlasakker CJ, et al. Association of intraoperative transcranial doppler monitoring variables with stroke from carotid endarterectomy. Stroke 2000;31:1817–23.

32. Al-Mubarak N, Roubin GS, Vitek JJ, et al. Effect of the distal-balloon protection system on microembolization during carotid stenting. Circulation 2001;104:1999–2002.

33. Reimers B, Corvaja N, Moshiri S, et al. Cerebral protection with filter devices during carotid artery stenting. Circulation 2001;104:12–15.

34. Macdonald S, Venables GS, Cleveland TJ, Gaines PA. Protected carotid stenting: safety and efficacy of the MedNova NeuroShield filter. J Vasc Surg 2002;35:966–72.

35. Al-Mubarak N, Colombo A, Gaines PA, et al. Multicenter evaluation of carotid artery stenting with a filter protection system. J Am Coll Cardiol 2002;39:841–6.

36. Henry M, Klonaris C, Henry I, et al. Protected renal stenting with the PercuSurge GuardWire device: a pilot study. J Endovasc Ther 2001;8:227–37.

37. Rogers C, et al. Size distribution and tissue composition of particulate retrieved with embolic protection filter is comparable to particulate retrieved with embolic protection balloon following SVG intervention. Circulation 2001;104(17 Suppl II):II-777.

14

Pathophysiology of restenosis

Stefan Verheye, Glenn Van Langenhove, Giuseppe M Sangiorgi

Introduction

Percutaneous coronary intervention (PCI) has revolutionized the treatment of obstructive coronary atherosclerosis, creating an alternative strategy to medical and surgical therapy. The concept is that PCI with different devices can fracture, remove, or ablate the atherosclerotic plaque. However, it quickly became clear that, following the intervention, a healing response, known as restenosis, significantly reduced the long-term success of the procedure.

Restenosis is a substantial medical problem both because it occurs in 40–50% of patients undergoing routine coronary revascularization procedures with increased patient morbidity and because of the significant burden of medical costs.[1,2] Restenosis may be effectively treated by repeat angioplasty, stent implantation, or intracoronary brachytherapy; however, further interventional procedures obviously entail additional costs.

It is therefore not surprising that in recent years there have been intense efforts to elucidate the pathophysiologic mechanisms of this process. Today, the cellular mechanisms and interactions involved in the pathophysiology of restenosis are better understood, and powerful effects have been obtained in some animal models with the use of different drugs and devices. Nevertheless, the search for successful therapeutic effects is ongoing, and very recently promising results have been obtained with the introduction of drug-eluting stents.

The goal of this chapter is to review the pathophysiology of restenosis. We will first define the problem and briefly review the mechanism of lumen expansion depending on the technique used, followed by a brief description of some animal models for studying restenosis, and we will then highlight the several steps of restenosis, including the early and late phases.

Defining the problem
Clinical and angiographic definition

Restenosis studies have suffered to various degrees from methodologic problems. Since native coronary atherosclerotic and restenotic lesions are both identified and treated using angiography, one would hope that a uniform angiographic definition of restenosis exists. Unfortunately, such a definition is currently lacking, representing a major limitation in comparing different studies.

The numerous angiographic definitions used in clinical studies,[3] and more recently, definitions based on absolute changes in minimal lumen diameter at follow-up,[4] have led to confusion and have hampered investigations in this field[5] (Table 14.1).

Using clinical criteria, restenosis may be defined by evidence of recurrent myocardial ischemia after the revascularization procedure discovered during clinical tests by the presence of symptoms (i.e. recurrence of angina and need for target vessel revascularization). However, discrepancies between angiography and clinical status occur, making clinical decision-making more difficult: a patient who is asymptomatic and/or has negative tests for ischemia but who might have a lesion fitting the angiographic criteria for restenosis will likely not be recatheterized on the basis of clinical criteria alone.

Table 14.1   Angiographic definitions of restenosis
1. An increase of ≥30% from immediate postangioplasty diameter stenosis to follow-up stenosis 2. An initial diameter of stenosis <50% after angioplasty, increasing to ≥70% at follow-up angiography 3. An increase in diameter of stenosis at follow-up angiography to within 10% of the preangioplasty value 4. A loss of >50% of the initial increase in diameter of stenosis achieved by angioplasty, from immediate postangioplasty to follow-up angiography 5. A postangioplasty diameter of stenosis <50% increasing to >50% at follow-up angiography 6. A decrease in the minimal lumen diameter at the lesion of >0.72 mm from immediate postangioplasty to follow-up angiography 7. Cumulative distribution of minimal lumen diameter

Moreover, restenosis has been previously characterized as an 'all or none' phenomenon and, by subsequent studies, as a continuous variable that occurs to a different extent in all treated lesions.[6] Many studies have been small, and the timing and methods of follow-up have been variable,[1,7] introducing selection biases and misleading interpretations of data.

It is clear that a more uniform definition, which includes a combination of angiographic and clinical criteria, and studies with more uniform groups of patients may provide a more accurate picture of the restenosis phenomenon.[8]

Mechanism of lumen expansion

To better understand the mechanisms of restenosis, it is useful to briefly review the potential mechanisms by which coronary interventional procedures increase lumen patency. Since the explanation given by Dotter and Judkins,[9] who described the enlargement of vessel lumen by balloon angioplasty as being due to compression of atheromatous plaque against the arterial wall, several morphologic and histologic observations have been made both in human necropsy studies[10,11] and in experimental models.[12] There are a number of different mechanisms that have been identified. The original concept of plaque compression is rather unlikely, because most of the plaques are composed of dense fibrocollageneous tissue with hard calcium deposits, which make them difficult to compress. Nevertheless, this mechanism plays a major role in the dilatation of newly formed atherosclerotic plaque (i.e. soft plaques) or recently formed thrombus.

Subsequent data suggest that the major mechanisms of action of coronary angioplasty are breaking, cracking, and splitting of the intimal plaque, with partial disruption of the media and vessel stretching of the plaque-free wall.[13,14] In particular, intravascular ultrasound (IVUS) studies have shown that those mechanisms may vary depending on the histologic plaque composition, with more plaque dissection in calcified lesions and more vessel expansion in non-calcified plaques.[15]

Conversely, directional and rotational coronary atherectomy improve lumen caliber by tissue removal, with little disruption and expansion of the vessel wall. Finally, the mechanism of laser angioplasty is related to atherosclerotic tissue photo-ablation and dissection associated with vessel expansion.

The mechanism of lumen expansion differs between balloon angioplasty and stenting, and so does the mechanism of restenosis. The predominant mechanism of lumen renarrowing after balloon angioplasty is constrictive vascular remodeling, with only a minor contribution from neointimal hyperplasia. This is in contrast with the mechanism of in-stent restenosis, which is explained by excessive neointimal hyperplasia; constrictive vascular remodeling is excluded due to the presence of the scaffolding stent struts.

Animal models of restenosis

Traditionally, animal models are the cornerstone to test strategies aimed at developing treatments for several pathologic conditions and for understanding pathophysiologic mechanisms. Restenosis is no exception, and several animal models have been developed during the last decade in an attempt to reproduce restenotic lesions and find a therapeutic strategy to reduce neointimal formation. Unfortunately, despite all efforts in developing a good model during the last 15 years, there is no perfect animal model for human restenosis. Common models include the rat carotid air desiccation or balloon endothelial denudation model,[16,17] the rabbit femoral or iliac artery balloon injury model with or without cholesterol supplementation,[18] and the porcine carotid and coronary artery model.[19]

The rat model, based on elastic arteries, does not develop severe stenotic neointimal lesions, and is therefore very permissive in term of efficacy of pharmacologic interventions. The cholesterol-fed rabbit model has been criticized for the high level of hyperlipidemia required for the development of lesions. This results in a large macrophage foam cell component, which resembles fatty streaks rather than human restenotic lesions. Conversely, the histopathologic features of neointima obtained in porcine models closely resemble those of human neointima, and the amount of neointimal thickening is proportional to injury severity.[20] This has allowed the creation of an injury–neointima relationship that can be used to evaluate the response to different therapies. However, the repair process in the pig coronary artery injury model using normal coronary arteries is certainly more rapid and may be different from the response to balloon angioplasty that characterizes human coronary atherosclerotic plaques.

The major limitation to the use of animal models of restenosis is that agents effective in reducing neointima in those models are ineffective when transferred to the clinical arena. Several explanations might support those differences. Different animal species, types of arteries, degrees of arterial injury, volumes of neointima, drug dosages and timing regimens, and atherosclerotic substrates might be considered. It is therefore believed that before transferring the results obtained in animal models to clinical trials, a standardization of injury type, method of measurement, and dose and timing of drug among different animal models should be the best solution to this problem.

Pathophysiology

Our understanding of restenosis evolved slowly, but major components in the evolution of the restenosis process have recently been identified. In the early 1990s, several pivotal studies distinguished basic restenosis mechanisms such as early recoil, negative remodeling, and proliferative response to injury.[21,22] Other landmark studies established the concept that the extent of luminal 'late loss' at follow-up is proportional to the amount of 'acute gain' achieved during the initial procedure.[23] Although this strategy provided incremental reduction in restenosis under the philosophy of 'bigger is better', the scientific community soon realized that restenosis could not be eliminated using only mechanical devices such as bare stents or atherectomy. Therefore, the battle against restenosis was ongoing and better understanding of the pathophysiology of restenosis was needed. This obviously required also the development of predictable animal models to allow precise, quantitative documentation of the in vivo response to injury.[24] Based on previous clinical and experimental observations, including molecular techniques, the presumed healing and repair processes leading to arterial restenosis are categorized as follows: an initial early phase (acute/subacute) characterized by elastic recoil, apoptosis, platelet aggregation, and inflammation, followed by a late phase (subacute/chronic) characterized by favorable or unfavorable arterial wall remodeling (Figure 14.1). These processes will be reviewed in depth.

Early phase
Elastic recoil

The vessel wall itself can participate in acute lumen loss observed in some patients just after coronary interventions by a mechanism termed 'recoil'. Elastic recoil occurs within minutes to hours following balloon angioplasty and seems to be the consequence of the 'spring-like' properties of the nondiseased vascular wall responding to its overstretching.[25,26] Other possible explanations are vasoconstriction due to vessel endothelial disruption[27] or platelet activation and thrombus formation with consequent release of vasoconstrictive substances.[28,29] Whenever the normal wall is significantly stretched, recoil may be the predominant mechanism of restenosis (Figure 14.2). Different studies, indeed, have shown that this very early vessel wall recoil increases the likelihood of subsequent restenosis with a rate of 73.6% for the lesions that had lumen loss greater than 10% and only 9.8% for lesions that diminished by less than 10%.[30,31] Early recoil may possibly have a significant importance in restenosis when the vessel has not been severely injured and the lesion consists of smooth muscle cells. When the vessel wall injury is more severe, thrombus formation with consequent activation of growth factors and release of cytokines may be, instead, the predominant mechanism of restenosis.

Apoptosis

Programmed cell death, which generally occurs when cells from multicellular eukaryotes are no longer needed or have become severely damaged, involves a genetically controlled cell suicide machinery, leading to characteristic morphologic changes that are broadly known as apoptosis and determined by in situ end-labeling techniques (TUNEL and ISNT). These morphologic changes, which include plasma membrane blebbing, DNA fragmentation, chromatin condensation, nuclear fragmentation, cell shrinkage, and budding-off of cellular fragments, are distinct from the cellular and organellar swelling and rupture that are typical of the setting of necrosis.[32] Apoptosis seems to play an important role in the pathogenesis of restenosis; however, there have been conflicting reports regarding the timing. One of the experiments investigating the balance between apoptosis and cellular proliferation in a pig model of coronary restenosis demonstrated that apoptotic cells were identified at all early time points, with a peak at 6 hours after overstretch injury as found by TUNEL labeling and confirmed by characteristic DNA ladders and transmission electron microscopic findings. In addition, a regional analysis showed that apoptosis within the media, adventitia, and neointima peaked at 18 hours, 6 hours, and 7 days after injury, respectively.[33] Another group reported also an early time point of apoptosis (1 week) and found in addition that there was a higher rate of apoptosis in the neointima after stent implantation compared with balloon angioplasty.[34] This was due to an increased rate of smooth muscle cell (SMC) and macrophage death; the authors concluded that macrophage accumulation and apoptosis in the early phase after stent implantation appear to play a role in extracellular

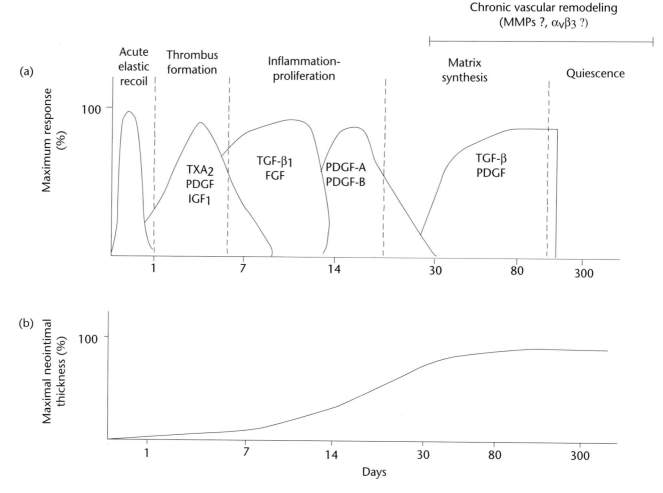

Figure 14.1
Different phases of the restenotic process. (a) Increase in neointimal thickening. (b) The associated expression of growth factors.

matrix secretion, which increases neointima formation after 4 and 12 weeks compared with balloon angioplasty.[34] In another model of vascular injury, Durand et al[35] found that cell proliferation preceded apoptosis 4 days earlier throughout the 4 weeks after angioplasty. Similar to the other findings, apoptosis was inversely correlated with restenosis and was also related to enlargement remodeling after balloon angioplasty.

Several mechanisms have been proposed to clarify the mechanism of apoptosis in the pathogenesis of restenosis. Nitric oxide (NO, 'endothelium-derived relaxing factor', EDRF) is known to induce apoptosis, but the signaling pathways still remain unclear. Protein kinase C (PKC) activation and nuclear transcription factor (NF-κB) binding activity, but not accumulation of p53, a tumor suppressor gene product regulating growth arrest and apoptosis after DNA damage, are possible signaling mechanisms of NO-induced apoptosis.[36] Other experiments have shown that inhibition of the ubiquitin–proteasome system, a major intracellular protein degradation pathway in eukaryotic cells, effectively reduces neointima formation in vivo,

which corresponds to strong antiproliferative, anti-inflammatory, and proapoptotic effects in vitro and in vivo.[37] Activation of tumor necrosis factor α (TNF-α) receptors is also known to induce cell death by apoptosis. Smooth muscle cells isolated from the neointima of injured rat aortas are characterized by increased expression of TNF-α in response to interleukin-1β (IL-1β) and interferon-γ (IFN-γ) compared with medial SMC. Incubation of intimal SMC with these cytokines also resulted in induction TUNEL-positivity and caspase–3 expression, suggesting cell death by apoptosis, whereas medial cells were markedly less sensitive in this respect.[38]

Platelet aggregation – thrombus formation

As an integral part of the dilatation mechanism, coronary angioplasty results in injury to the arterial wall, including

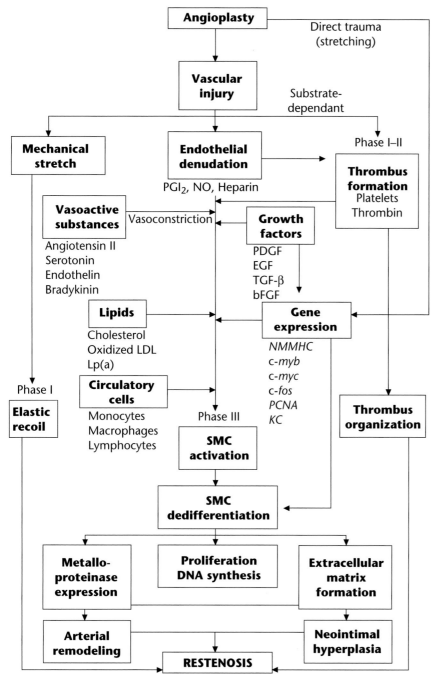

Figure 14.2
Sequence of events resulting in restenosis after vessel injury.

endothelial damage with loss of antithrombotic properties (NO, prostacyclin (PGI$_2$), and tissue-type plasminogen activator (t-PA)), induction of procoagulant factors (thrombin and tissue factor), and inflammatory infiltrates at the site of injury. In addition, fracture of the internal elastic lamina and medial disruption, with exposition to the blood elements of wall constituents such as collagen, von Willebrand factor (vWF), and extracellular matrix components, stimulates the interaction with platelet surface receptors (primarily glycoprotein Ib and IIb/IIIa integrins), resulting within minutes to hours after the intervention in platelet activation and deep mural thrombus formation[39–41] inaccessible to

the action of heparin.[42] Experimental and clinical studies have also shown that platelets are activated by contrast medium.[43,44] Activated platelets secrete several substances from their α-granules stimulating vasoconstriction, chemotaxis, and activation of adjacent platelets.[45,46] In addition, platelet aggregation releases or stimulates the production of several factors and cytokines, including thrombin, thromboxane A$_2$, serotonin, plasminogen activator inhibitor (PAI-1), platelet-derived growth factor (PDGF), transforming growth factor β (TGF-β), basic fibroblast growth factor (bFGF), epidermal growth factor (EGF), insulin-like growth factor (IGF-I), (IL-1), and monocyte

Table 14.2 Extracellular factors involved in restenosis

Angiotensin II
Collagen
Collagenase
Colony-stimulating factors (CSFs)
Elastic fibers
Endothelins (ETs)
Epidermal growth factor (EGF) / transforming growth
    factor α (TGF-α)
Fibroblast growth factors, acidic and basic (aFGF, bFGF)
Heparin
Heparin-binding epidermal growth factor (HB-EGF)
Insulin-like growth factor I (IGF-I)
Interferon-γ (IFN-γ)
Interleukin-1 (IL-1)
Low-density lipoprotein, oxidized (oxLDL)
Monocyte/macrophage colony-stimulating factor (M-CSF)
Monocyte chemoattractant protein 1 (monocyte
    chemotactic protein 1, MCP-1/MCAF-1)
Nitric oxide (NO) ('endothelium-derived relaxing factor',
    EDRF)
Plasmin
Plasminogen activator inhibitor (PAI-1)
Platelet-derived growth factor A (endothelium, PDGF-AA)
Platelet-derived growth factor B (smooth muscle cells,
    PDGF-BB)
Prostacyclin (PGI$_2$)
Prostaglandin E (PGE)
Proteoglycans
Thrombin
Thromboxane A$_2$ (TXA$_2$)
Tissue-type plasminogen activator (t-PA)
Transforming growth factor β (TGF-β)
Tumor necrosis factor α (TNF-α)

chemoattractant protein 1 (MCP-1)[47–49] (Table 14.2). These factors are believed to be responsible for neointimal growth by attracting and stimulating SMC migration and proliferation at the site of injury[50–53] (Figure 14.2). The severity of the thrombogenic response depends on the degree of vascular injury, the surface area of exposure, the type of substrate exposed in the underlying vessel wall, and the rheologic conditions, such as shear stress and time of exposure.

Platelet activation leads to the recruitment of glycoprotein IIb/IIIa integrin surface receptors, which mediate platelet aggregation and thrombus formation by binding fibrinogen molecules between adjacent receptors.[47,54,55] Aggregated platelets accelerate the conversion of prothrombin to thrombin, which in turn stimulates further platelet activation.[56] Thrombin is involved in thrombus formation, upregulation of E-selectin and P-selectin expression on endothelial cells, monocyte and neutrophil migration in the injured wall,[57] and stimulation of endothelin and tissue factor release from endothelial cells with a mitotic effect on SMC.[58] Of interest, there is also evidence

that monocyte/macrophage recruitment may contribute to a myofibrotic organization of thrombus.[59] Genes for the PDGF ligands and receptor components are expressed in normal and injured rat carotid arteries.[60] bFGF and FGF receptor type I are both expressed by endothelial and SMC after mechanical injury; inhibition of this growth factor reduces neointimal formation.[48,61,62] TGF-β seems to be the principal growth factor involved in the regulation and synthesis of proteoglycans, the major components of the extracellular matrix.[63,64] TGF-β induces both migration and proliferation of vascular cells, and there is evidence suggesting that is an important factor in the vascular remodeling process associated with restenosis.[65]

Ultimately, the extent of vessel wall injury, the amount of thrombus formation, and the likelihood of neointimal proliferation are interrelated. Although the relationship of thrombus formation to restenosis remains to be elucidated, evidence suggests that thrombus contributes directly to restenosis by vessel occlusion[66] and indirectly by mediating the release of several factors, which in turn are also involved in the third phase of the restenotic process.[67]

Inflammation

Following platelet activation, circulating inflammatory cells adhere to the site of injury and migrate into the thrombus. P-selectin, a protein stored in the α-granules of platelets and the Weibel–Palades bodies of endothelial cells, and binding to circulating monocytes and leukocytes, plays a crucial role in this early inflammatory response. Neutrophils, lymphocytes, and monocytes have been observed within the mural thrombus 1–5 days following angioplasty in an atherosclerotic rabbit model,[68] and scanning electron microscopy has demonstrated the presence of leukocytes and macrophages adherent to the luminal surface of stented arteries in different animal models.[69,70] In another study, peak monocyte adherence to the lumen surface was found 3 days after stenting, which correlated with intimal cellular proliferation.[71] Several players have been put forward as key regulators of inflammation in the pathogenesis of restenosis. First, nonspecific systemic stimulation of the innate immune system concurrently with arterial vascular injury may facilitate neointimal formation, and conditions associated with increased inflammation may increase restenosis.[72] Accordingly, C-reactive protein has been recently described as a useful preprocedure marker of risk of restenosis.[73] TNF-α is a pleiotropic proinflammatory cytokine involved in many aspects of inflammation. Recent data indicate that tissue TNF-α levels are markedly increased after balloon angioplasty. Anti-TNF-α treatment was sufficient to neutralize tissue TNF-α activity, and reduce inflammation. However, it did not inhibit neointimal formation following balloon angioplasty in a rabbit atherosclerotic model.[74] Other data implicate plasminogen in the migration of leukocytes in murine models. With numerous correlations between components and/or activation of the plasminogen system in restenosis and atherosclerosis, results derived from a study reported by Plow et al[75] also support a role of plasminogen in the corresponding human pathologies.

Inflammation in response to injury seems to occur predominantly in the intima and media; however, recent data suggest also a role for perivascular inflammatory cells in the pathogenesis of restenosis.[76] The authors hypothesized that these perivascular inflammatory cells are involved in the recruitment and/or proliferation of adventitial myofibroblasts, possibly through the release of reactive oxygen species and/or cytokines, and thus contribute to vascular remodeling associated with postangioplasty restenosis.

Stent deployment can also cause a foreign body reaction due to deeper arterial injury compared with balloon angioplasty.[34] Karas et al[77] found reactive inflammatory infiltrates and multinucleated giant cells surrounding the stent wires at 4 weeks follow-up in a porcine model of coronary injury. Farb et al[78] demonstrated in a large autopsy series that acute inflammation (mainly composed by neutrophils) was linked to the extent and location of vessel injury and that chronic inflammation (lymphocytes and macrophages) was frequently observed around metallic struts at different timepoints following stent placement in humans. Furthermore, it has been demonstrated that the extent of the inflammatory reaction is significantly correlated, both independently and in combination with the degree of arterial injury, with the amount of neointimal formation.[79] More recently, it was found that coronary stenting, accompanied by medial damage or penetration of the stent into a lipid core, induced increased arterial inflammation, which was associated with increased neointimal growth.[80] These observations of intermediate- to long-term stent implants are new – previously these effects were known to occur *early* after stenting: it appears from these findings that arterial medial disruption and lipid core penetration by stent struts are associated with chronic inflammation.[80] Finally, other important parameters with respect to the inflammatory response after stent deployment are the material, design, and surface of the stent.[81–83]

Late phase

Smooth muscle cell activation and synthesis of extracellular matrix

The final phase of vascular healing is predominantly characterized by neointimal formation due to SMC proliferation and extracellular matrix accumulation produced by the neointimal cells at the injury site.[84–86] The healing response is a normal process that is essential in maintaining vascular integrity after an injury to the vessel wall, but varies in the degree to which it occurs. One pathogenetic explanation of restenosis is, indeed, an exaggeration of this healing response (Figure 14.2).

This late phase can be further divided into three different waves.[87] In the first wave (days 1–4 after vessel injury), medial SMC from the site of injury and possibly from adjacent areas are activated and stimulated by the triggering factors mentioned earlier. In addition to mitogenic factors released by endothelial cells, stretching of the arterial wall is a potent stimulus for SMC activation and growth.[88] The second wave (3–14 days after vessel injury) and the third wave (14 days to months after vessel injury) are respectively characterized by the migration of SMC through breaks in the internal elastic lamina into the intima, local thrombus formation,[89] and further SMC proliferation.[90–92] Once activated, SMC undergo characteristic phenotypic transformation, from a 'contractile' to a 'synthetic' form,[85] which is responsible for the production of extracellular matrix rich in chondroitin sulfate and dermatan sulfate seen in the first 6 months after injury. These events are modulated by complex interactions between growth factors, second messengers, and gene-regulatory proteins (Table 14.2 and Figure 14.3).[50] The peak of proliferation is observed 4–5 days after balloon injury but the duration of migration is not known – nor is it known whether a phase of cellular replication is required before SMC migration. Few studies have been done to identify the matrix molecules involved in the migration into the intima. Osteopontin is expressed at sites of marked remodeling,[93] and antibodies to osteopontin inhibit SMC migration into the intima after balloon angioplasty.[94] Proteoglycans may also be important for the formation of neointima. CD44, a receptor for hyaluronic acid, seems to play a role in the migration of cells into fibrin or osteopontin.[95,96] SMC migration presumably requires degradation of the basement membrane surrounding the cells. Several metalloproteinases (MMPs), including tissue-type plasminogen activator (t-PA), plasmin, MMP-2, and MMP-9, may be responsible for this process;[97,98] besides, the administration of a protease inhibitor reduces SMC migration into the intima.[99] Cell migration is probably initiated by recognition of extracellular matrix proteins by a family of cell surface adhesion receptors known as integrins.[100,101] In vitro and in vivo studies have demonstrated that selective blockage of the $\alpha_v\beta_3$ integrin inhibits SMC migration and reduces neointimal formation.[102,103] Experimental studies have suggested that endothelin-1 and endothelin receptors may also be indirectly implicated in SMC migration and matrix synthesis.[104,105] Immunohistochemical studies have demonstrated a time-dependent increase in endothelin immunoreactivity after balloon angioplasty in the rat model.[106] The administration of endothelin receptor antagonists in different animal models of balloon injury has been shown to be effective in reducing neointimal formation.[105,107] Several in vitro studies have suggested that

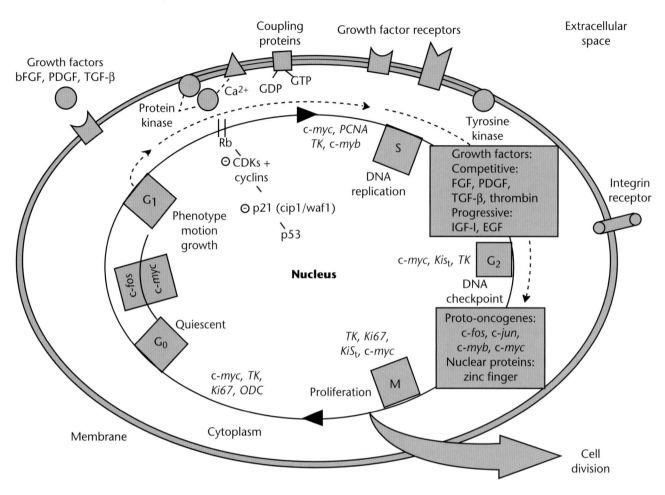

Figure 14.3
Cytoplasmatic and nuclear control points for SMC division and proliferation. CDKs, cyclin-dependent kinases; *TK*, tyrosine kinase gene; *ODC*, ornithine decarboxylase gene; Rb, retinoblastoma protein.

different growth factors, such as PDGF-AA, PDGF-BB, bFGF, IGF, EGF, TGF-β, and angiotensin II, may also play a major role in this process.[108–112]

Control of SMC proliferation is regulated by the actions of mitogens (e.g. PDGF) and the opposing effect of inhibitors (e.g. TGF-β). The growth factors bind to cell surface receptors and initiate a cascade of events leading to cell migration and division. Components of the cascade include different tyrosine kinases, coupling proteins, and membrane-associated and cytoplasmatic protein kinases (Figure 14.3). On stimulation by growth factors, proto-oncogenes are transiently activated and, together with other cell cycle-dependent proteins such as zinc-finger proteins, mediate the effects within the nucleus. Several studies have demonstrated that stimulation of SMC in vitro is associated with an increase in expression of the proto-oncogenes c-*myc*, c-*myb*, and c-*fos*.[113–115] The ornithine decarboxylase gene (*ODC*) and thymidine kinase (*TK*) messenger RNA are both expressed in stimulating cells and in continuously cycling cells.[115] Vascular cyclic guanosine monophosphate (cGMP) and cGMP-dependent protein kinase, a major cGMP effector in vascular smooth muscle,

play an important role in neointimal formation, and were found to be reduced after arterial injury.[116] Another contributor is phosphatidylinositol 3′-kinase (PI3-K) signaling, which also regulates proliferation and migration of SMC. The effectors of PI3-K are activated by the phospholipid products of PI3-K. A recent study hypothesized that over-expression of the tumor suppressor protein PTEN, an inositol phosphatase specific for the products of PI3-K, inhibited the SMC responses necessary for neointimal hyperplasia.[117] SMC proliferation may also result from a reduction in inhibitory factor, which normally prevents cell division. Proteins such as p21 are inhibitors of the cyclin-dependent kinases (CDKs), which regulate entry of the cell into the cell cycle (Figure 14.3). Stimulation of these proteins, indeed, inhibits SMC proliferation and neointimal formation after balloon injury.[118]

As smooth muscle cells decrease their proliferation rate, they begin to synthesize large quantities of proteoglycan matrix. The extracellular matrix production continues for up 20–25 weeks and is gradually replaced over time by collagen and elastin, while the SMC turn into quiescent mesenchymal cells. The resulting neointima is composed of a fibrotic extracellular matrix with few cellular constituents. The endothelial cells proliferate and cover the denuded area, resulting in a re-endothelialization process. The new endothelium begins to produce large quantities of heparan sulfate and NO, both of which inhibit SMC proliferation.[41] It remains unclear, though, whether SMC proliferation and extracellular matrix production cease after re-endothelialization.

Conclusions

Vascular restenosis after balloon angioplasty, stent implantation, or atherectomy has been a major problem for many years due to lack of knowledge of its pathophysiology. Only in recent years, thanks to ongoing experimental and clinical studies as well as to the introduction of molecular techniques, have better insights been acquired into the pathophysiology of this complex disease. However, the more we delve into it, the more complex and redundant this process appears. Moreover, it seems that not just one player is involved, but a multitude of factors account for the burden of restenosis. A selective approach attacking a single molecule or even phase of the pathophysiology may therefore not be sufficient. Restenosis remains an important problem involving a high number of patients worldwide, adding a considerable cost to the community. Restenosis rates are decreasing but have not yet reached zero. Research in both animal and human studies to explore the exact pathophysiology should therefore be ongoing.

References

1. Califf RM, Fortin DF, Frid DJ, et al. Restenosis after coronary angioplasty: an overview. J Am Coll Cardiol 1991;17:2B–13B.
2. Franklin SM, Faxon DP. Pharmacologic prevention of restenosis after coronary angioplasty: review of the randomized clinical trials. Coronary Artery Dis 1993;4:232–42.
3. Holmes DR, Vlietstra RE, Smith HC, et al. Restenosis after percutaneous transluminal coronary angioplasty (PTCA): a report from the PTCA registry of the National Heart, Lung, and Blood Institute. Am J Cardiol 1984;53:77C–81C.
4. Serruys PW, Luijten HE, Beat KJ, et al. Incidence of restenosis after successful coronary angioplasty: a time-related phenomenon. A quantitative angiographic study in 342 consecutive patients at 1,2,3,and 4 months. Circulation 1988;77:361–71.
5. Serruys PW, Rensing BJ, Hermans WRM, Beatt KJ. Definition of restenosis after percutaneous transluminal coronary angioplasty: a quickly evolving concept. J Interv Cardiol 1991;4:256–76.
6. Beatt KJ, Luijten HE, de Feyter PJ, et al. Change in diameter of coronary artery segments adjacent to stenosis after percutaneous transluminal coronary angioplasty: failure of percent diameter stenosis measurement to reflect morphologic changes induced by balloon dilation. J Am Coll Cardiol 1988;12:315–23.
7. Kuntz RE, Keaney KM, Senerchia C, Baim DS. A predictive method for estimating the late angiographic results of coronary intervention despite incomplete ascertainment. Circulation 1993;87:815–30.
8. Kuntz RE, Baim DS. Defining coronary restenosis: newer clinical and angiographic paradigms. Circulation 1993; 88:1310–23.
9. Dotter CT, Judkins MP. Transluminal treatment of atherosclerotic obstruction: desciption of new technique and a preliminary report of its application. Circulation 1964;30:654–70.
10. Block PC, Myler RK, Stertzer S, Fallon JT. Morphology after transluminal angioplasty in humans. N Engl J Med 1981;305:382.
11. Waller BF. Pathology of transluminal balloon angioplasty used in the treatment of heart disease. Hum Pathol 1987;18:476–84.
12. Sanborn TA, Faxon DP, Haudenschild C, et al. The mechanism of coronary angioplasty: evidence for formation of aneurysms in experimental atheroslerosis. Circulation 1983;68:1136–40.
13. Mizuno K, Kurita A, Imazeki N. Pathologic findings after percutaneous transluminal coronary angioplasty. Br Heart J 1984;52:588–90.
14. Kohchi K, Takebayashi S, Block PC, et al. Arterial changes after percutaneous coronary angioplasty: results at autopsy. J Am Coll Cardiol 1987;10:592–9.
15. Potkin BN, Keren GN, Mintz GS, et al. Arterial responses to balloon coronary angioplasty: an intravascular ultrasound study. J Am Coll Cardiol 1992;20:942–51.
16. Clowes AV, Karnovsky MJ. Suppression by heparin of smooth muscle cell proliferation in injured arteries. Nature 1977;265:625–6.
17. Olson LV, Clowes AW, Reidy MA. Inhibition of smooth muscle cell proliferation in injured rat arteries. J Clin Invest 1992;90:2044–9.
18. Faxon DP, Weber VJ, Haudenschild C, et al. Acute effect of transluminal angioplasty in three experimental models of atherosclerosis. Arteriosclerosis 1982;2:125–33.
19. Schwartz RS, Edwards WD, Huber KC, et al. Coronary restenosis: prospects for solution and new perspectives from a porcine model. Mayo Clin Proc 1993;68:54–62.
20. Schwartz RS, Huber KC, Murphy JG, et al. Restenosis and the proportional neointimal response to coronary artery injury: results in a porcine model. J Am Coll Cardiol 1992;19:267–74.
21. Glagov S. Intimal hyperplasia, vascular remodeling, and the restenosis problem. Circulation 1994;89:2888–91.
22. Mintz GS, Popma JJ, Pichard AD, et al. Arterial remodeling after coronary angioplasty: a serial intravascular ultrasound study. Circulation 1996;94:35–43.
23. Kuntz RE, Gibson CM, Nobuyoshi M, Baim DS. Generalized model of restenosis after conventional balloon angioplasty, stenting and directional atherectomy. J Am Coll Cardiol 1993;21:15–25.
24. Schwartz RS, Murpphy JG, Edwards WD, et al. Restenosis after balloon angioplasty: a practical proliferative model in porcine coronary arteries. Circulation 1990;82:2190–200.
25. Nobuyoshi M, Kimura T, Nosaka H, et al. Restenosis after successful percutaneous transluminal coronary angioplasty:

serial angiographic follow-up of 229 patients. J Am Coll Cardiol 1988;12:616–23.

26. Daniel WC, Pirwitz MJ, Willard JE, et al. Incidnce and treatment of elastic recoil occurring in the 15 minutes following successful percutaneous transluminal coronary angioplasty. Am J Cardiol 1996;78:253–9.

27. Fischell TA, Derby G, Tse TM, Stadius ML. Coronary artery vasoconstricitons routinely occurs after percutaneous transluminal angioplasty. Circulation 1988;78:1323–34.

28. Mabin TA, Holmes DR, Smith HC, et al. Intracoronary trombus: role in coronary occlusion complicating percutaneous transluminal coronary angioplasty. J Am Coll Cardiol 1985;5:198–202.

29. Arora RR, Platko WP, Bhadwar K, Simpfendorfer C. Role of intracoronary thrombus in acute complications during percutaneous transluminal coronary angioplasty. Cathet Cardiovasc Diagn 1989;16:226–9.

30. Rodriguez AE, Santaera O, Larribeau M, et al. Early decrease in minimal luminal diametr after successful percutaneous transluminal angioplasty predicts late restenosis. Am J Cardiol 1993;71:1391–5.

31. Rodriguez AE, Santaera O, Larribeau M, et al. Coronary stenting decreases restenosis in lesions with early loss in luminal diameter 24 hours after successful PTCA. Circulaton 1995;91:1397–402.

32. Kockx MM, Knaapen MW. The role of apoptosis in vascular disease. J Pathol 2000;190:267–80.

33. Malik N, Francis SE, Holt CM, et al. Apoptosis and cell proliferation after porcine coronary angioplasty. Circulation 1998;98:1657–65.

34. Kollum M, Kaiser S, Kinscherf R, et al. Apoptosis after stent implantation compared with balloon angioplasty in rabbits: role of macrophages. Arterioscler Thromb Vasc Biol 1997;17:2383–8.

35. Durand E, Mallat Z, Addad F, et al. Time courses of apoptosis and cell proliferation and their relationship to arterial remodeling and restenosis after angioplasty in an atherosclerotic rabbit model. J Am Coll Cardiol 2002;39:1680–5.

36. Ibe W, Bartels W, Lindemann S, et al. Involvement of PKC and NF-kappaB in nitric oxide induced apoptosis in human coronary artery smooth muscle cells. Cell Physiol Biochem 2001;11:231–40.

37. Meiners S, Laule M, Rother W, et al. Ubiquitin–proteasome pathway as a new target for the prevention of restenosis. Circulation 2002;105:483–9.

38. Niemann-Jönsson A, Ares MP, Yan Z-Q, et al. Increased rate of apoptosis in intimal arterial smooth muscle cells through endogeneous activation of TNF receptors. Arterioscler Thromb Vasc Biol 2001;21:1909–14.

39. Uchida Y, Hasegawa K, Kawarmura K, Shibuya I. Angioscopic observation of the coronary luminal changes induced by percutaneous transluminal coronary angioplasty. Am Heart J 1989;117:769–76.

40. Miller DD, Boulet AJ, Tio FO, et al. In vivo technetium-99m S12 antibody imaging of platelet alpha granules in rabbit endothelial neointimal proliferation after angioplasty. Circulation 1991;83:224–36.

41. Ip JH, Fuster V, Israel D, et al. The role of platelets, thrombin and hyperplasia in restenosis after coronary angioplasty. J Am Coll Cardiol 1991;17:77B–88B.

42. Weitz JI, Huboda M, Massel D, et al. Clot-bound thrombin is protected from inhibition by heparin–antithrombin III

but is susceptible to inactivation by antithrombin III-independent inhibitors. J Clin Invest 1990;86:385–91.

43. Chronos NAF, Goodall AH, Wilson DJ, et al. Profound platelet degranulation is an important side effect of some type of contrast media used in interventional coardiology. Circulation 1993;88:2035–44.

44. Kolarov P, Tschoepe D, Nieuwenhuis HK, et al. PTCA: periprocedal platelet activation. Part II of the Dusseldorf PTCA Platelet Study (DPPS). Eur Heart J 1996;17:1216–22.

45. Fukami MH, Salganicoff L. Human platelet storage organelles. Thromb Haemostas 1977;38:963–70.

46. Holmsen H. Secretable storage pools in platelets. Annu Rev Med 1979;30:119–34.

47. Le Breton H, Plow EF, Topol EJ. Role of platelets in restenosis after percutaneous coronary revascularization. J Am Coll Cardiol 1996;28:1643–51.

48. Lindner V, Reidy MA. Expression of basic fibroblast growth factor and its receptor by smooth muscle cells and endothelium in injured rat arteries: an enface study. Circ Res 1993;73:589–95.

49. Shimokawa H, Ito A, Fukumoto Y, et al. Chronic treament with interleukin-1 induces coronary intimal lesions and vasospastic responses in pigs in vivo. J Clin Invest 1996;97:769–76.

50. Casscells W. Migration of smooth muscle and endothelial cells. Critical events in restenosis. Circulation 1992;86:723–9.

51. Rekhter MD, O'Brien E, Shah N, et al. The importance of thrombus organization and stellate cell phenotype in collagen I gene expression in human coronary atherosclerosis and restenotic lesions. Cardiov Res 1996;32:496–502.

52. Poole JCF, Cromwell SP, Benditt EP. Behavior of smooth muscle cells and formation of extracellular structures in the reaction of the arterial walls to injury. Am J Pathol 1971;62:391–413.

53. Jeong MH, Owen WG, Staab ME, et al. Porcine model of stent thrombosis: platelets are the primary component of acute stent closure. Cathet Cardiovasc Diagn 1996;38:38–43.

54. Plow EF, McEver RP, Coller SW, et al. Related bunding mechanisms for fibrinogen, fibronectin, von Willebrand factor and thrombospondin on thrombin-stimulated human platelets. Blood 1985;66:724–7.

55. Weiss HG, Hawiger J, Ruggeri ZW, et al. Fibrinogen-independent platelet adhesion and thrombus formation on subendothelium mediated by glycoprotein IIb/IIIa complex at high share rate. J Clin Invest 1989;83:288–97.

56. Unterberg C, Sandrock D, Nebendhal K, Buchwald AB. Reduced acute thrombus formation results in decreased neointimal proliferation after coronary angioplasty. J Am Coll Cardiol 1995;26:1747–54.

57. Sugama Y, Malik A. Thrombin receptor 14-aminoacid peptide mediates endothelial hyperadhesivity and neutrophil adhesion by P-selectin-dependent mechanism. Circ Res 1992;71:1015–19.

58. Shi Y, Hutchinson HG, Hall DG, Zalewsky A. Down-regulation of c-*myc* expression by antisense oligonuleotides inhibits proliferation of human smooth muscle cells. Circulation 1993;88:1190–5.

59. Moreno P, Falk E, Palacios I, et al. Macrophage infiltration in acute coronary syndromes: implications for plaque rupture. Circulation 1994;90:775–8.

60. Majesky MW, Reidy MA, Bowen-Pope DF, et al. PDGF ligand and receptor genes expression during repair of arterial injury. J Cell Biol 1990;111:2149–58.

61. Nabel EG, Yang ZY, Plautz G, et al. Recombinant fibroblast growth factor-1 promotes intimal hyperplasia and angiogenesis in arteries in vivo. Nature 1993;362:844–6.

62. Lindner V, Reidy MA. Proliferation of smooth muscle cells after vascular injury is inhibited by an antibody against basic fibroblast growth factor. Proc Natl Acad Sci USA 1991;88:3739–43.

63. Chen JK, Hoshi H, McKeehan WL. Transforming growth factor type beta specifically stimulates synthesis of proteoglycan in human adult arterial smooth muscle cells. Proc Natl Acad Sci USA 1987;84:5287–91.

64. Nikol S, Weir L, Sullivan A, et al. Persistently increased expression of the transforming growth factor beta 1 gene in human vascular restenosis: analysis of 62 patients with one or more episodes of restenosis. Cardiovasc Pathol 1992;3:57–62.

65. Shi Y, Pieniek M, Fard A, et al. Adventitial remodeling after coronary arterial injury. Circulation 1996;93:340–8.

66. Violaris AG, Melkert R, Hermann JPR, Serruys PW. Role of angiographically identifiable thrombus on long-term luminal renarrowing after coronary angioplasty: a quantitative angiographic analysis. Circulation 1996;93:889–897.

67. Schwartz RS, Holmes DRJ, Topol EJ. The restenosis paradigm revisted: an alternative proposal for cellular mechanisms. J Am Coll Cardiol 1992;20:1284–93.

68. Wilensky RL, March KL, Gradus-Pizlo I, et al. Vascular injury, repair, and restenosis after percutaneous transluminal angioplasty in the atherosclerotic rabbit. Circulation 1995;92:2995–3005.

69. Rodgers GP, Minor ST, Robinson K, et al. Adjuvant therapy for intracoronary stents. Investigation in atherosclerotic swine. Circulation 1990;82:560–9.

70. Whelan DM, van der Giessen WJ, Krabbendam SC, et al. Biocompatibility of phosporylcholine coated stents in normal porcine coronary arteries. Heart 2000;83:338–45.

71. Rogers C, Welt FG, Karnovsky MJ, Edelman ER. Monocyte recruitment and neointimal hyperplasia in rabbits. Coupled inhibitory effects of heparin. Arterioscler Thromb Vasc Biol 1996;16:1312–18.

72. Danenberg HD, Welt FG, Walker M 3rd, et al. Systemic inflammation induced by lipopolysaccharide increases neointimal formation after balloon and stent injury in rabbits. Circulation 2002;105:2917–22.

73. Biasucci LM, Liuzzo G, Buffon A, Maseri A. The variable role of inflammation in acute coronary syndromes and in restenosis. Semin Interv Cardiol 1999;4:105–10.

74. Zhou Z, Lauer MA, Wang K, et al. Effect of anti-tumor necrosis factor-alpha polyclonal antibody on restenosis after balloon angioplasty in a rabbit atherosclerotic model. Atherosclerosis 2002;161:153–9.

75. Plow EF, Ploplis VA, Busuttil S, et al. A role of plasminogen in atherosclerosis and restenosis models in mice. Thromb Haemostas 1999;82:4–7.

76. Okamoto E, Couse T, De Leon H, et al. Perivascular inflammation after balloon angioplasty of porcine coronary arteries. Circulation 2001;104:2228–35.

77. Karas SP, Gravanis MB, Santoian EC, et al. Coronary intimal proliferation after balloon injury and stenting in swine: an animal model of restenosis. J Am Coll Cardiol 1992;20:467–74.

78. Farb A, Sangiorgi G, Carter AJ, et al. Pathology of acute and chronic coronary stenting in humans. Circulation 1999;99:44–52.

79. Kornowski R, Hong MK, Tio FO, et al. In-stent restenosis: contributions of inflammatory responses and arterial injury to neointimal hyperplasia. J Am Coll Cardiol 1998; 31:224–30.

80. Farb A, Weber DK, Kolodgie FD, et al. Morphological predictors of restenosis after coronary stenting in humans. Circulation 2002;105:2974–80.

81. Rogers C, Edelman E. Endovascular stent design dictates experimental restenosis and thrombosis. Circulation 1995;91:2995–3001.

82. McKenna CJ, Camrud A, Sangiorgi G, et al. Fibrin-film stenting in porcine coronary injury model:efficacy and safety compared with uncoated stents. J Am Coll Cardiol 1998;31:1434–8.

83. Edelman E, Seifert P, Groothuis A, et al. Gold-coated NIR stents in porcine coronary arteries. Circulation 2001;103:429–34.

84. Ueda M, Becker AE, Tsukada T, et al. Fibrocellular tissue response after percutaneous transluminal coronary angioplasty. An immunocytochemical analysis of the cellular composition. Circulation 1991;83:1327–32.

85. Nobuyoshi M, Kimura T, Ohishi H, et al. Morphologic studies: restenosis after percutaneous transluminal coronary angioplasty: pathologic observations in 20 patients. J Am Coll Cardiol 1991;17:433–9.

86. Garratt KN, Edwards WD, Kaufmann UP, et al. Differential histopathology of primary atherosclerotic and restenotic lesion in coronary arteries and saphenous vein bypass grafts: analysis of tissue obtained from 73 patients by directional atherectomy. J Am Coll Cardiol 1991;17:442–8.

87. Fuster V, Erling F, Fallon JT, et al. The three processes leading to post PTCA restenosis: dependence on the lesion substrate. Thromb Haemostas 1995;74:552–9.

88. Clowes A, Clowes M, Fingerle J, Reidy M. Kinetics of cellular proliferation after arterial injury V. Role of acute distension in the induction of smooth muscle proliferation. Lab Invest 1989;49:360–4.

89. Clowes AW, Schwartz SN. Significance of quiescent smooth muscle cell migration in the injured rat carotid artery. Circ Res 1985;56:139–45.

90. Clowes AW, Reidy MA, Clowes MM. Kinetics of cellular proliferation after arterial injury, I. Smooth muscle growth in the absence of endothelium. Lab Invest 1983;49:327–33.

91. Clowes A, Clowes M, Reidy M. Kinetics of cellular proliferation after arterial injury: endothelial and smooth muscle growth in chronically denuded vessels. Lab Invest 1986;54:295–303.

92. Clowes AW, Reidy MA, Clowes MM. Kinetics of cellular proliferation after arterial injury. Lab Invest 1987;49:327–33.

93. Thayer JM, Giachelli PM, Mirkes PE, Schartz SM. Expression of osteopontin in the head process late in gastrulation in the rat. J Exp Zool 1995;272:240–4.

94. Liaw L, Lombardi DM, Almeida MM, Schwartz SM. Neutralizing antibodies direct against osteopontin inhibit rat carotid neointimal thickening following endothelial denudation. Arterioscler Thromb Vasc Biol 1997;17:188–93.

95. Weber GF, Ashkar S, Glimcher MJ, Cantor H. Receptor–ligand interaction between CD44 and osteopontin (Eta-1). Science 1996;271:509–12.

96. Jain M, He Q, Lee WS, et al. Role of CD44 in the reaction of vascular smooth muscle cells to arterial wall injury. J Clin Invest 1996;97:596–603.

97. Bendeck M, Zempo N, Clowes A, et al. Smooth muscle cell migration and matrix metalloproteinase expression after injury in the rat. Circ Res 1994;75:539–545.

98. Schwartz SM. Smooth muscle migration in atherosclerosis and restenosis. J Clin Invest 1997;99:2814–17.

99. Bendeck MP, Irvin C, Reidy MA. Inhibition of matrix metalloproteinase activity inhibits smooth muscle cell migration but not neointimal thickening after arterial injury. Circ Res 1996;78:38–43.

100. Ruoslahti E. Integrins. J Clin Invest 1991;87:1–5.

101. Hynes RO. Integrins: versatility, modulation, and signalling in cell adhesion. Cell 1992;69:11–25.

102. Choi ET, Engel L, Callow AD, et al. Inhibition of neointimal hyperplasia by blocking $\alpha_v\beta_3$ integrin with a small peptide antagonist GpenGRGDSPCA. J Vasc Surg 1994;19:125–34.

103. Samanen J, Ali FE, Romoff T, et al. Development of a small RGD-peptide fibrinogen receptor antagonist with potent antiagrregatory activity in vitro. J Med Chem 1991; 34:3114–25.

104. Scott-Burden T, Resink TJ, Hahn AWA, Vanhoutte PM. Induction of endothelin secretion by angiotensin II: Effects on growth and synthetic activity of vascular smooth muscle cells. J Cardiovasc Pharmacol 1991;17:S96.

105. Douglas S, Ohlstein E. Endothelin–1 promotes neointima formation after balloon angioplasty in the rat. J Cardiovasc Pharmacol 1993;22(Suppl 8):S371–3.

106. Wang X, Douglas SA, Louden C, et al. Expression of endothelin-1, endothelin-3, endothelin-converting-enzyme-1, endothelin-A and endothelin-B receptor mRNA following angioplasty-induced neointima formation in the rat. Circ Res 1996;78:322–8.

107. Tsjuno M, Hirata Y, Eguchi S, et al. Nonselective ETA/ETB receptor antagonist blockes proliferation of rat vascular smooth muscle cells after balloon angioplasty. Life Sci 1995;56:PL449.

108. Ferns GA, Raines EW, Sprugel KH, et al. Inhibition of neointimal smooth muscle accumulation after angioplasty by an antibody to PDGF. Science 1991;253:1129–32.

109. Clowes AW, Clowes MM, Fingerle J, Reidy MA. Regulation of smooth muscle cell growth in injured artery. J Cardiovasc Pharmacol 1989;14:S12-15.

110. Nabel EG, Liptay S, Yang, et al. r-PDGF gene expression in porcine arteries induces intimal hyperplasia in vivo. J Clin Invest 1993;91:1822–9

111. Nabel EG, Yang Z, Plautz GE, et al. rFGF-1 gene expression in porcine arteries induces intimal hyperplasia and angiogenesis in vivo. Nature 1993;362:844–6.

112. Scott-Burden T, Vanhoutte PM. Regulation of smooth muscle cell growth by endothelium-derived growth factors. Tex Heart Inst J 1993;21:91–7.

113. Kindy MS, Sonenshein GE. Regulation of oncogene expression in cultured aortic smooth muscle cells: posttrascriptional control of c-myc m-RNA. J Biol Chem 1986;261:12865–8.

114. Simons M, Edelman ER, DeKeyser JL, et al. Antisense c-myb oligonucleotides ihibit intimal arterial smooth muscle cell accumulation in vivo. Nature 1992;359:67–70.

115. Campan M, Desgranges C, Gadeau AP, et al. Cell cycle dependent gene expression in quiescent stimulated and asynchronously cycling arterial smooth muscle cells in culture. J Cell Physiol 1992;150:493.

116. Sinnaeve P, Chiche JD, Gillijns H, et al. Overexpression of a constitutively active protein kinase G mutant reduces neointima formation and in-stent restenosis. Circulation 2002;105:2911–16.

117. Huang J, Kontos CD. Inhibition of vascular smooth muscle cell proliferation, migration, and survival by the tumor suppressor protein PTEN. Arterioscler Thromb Vasc Biol 2002;22:745–51.

118. Chang MW, Barr E, Lu MM, et al. Adenovirus-mediated over-expression of the cyclin/cyclin-dependent kinase inhibitor, p21 inhibits vascular smooth muscle cell proliferation and neointima formation in the rat carotid artery model of balloon angioplasty. J Clin Invest 1995;96:2260–8.

15

Pharmacological treatment of restenosis

Manel Sabaté

Introduction

Restenosis has been the main drawback of coronary angioplasty since its inception nearly 25 years ago. The only widely accepted means of reducing restenosis has been the coronary stent, following the demonstration of reduced restenosis rates compared with percutaneous transluminal coronary angioplasty (PTCA) alone for comparable lesions.[1,2] Currently, coronary stents are used in more than 77% of cases.[3] Coincident with this increased stent use has been the more widespread treatment of more complex lesions that has led to the development of increased in-stent restenosis rates. In the USA alone, in-stent restenosis occurred in 10–50% of cases currently treated in everyday practice, accounting for 150 000 patients in 1999.[4] Most pharmacological treatments failed to demonstrate improvement of restenosis rates after conventional balloon angioplasty or ablative techniques. In the current stent era, systemic pharmacological treatment has been tested, with controversial results. The aims of this chapter are to review the main trials designed to prevent restenosis with pharmacological treatment systemically administered during or after conventional balloon angioplasty and stent implantation, and to give pathophysiological insights into the effect of different drugs tested for the prevention of restenosis.

Types of drugs evaluated in trials (Table 15.1)

The mechanisms involved in the restenosis process after conventional balloon angioplasty are elastic recoil of the

Table 15.1 Types of drugs evaluated in trials of restenosis prevention

- Antithrombotic, anticoagulant, and antiplatelet agents
- Anti-inflammatory agents
- Antiproliferative agents
- Lipid-lowering agents
- ACE inhibitors
- Nitric oxide donors
- Calcium channel-blocking agents
- Beta-blockers
- Antioxidants and combination therapies
- Nucleic acid-based drugs
- Antibiotics

artery, local thrombus formation, vascular remodeling with shrinkage of the vessel, and an overactive healing process with neointimal hyperplasia.[5–8] Neointimal hyperplasia develops by migration and proliferation of smooth muscle cells and myofibroblasts after balloon-induced trauma of the arterial wall, and by deposition of extracellular matrix by the smooth muscle cells.[8–10]

In-stent restenosis is quite distinct from restenosis after balloon angioplasty. Since stenting virtually eliminates elastic recoil and negative remodeling, neointimal hyperplasia that occurs due to trauma of the arterial wall by the stent struts remains as the only process contributing to in-stent restenosis.[11] Neointima is composed principally of proliferating smooth muscle cells and extracellular matrix.[12,13] Persistent thrombus does not play an important role in neointima formation, although recent observations suggest that it may have some influence, particularly in the setting of hyperglycemia.[14]

By interacting with one or several of the processes involved in restenosis, several pharmacological agents have been evaluated after either conventional balloon angioplasty or stenting. The rationale for the use of these agents is summarized below.

Antithrombotic, anticoagulant, antiplatelet agents

Arterial injury triggers thrombus formation with the release of growth factors known to stimulate neointimal proliferation: platelet-derived growth factor (PDGF), transforming growth factor β (TGF-β), and fibroblast growth factor (FGF).[15,16] Thus, it was thought that antithrombotic and antiplatelet agents could modulate the stimuli for neointimal hyperplasia.

Anti-inflammatory agents

Inflammation has been involved in the pathogenesis of the atherosclerotic process. Furthermore, it has been detected early during balloon-induced or stent-induced injuries and it has been related to impairment of clinical outcome.[17] Thus, the use of anti-inflammatory agents could potentially reduce one of the triggers of the healing process that occurs after coronary interventions.

Antiproliferative agents

Some agents exhibit, both in vitro and in animal models, the property of inhibiting smooth muscle cell proliferation and migration. Thus, in-stent restenosis appears to be the main target of such agents.

Lipid lowering: statins, fish oils

Vascular effects of 3-hydroxy-3-methylglutaryl coenzyme A (HMG-CoA) reductase inhibitors (statins) – beyond serum cholesterol level reduction – include endothelial normalization, anti-inflammatory effects, stabilization of the atherosclerotic plaque, and reduction of the thrombogenic response.[18,19] ω-3 polyunsaturated fatty acids reduce serum triglycerides and very low-density lipoprotein (VLDL), and are associated with lower rates of atherosclerotic heart disease. Additionally, since these fish oils have vasodilatory and anti-platelet-aggregatory effects, alter smooth muscle cell proliferation and monocyte function,[20,21] and inhibit PDGF expression from endothelial cells,[22] they have been studied for restenosis prophylaxis.

ACE inhibitors

Inhibition of angiotensin I-converting enzyme (ACE) activity has anti-inflammatory, antiproliferative, and vasodilatory effects that can modulate this atherosclerotic process, from the earliest form of endothelial dysfunction to delay of lesion formation in primary atherosclerosis, and in myointimal proliferation after angioplasty.[23] The DD genotype for the ACE deletion allele (D) polymorphism is a possible genetic factor for restenosis after stenting.[24,25] Those individuals with raised concentrations of circulating and cellular ACE may show an accelerated growth response of smooth muscle cells, leading to restenosis.[26] In this context, ACE inhibition could modify the consequences of these increased ACE concentrations in DD carriers.

Nitric oxide donors

Nitric oxide donors, in addition to their vasodilator effect, decrease platelet aggregation and inhibit vascular smooth muscle cell proliferation. These actions could have beneficial effects on restenosis after coronary balloon angioplasty.[27]

Calcium channel blocking agents

Because the atherosclerotic plaque is marked by changes in calcium regulation, there has been interest in a potential antiatherosclerotic role for calcium channel blockers. In experimental studies, the growth factor-dependent proliferation and migration of smooth muscle cells was found to be inhibited by calcium channel blockers. Besides, calcium channel blockers also exhibit characteristics that may lead to a reduction in restenosis, such as inhibition of platelet aggregation, reduction of vasospasm, and inhibition of the action of mitogens that stimulate proliferation and migration of smooth muscle cells.[28]

Beta-blockers

Several in vivo and ex vivo studies have demonstrated antiproliferative and antiatherogenic effects of beta-blockers. Specifically, carvedilol, a competitive, nonselective β and α$_1$ receptor blocker, directly inhibits vascular myocyte migration and proliferation and exerts antioxidant effects that are considerably greater than those of vitamin E or probucol.[29]

Antioxidants and combination therapies

Total plasma homocysteine level appears to be an important predictor of cardiovascular risk[30] and correlates with the severity of coronary artery disease.[31] This has led to interest in its potential role in restenosis. Links between homocysteine and vascular damage includes promotion of vascular smooth muscle cell growth and impairment of endothelium-dependent vasodilation.[32–34] Oxidizing metabolites generated at the site of coronary angioplasty can induce chain reactions that may lead to restenosis. Antioxidants may counter oxidative stress and modify neointima formation and vascular remodeling.[35]

Nucleic acid-based drugs

The rationale behind the use of these agents is to specifically target and inhibit a regulatory gene that plays an important role in a pathogenic process, classically by creating a molecule of ribonucleic acid (RNA) or deoxyribonucleic acid (DNA) that undergoes complementary base-pairing with its endogenous target.[36] Nucleic acid-based drugs can broadly be divided into three main types: antisense, ribozymes, and DNAzymes. Antisense oligodeoxynucleotides targeting the proto-oncogenes c-myb and c-myc inhibit neointima formation in rat and pig models of injury[37,38] have recently been tested in humans.[39]

Antibiotics

Chlamydia pneumoniae has been detected in atherosclerotic plaques.[40] This has prompted the use of specific antibiotics against C. pneumoniae (e.g. roxithromycin) to prevent a potential inflammatory response induced by the microorganism as a trigger to restenosis.

Pharmacological trials in the pre-stent era

Antithrombotic, anticoagulant, and antiplatelet agents

(Table 15.2)

Aspirin and dipyridamole were evaluated in a randomized, double-blind, placebo-controlled trial.[41] An oral aspirin–dipyridamole combination failed to reduce the restenosis rate as compared with placebo.

Warfarin (International Normalized Ratio (INR) 2–2.5 times the control value) was compared with aspirin (325 mg) after successful PTCA in another randomized trial.[42] Patients randomized to warfarin exhibited a comparable restenosis rate to those assigned to aspirin.

The effect of postprocedural heparin was addressed in a prospective randomized trial.[43] Patients were randomized to receive either postprocedural dextrose or

Table 15.2 Trials using antithrombotic agents to prevent restenosis in the pre-stent era

| | | | Restenosis rate (%) | | |
Ref	Agent	N	Agent	Placebo/control	p-value
41	Aspirin 330 mg / dipyridamole 75 mg	376	38	39	NS
42	Warfarin / aspirin 325 mg	248	36	27	NS
43	18–24 h heparin	416	41	37	NS
44	Warfarin / aspirin	110	29	37	NS
45	Enoxaparin 40 mg	458	52	51	NS
46	Heparin s.c. × 4 mos	339	39	48	NS
47	Reviparin s.c. / 4 wks	625	34	33	NS
48	Ticlopidine	179	28	24	NS
50	Prostacyclin 5 ng/kg	270	27	32	NS
51	Prostacyclin 4 ng/kg	132	31	34	NS
52	Vapiprost 80 mg	649	21	19	NS
53	Sulotroban/aspirin	752	53	39	NS
54	Hirudin/heparin	1154	0.32[a]	0.26[a]	NS
55	Cilostazol/aspirin–ticlopidine	68	17	40	<0.05

[a] Mean late loss in mm.

18–24 hours of heparin infusion (no warfarin). No differences were observed between treatment regimens. In another study, Urban et al[44] randomized 110 patients to receive either warfarin or aspirin after uncomplicated PTCA. A prolonged (24-hour) infusion of heparin was given to all patients after angioplasty. There were no differences in the restenosis rate.

The efficacy of the low-molecular-weight heparin, *enoxaparin*, was assessed in a randomized, multicenter, double-blind trial (the ERA trial).[45] The restenosis rate was similar in patients randomized to enoxaparin as compared with those assigned to placebo. In two other large multicenter trials (SHARP and REDUCE), long-term administration of low-molecular-weight heparin failed to demonstrate any difference in restenosis as compared with placebo.[46,47]

Ticlopidine was assessed after balloon angioplasty, and showed no effect on restenosis as compared with placebo in another study.[48] A recent subanalysis from the TOSCA trial[49] evaluated the role of ticlopidine in addition to aspirin versus aspirin alone in the rate of reocclusion of previously occluded arteries treated with balloon angioplasty. Failure to sustain arterial patency was similar in both groups: 23% in the ticlopidine plus aspirin group versus 16% in the aspirin-alone group (*p*=NS).

The effect of short-term *prostacyclin* administration to inhibit restenosis was evaluated in two trials.[50,51] In both, the restenosis rate was comparable between patients treated with prostacyclin and control patients.

Thromboxane A2 receptor antagonists have been evaluated after conventional balloon angioplasty. The CARPORT trial[52] was a randomized, double-blind, placebo-controlled trial in which 522 compliant patients were randomly assigned to placebo versus the thromboxane A2 receptor inhibitor vapiprost. Late loss as a primary endpoint was similar in both groups at 6-month follow-up (0.31 ± 0.54 mm versus 0.31 ± 0.55 mm, respectively; *p*=NS). The more recent M-HEART II trial[53] compared the efficacy on restenosis prevention of long-term aspirin, the thromboxane A2 receptor blocker sulotroban, and placebo. Neither active treatment differed significantly from placebo in the rate of angiographic restenosis.

Hirudin, a highly selective inhibitor of thrombin with irreversible effects, was also tested in a multicenter, randomized, double-blind fashion (the HELVETICA trial).[54] Although early cardiac events were reduced in patients receiving hirudin, mean minimal luminal diameters were comparable between hirudin and heparin groups on follow-up angiography at 6 months.

Finally, *cilostazol*, a potent antiplatelet agent with antiproliferative properties, has been evaluated after PTCA.[55] A small cohort of 68 patients were randomized to receive cilostazol or aspirin/ticlopidine immediately after PTCA. The incidence of angiographic restenosis appeared to be reduced at 4–6 months of follow-up.

Anti-inflammatory agents

(Table 15.3)

The efficacy of *corticosteroids* on restenosis prevention was evaluated in the multicenter, double-blind, placebo-controlled M-HEART trial.[56] Either placebo or 1.0 g methylprednisolone was infused 2–24 hours before planned angioplasty. There was no significant difference in restenosis rate on comparing placebo- with steroid-treated patients.

Colchicine is also used for inflammatory disorders, but acts at a more molecular level by binding to tubulin and disrupting spindle formation during the metaphase of cell division. Although animal models of arterial injury showed dose-dependent reduction in neointimal formation by colchicine, in clinical PTCA trials it was ineffective in preventing restenosis.[57]

Table 15.3   Trials using anti-inflammatory and antiproliferative agents to prevent restenosis in the pre-stent era

| | | | Restenosis rate (%) | | |
Ref	Agent	N	Agent	Placebo/control	p-value
56	Methylprednisolone 1.0 g/placebo	915	40	39	NS
57	Colchicine 0.6 mg/placebo	197	46	47	NS
58	Angiopeptin 750 µg/375 µg/placebo	112	12	40	0.003
59	Angiopeptin 3 mg/6 mg/placebo	553	36	37	NS
60	Trapidil 100 mg TID	384	24	40	<0.01
63	Tranilast 600 mg/placebo	255	18	39	0.005
64	Tranilast 600 mg/placebo	297	26	42	0.01
65	Ketanserin 40 mg/placebo	658	32	32	NS

Antiproliferative agents

(Table 15.3)

Angiopeptin, a cyclic octapeptide analogue of somatostatin, has been shown to limit myointimal thickening of arteries in balloon injury models and also to restore the vasodilating response to acetylcholine. Several trials evaluated these properties in a randomized fashion to reduce restenosis rates after balloon angioplasty. One hundred and twelve patients were included in a pilot Scandinavian trial.[58] Angiopeptin (750 µg/day) or placebo was infused from the day before angioplasty and for the following 4 days. An additional 375 µg of angiopeptin or saline was infused immediately before angioplasty. Restenosis was significantly reduced in the angiopeptin group (12% versus 40%; $p=0.003$), as was late lumen loss (0.12±0.46 mm versus 0.52±0.64 mm; $p=0.003$).[58] This favorable effect was not confirmed in a large multicenter, randomized double-blind, placebo-controlled trial conducted in Europe,[59] in which 553 patients were included. Placebo or angiopeptin was subcutaneously administered 6–24 hours before angioplasty and for 4 days after the procedure (3 mg/24 h before the angioplasty followed by 6 mg/24 h after the angioplasty). A 1.5 mg bolus dose of placebo or angiopeptin was given at PTCA. Although clinical events were reduced at 12 months in the angiopeptin group, neither late loss nor restenosis rate were significantly different between the groups.

Trapidil (triazolopyrimidine) is an antiplatelet drug with specific PDGF antagonism and antiproliferative effects in the rat and rabbit models after balloon angioplasty. The STARC trial[60] was a multicenter randomized (trapidil versus aspirin), double-blind trial to assess the effects of trapidil (100 mg three times a day initiated 3 days before PTCA and for 6 months thereafter) in angiographic restenosis. Of the initial 384 patients, 254 were evaluable for restenosis analysis. Restenosis, defined as loss of initial percentage gain of at least 50%, was significantly reduced in the trapidil group.

Tranilast exhibits multiple effects, including inhibition of smooth muscle cell proliferation and migration, and reduces in-stent restenosis in a porcine model.[61,62] Additionally, it suppresses the release of cytokines such as PDGF, TGF-β1, and interleukin-1β (IL-1β), and prevents keloid formation after skin injury. The TREAT-1 and -2 trials evaluated this drug in restenosis prevention. The TREAT-1 trial[63] demonstrated that 600 mg/day of tranilast for 3 months markedly reduced the restenosis rate after PTCA in de novo lesions as compared with tranilast 300 mg/day for 3 months and placebo. Restenosis rates were 17.6% in the high-dose tranilast group, 38.6% in the low-dose tranilast group, and 39.4% in the placebo group ($p=0.005$ for 600 mg/day tranilast versus placebo). The TREAT-2 trial[64] evaluated this drug for 3 months after PTCA of either de novo or restenotic lesions. Results were similar to those of the TREAT-1 trial, with a reduction in restenosis rate in the tranilast group as compared with placebo.

Ketanserin, a serotonin 5-HT$_2$ receptor antagonist that inhibits the platelet activation and vasoconstriction induced by serotonin (5-hydroxytryptamine) and also inhibits the mitogenic effect of serotonin on vascular smooth muscle cells, was investigated in a multicenter, randomized, double-blind, placebo-controlled trial.[65] Six hundred and fifty-eight patients were entered in the study. Patients receiving ketanserin (loading dose 40 mg 1 hour before PTCA; maintenance dose 40 mg twice daily for 6 months) did not differ from those receiving placebo in either of the primary endpoints: major adverse cardiac events or late lumen loss.

Lipid-lowering therapy

(Table 15.4)

Several trials assessed the efficacy of *statins* on restenosis prevention after PTCA. Lovastatin was evaluated in a

Table 15.4 Trials using lipid-lowering agents to prevent restenosis in the pre-stent era

Ref	Agent	N	Restenosis rate (%)		p-value
			Agent	Placebo/control	
66	Lovastatin 20 mg/40 mg	156	12	44	<0.001
67	Lovastatin 80 mg	404	39	42	NS
68	Pravastatin 40 mg	695	39	44	NS
69	Fluvastatin 40 mg b.i.d.	1054	28	31	NS
70	ω3FA 4.5 g	119	31	48	0.03
71	ω3FA 3.2 g	82	16	36	0.02
72	ω3FA 6.9 g	551	52	46	NS
73	ω3FA 5.4 g	625	40	39	NS

ω3FA, ω-3 unsaturated fatty acids.

small, open-label, single-center randomized trial,[66] in which the restenosis rate was significantly reduced in the lovastatin group. However, the unblinded method and the low angiographic restudy rate reduce the value of such a study. A subsequent larger multicenter, double-blind, placebo-controlled trial[67] showed that restenosis was not decreased in patients receiving lovastatin, despite a greater than 40% reduction in the levels of LDL cholesterol. Further multicenter, randomized, double-blind, placebo-controlled trials (PREDICT and FLARE) failed to demonstrate benefit of other statins to prevent restenosis. In the PREDICT trial,[68] pravastatin 40 mg/day was compared with placebo in 695 patients. Either of angiographic and clinical parameters were comparable between groups. In the FLARE trial,[69] fluvastatin 40 mg twice daily initiated 2 weeks before the PTCA and continued after successful PTCA to follow-up angiography, was compared with placebo in 1054 patients. Again, restenosis rate was similar between both groups.

Assessment of the efficacy of *ω-3 unsaturated fatty acids* to prevent restenosis showed controversial results. The first small series of patients reported positive results,[70,71] whereas further larger multicenter trials conducted in the USA[72] and in Canada[73] were negative.

ACE inhibitors (Table 15.5)

Cilazapril was evaluated in several multicenter, randomized, double-blind, placebo-controlled trials. In the MERCATOR trial,[74] 595 out of 735 patients could be analyzed at 6-month angiographic control. Mean late luminal loss (primary endpoint) was similar between patients treated with cilazapril (2.5 mg in the evening before PTCA and then 5 mg twice daily for 6 months) and patients treated

with placebo. Higher doses of cilazapril (1 or 2.5 mg in the evening before PTCA and then 1, 5, or 10 mg twice daily for 6 months or matched placebo) were evaluated in the MARCATOR trial.[75] Mean late loss was again comparable between different dose groups: 0.35±0.51 mm for the placebo group; 0.37±0.52 mm, 0.45±0.52 mm, and 0.41±0.53 mm, respectively, for the 1, 5, and 10 mg twice daily cilazapril groups.

NO donors (Table 15.5)

In a prospective multicenter randomized trial,[27] 700 stable coronary patients scheduled for angioplasty received *direct NO donors* (infusion of linsidomine followed by oral molsidomine) or oral diltiazem. Although the restenosis rate was lower in the NO donor group, neither late luminal narrowing nor combined major clinical events differed significantly between groups. The improved angiographic result related predominantly to a better immediate procedural result in the NO donor group (minimal luminal diameter post PTCA: 1.94 mm versus 1.81 mm in the diltiazem group; $p=0.01$).

Calcium channel blockers
(Table 15.5)

Nifedipine was first evaluated in a double-blind, placebo-controlled, randomized study.[76] Restenosis were not significantly different between groups.

The efficacy of *diltiazem* was assessed in another randomized study.[77] But again this drug failed to demonstrate a reduction in the restenosis rate as compared with placebo.

Table 15.5 Trials using vasoactive drugs to prevent restenosis in the pre-stent era

Ref	Agent	N	Restenosis rate (%) Agent	Placebo/control	p-value
74	Cilazapril 10 mg	735	28	28	NS
75	Cilazapril 20 mg	1436	37	33	NS
27	Linsidomine vs diltiazem	700	38	46	0.02
76	Nifedipine 40 mg	241	28	30	NS
77	Diltiazem 270 mg	92	14	19	NS
78	Verapamil 480 mg	196	47	62	0.06
79	Amlodipine 10 mg	635	0.30[a]	0.29[a]	NS
80	Nisoldipine 40 mg	826	49	55	NS
81	Carvedilol 50 mg	406	23	24	NS
82	Metoprolol mg	192	57	44	NS

[a] Mean late loss in mm.

Verapamil was evaluated in a single-center, placebo-controlled, double-blind trial.[78] There was a trend to reduce restenosis rate after high-dose verapamil (480 mg) as compared with placebo.

Amlodipine failed to reduce restenosis in the CAPARES trial.[79] The mean loss in minimal luminal diameter was similar in both groups.

Finally, in the NICOLE trial,[80] *nisoldipine* was evaluated, showing no benefit with respect to placebo.

Beta-blocker agents

(Table 15.5)

The multicenter, double-blind, randomized placebo-controlled EUROCARE trial[81] evaluated the efficacy of *carvedilol* for the prevention of restenosis after directional coronary atherectomy. No differences in minimal luminal diameter as the primary endpoint (1.99±0.73 mm versus 2.00±0.74 mm), angiographic restenosis (23.4% versus 23.9%), target lesion revascularization (16.2% versus 14.5%), or event-free survival rate (79.2% versus 79.7%) were observed between the placebo and the carvedilol groups at 7 months.

Another drug, sustained-release *metoprolol*, did not reduce the restenosis rate following angioplasty in native coronary arteries in a single-center randomized trial.[82]

Antioxidants

The efficacy of drugs with antioxidant properties on the prevention of restenosis after PTCA was evaluated in a double-blind, randomized trial.[35] One month before angioplasty, 317 patients were randomly assigned to receive one of four treatments: placebo, probucol (500 mg), multivitamins (30 000 IU of β-carotene, 500 mg of vitamin C, or 700 IU of vitamin E), or both probucol and multivitamins. Patients were treated for 4 weeks before and 6 months after PTCA. The mean late loss was significantly lower in the probucol group as compared with the other three groups: 0.12±0.41 mm versus 0.22±0.46 mm in the combined treatment versus 0.33±0.51 mm in the multivitamin group, and 0.38±0.50 mm in the placebo group ($p=0.006$ for those receiving versus those not receiving probucol). In the same way, the restenosis rate was lower in the probucol group: 20.7% versus 28.9% in the combined treatment versus 40.3% in the multivitamin group, and 38.9% in the placebo group ($p=0.003$ for probucol versus no probucol). Figure 15.1 depicts cumulative curves of minimum luminal diameters between groups.

Summary

Only a few of the above-mentioned drugs showed efficacy of pharmacological treatment reducing restenosis rate in multicenter, randomized, double-blind trials. Some antiproliferative drugs (trapidil and tranilast) and probucol reduced the restenosis rate after conventional PTCA. These types of drugs interfere with the main contributors to restenosis after balloon angioplasty: intimal proliferation (trapidil and tranilast) and constrictive arterial remodeling (probucol). However, even in those favorable trials, the remaining restenosis rate ranged from 17% to 26%, which is roughly what one may achieve after stent implantation.[1,2] Among other things, this contributed to the worldwide expansion of stent use, creating a new problem: in-stent restenosis. To counterbalance this, the following pharmacological trials have been designed to prevent in-stent restenosis after stent placement.

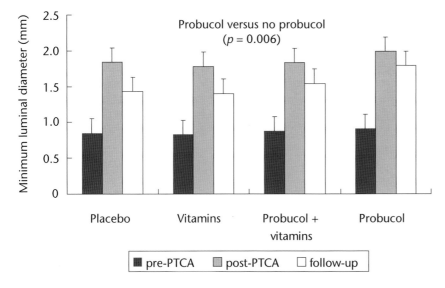

Figure 15.1
Minimum luminal diameters in the four groups evaluated in the probucol/multivitamin trial. (Adapted from Tardif J-C et al. N Engl J Med 1997;337:365–72.[35])

Table 15.6   Trials using antithrombotic agents to prevent restenosis in the stent era

| | | | Restenosis rate (%) | | |
| | | | Agent | Placebo/control | |
Ref	Agent	N	Agent	Placebo/control	p-value
83	Aspirin–ticlopidine vs phenprocoumon	517	27	29	NS
84	Warfarin/aspirin 100 mg	191	30	33	NS
85	Heparin 5000 u	179	12	13	NS
86	Enoxaparin 10 mg	100	10	24	<0.05
87	Abciximab	225	19	11	NS
89	Abciximab	401	31	31	NS
90	Cilostazol	409	23	27	NS

Pharmacological trials in the stent era

Antithrombotic, anticoagulant, and antiplatelet agents

(Table 15.6)

Combined *antiplatelet therapy* (*aspirin* plus *ticlopidine*) was tested against a conventional anticoagulant regimen (*phenprocoumon* with initial overlapping *heparin* plus *aspirin*) for 4 weeks after stenting.[83] The restenosis rate and late lumen loss were comparable between groups.

A recent study[84] evaluated the effect on restenosis prevention of postprocedural antithrombotic therapy with prolonged *heparin* infusion followed by 6 months of oral anticoagulation with *warfarin* in addition to aspirin. One hundred and ninety-one patients were randomized to aspirin or aspirin plus heparin followed by warfarin for 6 months. Stents were implanted in 33% and 36% of the patients in each group, respectively. No differences in the restenosis rate were observed. Unfractionated heparin delivered after predilatation and before stenting by means of a local delivery system has also been evaluated in the HIPS trial,[85] without any impact on restenosis and lumen loss.

Recently, *enoxaparin*, delivered by means of a microporous, local drug delivery/angioplasty catheter at predilatation before stenting, was evaluated in a propective, multicenter, unblinded, randomized trial of 100 patients.[86] Restenosis was significantly reduced in the locally administered enoxaparin group as compared with the conventional stenting plus heparin group.

The effect of *glycoprotein IIb/IIIa receptor blockers* on the prevention of restenosis has been evaluated in several trials. The ERASER trial[87] tested whether abciximab, administered for 12 or 24 hours after stenting, would reduce adverse clinical events as well as restenotic tissue volume as measured by intravascular ultrasound at 6 months as compared with placebo. Tissue volume did not differ between the three groups. These findings were confirmed on angiography, where neither loss index nor restenosis rate differed significantly between groups. A major multicenter, randomized trial of 2399 patients evaluated the efficacy of abciximab in improving long-term outcome after PTCA.[88] At 6 months, the clinical composite endpoint (death or myocardial infarction) was better in the abciximab after stenting group as compared with either the placebo plus stent group or the balloon angioplasty plus abciximab group. However, the rate of repeated revascularization of the target vessel as a surrogate of restenosis did not differ significantly between the groups. Among patients with diabetes, the combination of abciximab and stenting was associated with a lower rate of repeated target vessel revascularization (8.1%) than stenting plus placebo (16.6%; $p=0.02$) or angioplasty plus abciximab (18.4%; $p=0.008$). The ISAR-2 study[89] investigated the effect of abciximab on angiographic restenosis after acute myocardial infarction. Neither late lumen loss (primary endpoint) nor binary restenosis rates were significantly different between the groups (abciximab plus reduced-dose heparin versus standard-dose heparin).

Finally, *cilostazol* was investigated after stenting in a randomized study of 409 patients.[90] Patients receiving aspirin plus ticlopidine showed a comparable restenosis rate with those receiving aspirin plus cilostazol.

Anti-inflammatory agents

Corticosteroids were evaluated after stenting in a prospective randomized trial of 140 patients.[91] Pretreatment with single-dose (1 g) intravenous methylprednisolone 6–12 hours before angioplasty failed to reduce the in-stent restenosis rate as compared with placebo (17.5% in the steroid group versus 18.8% in the placebo group; $p=$NS).

Table 15.7 Trials using anti-inflammatory and antiproliferative agents to prevent restenosis in the stent era

			Restenosis rate (%)		
Ref	Agent	N	Agent	Placebo/control	p-value
91	Methylprednisolone 1.0 g / placebo	140	17	19	NS
92	Troglitazone 400 mg	52	5.3[a]	3.7[a]	0.0002[a]
93	Trapidil 600 mg	312	31	24	NS
94	Trapidil 400 mg	118	30	29	NS
95	Tranilast 600 mg/900 mg	11 500	NA	NA	NS

[a] In-stent mean lumen area (mm²) by IVUS at 6-month follow-up. NA, not available.

Antiproliferative agents

(Table 15.7)

Troglitazone appeared to reduce neointimal proliferation in a small series of 52 non-insulin dependent diabetic patients.[92]

Trapidil was investigated in a multicenter randomized trial (TRAPIST) of 303 patients after successful Wallstent implantation.[93] Oral trapidil 600 mg daily for 6 months did not reduce in-stent hyperplasia as assessed by intravascular ultrasound (IVUS) or improve clinical outcome after stent implantation. These findings corroborated those of previous small trial comparing trapidil with aspirin post Palmaz–Schatz stenting in 118 patients.[94]

Another agent that also showed positive effects after balloon angioplasty, *tranilast*, has been assessed in a large multicenter trial (PRESTO) of 11 500 patients.[95] Data were presented at the Euro-PCR 2002 (Paris, 21–24 May 2002). Randomization was blinded to one of the five treatment groups: placebo for 3 months, tranilast 300 mg twice daily for 1 month, tranilast 450 mg twice daily for 1 month, tranilast 300 mg twice daily for 3 months, and tranilast 450 mg twice daily for 3 months. The primary endpoint was major adverse cardiac events, and the secondary endpoints were quantitative coronary angiography of 2000 patients and intracoronary ultrasound data of 1000 patients. There were no significant differences between any of the five treatment groups in terms of major adverse cardiac events or restenosis rates.

Lipid-lowering therapies

In a retrospective analysis of 525 patients,[96] statin therapy was associated with reduced recurrence rates and improved clinical outcome after coronary stent implantation. Carriers of the Pl(A2) allele of the platelet glycoprotein IIIa gene have been associated with the occurrence of acute coronary syndromes and increased restenosis rates. Walter et al[97] evaluated the effect of statin therapy in this high-risk group of patients. Carriers of the Pl(A2) allele demonstrated significantly increased restenosis rates, which were abrogated by statin therapy (50.9% versus 28.6%; p=0.01). In addition, statin therapy was associated with a significant reduction of the occurrence of major adverse coronary events in the 6 months after intervention in patients with the Pl(A2) allele.

ACE inhibitors

The PARIS randomized, double-blind, placebo-controlled trial assessed the effect of high doses of *quinapril* to reduce restenosis after stent implantation in carriers of the DD genotype.[98] Late loss in minimum lumen diameter (as primary endpoint) was significantly higher in the quinapril group than in controls. Although not significant, differences in minimum lumen diameter at follow-up, percentage diameter stenosis at follow-up, and restenosis rate also showed a consistent trend towards increased restenosis in the quinapril group.

Plasma homocysteine-lowering therapy

A combination of folic acid (1 mg), vitamin B$_{12}$ (400 μg), and pyridoxine (10 mg), referred to as folate treatment, was compared with placebo after successful coronary angioplasty (57% of patients were treated with balloon and 43% with stent) in a prospective, double-blind, randomized trial.[99] Folate treatment significantly reduced homocysteine levels and decreased the rate of restenosis and the need for revascularization of the target lesion after coronary angioplasty (Figure 15.2).

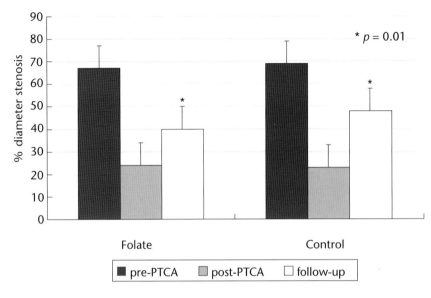

Figure 15.2
Comparison between percentage diameter stenosis in the two groups evaluated in the homocysteine lowering trial. (Adapted from Schnyder G et al. N Engl J Med 2001;345:1593–600.[99])

Nucleic acid-based drugs

To date, the only reported use of antisense to prevent in-stent restenosis in humans using a locally delivered antisense molecule targeting c-*myc* failed to demonstrate any benefit as compared with placebo.[39]

Antibiotics

The treatment of *Chlamydia pneumoniae* infection with roxithromycin to reduce restenosis rate after stent implantation has been investigated in a randomized, double-blind, placebo-controlled trial.[100] No differences in the rate of restenosis (primary endpoint) was observed between patients treated with antibiotic versus those without antibiotic (31% versus 29%, respectively; p=NS).

Summary

Adjunctive pharmacological treatment to prevent in-stent restenosis has so far been rather disappointing. Only folate treatment could reduce the restenosis rate after PTCA as compared with placebo, although 20% of treated patients still showed recurrence at 6 months. A few other small series of patients showed some benefit of active treatments (troglitazone, N=52; enoxaparin, N=100), which have to be established in larger multicenter, randomized trials.

References

1. Serruys PW, de Jaegere P, Kiemeneij F, et al. A comparison of balloon-expandable-stent implantation with balloon angioplasty in patients with coronary artery disease. Benestent Study Group. N Engl J Med 1994;331:489–95.

2. Fischman DL, Leon MB, Baim DS, et al. A randomized comparison of coronary-stent placement and balloon angioplasty in the treatment of coronary artery disease. Stent Restenosis Study Investigators. N Engl J Med 1994;331:496–501.

3. Hernández JM, Goicolea J, Durán JM, Augé JM. Registry of the working group on Hemodynamics and Interventional Cardiology of the Spanish Society of Cardiology for the year 2000. Rev Esp Cardiol 2001;54:1426–38.

4. Lowe HC, Oesterle SN, Khachigian LM. Coronary in-stent restenosis: current status and future strategies. J Am Coll Cardiol 2002;39:183–93.

5. Serruys PW, Luijten HE, Beatt KJ, et al. Incidence of restenosis after successful coronary angioplasty: a time-related phenomenon. A quantitative angiographic study in 342 consecutive patients at 1, 2, 3, and 4 months. Circulation 1988;77:361–71.

6. Schwartz RS, Holmes DR, Topol EJ. The restenosis paradigm revisited: an alternative proposal for cellular mechanisms. J Am Coll Cardiol 1992;20:1284–93.

7. Nobuyoshi M, Kimura T, Ohishi H, et al. Restenosis after percutaneous transluminal coronary angioplasty: pathologic observations in 20 patients. J Am Coll Cardiol 1991;17:433–9.

8. Mintz GS, Popma JJ, Pichard AD, et al. Arterial remodeling after coronary angioplasty: a serial intravascular ultrasound study. Circulation 1996;94:35–43.

9. MacLeod DC, Strauss BH, de Jong M, et al. Proliferation and extracellular matrix synthesis of smooth muscle cells cultured from human coronary atherosclerotic and restenotic lesions. J Am Coll Cardiol 1994;23:59–65.

10. Guarda E, Katwa LC, Campbell SE, et al. Extracellular matrix collagen synthesis and degradation following coronary balloon angioplasty. J Mol Cell Cardiol 1996;28:699–706.

11. Dussaillant GR, Mintz GS, Pichard AD, et al. Small stent size and intimal hyperplasia contribute to restenosis: a volumetric intravascular ultrasound analysis. J Am Coll Cardiol 1995;26:720–4.

12. Hoffman R, Mintz GS, Dussaillant RG, et al. Patterns and mechanisms of in-stent restenosis: a serial intravascular ultrasound study. Circulation 1996;94:1247–54.

13. Kearney M, Pieczek A, Haley L, et al. Histopathology of in-stent restenosis in patients with peripheral artery disease. Circulation 1997;95:1998–2002.

14. Carter AJ, Bailey L, Devries J, Hubbard B. The effects of uncontrolled hyperglycemia on thrombosis and formation of neointima after coronary stent placement in a novel porcine model of restenosis. Coron Artery Dis 2000;11:473–9.

15. Dinbergs ID, Brown L, Edelman ER. Cellular response to transforming growth factor-beta1 and basic fibroblast growth factor depends on release kinetics and extracellular matrix interactions. J Biol Chem 1996;271:29822–9.

16. Unterberg C, Meyer T, Wiegand V, et al. Proliferative response of human and minipig smooth muscle cells after coronary angioplasty to growth factors and platelets. Basic Res Cardiol 1996;91:407–17.

17. Libby P, Ridker PM, Maseri A. Inflammation and athero-sclerosis. Circulation 2002;105:1135–43.

18. LaRosa JC. Pleitropic effects of statins and their clinical significance. Am J Cardiol 2001;88:291–3.

19. Rosenson RS, Tangney CC. Antiatherothrombotic proper-ties of statins: implications for cardiovascular event reduc-tion. JAMA 1998;279:1643–50.

20. Knapp HR, Reilly IAG, Alessandrini P, Fitzgerald GA. In vivo indexes of platelet and vascular function during fish-oil administration in patients with atherosclerosis. N Engl J Med 1986;314:937–42.

21. Kromhout D, Bosschieter EB, de Lezemer Coulander C. The inverse relationship between fish consumption and 20-year mortality from coronary heart disease. N Engl J Med 1985;312:1205–9.

22. Bairati I, Roy L, Meyer F. Double-blind, randomized, con-trolled trial of fish-oil supplements in prevention of recur-rence of stenosis after coronary angioplasty. Circulation 1992;85:950–6.

23. Curzen NP, Fox KM. Do ACE inhibitors modulate athero-sclerosis? Eur Heart J 1997;18:1530–5.

24. Amant C, Bauters C, Bodart JC, et al. D allele of the angiotensin I converting enzyme is a major risk for restenosis after coronary stenting. Circulation 1997;96:56–60.

25. Ribichini F, Steffenino G, Dellavalle A, et al. Plasma activity and insertion/deletion polymorphism of angiotensin I-converting enzyme: major risk and a marker of risk for coronary stent restenosis. Circulation 1998;97:147–54.

26. Rigat B, Hubert C, Alhenc-Gelas F, et al. An insertion/dele-tion polymorphism in the angiotensin-converting enzyme gene accounting for half the variance of serum enzyme levels. Clin Invest 1990;86:1343–6.

27. Lablanche JM, Grollier G, Lusson JR, et al. Effect of the nitric oxide donors linsidomine and molsidomine on angio-graphic restenosis after coronary balloon angioplasty. The ACCORD study. Angioplastic Coronaire Corvasal Diltiazem. Circulation 1997;95:83–9.

28. Thaulow E, Jorgensen B. Clinical promise of calcium antagonists in the angioplasty patient. Eur Heart J 1997;18(Suppl B):B21–6.

29. Sung CP, Arleth AJ, Ohlestein EH. Carvedilol inhibits vascular smooth muscle cell proliferation. J Cardiovasc Pharmacol 1993;21:221–7.

30. Boushey CJ, Beresford SAA, Omenn GS, Motulsky AG. A quantitative assessment of plasma homocysteine as a risk factor for vascular disease: probable benefits of increasing folic acid intakes. JAMA 1995;274:1049–57.

31. Schnyder G, Pin R, Roffi M, et al. Association of plasma homocysteine with the number of major coronary arteries severely narrowed. Am J Cardiol 2001;88:1027–30.

32. Tsai JC, Perrella MA, Yoshizumi M, et al. Promotion of vascular smooth muscle cell growth by homocysteine: a link to atherosclerosis. Proc Natl Acad Sci USA 1994;91:6369–73.

33. Tang L, Mamotte CD, van Bockxmeer FM, Taylor RR. The effect of homocysteine on DNA synthesis in cultured human vascular smooth muscle. Atherosclerosis 1998;136:169–73.

34. Tawakol A, Omland T, Gerhard M, et al. Hyper-homocyteinemia is associated with impaired endothelium-dependent vasodilation in humans. Circulation 2000; 101:E116.

35. Tardif J-C, Cote G, Lesperance J, et al. Probucol and mul-tivitamins in the prevention of restenosis after coronary angioplasty. N Engl J Med 1997;337:365–72.

36. Khachigian LM. Catalytic DNAs as potential therapeutic agents and sequence-specific molecular tools to dissect biologic function. J Clin Invest 2000;106:1189–95.

37. Simons M, Edelman ER, DeKeyser JL, et al. Antisense c-myb oligonucleotides inhibit intimal smooth muscle cell accumulation in vivo. Nature 1992;359:67–73.

38. Gunn J, Holt CM, Francis SE, et al. The effect of oligonu-cleotides to c-myb on vascular smooth muscle cell prolif-eration and neointima formation after porcine coronary angioplasty. Circ Res 1997;80:520–31.

39. Kutryk MJB, Foley DP, van den Brand M, et al. Local intra-coronary administration of antisense oligonucleotide against c-myc for the prevention of in-stent restenosis. Results of the randomized investigation by the Thoraxcenter of antisense DNA using local delivery and IVUS after coronary stenting (ITALICS) trial. J Am Coll Cardiol 2002;39:281–7.

40. Muhlestein JB, Hammond EH, Carlquist JF, et al. Increased incidence of Chlamydia species within the coronary arter-ies of patients with symptomatic atherosclerotic versus other forms of cardiovascular disease. J Am Coll Cardiol 1996;27:1555–61.

41. Schwartz L, Bourassa MG, Lesperance J, et al. Aspirin and dipyridamole in the prevention of restenosis after percu-taneous transluminal coronary angioplasty. N Engl J Med 1988;318:1714–19.

42. Thornton MA, Gruentzig AR, Hollman J, et al. Coumadin and aspirin in prevention of recurrence after transluminal coronary angioplasty: a randomized study. Circulation 1984;69:721–7.

43. Ellis SG, Roubin GS, Wilentz J, et al. Effect of 18- to 24-hour heparin administration for prevention of restenosis after uncomplicated coronary angioplasty. Am Heart J 1989;117:777–82.

44. Urban P, Buller N, Fox K, et al. Lack of effect of warfarin on the restenosis rate or on clinical outcome after balloon coronary angioplasty. Br Heart J 1988;60:485–8.

45. Faxon DP, Spiro TE, Minor S, et al. Low molecular weight heparin in the prevention of restenosis after angioplasty: results of the Enoxaparin Restenosis (ERA) trial. Circulation 1994;90:908–14.

46. Brack MJ, Ray S, Chauhan A, et al. The Subcutaneous Heparin and Angioplasty Restenosis Prevention (SHARP) trial. J Am Coll Cardiol 1995;26:947–54.

47. Karsch KR, Preisack MB, Baildon R, et al. Low molecular weight heparin (reviparin) in percutaneous transluminal coronary angioplasty: results of a randomized, double-blind, unfractionated heparin and placebo-controlled multicenter trial (REDUCE). J Am Coll Cardiol 1996;28:1436–43.

48. Iñiguez A, Macaya C, Hernández-Antolín R, et al. The effects of ticlopidine administration at low doses on the incidence of restenosis following percutaneous transluminal coronary angioplasty. Rev Esp Cardiol 1991; 44:366–74.

49. Berger PB, Dzavik V, Penn IM, et al. Does ticlopidine reduce reocclusion and other adverse events after successful balloon angioplasty of occluded coronary arteries? Results from the Total Occlusion Study of Canada (TOSCA). Am Heart J 2001;142:776–81.

50. Knudtson ML, Flintoft VF, Roth DL, et al. Effect of short-term prostacyclin administration on restenosis after percuatenous transluminal coronary angioplasty. J Am Coll Cardiol 1990;15:691–7.

51. Gershlick AH, Spriggins D, Davies SW, et al. Failure of epoprostenol (prostacyclin PGI2) to inhibit platelet aggregation and to prevent restenosis after coronary angioplasty: results of a randomised, placebo controlled trial. Br Heart J 1994;71:7–15.

52. Serruys PW, Rutsch W, Heyndrickx GR, et al, for the Coronary Artery Restenosis Prevention on Repeated Thromboxane-Antagonism Study Group (CARPORT). Prevention of restenosis after percutaneous transluminal coronary angioplasty with thromboxane A2-receptor blockade: a randomized, double-blind, placebo-controlled trial. Circulation 1991;84:1568–80.

53. Savage MP, Goldberg S, Bove AA, et al. Effect of thromboxane A2 blockade on clinical outcome and restenosis after successful coronary angioplasty: Multihospital Eastern Atlantic Restenosis Trial (M-HEART II). Circulation 1995;92:3194–200.

54. Serruys PW, Herrman JP, Simon R, et al., Investigators for the HELVETICA. A comparison of hirudin with heparin in the prevention of restenosis after coronary angioplasty. N Engl J Med 1995;333:757–63.

55. Take S, Matsutani M, Ueda H, et al. Effect of cilostazol in preventing restenosis after percutaneous transluminal coronary angioplasty. Am J Cardiol 1997;79:1097–9.

56. Pepine CJ, Hirshfeld JW, Macdonald RG, et al. A controlled trial of corticosteroids to prevent restenosis after coronary angioplasty. Circulation 1990;81:1753–61.

57. O'Keefe JH Jr, McCallister BD, Bateman TM, et al. Ineffectiveness of colchicine for the prevention of restenosis after coronary angioplasty. J Am Coll Cardiol 1992;19:1597–600.

58. Eriksen UH, Amtorp O, Bagger JP, et al. Randomized double-blind Scandinavian trial of angiopeptin versus placebo for the prevention of clinical events and restenosis after coronary balloon angioplasty. Am Heart J 1995;130:1–8.

59. Emanuelsson H, Beatt KJ, Bagger JP. Long-term effects of angiopeptin treatment in coronary angioplasty. Circulation 1995;91:1689–96.

60. Maresta A, Balducelli M, Cantini L, et al, for the STARC Investigators. Trapidil (triazolopyrimidine), a platelet-derived growth factor antagonist, reduces restenosis after percutaneous transluminal coronary angioplasty. Results of the randomized, double-blind STARC study. Circulation 1994;90:2710–15.

61. Muranaka Y, Yamasaki Y, Nozawa Y, et al. TAS-301, an inhibitor of smooth muscle cell migration and proliferation, inhibits intimal thickening after balloon injury to rat carotid arteries. J Pharmacol Exp Ther 1998;285:1280–6.

62. Ishiwata S, Verheye S, Robinson KA, et al. Inhibition of neointima formation by tranilast in pig coronary arteries after balloon angioplasty and stent implantation. J Am Coll Cardiol 2000;35:1331–7.

63. Tamai H, Katoh O, Suzuki S, et al. Impact of tranilast on restenosis after coronary angioplasty: Tranilast Restenosis following Angioplasty Trial (TREAT). Am Heart J 1999;138:968–75.

64. Tamai H, Katoh K, Yamaguchi T, et al. The impact of tranilast on restenosis after coronary angioplasty: the Second Tranilast Restenosis following Angioplasty Trial (TREAT-2). Am Heart J 2002;143:506–13.

65. Serruys PW, Klein W, Tijssen JP, et al. Evaluation of ketanserin in the prevention of restenosis after percutaneous transluminal coronary angioplasty: a multicenter randomized, double-blind, placebo-controlled trial. Circulation 1993;88:1588–601.

66. Sahni R, Maniet AR, Voci G, Banka VS. Prevention of restenosis by lovastatin after successful coronary angioplasty. Am Heart J 1991;121:1600–8.

67. Weintraub WS, Boccuzzi SJ, Klein JL, et al. Lack of effect of lovastatin on restenosis after coronary angioplasty. N Engl J Med 1994;331:1331–7.

68. Bertrand ME, McFadden EP, Fruchart JC, et al. Effect of pravastatin on angiographic restenosis after coronary balloon angioplasty. The PREDICT Trial Investigators. Prevention of restenosis by Elisor after transluminal coronary angioplasty. J Am Coll Cardiol 1997;30:863–9.

69. Serruys PW, Foley DP, Jackson G, et al. A randomized placebo-controlled trial of fluvastatin for prevention of restenosis after successful coronary balloon angioplasty: final results of the Fluvastatin Angiographic Restenosis (FLARE) trial. Eur Heart J 1999;20:58–69.

70. Bairati I, Roy L, Meyer F. Double-blind, randomized, controlled trial of fish oil supplements in prevention of recurrence of stenosis after coronary angioplasty. Circulation 1992;85:950–6.

71. Dehmer GJ, Popma JJ, van den Berg EK, et al. Reduction in the rate of early stenosis after coronary angioplasty by a diet supplemented with $\varphi3$ fatty acids. N Engl J Med 1988;319:733–40.

72. Leaf A, Jorgensen MB, Jacobs AK, et al. Does fish oil prevent restenosis after coronary angioplasty? Circulation 1994;90:2248–57.

73. Cairns JA, Gill J, Morton B, et al, for the EMPAR Collaborators. Fish oils and low-molecular-weight heparin for the reduction of restenosis after percutaneous transluminal coronary angioplasty: the EMPAR study. Circulation 1996;94:1553–60.

74. Multicenter European Research Trial with Cilazapril after Angioplasty to Prevent Transluminal Coronary Obstruction and Restenosis (MERCATOR) Study Group. Does the new angiotensin converting enzyme inhibitor cilazapril prevent restenosis after percutaneous transluminal coronary angioplasty? Results of the MERCATOR

study: a multicenter, randomized, double-blind placebo-controlled trial. Circulation 1992;86:100–10.

75. Faxon DP. Effects of high dose angiotensin-converting enzyme inhibition on restenosis: final results of the MARCATOR study, a multicenter, double-blind, placebo-controlled trial of cilazapril. The Multicenter American Research Trial with Cilazapril After Angioplasty to Prevent Transluminal Coronary Obstruction and Restenosis (MARCATOR) Study Group. J Am Coll Cardiol 1995;25:362–9.

76. Whitworth HB, Roubin GS, Hollman J, et al. Effect of nifedipine on recurrent stenosis after percutaneous transluminal coronary angioplasty. J Am Coll Cardiol 1986;8:1271–6.

77. Corcos T, David PR, Val PG, et al. Failure of diltiazem to prevent restenosis after percutaneous transluminal coronary angioplasty. Am Heart J 1985;109:926–31.

78. Hoberg E, Dietz R, Frees U, et al. Verapamil treatment after coronary angioplasty in patients at high risk of recurrent stenosis. Br Heart J 1994;71:254–60.

79. Jorgensen B, Simonsen S, Endresen K, et al. Restenosis and clinical outcome in patients treated with amlodipine after angioplasty: results from the Coronary Angioplasty Amlodipine Restenosis Study (CAPARES). J Am Coll Cardiol 2000;35:592–9.

80. Dens JA, Desmet WJ, Coussement P, et al. Usefulness of nisoldipine for prevention of restenosis after percutaneous transluminal coronary angioplasty (results of the NICOLE study). Nisoldipine in coronary artery disease in Leuven. Am J Cardiol 2001;87:28–33.

81. Serruys PW, Foley DP, Hofling B, et al. Carvedilol for prevention of restenosis after directional coronary atherectomy: final results of the European Carvedilol Atherectomy Restenosis (EUROCARE) trial. Circulation 2000;101:1512–18.

82. Franzen D, Seifert N, Metha A, Hopp HW. Metoprolol treatment to prevent restenosis following percutaneous transluminal coronary angioplasty. Cardiology 2002;97:94–8.

83. Kastrati A, Schuhlen H, Hausleiter J, et al. Restenosis after coronary stent placement and randomization to a 4-week combined antiplatelet or anticoagulant therapy: six-month angiographic follow-up of the intracoronary stenting and antithrombotic regimen (ISAR) trial. Circulation 1997;96:462–7.

84. Garachemani AR, Fleisch M, Windecker S, et al. Heparin and Coumadin versus acetylsalicylic acid for prevention of restenosis after coronary angioplasty. Cathet Cardiovasc Interv 2002;55:315–20.

85. Wilensky R, Tanguay J-F, Ito S, et al. The heparin infusion prior to stenting (HIPS) trial: procedural, in-hospital, 30 day, and six month clinical, angiographic and IVUS results. Am Heart J 2000;139:1061–70.

86. Kiesz RS, Buszman P, Martin JL, et al. Local delivery of enoxaparin to decrease restenosis after stenting: results of initial multicenter trial. Polish–American Local Lovenox NIR Assessment study (the POLONIA study). Circulation 2001;103:26–31.

87. The Eraser Investigators. Acute platelet inhibition with abciximab does not reduce in-stent restenosis (ERASER study). Circulation 1999;100:799–806.

88. Lincoff AM, Califf RM, Moliterno DJ, et al. Complementary clinical benefits of coronary artery stenting and blockade of platelet glycoprotein IIb/IIIa receptors. Evaluation of platelet IIb/IIIa inhibition in stenting investigators. N Engl J Med 1999;341:319–27.

89. Neumann FJ, Kastrati A, Schmitt C, et al. Effect of glycoprotein IIb/IIIa receptor blockade with abciximab on clinical and angiographic restenosis rate after the placement of coronary stents following acute myocardial infarction. J Am Coll Cardiol 2000;35:915–21.

90. Park SW, Lee CW, Kim HS, et al. Effects of cilostazol on angiographic restenosis after coronary stent placement. Am J Cardiol 2000;86:499–503.

91. Lee CW, Chae JK, Lim HY, et al. Prospective randomized trial of corticosteroids for the prevention of restenosis after intracoronary stent placement. Am Heart J 1999;138:60–3.

92. Takagi T, Akasaka T, Yamamuro A, et al. Troglitazone reduces neointimal tissue proliferation after coronary stent implantation in patients with noninsulin dependent diabetes mellitus. J Am Coll Cardiol 2000;36:1529–35.

93. Serruys PW, Foley DP, Pieper M, et al. The TRAPIST study. A multicenter randomized placebo controlled clinical trial of trapidil for prevention of restenosis after coronary stenting, measured by 3-D intravascular ultrasound. Eur Heart J 2001;22:1938–47.

94. Galassi AR, Tamburino C, Nicosia A, et al. A randomized comparison of trapidil (triazolopyrimidine), a platelet derived growth factor antagonist, versus aspirin in prevention of angiographic restenosis after coronary artery Palmaz–Schatz stent implantation. Cathet Cardiovasc Interv 1999;46:162–8.

95. Holmes D, Fitzgerald P, Goldberg S, et al. The PRESTO (Prevention of Restenosis with Tranilast and its Outcomes) protocol: a double-blind, placebo-controlled trial. Am Heart J 2000;139:23–31.

96. Walter DH, Schachinger V, Elsner M, et al. Effect of statin therapy on restenosis after coronary stent placement. Am J Cardiol 2000;85:962–8.

97. Walter DH, Schachinger V, Elsner M, et al. Statin therapy is associated with reduced restenosis rates after coronary stent implantation in carriers of the PI(A2) allele of the platelet glycoprotein IIIa gene. Eur Heart J 2001;22:587–95.

98. Meurice T, Bauters C, Hermant X, et al. Effect of ACE inhibitors on angiographic restenosis after coronary stenting (PARIS): a randomised, double-blind, placebo-controlled trial. Lancet 2001;357:1321–4.

99. Schnyder G, Roffi M, Pin R, et al. Decreased rate of coronary restenosis after lowering of plasma homocysteine levels. N Engl J Med 2001;345:1593–600.

100. Neumann F, Kastrati A, Miethke T, et al. Treatment of *Chlamydia pneumoniae* with roxithromycin and effect on neointima proliferation after coronary stent placement (ISAR-3): a randomised, double-blind, placebo-controlled trial. Lancet 2001;357:2085–9.

16

Mechanical treatment of in-stent restenosis

Fernando Alfonso, María-José Pérez-Vizcayno

Introduction

Coronary stenting is increasingly used during coronary interventions, and currently stents are implanted in most patients undergoing percutaneous catheter-based procedures.[1–3] New stent designs may be readily delivered to the target lesion, are easily deployed, and can match almost every potential anatomic demand.[3] The widespread adoption of coronary stenting relies on its ability to guarantee an optimal immediate angiographic result. Seminal studies both from Europe and from America demonstrated that stents are able to reduce the risk of restenosis when compared with balloon angioplasty.[1,2] Some patients, however, still develop restenosis after stent implantation. In fact, coronary stenting elicits a more profound neointimal response than conventional balloon angioplasty.[1] Restenosis after balloon angioplasty is the result of acute vessel recoil, vascular remodeling, and neointimal proliferation.[4] Conversely, in-stent restenosis is largely dependent on severe neointimal tissue growth, which eventually obstructs the stent lumen.[5] Therefore, treatment of in-stent restenosis is not an easy task, representing a technical and clinical challenge affecting a significant number of patients.[6] Currently, in-stent restenosis constitutes a major health problem affecting up to 150 000 patients annually in the USA alone.[6] In other words, restenosis, the main drawback of balloon angioplasty since its inception 25 years ago, still persist as the Achilles' heel of the technique in the stent era.

In patients with in-stent restenosis, satisfactory initial results are usually obtained with conventional balloon angioplasty, but the risk of recurrent restenosis remains high.[7–16] Of interest, studies using both angiography[7–16] and intravascular ultrasound (IVUS)[17–21] suggested that most repeated coronary interventions do not obtain the same results that were initially achieved during initial stent implantation. Accordingly, the suboptimal results of the repeated treatment could explain, at least in part, the unsatisfactory course of some of these patients. Therefore, the use of alternative mechanical approaches, such as debulking techniques (laser, rotational atherectomy, and directional atherectomy) have been advocated.[22–38] In addition, other techniques such as the 'cutting balloon' have also been suggested as being potentially useful in this setting.[39–45] Finally, some reports[46–54] have suggested the potential value of 'elective' re-stenting (used as the primary strategy) in these patients. Compared with other mechanical techniques, repeat stenting is able to ensure optimal immediate angiographic results in this adverse anatomic scenario.[46–54] Besides, the potential benefit of drug-eluting stents in this adverse anatomic setting is currently being actively investigated.

Several multicenter, large-scale, controlled studies have convincingly demonstrated the usefulness of intracoronary brachytherapy in patients with in-stent restenosis.[6,55–58] This technique, and particularly its value for patients with in-stent restenosis, are reviewed in detail in Chapter 17 of this book. Although brachytherapy has the unique ability to inhibit neointimal proliferation, it is not widely available (it requires adequate logistics and is relatively cumbersome to implement) and also has inherent problems and limitations.[59–61] Therefore, mechanical coronary interventions are used worldwide in most patients presenting with symptomatic in-stent restenosis. Most mechanical interventions, however, have so far failed to consistently demonstrate a reduction in the rate of recurrent restenosis or an improvement in the long-term clinical outcome of these patients. Accordingly, the mechanical intervention of choice for patients with in-stent restenosis still remains uncertain.

In this chapter, we will review the use of currently available mechanical techniques for the management of patients with in-stent restenosis.

Classification and mechanism

The Washington group[62] has put forward a classification of in-stent restenosis that provides important therapeutic and prognostic clues and has gained widespread acceptance. Four major categories have been suggested:

(I)   focal in-stent restenosis (≤ 10 mm in length);
(II) diffuse restenosis (length >10 mm within the stent boundaries);
(III) proliferative restenosis (length >10 mm but extending outside the stented segment);
(IV) occlusive pattern (in-stent restenosis presenting as a total occlusion).

In addition, type I (or focal) restenosis has been further divided into four subgroups according to its location with respect to the stent: (IA) articulation gap; (IB) margin; (IC) stent body; (ID) multifocal. See Figures 16.1 and 16.2. Although different techniques have been used to treat these patients, the requirement for target vessel revascularization increased progressively from classes I to IV: 19%, 35%, 50%, and 83%, respectively.[62]

In contrast to restenosis after balloon angioplasty, in-stent restenosis is almost exclusively attributable to neointimal hyperplasia, because stents virtually eliminate elastic recoil and vessel remodeling.[5] Pathologic studies[63–65] have revealed that the process of in-stent restenosis parallels wound healing responses. Initially, stent deployment results in early thrombus deposition and acute inflammation with granulation development. Ultimately, the exuberant proliferation of neointima mainly consists of smooth muscle cell proliferation and extracellular matrix synthesis and accumulation.[65] In addition, it is well established that the severity of arterial injury during coronary stenting correlates with the inflammatory response and later with neointimal growth.

IVUS is a unique tool able to visualize a significant proportion of suboptimally expanded stents in many patients with in-stent restenosis, typically not visible on fluoroscopy. In a recent study, Castagna et al[66] analyzed ultrasound findings in 1090 consecutive in-stent restenosis lesions. Major morphologic problems (including stent 'crush' and stents missing the lesion) were identified in 4.5% of patients. Besides, stent underexpansion – defined as a stent cross-sectional area less than 80% of the average (proximal and distal) reference segment lumen area – was found in 20% of cases. In addition, 38% of stents had a minimal lumen area less than 6 mm². Finally, in 24% of stents, the intimal hyperplasia burden was less than 60%. These findings emphasize that although neointimal hyperplasia obstructing the stent is the leading mechanism accounting for in-stent restenosis,[5] other morphologic problems should be ruled out.[66]

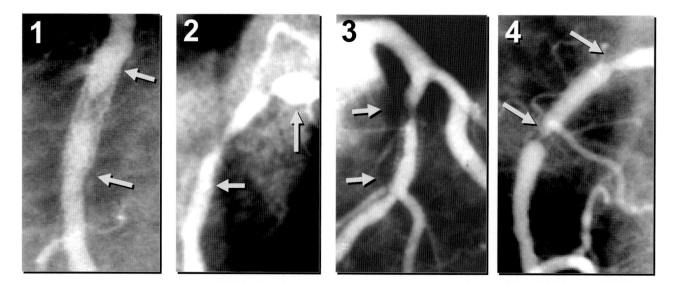

Figure 16.1
Morphologic patterns of focal in-stent restenosis. The location of the underliying stent is indicated by the arrows.
(1) Focal in-stent restenosis in the mid-portion (stent body) of a stent implanted in the right coronary artery (lateral view).
(2) Multifocal in-stent restenosis in the proximal right coronary artery. (3) Edge-in-stent restenosis (proximal margin) of a long stent implanted in the left anterior descending coronary artery (left anterior oblique view with cranial angulation).
(4) In-stent restenosis at the proximal and distal margins of the stent ('candy-wrapper' phenomenon).

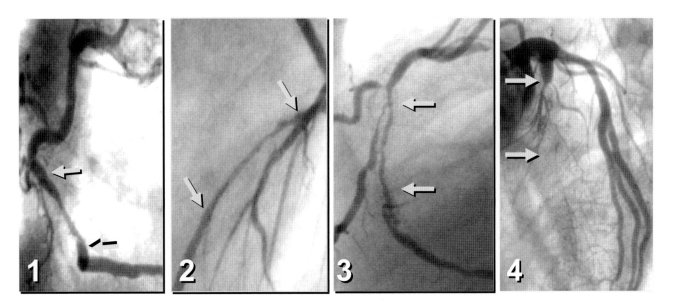

Figure 16.2
Challenging patterns of in-stent restenosis. The arrows indicate the location of the stent. (1) Difuse (>10 mm) in-stent restenosis at the distal right coronary artery (left anterior oblique view). (2) Diffuse in-stent restenosis in a long stent on the left anterior descending (LAD) coronary artery (lateral view). (3) Proliferative in-stent restenosis on the right coronary artery (lateral view). Note the narrowing extending to some extent out from the underlying stent. (4) Total occlusion of a stent in the proximal LAD coronary artery. This patient had previously had an anterior myocardial infarction and was asymptomatic at the time of angiographic follow-up.

Patient selection and adjunctive treatment

Patient selection

Not every patient with in-stent restenosis requires treatment. First of all, a significant lumen narrowing (typically over 50% diameter stenosis) must be documented before a new percutaneous treatment is considered.[10,67] It is important to keep in mind that the degree of intimal hyperplasia may decrease during long-term follow-up[68] (Figure 16.3). An analogy with the healing process that may occur with some skin scars could help to explain this finding. This spontaneous increase in lumen size appears to be especially prevalent among patients presenting with mild to moderate lumen narrowing at the stented site, where an increase in minimal lumen diameter at follow-up was demonstrated by Kimura et al[68] (Figure 16.4). Second, in-stent restenosis should be associated with either angina or myocardial ischemia before considering re-intervention.[10,67] In fact, every effort should be made to avoid the oculo-stenotic reflex in these patients. The rationale behind this approach is that several reports have demonstrated that the long-term clinical outcome of asymtomatic patients with in-stent restenosis (mainly in the absence of inducible ischemia) is favorable with medical management only. In the study by Lee et al,[69] the event-free survival rate in patients with asymptomatic, noncritical stenosis (mean follow-up 26±15 months), in whom rein-

tervention was deferred, was 87%, which is similar to that of patients without restenosis. Accordingly, as a general rule, patients should have angina or inducible ischemia before undergoing repeated percutaneous treatment.

In the real world, one end of the spectrum will be the asymptomatic patient presenting 6 months after a large Q-wave inferior myocardial infarction with an occluded stent in the right coronary artery. Not only is this a challenging technical scenario acutely (during the repeated intervention), but also it will be associated with a high rate of recurrence and very little – if any – clinical benefit. The other end of the spectrum will be the patient with three-vessel disease and recurrent in-stent restenosis in the proximal left anterior descending coronary artery, where coronary surgery should be contemplated. Finally, nowadays it is quite clear that mechanical interventions should be associated with the use of brachytherapy in patients with recurrent, diffuse, in-stent restenosis presenting as a single lesion.

Adjunctive therapy

Patients undergoing reinterventions for in-stent restenosis are managed in a way similar to other patients subjected to coronary interventions.[10,67] Some investigators claim that ticlopidine or clopidogrel should be used systematically in these patients because after the procedure some areas of the initial stent may be exposed to the flowing

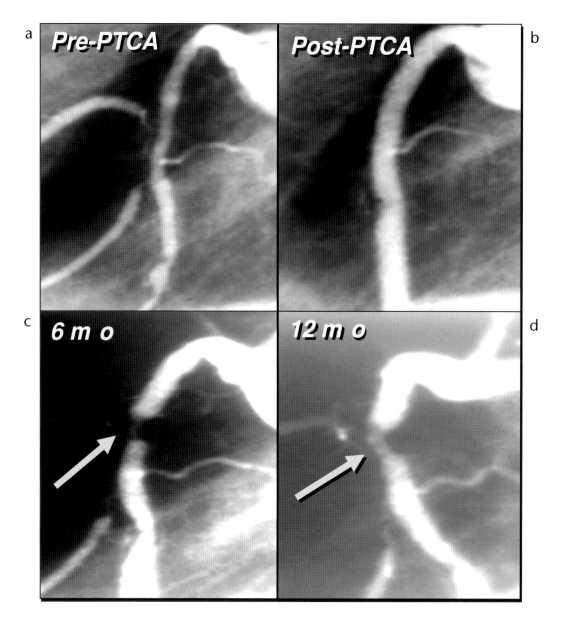

Figure 16.3
Spontaneous improvement in severity of stenosis in a patient with asymptomatic in-stent restenosis. (a) Before intervention, diffuse in-stent restenosis is visualized. (b) After the procedure, an excellent angiographic result is obtained (balloon angioplasty), but some right ventricular branches are lost. (c) At follow-up, recurrent restenois was demonstrated, although the patient was asymptomatic and no intervention was performed. (d) One year later, spontaneous improvement of the angiographic result was seen.

blood. The potential benefit of using GP IIb/IIIa receptor inhibitors in patients with in-stent restenosis remains controversial. An initial report from the Cleveland Clinic[70] suggested that the adjunct administration of these drugs was associated with a lower incidence of myocardial infarction and, unexpectedly, a lower mortality at 1-year follow-up. However, a more recent report from the University of Texas[71] failed to find any significant beneficial effect of abciximab administration (use based on operator discretion) in a large cohort of patients with in-stent restenosis.

Balloon angioplasty

Repeat balloon angioplasty is the most commonly used technique for patients with in-stent restenosis. The procedure is technically straightforward, and redilating the narrowed part of the stent is usually achieved using the same strategy as in 'de novo' lesions (namely a balloon-to-artery ratio of 1.1:1 and pressures up to 14 atmospheres).[10] IVUS studies demonstrated that nearly half of the total lumen gain after balloon dilation is obtained as the result of tissue extrusion (or reduction/compression), while the remaining gain is

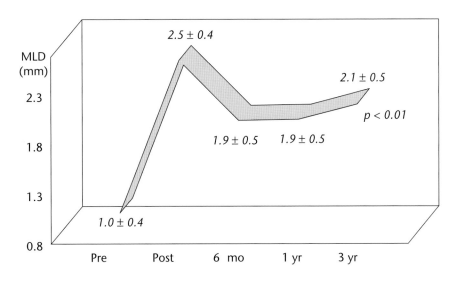

Figure 16.4
Long-term analysis of minimal lumen diameter (MLD) after stent implantation. A significant improvement in lumen diameter occurs between 1 and 3 years. (Adapted from Kimura T et al. N Engl J Med 1996;334:561–6.[68])

achieved by further stent expansion[20,21] (Figure 16.5). In fact, when a stepwise protocol (progressive increase in pressures) was followed, it could be demonstrated that when relatively low pressures are selected, both the reduction in neointimal tissue and stent overexpansion explain the lumen enlargement. However, with the use of higher pressures, only additional stent overexpansion is observed.[19] Nevertheless, the acute results are never as good as those obtained during original stenting. Both angiographic data[7–16] and IVUS studies[17–21] have demonstrated significant residual lumen stenosis due to residual tissue within the stent after balloon dilation. This is true in spite of the use of larger balloons or higher pressures than those employed at the time of the original stent implantation (Figure 16.6).

Initial studies reported relatively high clinical and angiographic restenosis rates (31–54%) after repeat balloon angioplasty for in-stent restenosis. It soon became evident that the rate of recurrent restenosis was especially high in patients with diffuse (>10 mm) in-stent restenosis. Eltchaninoff et al[8] emphasized the importance of lesion length for the appearance of recurrent restenosis after balloon angioplasty. In that series, the recurrent restenosis rate was 63% for patients with diffuse in-stent restenosis and was halved (31%) in patients with focal in-stent restenosis. Other clinical and angiographic factors associated with recurrence are basically the same as those reported after the treatment of de novo lesions, as summarized in Table 16.1.

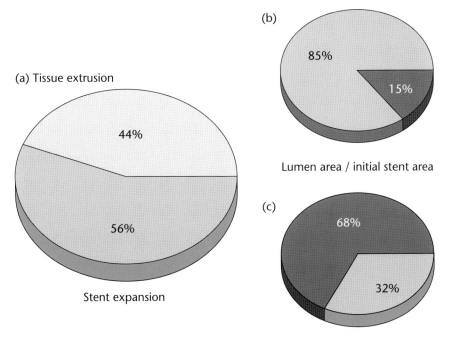

Figure 16.5
Intravascular ultrasound analysis of the mechanisms of lumen enlargement after balloon dilation of in-stent restenosis. (a) Diagram showing the relative contribution of tissue extrusion and further stent dilation. (b,c) The lumen obtained is frequently not as large as that previously obtained with initial stent implantation, and some obstructive tissue always remains within the stent struts. (Adapted from Mehran R et al. Am J Cardiol 1996;78:618–22[20] with permission from Excerpta Medica Inc.)

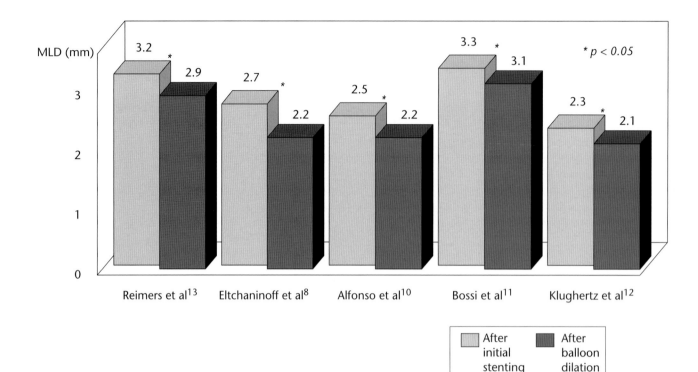

Figure 16.6
Angiographic studies comparing minimal lumen diameter (MLD) after initial stenting with that obtained after balloon dilation for in-stent restenosis in the same patients. Results of repeated interventions are never as good as initial results of the first stent. (Adapted from references 8–13.)

Table 16.1   Predictors of long-term clinical and angiographic outcome after balloon dilation of in-stent restenosis: the numbers indicate the reference reporting the study in which the variable was found to predict the event

	Angiographic restenosis	TVR	MACE/TVR
Diabetes		12	10, 12
HBP		12	12
Unstable angina		11	
Early restenosis		11, 12	10, 12, 13
Diffuse restenosis	8, 9	11	
Severe restenosis	9		
SVG location			13
Low LVEF			13
Multivessel disease			13
Reference MLD		11	
Final MLD		11	

TVR, target vessel revascularization; MACE, major adverse cardiac events; SVG, saphenous vein graft; LVEF, left ventricular ejection fraction; HBP, high blood pressure; MLD, minimal lumen diameter.
[a] Independent predictors after adjustment.

In our own experience, most patients with in-stent restenosis treated with balloon angioplasty have a favorable clinical outcome. In a previous study,[10] we found that the rate of event-free survival (freedom from death, myocardial infarction, and target vessel revascularization) was 80% at 1 year and 77% at 2 years. In this series, the recurrent restenosis rate was 40%, but angiographic follow-up was not systematic (driven just by angina or myocardial ischemia). Patients with a short time interval (<4 months) from stenting to repeat angioplasty and those with diabetes experienced adverse cardiac events more frequently (a threefold risk increase) at follow-up. Other angiographic factors were less important in our series, but this was probably explained by a selection bias where the more complex cases (including very diffuse in-stent restenosis) were preferentially treated with debulking strategies.

Other investigators have also reported a favorable outcome after balloon angioplasty. In the study by Reimers et al,[13] the event-free survival rate at 2 years was 81%. This study also stressed the importance of clinical factors (namely interval from stenting to repeat intervention) as predictive of recurrent events in these patients. In addition, in the study by Bauters et al[9] with an 85% rate of late angiographic follow-up, the restenosis rate was only 22%, and only 17% required target vessel revascularization. In some studies, angiographic factors, including left ventricular ejection fraction, multivessel disease, saphenous vein graft location, and restenosis length and severity, emerged as major determinants of long-term outcome.[9–13] As previously stated, selection criteria could help to explain some of these differences (Table 16.1).

Complications of balloon angioplasty in this setting are rare. In some cases with overtly aggressive dilation, a dissection flap, typically at the stent margin, may complicate the procedure (Figure 16.7). In other cases, the dissected neointima may result in a suboptimal hazy appearance within the stent body (Figure 16.8). Nowadays, repeat stenting is indicated to deal with these situations.[46–48] Some authors still recommend the use of prolonged inflations in this scenario in an attempt to improve angiographic findings. Nevertheless, in some patients, this strategy can just promote further extension of the dissection flap, resulting in a worsening of the problem that could eventually require stenting large coronary segments. Another peculiar problem in this setting is the 'watermelon-seeding' phenomenon (Figure 16.9). This factor appears to be more frequent in cases with severe and diffuse in-stent restenosis.[72] Vessel trauma outside the stented segment can increase procedure-related complications acutely, as well as the risk of restenosis. In a recent study,[72] we have demonstrated that patients with in-stent restenosis presenting the 'watermelon-seeding' phenomenon had poorer immediate angiographic results and, more importantly, were eventually associated with a poorer long-term clinical outcome. The cutting balloon appears especially

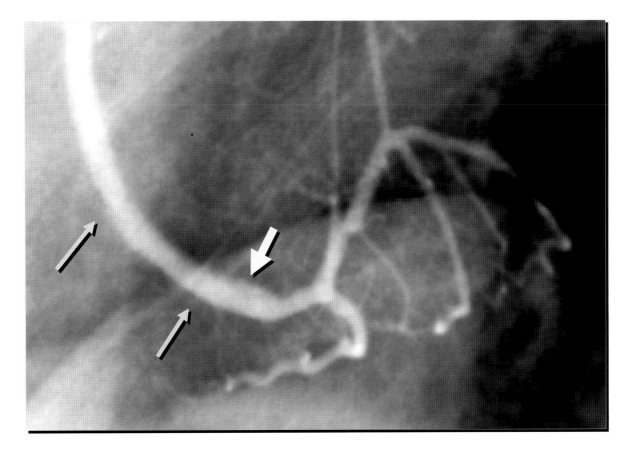

Figure 16.7
Residual type A dissection after relatively aggressive balloon dilation of an in-stent restenosis in the distal right coronary artery (thick arrow). Usually, these residual dissections are no longer present at follow-up.

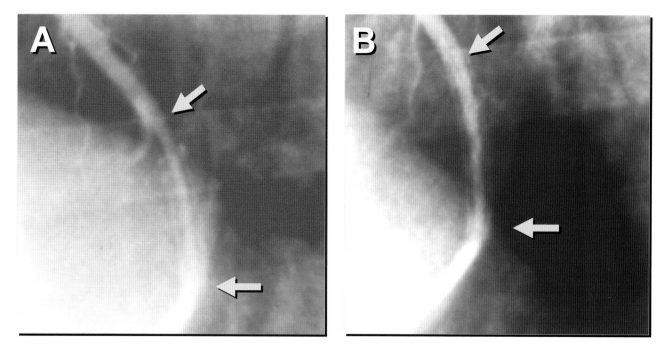

Figure 16.8
Suboptimal results after balloon dilation of in-stent restenosis (A and B). Arrows indicate the stent location. Note the residual narrowing and hazy appearance of the treated segment.

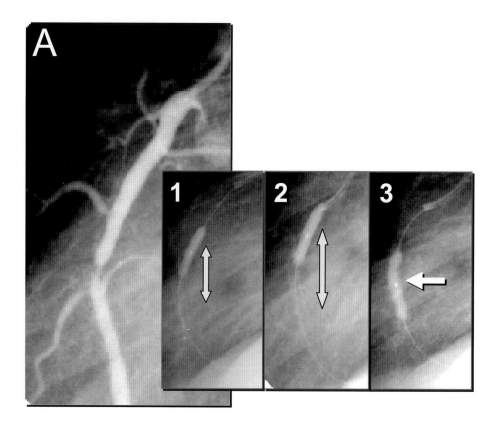

Figure 16.9
The 'watermelon-seeding' phenomenon. (A) Focal in-stent restenosis in the middle right coronary artery. A cranial displacement (slippage) of the balloon occurred during multiple inflation attemps (1 and 2). Eventually (3), the balloon could be stabilized at the lesion site.

suited to prevent this phenomenon.[40,41] Furthermore, avoiding damage to the coronary segment adjacent to the site of in-stent restenosis is crucial during intracoronary radiation, since this problem has been associated with geographic miss[60] and secondarily with a characteristic form of edge restenosis, yielding a 'candy-wrapper' appearance at follow-up.

Another potential caveat is management of side branches (Figure 16.10). Since most stents do not cover large side branches, this problem seldom complicates repeat interventions. To determine the fate of stent-related side branches, we analyzed 100 consecutive patients with in-stent restenosis undergoing repeat coronary interventions.[73] A total of 226 side branches (mostly relatively small branches) spanned by the stent were identified. Occlusion (TIMI 0 flow) was seen in 24 branches (10%), whereas

some degree of flow compromise during or after the procedure was observed in 25% of these side branches. Diabetes mellitus, side-branch ostium involvement, baseline side-branch flow, and restenosis length were identified as independent predictors of side-branch occlusion. Most side-branch occlusions were clinically silent, and only two patients with side-branch occlusion (relatively large side branches) developed a non-Q-wave myocardial infarction. Of interest, at late angiography, 90% of side branches that became occluded during the procedure were patent again.[73] Large side branches jailed by the initial stent, mainly in patients with those risk characteristics, will require adequate protection and eventual treatment should a vessel occlusion occur.

Finally, we need to discuss the so-called 'early lumen loss' phenomenon. Shiran et al[74] demonstrated that

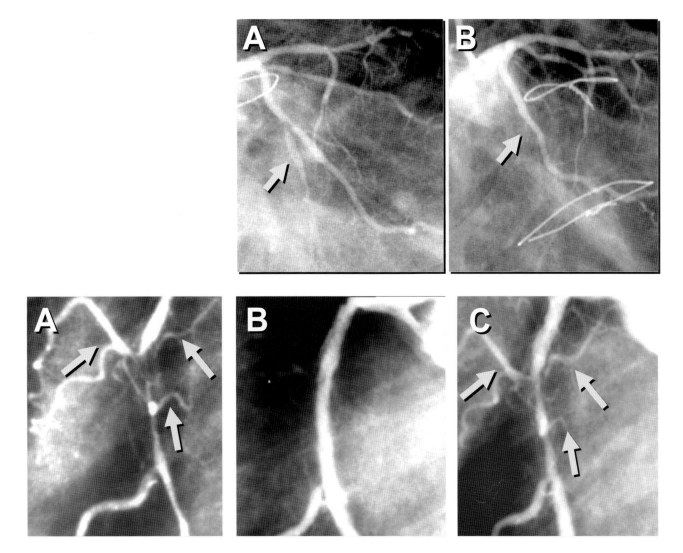

Figure 16.10
The problem of side branches emerging from the stent. Top row: A relatively large circumflex coronary artery (A) is lost (B) after dilating the stent on the marginal branch. Bottom row: Multiple small right ventricular branches (arrows) disappear after treatment of a severe in-stent restenosis in the proximal right coronary artery (A, B). However, when the patient returned back with moderate recurrent in-stent restenosis, all these branches were patent again (C).

early after balloon angioplasty (and also after debulking), significant tissue reintrusion (back into the stent lumen) may be detected by IVUS in patients treated for in-stent restenosis. This 'early lumen loss' phenomenon was actually observed after the 'dwell time' interval required for intracoronary gamma radiation (mean delay time 42 minutes) in these patients. In nearly one-third of patients, the reduction in cross-sectional area was significant (≥ 2.0 mm^2). This acute lumen loss was readily detected by IVUS, resulted from increased tissue within the stent, and correlated with lesion length and preintervention in-stent tissue (neointimal burden).[74] During this waiting time, stent recoil was absent. Probably the main clinical implication of this finding is that – at least in some patients – it might contribute to late recurrence. As we will discuss later in this chapter, this phenomenon may be prevented by repeat stenting.

Directional atherectomy

Directional atherectomy is the most effective means to debulk plaque burden in patients undergoing coronary interventions. In fact, since both pre-existing and residual plaque burden after intervention contribute to in-stent restenosis,[75–78] some investigators have suggested the potential use of debulking to reduce the risk of subsequent in-stent restenosis. The same concept is behind the use of debulking to remove neointimal tissue within the stent in an attempt to optimize the final result and reduce recurrences. Directional atherectomy has the unique ability to obtain the specimen of tissue responsible for in-stent restenosis, thus opening the way to other avenues of research.[22–24]

The Boston group has a relatively wide experience with the use of directional atherectomy in this setting.[22,23] They suggested that debulking of restenotic tissue within stents using directional coronary atherectomy may offer a therapeutic advantage over the disappointing results of balloon angioplasty in some patients. In a series of 45 patients with Palmaz–Schatz in-stent restenosis,[22] they had an inicidence of non-Q-wave myocardial infarction of 9%. At follow-up (mean 10±4 months) the event-free survival rate was 71% and 45% at 6 and 12 months after the procedure respectively. Target vessel revascularization was the most frequent event, occurring in 28% of patients. Angiographically, this technique provided an excellent result (a postprocedural minimal lumen diameter of 2.7±0.7 mm), which compared favorably with the results obtained by balloon angioplasty. In keeping with previous studies, longer lesion length, saphenous vein graft location, and a short time interval from stenting to restenosis were independent predictors of target vessel revascularization.[22]

Although all of these results are encouraging and new more user-friendly catheters (Flexicut, 8 Fr-compatible)[24] are currently available, the use of directional atherectomy

is currently rather limited since (I) it is still more technically demanding than other available alternatives, (II) the technique has an inherent risk of minor procedural related complications, (III) anecdotal cases of strut damage (fracture or disruption) have been reported (mainly in patients with coil-design stents), and (IV) likewise, occasional microscopic stent particles in tissue specimens have also been demonstrated.[24] Such concerns have hindered wider adoption of this strategy in patients with in-stent restenosis.

Finally, alternative atherectomy modalities (transluminal extraction atherectomy and pullback atherectomy)[25] have also been used in patients with in-stent restenosis, but currently the available experience with these techniques is still rather limited.

Rotational atherectomy

Debulking of in-stent tissue with high-speed rotational atherectomy constitute a very attractive strategy for patients with in-stent restenosis. With this approach, we can remove (athero-ablation) to some extent the neointima obstructing the stent with the aim of optimizing procedural results.[26–31] The idea is to increase the final lumen size by reducing in-stent residual neointima. Usually, a bur-to-artery ratio of 0.7–0.8 and a speed of 140 000–160 000 rpm is selected. Falls in speed greater than 5000 rpm should be avoided. In addition, the systematic use of vasodilator drugs and a progressive/conservative approach (allowing some time during the procedure to ensure satisfactory anterograde blood flow) have been advocated. This is especially important in patients with very diffuse or proliferative patterns of in-stent restenosis, where every attempt should be made to prevent the no-reflow phenomenon. In addition, Cho et al[32] have suggested that side-branch occlusion may explain some non-Q-wave myocardial infarctions in patients with in-stent restenosis treated with rotational atherectomy. In this series, the presence of ostial disease at the side branch was found to be an important predisposing factor for this complication.[32] Eventually, once debulking with rotational atherectomy is finished, adjunct conventional balloon angioplasty should be performed to optimize procedural results. Early studies suggested the potential benefit of using low pressures during this adjunctive dilation. Theoretically, this approach should reduce the stimulus for recurrent neointimal proliferation. When such a strategy is followed, most of the lumen gain is obtained from true tissue debulking or neointimal redistribution, whereas further stent expansion plays a minor role. More recently, however, higher pressures have been advocated to improve the final results in an attempt to reduce recurrences.

Initial data from single-center studies demonstrated the feasibility and safety of rotational atherectomy in patients with in-stent restenois.[26–29] Furthermore, early studies using quantitative angiography and IVUS confirmed the effectiveness of rotational atherectomy in debulking neointima. A significant increase in debulking efficiency could be accomplished with the stepped-burr approach. Nevertheless, compared with directional atherectomy, the debulking capacity of rotational atherectomy is relatively modest. Observational (nonrandomized) studies, mainly involving patients with diffuse in-stent restenosis, also suggested that the use of rotational atherectomy was associated with a lower recurrence of angina, requirement for clinically driven reinterventions, and angiographic restenosis as compared with balloon angioplasty. Dauerman et al[27] suggested that mechanical debulking with rotational atherectomy in patients with diffuse in-stent retenosis resulted in a better immediate final result after the procedure. Likewise, the study by Lee et al[28] in patients with diffuse in-stent restenosis suggested that the acute angiographic result was better and the clinical recurrence significantly lower in patients undergoing debulking as compared with those treated with conventional angioplasty. Predictors of recurrent restenosis after rotational atherectomy in various studies[27–30] have included a short time to restenosis, lesion length and severity, a bur-to-artery ratio less than 0.6, and the presence of acute neointimal recoil.

In an elegant, large randomized study, the ARTIST trial, von Dahl et al[31] compared rotational atherectomy ($n = 152$) with balloon angioplasty ($n = 146$) in patients with diffuse in-stent restenosis. They found that rotational atherectomy did not reduce the risk of recurrent in-stent restenosis, and, unexpectedly, in fact a better long-term clinical and angiographic outcome was obtained in the balloon arm. The restenosis rate (65% versus 51%, $p = 0.039$) was higher and the event-free survival rate (79.6% versus 91.1%; $p = 0.005$) poorer in the rotational atherectomy group.[31] Moreover, these investigators reported a higher incidence of vessel spasm and slow flow in the rotational atherectomy group. In an IVUS substudy (involving 86 [29%] of the 298 randomized patients), they further demonstrated that effective debulking was indeed achieved with rotational atherectomy, whereas adjunctive low-pressure balloon inflation (selected to minimize vessel trauma and prevent recurrent neointimal proliferation) failed to enlarge stent cross-sectional area in this group. Conversely, additional stent overexpansion was obtained with the high-pressure dilations performed in the balloon arm. At follow-up, IVUS demonstrated that neointimal tissue growth and final minimal lumen area were similar in both groups.[31] These investigators suggested that higher-pressure inflations in the rotational atherectomy group could lead to larger stent diameters, which, associated with a similar amount of neointimal proliferation, might reduce the restenosis rate. Although this is an attractive speculation, it important to keep in mind the fact that in the ARTIST trial the angiographic late loss was actually larger in the rotational atherectomy group (0.91 ± 0.5 mm versus 0.67 ± 0.5 mm; $p = 0.0019$). Finally, von Dahl et al[31] also suggested that in patients with in-stent restenosis undergoing rotational atherectomy, the systematic use of IVUS and glycoprotein IIb/IIIa inhibitors could be particularly advantageous. Figure 16.11 illustrates the value of IVUS in this setting.

In the smaller, single-center, ROSTER study[79] (a randomized trial of angioplasty versus rotational atherectomy for diffuse in-stent restenosis), patients undergoing rotational atherectomy ($n = 75$) had a more favorable outcome than patients allocated to the balloon arm ($n = 75$): clinical restenosis rates of 20% and 43% ($p < 0.01$), respectively. In this study, baseline IVUS was required by protocol before randomization. This resulted in an exclusion rate (due to major stent subexpansion) of 30% of all screened patients. Again, this information further emphasizes the value of readily identifying cases with severe stent underexpansion when the use of relatively aggressive strategies – such as rotational atherectomy – is contemplated. Other differences from the ARTIST trial included the use of higher pressures in the rotational atherectomy arm and the fact that up to 31% of patients in the balloon arm eventually required additional stenting.[31,79]

Coronary laser

In vitro and in vivo studies have clearly demonstrated that excimer lasers can precisely cut and ablate atheroma without harmful thermal injury to the vessel wall. The rationale behind using laser angioplasty in patients with in-stent restenosis is, once again, trying to improve procedural results by effectively ablating the in-stent tissue. Subsequently, an adjunct balloon angioplasty should be performed to optimize the final result (Figure 16.12). The use of a laser fiber catheter of 2 mm enables more efficient ablation of the in-stent tissue than that obtained with smaller catheters. More recently, the use of a multiple-pass technique and optimally spaced catheters and the advent of the eccentric laser catheter has permitted even greater ablation efficacy. On the other hand, the 'saline flush' technique has also been advocated to clean-up the distal end of the laser fiber from blood and debris, increasing the safety and efficacy of the technique.

Preliminary single-center studies[37] suggested the safety and efficacy of excimer lasers in the treatment of patients with in-stent restenosis. In addition, early IVUS studies[33] demonstrated that tissue ablation contributed to 29%, tissue extrusion to 31%, and additional stent expansion to 16% of the overall lumen gain. Of interest, compared with balloon angioplasty alone, laser plus adjunctive angioplasty achieved better immediate results.[33]

The LARS (Laser Angioplasty of Restenosed Stents) Registry was a large multicenter study (440 patients, 527 stents) designed to evaluate the safety and efficacy of laser angioplasty for restenosed or occluded stents.[34,35] In this registry, the procedural success rate was 91% and better results were obtained with large or eccentric laser catheters. Perforations occurred in 0.9% of patients after laser treatment and in 0.2% after balloon angioplasty.

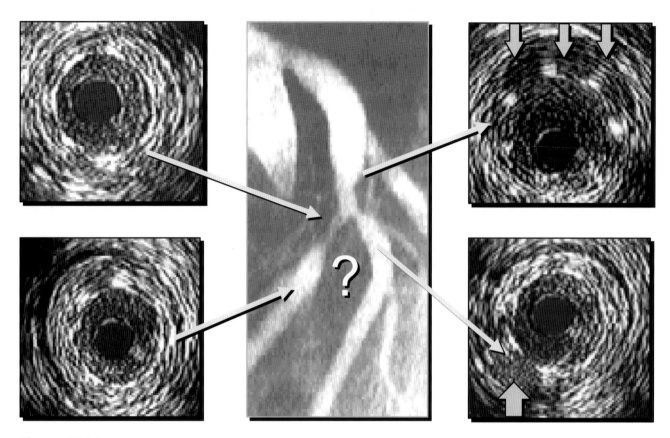

Figure 16.11
Value of intravascular ultrasound (IVUS) in the assessment of in-stent restenosis. In this patient, the exact location of the stent could not be elucidated by angiography alone. IVUS revealed the exact location of the stent with regard to lumen narrowing, the severity of the lesion (top left), that the large diagonal branch was jailed by the stent (bottom right), and malapposition of the most proximal part of the stents (top right).

Cardiac tamponade occurred in 0.5% of cases and stent damage in 0.5%. These results from a multicenter study suggested that laser angioplasty was a safe and effective technique for patients with in-stent restenosis.[34,35] However, this registry provided no data on late angiographic outcome.

In a mechanistic study, Mehran et al[36] compared the ablation efficiency of excimer laser coronary angioplasty with that of rotational atherectomy in patients with diffuse in-stent restenosis. In this study, 158 lesions were treated by laser and 161 by rotational atherectomy. Baseline characteristics were comparable in the two groups. Similar, relatively high pressures and balloon-to-artery ratio were subsequently used during adjunct balloon angioplasty in both groups. Eventually, similar final angiographic results were obtained with the two strategies. Laser treatment, however, resulted in a lower reduction of intimal hyperplasia volume than rotational atherectomy (19 mm^3 versus 43 mm^3; $p < 0.001$), as demonstrated by serial IVUS studies. Ablation efficiency (lumen volume post ablation/device volume) was 77% after laser and 90% after rotational atherectomy. The tissue-ablation capability of the technique is thus limited. Nevertheless, adjunct balloon angioplasty was responsible for over 50% of lumen gain in both

groups, and the final lumen dimensions were equal. In addition, the long-term clinical outcome was similar in the two populations, with a 1-year target vessel revascularization rate of 26% and 28%, respectively. The authors concluded that, despite certain differences in mechanisms of lumen enlargement, both techniques can be used to treat patients with diffuse in-stent restenosis, with similar clinical results.[36]

Other more recent studies, however, have yielded poorer results. Köster et al[37] successfully used an excimer laser in 96 consecutive patients with in-stent restenosis. Follow-up angiography (available in 93% of patients) revealed a restenosis rate of 65% (54% of patients with residual stenosis greater than 50% and an additional 11% of total occlusions). These investigators suggested that this technique was unlikely to reduce recurrent restenosis in this scenario and that other approaches were necessary. Along the same lines, Hamburger et al[38] reported systematic follow-up in 16 patients with very diffuse (mean lesion length 32 mm) in-stent restenosis treated with excimer laser. Despite adjunct high-pressure balloon angioplasty, the minimal lumen diameter after the procedure remained smaller than that after initial stent implantation. After 6 months of follow-up, there was recurrence of angina in all

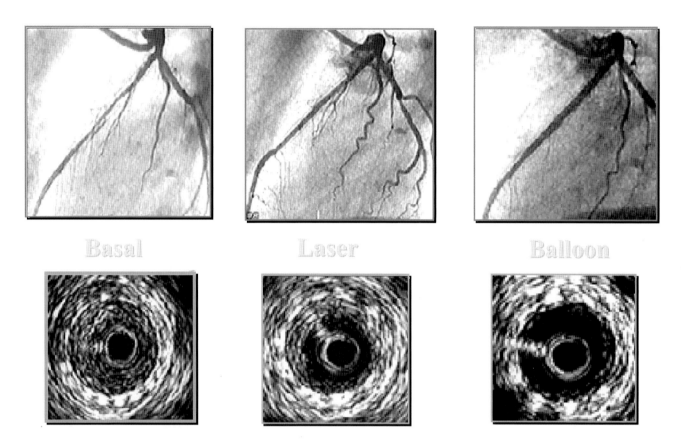

Figure 16.12
Excimer laser for in-stent restenosis. Angiographic and intravascular ultrasound (IVUS) findings. Left top: Diffuse in-stent restenosis on the left anterior descending coronary artery. Left bottom: IVUS revealing the characteristic appearance of neointimal hyperplasia (soft material) obstructing the stent and causing wedging of the imaging catheter. Middle: Angiographic and IVUS results after laser treatment. Right: Final result after adjunctive balloon dilation. Despite a beautiful angiographic and IVUS result, this patient subsequently developed once again recurrent diffuse in-stent restenosis.

patients, six presented with occluded vessels, and six additional patients had non-occlusive restenosis. Due to this adverse long-term clinical and angiographic outcome, it was concluded that excimer laser plus adjunct angioplasty should not be recommended for patients with diffuse in-stent restenosis of long-stented segments.

Cutting balloon

This device is potentially able to reduce vessel wall stretch and resultant injury by inducing controlled disruption of the atheromatous material. The atherotomes (blades) provide a controlled fault-line to ensure uniform dilation. Then, a low-pressure inflation will (theoretically) decrease the risk of a severe neoproliferative response. Although initial studies suggested that the optimal strategy with this device was just to perform one or two low-pressure inflations, some investigators are currently using higher pressures to improve procedural results. The blades of the device help to provide longitudinal cuts into the tissue obstructing the stent, which in turn could facilitate the

extrusion of the neointima during maximal balloon inflation. Another unique characteristic of the cutting balloon is the avoidance of the 'watermelon-seed' phenomenon. As described above, this technical problem may be associated with suboptimal procedural results after conventional balloon, which may be translated into an untoward clinical course.[72] The blades (three or four) of the cutting balloon not only are potentially helpful to excise in-stent neointimal hyperplasia in a more controlled fashion, but also can 'anchor' the device at the target site during inflation, preventing balloon slippage and vessel trauma out of the region of interest.[39–43] This explains why this technique is highly appreciated by physicians involved in brachytherapy procedures, since it can avoid the 'geographic miss' phenomenon and the subsequent appearance of late 'edge restenosis'.

In a large matched comparison of cutting balloon, conventional balloon, rotational atherectomy, and additional stent implantation in 258 patients with in-stent restenosis, Adamian et al[41] confirmed the usefulness of the cutting balloon in this setting. Among these different procedures, acute luminal gain was higher after stenting, but, interestingly, late lumen loss and the restenosis rate were lower in the cutting balloon group. Moreover, on multivariate analysis, the use of a cutting balloon (odds ratio (OR) 0.17) and a diffuse restenosis pattern (OR 2.1) were identified as independent predictors of target vessel revascularization at follow-up.

Since the length of the cutting balloon is limited to 10–15 mm, it would appear that the device is not well suited to the management of long lesions. However, many investigators have used a stepwise approach in order to treat diffuse lesions. Braun et al[39] compared cutting balloon with rotational atherectomy in the treatment of patients with 'diffuse' in-stent restenosis (51 patients treated with rotational atherectomy and 76 with cutting balloon). Demographics and clinical and angiographic data were comparable in the two groups. At follow-up, the restenosis rate (27% versus 63%; $p < 0.01$) and the need for target vessel revascularization (43% versus 19%; $p < 0.05$) were significantly lower in the group treated with a cutting balloon.

IVUS has been used to determine the mechanisms of lumen enlargement after use of a cutting balloon in patients with in-stent restenosis. However, the results have been controversial. In a preliminary study, Ahmed et al[42] analyzed 10 patients treated with this technique and suggested that the mechanism of lumen dilation may differ from that of conventional balloon angioplasty, since most of the lumen enlargement is intimal hyperplasia extrusion, with very little additional stent expansion. Axial redistribution of neointimal hyperplasia also contributed to lumen gain, but to a lesser extent. These authors speculated that the microsurgical incisions of the device would facilitate tissue extrusion. However, as they acknowledged, another potential explanation was that they used relatively low inflation pressures (maximum 10 atmospheres). In the study by Schiele et al,[43] 39 patients treated with a cutting balloon were compared with 19 undergoing balloon angioplasty. In this study, most of the acute lumen gain with both techniques was the result of additional stent expansion (72% in the cutting balloon group and 66% in the conventional balloon group). In addition, the qualitative characteristics of the retained plaque were similar in both groups. The decrease in neointimal tissue (compression and longitudinal redistribution) played a minor role.

Finally, the potential advantages of the cutting balloon, suggested by many observational single-center studies and also some pilot randomized studies, stimulated the design of a larger controlled study. The RESCUT trial (Restenosis Cutting Balloon Evaluation) was a randomized comparison (including 428 patients from 23 European sites) of traditional balloon angioplasty with the cutting balloon in patients with in-stent restenosis. In this study, hospital complications (1.4% versus 2.8%; $p = 0.5$), restenosis rate (31.3% versus 29.3%; $p = 0.82$), and event-free survival rate (82% versus 81%; $p = NS$) were similar in the balloon and cutting balloon groups, respectively. However, the number of balloons used (more than one balloon: 18% versus 25%; $p < 0.05$) and the incidence of the 'water-

melon-seeding' phenomenon (balloon slippage: 6.5% versus 25.1%; $p < 0.01$) were lower in the cutting balloon group. In addition, a similar – but not significant – trend to a lower incidence of type $\geq$ D dissections and stent requirements were seen in this group.

Complications secondary to the use of the cutting balloon in patients with in-stent restenosis are exceedingly rare. However, occasional reports have described the possibility of entrapment of the cutting balloon because of blade fracture[45] and even the occurrence of stent avulsion during withdrawal of the deflated balloon catheter.[44]

Stenting the stent

Stenting the stent was initially reserved for patients with suboptimal results or complications after the failure of another primary strategy in patients with in-stent restenosis.[46–50] However, it soon became clear that, even in these patients (probably the worst-case scenario) restenting could achieve an excellent angiographic result in most cases (Figure 16.13). In fact, several reports suggested that, despite this negative patient selection bias, repeat stenting was the only technique able to provide acute results similar to or approaching those initially obtained during the original stent implantation.[46–50] In addition, stenting the stent is readily performed with a straightforward technique that basically is quite similar to stenting in 'de novo' lesions. Accordingly, all cardiac catheterization laborartories worldwide, even those with limited experience with complex techniques, can use this strategy. Conventional stents provided the best results, whereas covered stents appeared to be associated with a higher risk of recurrences.[53] Early reports, however, suggested that both clinical and angiographic restenosis rates were significant after 'non-elective' restenting, but it was difficult to deny that the selection of adverse cases may indeed have played a role in these results.

To evaluate the potential role of a second stent implantation in patients with in-stent restenosis, 65 patients from four Spanish centers were enrolled in a pilot study.[50] Restenting was 'elective' in 42 patients, whereas in the remaining 23, stents were implated 'non-electively' following complications or suboptimal results after the use of another strategy. Two-thirds of the patients presented with diffuse in-stent restenosis. The angiographic success rate was 100%. During a mean clinical follow-up of 17 months, only 14% of patients required target vessel revascularization. The event-free survival rate was 84% and patients with (a) unstable symptoms, (b) a short time to restenosis, (c) 'non-elective' stenting, and (d) B2-C lesions were associated with a poorer clinical outcome. Recurrent restenosis was demonstrated in 30% of patients, and time to restenosis and restenosis length emerged as the only independent predictors of recurrent restenosis.

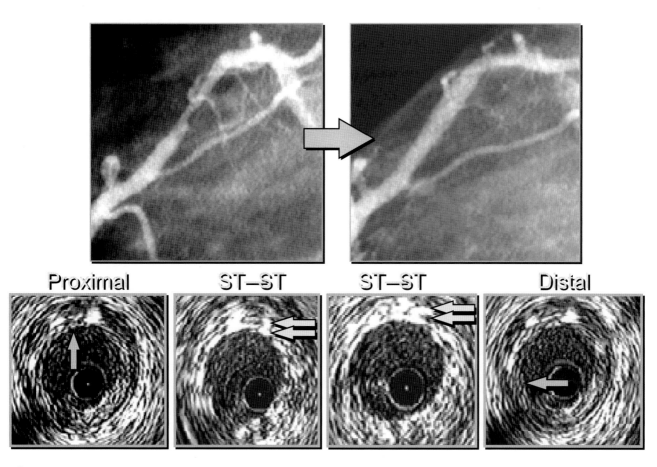

Figure 16.13
Diffuse in-stent restenosis in the right coronary artery. Repeat stenting was able to readily ensure optimal angiographic results in this patient. In this particular case, the restenosis involved most of the previous stent, but not its entire length. Restenting was aimed at treating the narrowing (the lesion). Intravascular ultrasound was able to visualize the in-stent restenosis, and then the two layers of bare metal at the target site (ST–ST) (double arrow). Residual mild intimal thickening of the previous stent is also visualized (single arrow).

Stents not only are able to guarantee an excellent immediate result in these patients but may also confer additional mechanistic advantages. As described at the beginning of this chapter, an important problem during treatment of in-stent restenosis is that some tissue reintrusion back into the stent may occur shortly after treatment.[74] Preliminary data suggested that this early lumen loss phenomenon could be prevented by repeat stenting.[80] In a prospective and randomized study[81] dedicated to studying this phenomenon in patients with in-stent restenosis (20 patients allocated to balloon angioplasty and 20 patients allocated to restenting), we found that early lumen loss is significant after balloon angioplasty (after a mean delay time interval of 45 minutes). This finding can be detected both by IVUS and by quantitative angiography. Repeat stenting can abolish this early lumen loss phenomenon.[81]

Finally, to properly compare elective restenting with balloon angioplasty, we designed the RIBS trial (Restenosis Intra-stent: Balloon angioplasty versus elective Stenting). In this study,[54] 450 patients with in-stent restenosis (24 sites from Spain and Portugal) were randomized to either con-

ventional balloon angioplasty ($n = 226$) or repeat stenting ($n = 224$). All patients had angina or objective evidence of myocardial ischemia and lesions amenable to both interventional strategies. Altogether, there was a lower number of major in-hospital complications in the stent group (relative risk 0.27; 95% confidence interval 0.07–0.97). Furthermore, after the procedure, angiographic results were significantly better in the stent group. Patients in the stent group had a larger final minimal lumen diameter and a greater acute gain, compared with those in the balloon group. The restenosis rate per segment analysis (the primary study endpoint) was similar in the two groups: 38% in the stent group and 39% in the balloon group. Of interest, a major interaction was found between vessel size and treatment effect. In patients with large vessels (reference diameter >3 mm), the binary restenosis rate was significantly reduced after stenting (27% versus 49%; $p = 0.007$). In clinical terms, four patients with in-stent restenosis in large vessels would need to be treated by repeat stenting to prevent one episode of recurrent restenosis. Moreover, long-term clinical follow-up results were also improved with repeat stenting in these patients. Conversely, in patients with small vessels, the restenosis rate was higher in the stent group, and therefore restenting probably should be avoided in such patients.[54] Another important subgroup of patients identified in the RIBS trial comprised those with edge restenosis[82] (i.e. restenosis affecting the stent margin and extending to some extent to the unstented adjacent vessel). In these patients, restenting also reduced the restenosis rate and improved the long-term clinical outcome as compared with balloon angioplasty.[82]

On the other hand, an important subgroup of patients among whom restenting appears to be harmful comprises those receiving brachytherapy procedures.[58] Accordingly, every effort should be made to avoid restenting in this situation, because delayed endothelization and/or positive vessel remodeling may trigger late stent thrombosis. In fact, many late thromboses after brachytherapy (frequently presenting as myocardial infactions during follow-up) appear to be associated either with restenting during the procedure or with clopidogrel withdrawal.[58]

Finally, the use of drug-eluting stents in patients with in-stent restenosis has generated a great deal of enthusiasm. Since these stents effectively inhibit neointimal proliferation, they are especially attractive for patients presenting with in-stent restenosis.[83–90] All the advantages of repeat stenting in this setting will be preserved – but hopefully without the limitations of the technique (excessive neointimal proliferation). Although this strategy is highly appealing, it should be kept in mind that the results of drug-eluting stents in patients with in-stent restenosis do not appear to be as good as those reported in de novo lesions.[87–90] In fact – at least with one type of drug-eluting stent that used a particular polymer – high rates of late clinical and angiographic recurrences have been reported.[87] In addition, other studies suggest the need for caution when multiple overlapping drug-eluting stents are implanted, when drug-eluting stents are associated with bare-metal stents, and also when stent coverage of the restenotic lesions is not perfect.[89] All this emerging information emphasizes the need to prospectively evaluate the results of drug-eluting stents in a large trial focused on patients with in-stent restenosis, which is currently ongoing (RIBS-II).

Conclusions

In-stent restenosis represents a technical and clinical challenge. Only patients with severe restenosis with either angina or evidence of ischemia should be considered for repeated interventions. Most patients with a 'focal' pattern of in-stent restenosis have good long-term clinical and angiographic outcome after a new percutaneous intervention. Conventional balloon angioplasty is usually selected in these patients. The use of debulking techniques, although very attractive from a mechanical point of view, has not

resulted in better results than conventional angioplasty. Therefore, if they are used, they should be reserved for selected patients with diffuse in-stent restenosis and only in institutions with wide experience with the technique, optimizing the procedure with relatively aggressive balloon angioplasty. Cutting balloon angioplasty appears to be particularly advantageous to prevent the 'watermelon-seeding' phenomenon, and accordingly is an attractive technique for patients undergoing intracoronary brachytherapy. Repeat stenting is able to guarantee excellent angiographic results after the procedure, and should be used whenever suboptimal results or significant residual dissections are produced with other techniques. Elective restenting appears to provide superior long-term results to conventional balloon angioplasty in patients with large vessels and also in patients with edge in-stent restenosis. Repeat stenting, however, should probably be used with great caution in small vessels or during intracoronary irradiation procedures. The potential use of drug-eluting stents in this setting is very attractive, but warrants definitive confirmation. Currently, brachytherapy remains the cornerstone of therapy for patients with diffuse in-stent restenosis (where, to date, all the available mechanical strategies have systematically failed) to ensure a satisfactory long-term outcome.

References

1. Serruys PW, De Jaegere P, Kiemeneij F, et al. A comparison of balloon-expandable-stent implantation with balloon angioplasty in patients with coronary artery disease. N Engl J Med 1994;331:489–95.
2. Fischman DL, Leon MB, Baim DS, et al. A randomized comparison of coronary-stent placement and balloon angioplasty in the treatment of coronary artery disease. N Engl J Med 1994;331:496–501.
3. Rankin JM, Spinelli JJ, Carere RG, et al. Improved clinical outcome after widespread use of coronary stenting in Canada. N Engl J Med 1999;341:1957–65.
4. Mintz GS, Popma JJ, Pichard AD, et al. Arterial remodeling after coronary angioplasty: a serial intravascular ultrasound study. Circulation 1996;94:35–43.
5. Hoffman R, Mintz GS, Dusaillant GR, et al. Patterns and mechanisms of in-stent restenosis. A serial intravascular ultrasound study. Circulation 1996;94:1247–54.
6. Leon MB, Teirstein PS, Moses JW, et al. Localized intracoronary gamma-radiation therapy to inhibit the recurrence of restenosis after stenting. N Engl J Med 2001;344:250–6.
7. Baim DS, Levine MJ, Leon MB, et al. Management of restenosis within the Palmaz–Schatz coronary stent (the U.S. multicenter experience). Am J Cardiol 1993;71:364–66.
8. Eltchaninoff H, Koning R, Tron Ch, et al. Balloon angioplasty for the treatment of coronary in-stent restenosis: immediate results and 6-months angiographic recurrent restenosis rate. J Am Coll Cardiol 1998;32:980–4.
9. Bauters C, Banos JL, Van Belle E, et al. Six-month angiographic outcome after successful repeat percutaneous

intervention for in-stent restenosis. Circulation 1998; 97:318–21.

10. Alfonso F, Pérez-Vizcayno MJ, Hernandez R, et al. Long-term outcome and determinants of event-free survival in patients treated with balloon angioplasty for in-stent restenosis. Am J Cardiol 1999;83:1268–70.

11. Bossi I, Klersy C, Black AJ, et al. In-stent restenosis: long-term outcome and predictors of subsequent target lesion revascularization after repeat balloon angioplasty. J Am Coll Cardiol 2000;35:1569–76.

12. Klughertz BD, Meneveau NF, Kolansky DM, et al. Predictors of clinical outcome following percutaneous intervention for in-stent restenosis. Am J Cardiol 2000;85;1427–31.

13. Reimers B, Moussa I, Akiyama T, et al. Long-term clinical follow-up after successful repeat percutaneous intervention for in-stent restenosis. J Am Coll Cardiol 1997;30:186–92.

14. Macander PJ, Roubin GS, Agrawal SK, et al. Balloon angioplasty for treatment of in-stent restenosis: feasibility, safety and efficacy. Cathet Cardiovasc Diagn 1994;32:125–31.

15. Gordon PC, Gibson CM, Cohen DJ, et al. Mechanisms of restenosis and redilation within coronary stents – quantitative angiographic assessment. J Am Coll Cardiol 1993;21:1166–74.

16. Carroza JP. In-stent restenosis: Should an old device treat a new problem? J Am Coll Cardiol 2000;35:1577–9.

17. Sakamoto T, Kawarabayashi T, Taguchi H, et al. Intravascular ultrasound-guided balloon angioplasty for treatment of in-stent restenosis. Cathet Cardiovasc Interv 1999;47: 298–303.

18. Schiele F, Meneveau N, Seronde M, et al. Predictors of event-free survival after repeat intracoronary procedure for in-stent restenosis. Study with angiography and intravascular ultrasound imaging. Eur Heart J 2000;21:754–62.

19. Schiele F, Vuillemenot A, Meneveau N, et al. Effects of increasing balloon pressure on mechanism and results of balloon angioplasty for treatment of restenosis after Palmatz–Schatz stent implantation: an angiographic and intravascular ultrasound study. Cathet Cardiovasc Interv 1999;46:314–21.

20. Mehran R, Mintz GS, Popma JJ, et al. Mechanisms and results of balloon angioplasty for the treatment of in-stent restenosis. Am J Cardiol 1996;78:618–22.

21. Mintz GS, Hoffmann R, Mehran R, et al. In-stent restenosis: the Washington Hospital Center experience. Am J Cardiol 1998;81(7A):7E–13E.

22. Mahdi NA, Pathan AZ, Harrell L, et al. Directional coronary atherectomy for the treatment of Palmaz–Schatz in-stent restenosis. Am J Cardiol 1998;82;1345–51.

23. Palacios IF, Sanchez PL, Mahdi NA. The place of directional coronary atherectomy for the treatment of in-stent restenosis. Semin Interv Cardiol 2000;5:209–16.

24. O'Brien ER, Glover C, Labinaz M. Acute outcome with the Flexicut directional coronary atherectomy catheter for the treatment of coronary in-stent restenosis. J Invasive Cardiol 2001;13:618–22.

25. Lins M, Fu GH, el-Mokhtari N, et al. Pull-back atherectomy. An alternative procedure in the treatment of coronary stenoisis and in-stent restenosis. Z Kardiol 2002;91:40–8.

26. von Dahl J, Radke PW, Haager PK, et al. Clinical and angiographic predictors of in-stent restenosis after percutaneous transluminal rotational atherectomy for treatment of diffuse in-stent restenosis. Am J Cardiol 1999;83:862–7.

27. Dauerman HL, Baim DS, Cutlip DE, et al. Mechanical debulking versus balloon angioplasty for the treatment of diffuse in-stent restenosis. Am J Cardiol 1998;82:277–84.

28. Lee SG, Lee CW, Cheong SS, et al. Immediate and long-term outcomes of rotational atherectomy versus balloon angioplasty alone for treatment of diffuse in-stent restenosis. Am J Cardiol 1998;82:140–3.

29. Radke W, Klues HG, Haager PK, et al. Mechanisms of acute lumen gain and recurrent restenosis after rotational atherectomy of diffuse in-stent restenosis. J Am Coll Cardiol 1999;34:33–9.

30. Sharma SK, Duvuri S, Dangas G, et al. Rotational atherectomy for in-stent restenosis: acute and long-term results of the first 100 cases. J Am Coll Cardiol 1998;32:1358–65.

31. von Dahl J, Dietz U, Haager PK, et al. Rotational atherectomy does not reduce recurrent in-stent restenosis. Results of the Angioplasty versus Rotational atherectomy for Treatment of diffuse In-Stent restenosis Trial (ARTIST). Circulation 2002;105:583–8.

32. Cho GY, Lee CW, Hong MK, et al. Side-branch occlusion after rotational atherectomy of in-stent restenosis: incidence predictors and clinical significance. Cathet Cardiovasc Interv 2000;50:406–10.

33. Mehran R, Mintz GS, Satler LF, et al. Treatment of in-stent restenosis with excimer laser coronary angioplasty: mechanisms and results compared with PTCA. Circulation 1997;96:2183–9.

34. Giri S, Lansky AJ, Mehran R, et al. Clinical and angiographic outcome in the Laser Angioplasty for Restenostic Stents (LARS) multicenter registry. Cathet Cardiovasc Interv 2001;52:24–34.

35. Köster R, Hamm CW, Seabra-Gomes R, et al. Laser angioplasty of restenosed coronary stents: results of a surveillance trial. The Laser Angioplasty of Restenosed Stent Investigators. J Am Coll Cardiol 1999;34:25–32.

36. Mehran R, Dangas G, Mintz GS, et al. Treatment of in-stent restenosis with excimer laser coronary angioplasty versus rotational atherectomy: comparative mechanisms and results. Circulation 2000;101:2484–9.

37. Köster R, Kalher J, Terres W, et al. Six-month clinical and angiographic outcome after successful excimer laser angioplasty for in-stent restenosis. J Am Coll Cardiol 2000;36:69–74.

38. Hamburger JN, Foley DP, de Feyter PJ, et al. Six-month outcome after excimer laser coronary angioplasty for diffuse in-stent restenosis in native coronary arteries. Am J Cardiol 2000;86:390–4.

39. Braun P, Stroh E, Heinrich KW. Rotablator versus cutting balloon for the treatment of long stent restenosis. J Invasive Cardiol 2002;14:291–6.

40. Albiero R, Nishida T, Karvoini E, et al. Cutting balloon angioplasty for treatment of in-stent restenosis. Cathet Cardiovasc Interv 2000;50:452–9.

41. Adamian M, Colombo A, Briguori C, et al. Cutting balloon angioplasty for the treatment of in-stent restenosis: a matched comparison with rotational atherectomy, additional stent implantation and balloon angioplasty. J Am Coll Cardiol 2001;38:672–9.

42. Ahmed JM, Mintz GS, Castagna M, et al. Intravascular ultrasound assessment of the mechanism of lumen enlargement during cutting balloon angioplasty treatment of in-stent restenosis. Am J Cardiol 2001;88:1032–4.

43. Schiele TM, Koning A, Reiber J, et al. Comparison of volumetric ultrasound analysis of acute results and underlying mechanism from cutting balloon and conventional balloon angioplasty for the treatment of coronary in-stent restenotic lesions. Am J Cardiol 2002;90:539–42.

44. Wang HJ, Kao HL, Liau CS, Lee YT. Coronary stent strut avulsion in aorto-ostial in-stent restenosis. A potential complication after cutting balloon angioplasty. Cathet Cardiovasc Interv 2002;56:215–19.

45. Kawamura A, Asakura Y, Ishikawa S, et al. Extraction of previously deployed stent by an entrapped cutting balloon due to blade fracture. Cathet Cardiovasc Interv 2002;57:239–43.

46. Moris C, Alfonso F, Lambert JL, et al. Stenting for coronary dissection after balloon dilation of in-stent restenosis: stenting a previously stented site. Am Heart J 1996;131:834–6.

47. Elezi S, Kastrati A, Hadamitzky M, et al. Clinical and angiographic follow-up after balloon angioplasty with provisional stenting for coronary in-stent restenosis. Cathet Cardiovasc Interv 1999;48:151–6.

48. Alsergani HS, Ho PC, Nesto RW, et al. Stenting for in-stent restenosis: a long-term clinical follow-up. Cathet Cardiovasc Interv 1999;48:143–8.

49. Antoniucci D, Valenti R, Moschi G, et al. Stenting fort in-stent restenosis. Cathet Cardiovasc Interv 2000;49:376–81.

50. Alfonso F, Cequier A, Zueco J, et al. Stenting the stent: initial results and long-term clinical and angiographic outcome of coronary stenting for patients with in-stent restenosis. Am J Cardiol 2000;85:327–32.

51. Mehran R, Dangas G, Abizaid A, et al. Treatment of focal in-stent restenosis with balloon angioplasty alone versus stenting. Short- and long-term results. Am Heart J 2001;14:610–14.

52. Morino Y, Limpijankit T, Honda Y, et al. Late vascular response to repeat stenting for in-stent restenosis with and without radiation. An intravascular ultrasound volumetric analysis. Circulation 2002;105:2465–8.

53. Elsner M, Auch-Schwelk W, Briten M, et al. Coronary stent grafts covered by a polytetrafluoroethylene membrane. Am J Cardiol 1999;84:335–8.

54. Zueco J, Mainar V, Tascón J, et al. Predictors of event-free survival in patients treated for in-stent restenosis. Insight from the RIBS randomized study. Circulation 2002;106(Suppl):II-482.

55. Teirstein PS, Massullo V, Jani S, et al. A double-blinded randomized trial of catheter based radiotherapy to inhibit restenosis after coronary stenting. N Engl J Med 1997;336:1697–703.

56. King SB III, Williams DO, Chougule P, et al. Endovascular beta-radiation to reduce restenosis after coronary balloon angioplasty: results of the Beta Energy Restenosis Trial (BERT). Circulation 1998;97:2025–30.

57. Waksman R, White RL, Chan RC, et al. Intracoronary gamma-radiation therapy after angioplasty inhibits recurrence in patients with in-stent restenosis. Circulation 2000;101:2165–71.

58. Waksman R, Bhargava B, Mintz GS, et al. Late total occlusion after intracoronary brachytherapy for patients with in-stent restenosis. J Am Coll Cardiol 2000;36:65–8.

59. Kozuma K, Costa MA, Sabate M, et al. Late stent malapposition occurring after coronary beta irradiation detected by intravascular ultrasound. J Invasive Cardiol 1999;11:651–5.

60. Sabaté M, Costa MA, Kozuma K, et al. Geographic miss: a cause of treatment failure in radio-oncology applied to intracoronary radiation therapy. Circulation 2000;101:2467–71.

61. Sabate M. Current status of intracoronary brachytherapy. Rev Esp Cardiol 2001;54:1197–209.

62. Mehran R, Dangas G, Abizaid AS, et al. Angiographic patterns of in-stent restenosis. Classifications and implications for long-term outcome. Circulation 1999;100:1872–8.

63. Moreno PR, Palacios IF, Leon MN, et al. Histopathologic comparison of human coronary in-stent and post-balloon angioplasty restenotic tissue. Am J Cardiol 1999;84:462–6.

64. Glover C, Ma X, Chen YZ, et al. Human in-stent restenosis tissue obtained by means of coronary atherectomy consists of abundant proteoglycan matrix with a paucity of cell proliferation. Am Heart J 2002;144:702–9.

65. Virmani R, Farb A. Pathology of in-stent restenosis. Curr Opin Lipidol 1999;10:499–506.

66. Castagna NG, Mintz GS, Weissman NJ, et al. The contribution of 'mechanical' problems to in-stent restenosis: an intravascular ultrasonographic analysis of 1090 consecutive in-stent restenosis lesions. Am Heart J 2001;142:970–4.

67. Lowe HC, Oesterle SN, Khachigian LM. Coronary in-stent restenosis: current status and future strategies. J Am Coll Cardiol 2002;39:183–93.

68. Kimura T, Yokoi H, Nakagawa Y, et al. Three-year follow-up after implantation of metallic coronary-artery stents. N Engl J Med 1996;334:561–6.

69. Lee JH, Lee CW, Park SW, et al. Long-term follow-up after deferring angioplasty in asymptomatic patients with moderate non-critical in-stent restenosis. Clin Cardiol 2001;24:551–55.

70. Mukherjee D, Reginelli JP, Moliterno DJ, et al. Unexpected mortality reduction with abciximab for in-stent restenosis. J Invasive Cardiol 2000;12:545–6.

71. Moustapha A, Assali AR, Sdringola S, et al. Abciximab administration and clinical outcomes after percutaneous intervention for in-stent restenosis. Cathet Cardiovasc Interv 2002;56:184–7.

72. Gómez-Recio M, Calvo I, Bullones JA, et al. Implications of the watermelon seeding phenomenon during treatment of patients with in-stent restenosis. Am J Cardiol 2002;90(Suppl 6A):83H.

73. Alfonso F, Hernández C, Pérez-Vizcayno MJ, et al. Fate of stent-related side-branches after coronary interventions in patients with in-stent restenosis. J Am Coll Cardiol 2000;36:1549–56.

74. Shiran A, Mintz GS, Waksman R, et al. Early lumen loss after treatment of in-stent restenosis. An intravascular ultrasound study. Circulation 1998;98:200–3.

75. Moussa I, Moses J, Di Mario C, et al. Stenting after Optimal Debulking (SOLD) Registry. Angiographic and clinical outcome. Circulation 1998;98:1604–9.

76. Prati F, Di Mario C, Moussa I, et al. In-stent neointimal proliferation correlates with the amount of residual plaque burden outside the setnt. An intravascular ultrasound study. Circulation 1999;1011–14.

77. Alfonso F. Residual plaque burden after stenting. Does it matter? Am J Cardiol 2002;90:910.

78. Alfonso F, García P, Pimentel G, et al. Predictors and implications of residual plaque burden after coronary stenting: an intravascular ultrasound study. Am Heart J 2003;145:254–61.

79. Sharma SK, Annapoorna SK, King T, et al. Multivariate predictors of target lesion revascularization in the randomized trial of PTCA vs Rotablator for diffuse in-stent restenosis (ROSTER). J Am Coll Cardiol 2001;37:55A.

80. Malhotra S, Sweeny J, Anderson J, et al. Early lumen loss after repeat coronary intervention for in-stent restenosis. Cathet Cardiovasc Interv 2001;52:35–8.

81. Alfonso F, García P, Fleites H, et al. Early lumen loss after coronary interventions for in-stent restenosis. A randomized comparison of repeat stenting and balloon angioplasty. Circulation 2002;106:II-390.

82. Angel J, Moris C, Zueco J, et al. Therapeutic implications of in-stent restenosis located at the stent edge. Circulation 2002;106:II-481.

83. Sousa JE, Costa MA, Abizaid A, et al. Lack of neointimal proliferation after implantation of a sirolimus-coated stents in human coronary arteries: a quantitative coronary angiography and three-dimensional intravascular ultrasound study. Circulation 2001;103:192–5.

84. Rensing BJ, Vos J, Smits PC, et al. Coronary restenosis elimination with a sirolimus eluting stent. European human experience with 6-month angiographic and intravascular ultrasonic follow-up. Eur Heart J 2001;22:2125–30.

85. Degertekin M, Serruys PW, Foley DP, et al. Persistent inhibition of neointimal hyperplasia after sirolimus-eluting stent implantation. Long-term (up to two years) clinical angiographic and intravascular ultrasound follow-up. Circulation 2002;106;1610–13.

86. Tanabe K, Serruys PW, Degertekin M, et al. Fate of side branches after coronary arterial sirolimus eluting stent implantation. Am J Cardiol 2002;90:937–41.

87. Moses A, Leon MB, Popma J, et al. A multicenter randomized clinical study of the sirolimus eluting stent in native coronary lesions: clinical outcomes. Circulation 2002;106: II-392.

88. Liistro F, Stankovic G, Di Mario C, et al. First clinical experience with a paclitaxel derivate-eluting polymer stent system implantation for in-stent restenosis. Immediate and long-term clinical and angiographic outcome. Circulation 2002;105:1883–6.

89. Tanabe K, Degertekin M, de Feyter P, et al. Paclitaxel-eluting stent for the treatment of in-stent restenosis: TAXUS III trial. Circulation 2002;106:II-355.

90. Sousa JE, Abizaid A, Costa MA, et al. Late (1-year) follow-up after sirolimus-eluting stent implantation to treat in-stent restenosis. Circulation 2002;106:II-393.

17

Restenosis and brachytherapy

I Patrick Kay, Mand Sabaté

Introduction

Intracoronary radiation therapy has been developed in an attempt to decrease restenosis after balloon angioplasty and stent implantation. Two parallel techniques – one employing catheter-based radiation (using either β- or γ-emitters), the other using radioactive stents – have been the subject of both animal and human studies. In vivo intravascular ultrasound (IVUS) imaging studies have helped us to determine the effect of brachytherapy on the vessel wall. This chapter is aimed at reviewing the potential and limitations of this technique, summarizing the results of the currently reported clinical trials.

Percutaneous transluminal coronary angioplasty (PTCA) is an accepted treatment for coronary artery disease. However, angiographic restenosis is reported in 40–60% of patients after a successful PTCA.[1,2] Mechanisms involved in the restenosis process are elastic recoil of the artery, local thrombus formation, vascular remodeling with shrinkage of the vessel, and an overactive healing process with neointimal hyperplasia.[2–5] Neointimal hyperplasia develops by migration and proliferation of smooth muscle cells and myofibroblasts after balloon-induced trauma of the arterial wall and by deposition of extracellular matrix by smooth muscle cells.[5–7] The introduction of the stent into the arsenal of the interventional cardiologist has reduced the restenosis rate to 15–20%,[8,9] by preventing elastic recoil and negative remodeling.[10] However, the occurrence of restenosis after stent implantation remains unresolved, especially in small vessels and long lesions, where it may exceed 30% of cases.[11] It is primarily caused by neointimal hyperplasia, which occurs due to trauma of the arterial wall by the stent struts. The treatment of in-stent restenosis with conventional techniques (balloon angioplasty or debulking) is rather disappointing, with restenosis rates of 27–63%, which increases with the number of re-interventions.[12–14] Since radiation therapy had proven to be effective in treating the exuberant fibroblastic activity of keloid scar formation and other nonmalignant processes such as ocular pterygia,[15,16] it was assumed that this adjunctive therapy would also inhibit coronary restenosis.

The first experimental study in this field was carried out in 1964 by Friedman et al,[17] with the use of iridium-192 (^{192}Ir) in the cholesterol-fed rabbit. In 1992, in Frankfurt, Liermann et al[18] performed the first four cases of brachytherapy, in patients who had undergone a femoral percutaneous angioplasty. A second wave of experimental work was carried out in the USA by Wiedermann and Weinberger in New York,[19] Waksman and Crocker in Atlanta,[20] and Mazur and Raizner in Houston.[21] In parallel, Verin and Popowski in Geneva[22] conducted experimental studies with the pure β-emitter yttrium-90 (^{90}Y) in carotid and iliac arteries of rabbits. The first clinical experience in coronary arteries in humans was obtained by Condado et al,[23] using a hand-delivered ^{192}Ir wire in a noncentered, closed-end lumen catheter, and by Verin et al,[24] using a β-source and a centered device. Both studies demonstrated that the delivery of radiation in the coronary artery was feasible and safe, although the restenosis rate remained relatively high. The positive results of the first randomized trials, aiming to determine the effectiveness of γ-radiation for the treatment of restenotic lesions,[25] encouraged subsequent studies.

Radiation therapy systems

Radiation therapy can be delivered to the coronary arteries by external radiation or by brachytherapy methods, using either catheter-based systems or radioactive stents.[26] Catheter-based systems employ either β- or γ-emitters, which can deliver the prescribed dose at either a high- or a low-dose rate, manually or automatically. Radioactive stents utilize mainly pure β-emitters at a very low dose rate, although the use of γ-stents (with palladium-103, [103]Pd) has also been investigated. A list of the isotopes most commonly used in clinical practice for vascular brachytherapy is presented in Table 17.1.

Pathophysiology of intracoronary radiation therapy

Target tissue and target cell

Numerous experimental studies demonstrated a significant reduction in the size of the neointima when balloon angioplasty is immediately preceded or followed by intracoronary β- or γ-radiation.[19,22] However, the mechanism by which radiation may prevent restenosis is not completely understood. The potential role of the adventitia in restenosis has been identified.[27] In this regard, cell proliferation and growth factor synthesis appeared to be greater at the level of the adventitia as compared with the medial wall early after angioplasty. These adventitial cells migrated from their position in the adventitia to the media and contributed to the cellular mass in the neointima.[27] Further experiments[28] demonstrated that the number of proliferating adventitial cells was significantly reduced when ionizing radiation (using either a strontium-90 (^{90}Sr)/^{90}Y or a ^{192}Ir source) was delivered. Similarly, the migration of these proliferating cells was also inhibited. In addition, the recruitment of α-actin-positive myofibroblasts in the adventitia 14 days after balloon overstretch injury was reduced, suggesting an inhibition of adventitial fibrosis and subsequently an inhibition of constrictive vascular remodeling.[28] From all the above experimental observations, the target tissue of intracoronary radiation therapy is likely to be the surrounding adventitia. More

controversial is the identification of the target cell within this adventitial layer. A plausible candidate has been proposed in the *unified hypothesis for vascular restenosis*:[29] the dominant cell responsible for restenosis after angioplasty is the same as the cell that initiates the atherosclerotic plaque, namely the monocyte-derived macrophage. These cells appear to be the most radiosensitive family of cells in the arterial wall, and act as a trigger for adventitial fibroblasts to proliferate and migrate, undergoing phenotypic conversion to myofibroblasts.[29]

The vascular effects of brachytherapy: feasibility studies

The routine use of IVUS imaging in the first feasibility trials helped us to define the effect of brachytherapy on vessel structures after balloon angioplasty with or without conventional stent implantation or after radioactive stent implantation.

The effect of intracoronary radiation therapy on vascular remodeling has been clinically demonstrated in the Beta Energy Restenosis Trial (BERT). In this trial, radiation therapy was delivered via a noncentered device (BetaCath system, Novoste Corporation) that used the pure β-emitter ^{90}Sr/^{90}Y with the dose prescribed to 2 mm from the source and randomly assigned to 12, 14, or 16 Gy.[30] In a careful volumetric analysis of the irradiated coronary segment following successful balloon angioplasty, vessel size (i.e. the volume encompassed by the external elastic membrane) increased significantly during the 6-month follow-up. This vessel enlargement (i.e. positive remodeling) accommodated a parallel increase in plaque volume. As a result, the luminal volume remained unchanged at follow-up.[31] This morphologic evolution was not blunted by the implantation of a conventional stent at the site of radiation therapy as observed in a cohort of patients treated by means of a centered system (the Guidant system, Santa Clara, CA) that used the pure β-emitter phosphorus-32 (^{32}P).[32]

Table 17.1 Isotopes most commonly used for intravascular brachytherapy

Isotope	Emission	Maximum energy (MeV)	Average energy (MeV)	Half-life
Iridium-192 (^{192}Ir)	γ	0.6	0.37	74 days
Phosphorus-32 (^{32}P)	β	1.7	0.60	14 days
Strontium-90 (^{90}Sr)	β	0.5	0.20	28 years
Yttrium-90 (^{90}Y)	β	2.3	0.90	64 hours
Rhenium-188 ([188]Re)	β	2.2	0.79	17 hours
Tungsten-188 ([188]W)	β	0.5	0.17	60 days

A distinct pattern of remodeling was observed after radioactive stent implantation.[33] In both low-activity (0.75–1.5 μCi) and high-activity (6–12 μCi) radioactive Isostents, vessel remodeling was unchanged within the boundaries of the stent, and neointimal hyperplasia was inhibited in a dose-dependent manner.[33,34] Differences in activity and dose rate (catheter-based system: high activity–high dose rate; radioactive stent: low activity–low dose rate) may account for this distinct morphologic change in vessel structures between both systems.

The functional effect of brachytherapy on coronary vasomotion was assessed in irradiated coronary segments following successful balloon angioplasty.[35] At 6-month follow-up, endothelium-dependent coronary vasomotion was restored in most of the irradiated segments, in contrast to those treated only with balloon angioplasty and also to those that were not injured and not irradiated. It is important to note that in this cohort, the dose calculated at the level of the luminal surface was rather low (8.2±3 Gy). Thus, the functional effect of a higher dose or of different devices that allow a more homogeneous dose distribution remains to be elucidated. However, these clinical findings were concordant with previous experimental work in which endothelial function after high-dose (20 Gy) γ-radiation was restored at follow-up.[36] A plausible explanation for this protective effect of brachytherapy may be obtained from the experimental model of porcine coronary arteries subjected to balloon overstretch injury and either placebo or radiation.[37] In this model, the expression of enzyme-inducible nitric oxide synthase (iNOS), responsible for NO production, was enhanced, whereas expression of the cytokine transforming growth factor β1 (TGF- β1) was suppressed in the irradiated group. iNOS is potentially responsible for inhibition of neointimal hyperplasia and stimulation of re-endothelialization, whereas TGF-β1 expression would enhance intimal hyperplasia and fibrosis by negatively modulating the expression of iNOS.[37] In contrast to the above findings, an experimental study[38] reported that the combination of transluminal coronary angioplasty and intracoronary radiation therapy reduced the substance P-induced NO-dependent relaxation. Whether this finding, as opposed to previous observations, is a common phenomenon in clinical practice remains to be established.

Potential limitations of intracoronary brachytherapy

Aneurysm formation

Theoretically, the early beneficial effect of intravascular brachytherapy on arterial remodeling could lead to undesired aneurysm formation. The incidence of coronary aneurysm formation (coronary dilatation that exceeded the diameter of normal adjacent segments by a factor of 1.5) after balloon angioplasty or stenting ranges between 3.4% and 5.4% and has not been associated with angiographic restenosis or unfavorable clinical outcomes.[39] The incidence of aneurysm formation after radiation therapy is unknown. Condado et al[23] reported four cases (20%) within 2 months after γ-radiation. A further increase in size was observed in two cases at 6 and 8 months, respectively, and remained unchanged at 2, 3, and 5 years. This undesirable phenomenon was probably related to the high dose received by these coronary segments. Since the prescribed dose was 20–25 Gy to 1.5 mm depth, the actual dose calculated a posteriori ranged between 19 and 55 Gy.[23] In our cohort of patients included in the Rotterdam arm of the BERT-1.5 trial, we observed one case of aneurysm formation within the irradiated segment. Interestingly, this was accompanied by a focal increase in plaque burden, which led to restenosis.[31] Subsegmental analysis of the delivered dose demonstrated a clear inhomogeneity in dose distribution in both regions: the segment that became restenotic received a low dose at the level of the adventitia as compared with that received by the region that was excessively dilated (4.6 Gy versus 8.6 Gy, respectively). The presence of a coronary dissection at the treated site may have precipitated the development of the coronary aneurysm in the context of a relatively high dose.

Late thrombotic occlusion

The occurrence of coronary thrombosis beyond 1 month after conventional angioplasty or stenting under aspirin and ticlopidine or clopidogrel (for 15 days to 1 month) regimens was anecdotal.[40] However, this undesirable phenomenon became apparent in the first series of patients treated with brachytherapy worldwide. In the first 92 patients treated with intracoronary brachytherapy in Rotterdam, we observed a higher-than-expected incidence (6.6%) of thrombotic clinical events 2–15 months after treatment.[41] This finding was subsequently confirmed in the American series of patients treated with γ-radiation. Data pooled from the WRIST, Long-WRIST, SVG-WRIST, GAMMA-1, and BETA-WRIST trials demonstrated an incidence of late thrombotic occlusion of 9.1% as compared with 1.2% in the placebo groups at 5.4±3 months after the procedure.[42,43]

The implantation of a conventional stent within the irradiated segment has been considered a main contributor to this phenomenon. In this regard, considering only the cohort of stented patients, the rate of late thrombosis increased to 8.8% in the Rotterdam series and 14.6% in the American series. The delay in stent re-endothelialization has been considered as a trigger mechanism for this event.[44] In addition, the possibility that brachytherapy may induce late stent malapposition, by causing positive remodeling, has been advocated with regard to this process.[45,46] In patients treated only with balloon angioplasty followed by intracoronary brachytherapy, the presence of unhealed dissections at 6-month follow-up was a common phenomenon.[47] Whether persistent dissection is related to late thrombosis in nonstented patients remains to be elucidated.

This clinical evidence was confirmed in an experimental model.[48] A retrospective analysis of tissue sections from 51 juvenile swine (76 coronary arteries) subjected to overstretch balloon injury followed by irradiation with doses of 0–18 Gy demonstrated a dose-dependent increase in thrombus rate when examined 14 days after treatment. However, this increased thrombus rate appeared to be at the expense of mural thrombus rather than luminal thrombus.

Late stent thrombosis has also been reported after radioactive stent implantation in the Milan Dose–Response Study.[34] This registry included 122 ^{32}P β-emitting stents implanted in 91 lesions in 82 patients. Three levels of stent activity were studied: 0.75–3.0 μCi ($n = 23$), 3.0–6.0 μCi ($n = 29$), and 6.0–12 μCi ($n = 30$). One of the patients from the high-activity group presented with late stent thrombosis at 3-month follow-up, 1 week after stopping both aspirin and ticlopidine. Pathologic studies demonstrated that neointima of high activity (3.0–23 μCi) stents consisted of fibrin, erythrocytes, occasional inflammatory cells, and smooth muscle cells with partial endothelialization of the luminal surface.[49] The correlation of these pathologic findings with long-term clinical follow-up remains to be established.

To overcome this drawback, long-term use (>6 months) of double antiplatelet therapy (aspirin and clopidogrel or ticlopidine) is clearly appropriate when intracoronary radiation therapy is performed.

Edge effect (the 'candy wrapper' effect)

A potential limitation of intracoronary brachytherapy is the development of new stenotic lesions at both edges of the irradiated segments. This so-called edge effect or 'candy wrapper' effect was originally described after high-activity (>3 μCi) radioactive stent implantation[34] (Figure 17.1). However, this phenomenon is not exclusive to radioactive stents but may also affect coronary segments treated by means of catheter-based systems.[31] Vessel wall injury[48,50] concomitant with low-dose radiation at the edge of the irradiated segment[51] may be involved in the pathophysiology of this phenomenon. To integrate both components, we proposed a new concept in interventional cardiology: the *geographic miss*.[52] This concept is translated from a

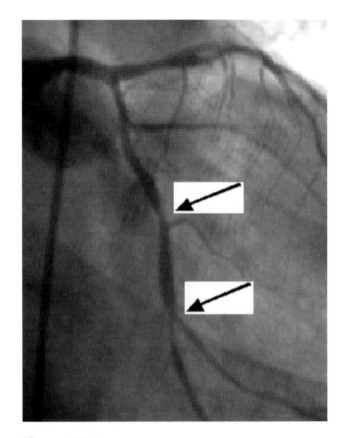

Figure 17.1
The 'candy wrapper' effect. Angiography shows the luminogram 6 months after radioactive stent implantation. Two narrowings, at each edge of the stent, are clearly visible, whereas the stented segment remains without signs of restenosis.

term that in radio-oncology defines a cause of treatment failure due to a low dose. In such cases, a small part of the treatment zone either has escaped radiation or has been inadequately irradiated because the total volume of the tumor was not appreciated and hence an insufficient margin was taken.[53] In interventional cardiology, this phenomenon occurs by injuring the edges of the irradiated segment, where, by definition, the dose received is rather low. In a retrospective analysis[52] of 50 consecutive patients treated with β-radiation after balloon angioplasty or stent, the incidence of this event was 32%. The following reasons were responsible for this phenomenon: (1) development of procedural complications that extended the treatment zone beyond the margins of the irradiated segment; (2) lack of availability of longer radiation sources to cover the treatment zone; and (3) lack of accurate matching between the injured segment and the irradiated region. In those geographic miss edges, a quantitative coronary analysis demonstrated a significantly higher late loss (0.84±0.6) as compared with both the irradiated segment (0.15±0.4) and the uninjured edges (0.09±0.4; $p < 0.0001$). Similarly, binary restenosis was significantly higher in the geographic miss edges (Figure 17.2).

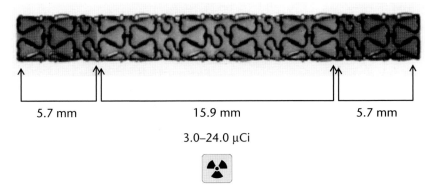

Figure 17.2
Comparison of late loss between irradiated segments, segments of geographic miss, and uninjured segments.

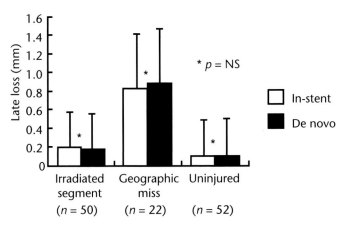

5.7 mm   15.9 mm   5.7 mm

3.0–24.0 μCi

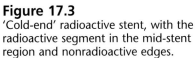

Figure 17.3
'Cold-end' radioactive stent, with the radioactive segment in the mid-stent region and nonradioactive edges.

Conceptually, after radioactive stent implantation, the incidence of geographic miss is 100%, since the length of the balloon used to deliver the stent is always longer than the radioactive stent. Thus, both edges are always injured and receive low-dose radiation. This would explain the fact that in the Milan Dose–Response Study the incidence of restenosis was high, but mostly at the expense of edge restenosis ('candy wrapper') (36% for 1.5–3.0 μCi, 38% for 3.0–6.0 μCi, 39% for 6.0–12 μCi, and 30% for 12–20 μCi stent activities).[34] In addition, the authors identified the final balloon-to-artery ratio as a factor associated with the development of edge restenosis.[34] Volumetric IVUS studies demonstrated that lack of positive remodeling or vessel shrinkage together with plaque increase were the contributors to the lumen shrinkage at both edges of the irradiated segment either after catheter-based brachytherapy[31] or after radioactive stent implantation.[33,34]

To prevent edge restenosis, two strategies were proposed. The first was the use of a 'cold-end' radioactive stent (Figure 17.3). This approach aimed to decrease edge restenosis by preventing remodeling at the injured extremities. The cold-end stents had an activity of 3–12 μCi at implantation. Forty-three stents were implanted in 43 patients with de novo native coronary artery disease. A restenosis rate of 22% was observed, with a shift of restenosis from the stent edges to the area of radiation fall-off within the cold-end stent (Figure 17.4).

'Hot-end' radioactive stents have increased radioactive activity at the stent edges. (Figure 17.5). Theoretically, this activity should decrease the chance of injury occurring without adequate radiation coverage (geographic miss).

In the Milan study, the hot-end stent had a length of 18 mm. The initial radioactivity level was 2.6 μCi/mm in the proximal and distal 2 mm of the stent, and 0.57 μCi/mm in the central 14 mm of the stent. The initial total radioactivity of the stent was approximately 18.5 μCi. From July until November 1999, 53 patients with 56 lesions were treated by implantation of 56 hot-ends ^{32}P radioactive stents. At 6-month angiographic follow-up, performed in 51 patients with 54 lesions (96%), the intralesion binary restenosis rate was 33% (19% at the proximal edge, 7% at the distal edge, and 7% at both edges) (Figure 17.6). Thus, radioactive ^{32}P hot-ends stents did not solve the problem of edge restenosis.

The black hole

A new observation was noted using IVUS at 6-month follow-up[54] mainly after radioactive stent implantation (Figure 17.7). We analyzed 128 consecutive patients enrolled in

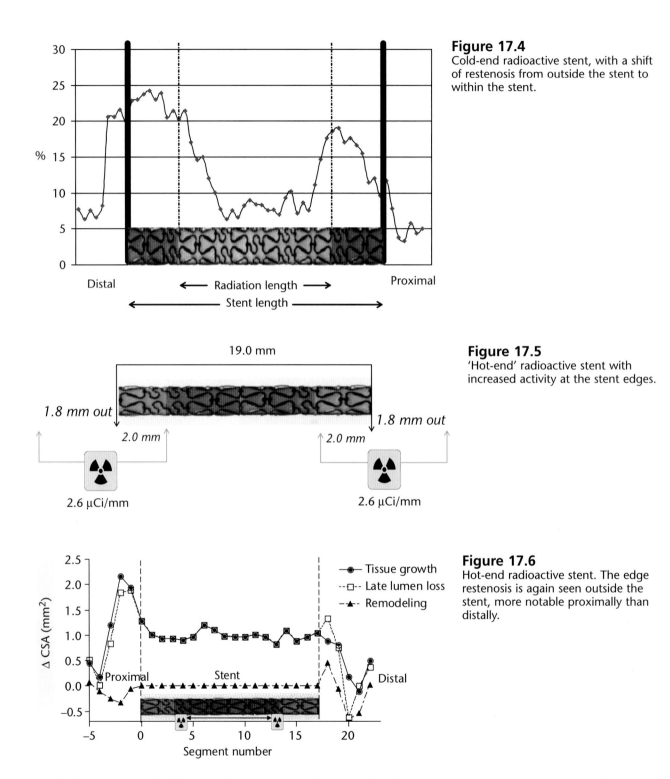

Figure 17.4
Cold-end radioactive stent, with a shift of restenosis from outside the stent to within the stent.

Figure 17.5
'Hot-end' radioactive stent with increased activity at the stent edges.

Figure 17.6
Hot-end radioactive stent. The edge restenosis is again seen outside the stent, more notable proximally than distally.

brachytherapy protocols. The control group consisted of individuals who underwent PTCA with ($n = 48$) and without ($n = 22$) stent implantation. Radiation groups included those who underwent low-activity ($n = 18$), high-activity ($n = 26$) and cold-end ($n = 18$) radioactive stenting. The Novoste BetaCath ($n = 39$) and Guidant ($n = 27$) catheter-based radiation systems were also employed. At 6-month follow-up, echo-lucent tissue was identified in a total of 28 cases (22%). Angiographic restenosis occurred in 17 cases (61%).

No echo-lucent tissue was seen in the control group or in the low-activity group. High-activity and cold-end radioactive stents were most commonly associated with echo-lucent tissue. Echo-lucent tissue was seen in all groups treated with catheter-based radiation with and without stenting. Pathology after atherectomy demonstrated smooth muscle cells scattered in extracellular matrix containing abundant proteoglycans and an absence of elastin and mature collagen (Figure 17.8).

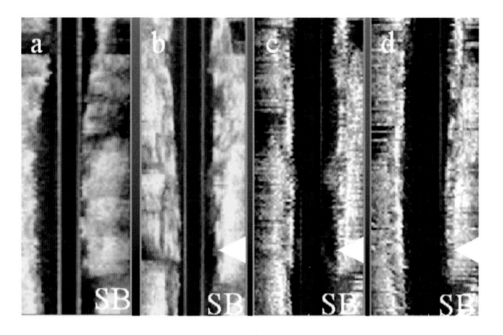

Figure 17.7
(a) Baseline longitudinal IVUS reconstruction of a freshly implanted 6.0 µCi activity radioactive stent. (b) Six-month follow-up. This confirms the presence of a uniform black semicircular structure with a thin cap. Note the adjacent side branch (SB). (c) The same image seen at 1 year, with echo-lucent tissue in a similar position, as verified by the location of the side branch. Note the greater reflectivity of the echo-lucent tissue and the thicker fibrous cap that is present. (d) Post-atherectomy image showing complete removal of tissue adjacent to the side branch.

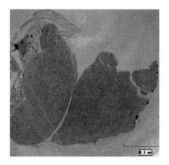

Figure 17.8
Alcian Blue stain showing that the extracellular matrix contains large amounts of proteoglycans.

Delayed restenosis

Catheter-based radiation

From a theoretical point of view, intracoronary brachytherapy may induce a delay of the restenotic process rather than a permanent inhibition of restenosis.[55,56] Considering that a single acute dose of 12 or 16 Gy would result in a depopulation of smooth muscle cells of about 10^{-3} to 10^{-6} (about 1 cell in 1000 to 1 million would survive), the number of doublings of the surviving cells to produce enough progeny to block the artery would be between 12 and 20, which would take between 12 and 24 months. Although smooth muscle cells are not malignant and therefore do not have the capacity for indefinite proliferation – at least theoretically – one cannot assume that the restenosis process would come to an end after 6 months.[56] This concept has been observed in clinical trials. In the SCRIPPS trial, the mean minimal luminal diameter decreased from

2.49±0.81 mm at 6 months to 2.12±0.73 mm at 3 years in the ^{192}Ir group, whereas there was no significant change in the placebo group.[56] Similarly, in the Washington Radiation for In-Stent Restenosis Trial (WRIST), target lesion revascularization increased from 13.8% at 6 months to 26.2% at 2-year follow-up.[57–59]

Radioactive stents

This 'catch-up' phenomenon occurred earlier after radioactive stenting. Significant luminal deterioration was observed within the stents between 6 months and 1 year, as evidenced by a decrease in the angiographic minimum lumen diameter (-0.43 ± 0.56 mm; $p = 0.028$) and in the mean lumen diameter in the stent (-0.55 ± 0.63 mm; $p = 0.001$); a significant increase in in-stent neointimal hyperplasia by IVUS (18.16 ± 12.59 mm^3 at 6 months to 27.75 ± 11.99 mm^3 at 1 year; $p = 0.001$) was also observed. Target vessel revascularization was performed in 5 patients (23%). By 1 year, 21 of the initial 40 patients (53%) remained event-free.

Therefore, we considered that, in contrast to previous historical trials, the efficacy of intracoronary radiation should be determined at long-term (≥ 1 year) follow-up.

Dose inhomogeneity

This phenomenon is inherent to the presence of a variable degree of vessel curvature, tortuosity, tapering, remodeling, and plaque extent and distribution. Further, the position of the radiation source in the lumen of a coronary segment is not fixed during the cardiac cycle, and may vary in either axial or perpendicular direction during the dwell time, leading to some degree of dose inhomogeneity. Finally, both the isotope (β- or γ-emitter) and the system used to deliver radiation (centered or noncentered device, radioactive stent) may influence the dose distribution. Using dose–volume histograms, Carlier et al[60] demonstrated in 23 patients enrolled in the BERT-1.5 trial that 90% of the adventitial volume received only 37% of the prescribed dose. By simulating a centering of the source and the use of a γ-emitter, this percentage of dose received by the adventitia would increase to 49% and 67% of the prescribed dose, respectively. Further, in a subsegmental analysis of irradiated coronary segments by means of a noncentered device and the β-emitter ^{90}Sr/^{90}Y, the delivered dose to the adventitia appeared to vary considerably between subsegments, ranging from less than 2 Gy to 12 Gy.[61] The delivered dose appeared to be an independent predictor of plaque volume at follow-up, and the significant relationship demonstrated between both variables was best described as polynomial with linear and nonlinear components. Clearly, dose uniformity is strongly related to the outcome, and radiation systems must be capable of delivering the prescribed dose to the target in a homogeneous manner.

Results of clinical trials

(Table 17.2)

Catheter-based γ-radiation trials

Condado et al[23] reported for the first time the use of γ-radiation for the treatment of de novo coronary stenoses after balloon angioplasty. Twenty-one patients (22 coronaries) were included. Angiographic follow-up at 5 years has been reported. The mean minimal luminal diameter remained stable from 6-month to 5-year follow-up (1.97 mm post procedure, 1.77 at 6 months, and 1.68 at 2, 3, and 5 years). The restenosis rate was 23.8% at 5 years. No additional aneurysm formation was reported, nor any cases of late thrombosis.

Teirstein et al[25] designed the first randomized trial with γ-radiation for the treatment of *restenotic* lesions. In the SCRIPPS I trial, 55 patients were enrolled who had restenosis after balloon angioplasty ($n = 20$) or after stent implantation ($n = 35$). Angiographic indices of restenosis were markedly different in the irradiated arm as compared with the placebo group: late loss was 0.38 ± 1.06 mm in the ^{192}Ir group as compared with 1.03 ± 0.97 mm in the placebo group ($p = 0.009$); the restenosis rate (including the stent and the border) was 16.7% in the irradiated group and 53.6% in the placebo group ($p = 0.025$). Further, the IVUS study demonstrated a 60% reduction in in-stent tissue growth after brachytherapy (15.5 mm^3 versus 45.1 mm^3; $p=0.01$). Despite the above late reduction in minimal lumen diameter during long-term follow-up, the global beneficial effect in the ^{192}Ir group was maintained at 3-year follow-up:[57] target lesion revascularization was 15.4% in the ^{192}Ir group and 48.3% in the placebo group ($p < 0.01$); the restenosis rate was 33% in the irradiated group versus 64% in the non-irradiated group ($p < 0.05$). A particular benefit was witnessed in the subgroup of diabetic patients and in those receiving more than 8 Gy.[62]

WRIST[57] was a single-center, double-blind, randomized trial for patients presenting with in-stent restenosis. One hundred and thirty patients (100 native coronary arteries and 30 saphenous vein grafts) were randomized to either placebo or radiation with ^{192}Ir at a prescribed dose of 14 Gy at 2 mm from the source. In this trial, all debulking devices were used prior to radiation: rotational atherectomy (45%), laser (35%), stent (35%), and balloon (7%).[63] At 6-month follow-up, significant reductions in restenosis rate, late loss, and target lesion revascularization were demonstrated in the ^{192}Ir group. Further, device selection did not influence the outcome in either irradiated or non-irradiated groups, although stent implantation was associated with higher rates of late thrombosis. Although the ^{192}Ir group presented with more late recurrences than the placebo group between 6 months and 2 years (9.3% versus 0%), the need for repeat target vessel revascularization was still markedly lower in the ^{192}Ir

Table 17.2   Results of pivotal trials and registries for coronary in-stent restenosis

Trial	% TVR: placebo vs radiation	% MACE: placebo vs radiation	% in-stent restenosis: placebo vs radiation	% in-lesion restenosis: placebo vs radiation	In-stent late loss: placebo vs radiation
SCRIPPS I	45 vs 12	62 vs 19	36 vs 8	54 vs 17	1.03 vs 0.38
WRIST	63 vs 14	68 vs 29	58 vs 19	60 vs 22	1.0 vs 0.22
GAMMA I	44 vs 25	46 vs 29	51 vs 22	55 vs 32	1.14 vs 0.73
GAMMA II	23	30	25	34	0.61
START	24 vs 16	26 vs 18	41 vs 14	45 vs 29	0.67 vs 0.21
INHIBIT	29 vs 11	33 vs 22	48 vs 16	52 vs 26	0.62 vs 0.41

TVR, target vessel revascularization; MACE, major adverse cardiac events.

group (26.2% versus 63.1% in the placebo group; $p=0.001$) at 2 years.[59]

As an extension of the original WRIST trial, two trials evaluated the effectiveness of γ-radiation in patients with in-stent restenosis in the subset of long lesions (>36–<80 mm; Long-WRIST) and in vein grafts (SVG-WRIST).

Long WRIST was a two-instituition, 120-patient randomized trial. Lesion length was 36–80 mm. There was a statistically significant decrease in angiographic restenosis in favor of radiation (71% versus 32%). The Long WRIST HD study attempted to improve the relatively high restenosis rate seen in the original sudy. By increasing the dose at 2 mm from 15 to 18 Gy, the restenosis rate was decreased to 24%.[64]

SVG-WRIST assessed the effects of intravascular γ-radiation in patients with in-stent restenosis of saphenous vein bypass grafts.[57] A total of 120 patients with in-stent restenosis of saphenous vein grafts, the majority of whom had diffuse lesions, underwent balloon angioplasty, atherectomy, additional stenting, or a combination of these procedures. If the intervention was successful, the patients were randomly assigned in a double-blind fashion to intravascular treatment with a ribbon containing either ^{192}Ir or nonradioactive seeds. The prescribed dose, delivered at a distance of 2 mm from the source, was 14–15 Gy in vessels that were 2.5–4.0 mm in diameter and 18 Gy in vessels with a diameter exceeding 4.0 mm.

At 6 months, the restenosis rate was lower in the 60 patients assigned to the ^{192}Ir group than in the 60 assigned to the placebo group (21% versus 44%; $p = 0.005$). At 12 months, the rate of revascularization of the target lesion was 70% lower in the ^{192}Ir group than in the placebo group (17% versus 57%; $p < 0.001$), and the rate of major cardiac events was 49% lower (32% versus 63%; $p < 0.001$).[65]

The GAMMA-1 trial[66] was a multicenter, double-blind, randomized placebo-controlled trial aimed at demonstrating the effectiveness of γ-radiation (^{192}Ir) in patients with in-stent restenosis. In comparison with the WRIST trial, 80% of the lesions were restented. Radiation groups showed a reduction in 6-month follow-up restenosis rate (50.5% in the placebo group versus 22% in the ^{192}Ir group). The late thrombosis rate was also significantly higher in the irradiated group (5.3% versus 0% in the placebo group; $p = 0.02$). This was associated with new stent implantation. Similar to the SCRIPPS trial, diabetic patients had a particularly good response to brachytherapy (36.1% restenosis in the ^{192}Ir group versus 76% in the placebo group; $p = 0.01$).[62] The Washington group have recently published data on their experience in diabetic patients. The study group consisted of 749 consecutive patients with in-stent restenosis who were treated with either intracoronary radiation or placebo in randomized trials and registries at our center. Diabetic patients (252 radiation and 51 placebo) were compared with nondiabetic patients (371 radiation and 75 placebo). In-hospital outcomes were similar between diabetic and nondiabetic patients treated with and without radiation. At 6-month clinical and angiographic follow-up, there was a significant reduction in the binary restenosis (63.8% versus 15.7%; $p < 0.0001$), target lesion revascularization (66.7% versus 17.6%; $p < 0.0001$) and target vessel revascularization (70.6% versus 22.9%; $p < 0.0001$) rates in diabetic patients treated with radiation compared with placebo. Comparisons between the placebo arms detected a trend towards higher restenosis (63.8% versus 48.4%; $p = 0.13$) and target vessel revascularization (70.6% versus 56.0%; $p = 0.14$) rates in diabetic versus nondiabetic patients. In contrast, diabetic and nondiabetic patients treated with intracoronary radiation experienced similar restenosis (15.6% versus 10.7%; $p = 0.33$) and target vessel revascularization (22.9% versus 28.2%; $p = 0.41$) rates.[67]

Catheter-based β-radiation trials

The GENEVA Pilot Clinical Experience was the first feasibility study performed in Europe and also the first in the world to use intracoronary β-radiation in humans.[24] A pure β-emitter ^{90}Y source delivered via a centering catheter (Schneider Endovascular Radiation System, Schneider Worldwide, Büllach, Switzerland) was used to deliver 18 Gy at the surface of the balloon in 15 patients with de novo coronary stenoses treated with balloon angioplasty. At follow-up, the restenosis rate was 40%. The investigators considered these unfavorable results to be due to an insufficient dose administered at the adventitia (<4 Gy).

Beta-WRIST[69] was an extension of the original WRIST trial using the Schneider pure β-emitter ^{90}Y and a centering device to treat patients with in-stent restenosis. The control group was taken from the original WRIST trial. Angiographic and IVUS results were comparable to those obtained with γ-radiation.

The Stents and Radiation Therapy (START) trial[70] was the first trial to randomized to either β-radiation using the β-emitter ^{90}Sr/^{90}Y and the Beta-Cath system (16 or 20 Gy according to the reference vessel diameter by quantitative coronary analysis) or placebo for patients with in-stent restenosis. After successful catheter-based treatment of in-stent restenosis, 476 patients were randomly assigned to receive an intracoronary catheter containing either ^{90}Sr/[90]Y ($n = 244$) or placebo ($n = 232$) sources. The prescribed dose 2 mm from the center of the source was 18.4 Gy for vessels between 2.70 and 3.35 mm in diameter and 23.0 Gy for vessels between 3.36 and 4.0 mm. Clinically driven target-vessel revascularization at 8 months was observed in 56 (26.8%) of the patients assigned to placebo and 39 (17.0%) of the patients assigned to radiation ($p = 0.015$). The incidence of the composite endpoint (death, myocardial infarction, or target vessel revascularization) was observed in 60 (28.7%) of the patients assigned to placebo and 44 (19.1%) of the patients assigned to radiation ($p = 0.024$). Binary 8-month angiographic restenosis ($\geq 50\%$ diameter stenosis) within the entire segment treated with radiation was reduced from 45.2% in the placebo-treated patients to 28.8% in the ^{90}Sr/^{90}Y-treated patients ($p = 0.001$). Stent thromboses occurred in one patient assigned to placebo less than 24 hours after the procedure and in one patient assigned to ^{90}Sr/^{90}Y at day 244.

The START 40/20 trial[71] was a registry of 207 patients with the same entry criteria as START, except that the source train was 40 mm long so as to minimize geographic miss. The frequency of geographic miss was decreased from 15% to 6%. The 8-month restenosis rate was 16%; analysis segment failure was reduced from 29% (30 mm) to 22% (40 mm).

The Intimal Hyperplasia Inhibition with Beta In-stent Trial (INHIBIT),[72] a randomized multicenter, double-blind, sham-controlled trial, was designed to demonstrate the clinical safety and efficacy of the Guidant β-radiation system for treatment of in-stent restenosis; 332 patients with in-stent restenosis underwent successful coronary intervention, and were then randomly allocated to intracoronary β-radiation with a ^{32}P source ($n = 166$) or placebo ($n = 166$) delivered into a centering balloon catheter through an automatic afterloader. Longer lesions (>22 mm of dilated length) were treated with tandem positioning of the study wire. At 9 months, 24 (15%) patients in the radiated group experienced the primary safety endpoint of death, myocardial infarction, or repeat target vessel revascularization compared with 15 (31%) in the placebo group (difference 16%; 95% confidence interval (CI) 7–25%; $p = 0.0006$). The binary angiographic restenosis rate was lower in the radiated group than the placebo group for the entire analyzed segment (difference 25%; 95% CI 14–37%; $p < 0.0001$).

β-radiation for de novo lesions

BERT

BERT[30] was a feasibility study designed to test the ^{90}Sr/^{90}Y source delivered by a hydraulic system (BetaCath system). At 6 months, the reported restenosis rate was 15%. This trial had two extensions: a Canadian arm[67] and a European arm. The results of the Canadian arm were comparable to those of the original BERT trial,[62] whereas the restenosis rate in the European arm was higher (28%).

PREVENT

The Proliferation Reduction with Vascular Energy Trial (PREVENT)[73] was a prospective, randomized, blinded,

multicenter study aimed to determine the safety of the Guidant β-radiation system in human coronary arteries following balloon angioplasty or stent implantation. Seventy-two patients were randomized to 16, 20, or 24 Gy prescribed to 1 mm from the source. At 6-month follow-up, the restenosis rate (including the edges of the irradiated segment) showed a 58% reduction in the irradiated group (22% versus 52% in the placebo group; $p < 0.01$). However, an increased rate of late thrombosis in the ^{32}P group (7 cases) led to nonsignificant differences in major adverse cardiac events (27% in the irradiated group versus 32% in the placebo group; $p = $ NS).

BETACATH

The BETACATH trial[74] was a multi-instituition double-blind randomized study with 1456 patients with de novo lesions. The doses delivered were 18 and 23 Gy, depending on vessel diameter and stenting. This was a negative trial with no improvement in primary endpoints.

GENEVA

The Boston Scientific/Schneider Dose-Finding Study[75] was a multicenter, prospective, randomized, noncontrolled study aimed at determining the effect of four different doses of β-radiation, using the ^{90}Y pure β-emitting source via a centering catheter (Schneider Irradiation Therapy System, Büllach, Switzerland) on de novo coronary stenoses. In five European centers, 181 patients were randomized to receive 9, 12, 15, or 18 Gy at 1 mm of tissue depth. The preliminary analysis (93% with 6-month follow-up) demonstrated a dose-dependent reduction in angiographic restenosis with an extremely low restenosis rate in patients treated with balloon alone and a prescribed dose of 18 Gy (3.9%). However, this benefit was not maintained in patients receiving a stent ($n=49$), in whom the restenosis rate was high regardless of the prescribed dose (30% in the 9 Gy group, 33.3% in the 12 Gy group, 35.4% in the 15 Gy group, and 35.7% in the 18 Gy group). The target vessel occluded at 6 months in four patients treated with balloon alone (3.3%) and in seven patients receiving a stent (14.2%). Five patients presented with Q-wave myocardial infarction (2.9%) and target lesion revascularization was performed in 19 patients (11.2%).

Conclusions

The use of intracoronary radiation therapy is established as an efficacious treatment for in-stent restenosis, particularly in diabetics. Two major concerns came from the first randomized trials in in-stent restenosis: edge restenosis and late thrombotic occlusion. The avoidance of geographic miss and long-term use of antiplatelet agents have significantly decreased the incidence of these problems. Despite promising results using ^{90}Y in de novo lesions, subsequent large randomized studies using ^{90}Sr have not proven to be efficacious.

Research into drug-eluting stents will progress rapidly on the basis of concepts established during the brachytherapy era. One could argue that for 'nonresponders' to drug-eluting stents, brachytherapy may remain a viable niche option.

References

1. Holmes DR Jr, Vlietstra RE, Smith HC, et al. Restenosis after percutaneous transluminal coronary angioplasty (PTCA): a report from the PTCA Registry of the National Heart, Lung, and Blood Institute. Am J Cardiol. 1984;53:77C–81C.

2. Serruys PW, Luijten HE, Beatt KJ, et al. Incidence of restenosis after successful coronary angioplasty: a time-related phenomenon. A quantitative angiographic study in 342 consecutive patients at 1, 2, 3, and 4 months. Circulation 1988;77:361–71.

3. Schwartz RS, Holmes DR, Topol EJ. The restenosis paradigm revisited: an alternative proposal for cellular mechanisms. J Am Coll Cardiol 1992;20:1284–93.

4. Nobuyoshi M, Kimura T, Ohishi H, et al. Restenosis after percutaneous transluminal coronary angioplasty: pathologic observations in 20 patients. J Am Coll Cardiol 1991; 17:433–9.

5. Mintz GS, Popma JJ, Pichard AD, et al. Arterial remodeling after coronary angioplasty: a serial intravascular ultrasound study. Circulation 1996;94:35–43.

6. MacLeod DC, Strauss BH, de Jong M, et al. Proliferation and extracellular matrix synthesis of smooth muscle cells cultured from human coronary atherosclerotic and restenotic lesions. J Am Coll Cardiol 1994;23:59–65.

7. Guarda E, Katwa LC, Campbell SE, et al. Extracellular matrix collagen synthesis and degradation following coronary balloon angioplasty. J Mol Cell Cardiol 1996;28:699–706.

8. Serruys PW, de Jaegere P, Kiemeneij F, et al. A comparison of balloon-expandable-stent implantation with balloon angioplasty in patients with coronary artery disease. Benestent Study Group. N Engl J Med 1994;331:489–95.

9. Fischman DL, Leon MB, Baim DS, et al. A randomized comparison of coronary-stent placement and balloon angioplasty in the treatment of coronary artery disease. Stent Restenosis Study Investigators. N Engl J Med 1994;331:496–501.

10. Haude M, Erbel R, Issa H, Meyer J. Quantitative analysis of elastic recoil after balloon angioplasty and after intracoronary implantation of balloon-expandable Palmaz–Schatz stents. J Am Coll Cardiol 1993;21:26–34.

11. Dussaillant GR, Mintz GS, Pichard AD, et al. Small stent size and intimal hyperplasia contribute to restenosis: a volumetric intravascular ultrasound analysis. J Am Coll Cardiol 1995;26:720–4.

12. Sharma SK, Duvvuri S, Dangas G, et al. Rotational atherectomy for in-stent restenosis: acute and long-term results of the first 100 cases. J Am Coll Cardiol 1998;32:1358–65.

13. Eltchaninoff H, Koning R, Tron C, et al. Balloon angioplasty for the treatment of coronary in-stent restenosis: immedi-

14. Bauters C, Banos JL, Van Belle E, et al. Six-month angiographic outcome after successful repeat percutaneous intervention for in-stent restenosis. Circulation 1998; 97:318–21.

15. Kovalic JJ, Perez CA. Radiation therapy following keloidectomy: a 20-year experience. Int J Radiat Oncol Biol Phys 1989;17:77–80.

16. Walter WL. Another look at pterygium surgery with postoperative beta radiation. Ophthal Plast Reconstr Surg 1994;10:247–52.

17. Friedman M, Felton L, Byers S. The antiatherogenic effect of iridium 192 upon the cholesterol-fed rabbit. J Clin Invest 1964;43:186–92.

18. Liermann D, Bottcher HD, Kollath J, et al. Prophylactic endovascular radiotherapy to prevent intimal hyperplasia after stent implantation in femoropopliteal arteries. Cardiovasc Interv Radiol 1994;17:12–16.

19. Wiedermann JG, Marboe C, Amols H, et al. Intracoronary irradiation markedly reduces neointimal proliferation after balloon angioplasty in swine: persistent benefit at 6-month follow-up. J Am Coll Cardiol 1995;25:1451–6.

20. Waksman R, Robinson KA, Crocker IR, et al. Intracoronary low-dose beta-irradiation inhibits neointima formation after coronary artery balloon injury in the swine restenosis model. Circulation 1995;92:3025–31.

21. Mazur W, Ali MN, Khan MM, et al. High dose rate intracoronary radiation for inhibition of neointimal formation in the stented and balloon-injured porcine models of restenosis: angiographic, morphometric, and histopathologic analyses. Int J Radiat Oncol Biol Phys 1996;36:777–88.

22. Verin V, Popowski Y, Urban P, et al. Intraarterial beta-irradiation prevents neointimal hyperplasia in a hypercholesterolemic rabbit restenosis model. Circulation 1995;92:2284–90.

23. Condado JA, Waksman R, Gurdiel O, et al. Long-term angiographic and clinical outcome after percutaneous transluminal coronary angioplasty and intracoronary radiation therapy in humans. Circulation 1997;96:727–32.

24. Verin V, Urban P, Popowski Y, et al. Feasibility of intracoronary beta-irradiation to reduce restenosis after balloon angioplasty. A clinical pilot study. Circulation 1997;95:1138–44.

25. Teirstein PS, Massullo V, Jani S, et al. Catheter-based radiotherapy to inhibit restenosis after coronary stenting. N Engl J Med 1997;336:1697–703.

26. Waksman R. Vascular Brachytherapy, 2nd edn. Armonk, NY: Futura, 1999.

27. Scott NA, Ross C, Dunn B, et al. Identification of a potential role for the adventitia in vascular lesion formation after balloon overstretch injury of porcine coronary arteries. Circulation 1996;93:2178–87.

28. Waksman R, Rodriguez JC, Robinson KA, et al. Effect of intravascular irradiation on cell proliferation, apoptosis and vascular remodeling after balloon overstretch injury of porcine coronary arteries. Circulation 1997;96:1944–52.

29. Rubin P, Williams JP, Kinkelstein J, et al. Radiation inhibition versus induction of vascular restenosis: the role of the monocyte-derived macrophage. In: Vascular Brachytherapy, 2nd edn (Waksman R, ed). Armonk, NY: Futura, 1999:103–25.

30. King SB III, Williams DO, Chogule P, et al. Endovascular β-radiation to reduce restenosis after coronary balloon

angioplasty. Results of the Beta Energy Restenosis Trial (BERT). Circulation 1998;97:2025–30.

31. Sabaté M, Serruys PW, van der Giessen WJ, et al. Geometric vascular remodeling after balloon angioplasty and beta-radiation therapy: a three-dimensional intravascular ultrasound study. Circulation 1999;100:1182–8.

32. Costa M, Sabaté M, Serrano P, et al. The effect of P^{32} beta-radiotherapy on both vessel remodeling and neointimal hyperplasia after coronary balloon angioplasty and stenting. A three-dimensional intravascular ultrasound investigation. J Invas Cardiol 2000;12:113–20.

33. Kay IP, Sabaté M, Costa M, et al. Positive geometric vascular remodeling is seen after catheter-based radiation followed by conventional stent implantation, but not after radioactive stent implantation. Circulation 2000;102:1434–9.

34. Albiero R, Adamian M, Kobayashi N, et al. Short- and inter-mediate-term results of P^{32}radioactive β-emitting stent implantation in patients with coronary artery disease. The Milan dose–response study. Circulation 2000;101:18–26.

35. Sabaté M, Kay IP, van der Giessen WJ, et al. Preserved endothelium-dependent vasodilation in coronary segments previously treated with balloon angioplasty and intra-coronary irradiation. Circulation 1999;100:1623–9.

36. Wiederman JG, Leavy JA, Amols H, et al. Effects of high-dose intracoronary irradiation on vasomotor function and smooth muscle histopathology. Am J Physiol 1994; 267:H125–32.

37. Vodovotz Y, Waksman R. Potential roles for nitric oxide and transforming growth factor β$_1$ in endovascular brachytherapy. In: Vascular Brachytherapy (Waksman R, ed). Armonk, NY: Futura, 1999:139–46.

38. Thorin E, Meerkin D, Bertrand OF, et al. Influence of postangioplasty β-irradiation on endothelial function in porcine coronary arteries. Circulation 2000;101:1430–5.

39. Bal ET, Plokker T, van den Berg EMJ, et al. Predictability and prognosis of PTCA-induced coronary aneurysms. Cathet Cardiovasc Diagn 1991;22:85–8.

40. Colombo A, Hall P, Nakamura S, et al. Intracoronary stent-ing without anticoaguation accomplished with intravascular ultrasound guidance. Circulation 1995;91:1676–88.

41. Costa M, Sabaté M, van der Giessen WJ, et al. Late coronary occlusion after intracoronary brachytherapy. Circulation 1999;100:789–92.

42. Waksman R, Bhargava B, Leon MB. Late thrombosis follow-ing intracoronary brachytherapy. Cathet Cardiovasc Interv 2000;49:344–7.

43. Waksman R, Ajani AE, Pinnow E, et al. Twelve versus six months of clopidogrel to reduce major cardiac events in patients undergoing gamma-radiation therapy for in-stent restenosis: Washington Radiation for In-Stent restenosis Trial (WRIST) 12 versus WRIST PLUS. Circulation 2002;106:776–8.

44. Farb A, Tang A, Virmani R. The neointima is reduced but endothelialization is incomplete 3 months after ^{32}P β-emitting stent placement. Circulation 1998;98(Suppl I): I-770 (abst).

45. Sabaté M, van der Giessen WJ, Deshpande NV, et al. Late thrombotic occlusion of a malapposed stent 10 months after intracoronary brachytherapy. Int J Cardiovasc Interv 1999;2:55–9.

46. Kozuma K, Costa MA, Sabaté M, et al. Late stent malap-position occurring after intracoronary beta-irradiation detected by intravascular ultrasound. J Invas Cardiol 1999;11:651–5.

47. Kay IP, Sabaté M, van Langenhove G. The outcome from balloon-induced coronary artery dissection after intra-coronary β-radiation. Heart 2000;83:332–7.

48. Vodovotz Y, Waksman R, Kim WH, et al. Effects of intra-coronary radiation on thrombosis after balloon overstretch injury model. Circulation 1999;100:2527–33.

49. Carter AJ, Laird JR, Bailey LR, et al. Effects of endovascular radiation from a β-particle-emitting stent in a porcine coro-nary restenosis model: a dose–response study. Circulation 1996;94:2364–8.

50. Schwartz RS, Huber KC, Murphy JG, et al. Restenosis and proportional neointimal response to coronary artery injury: results in a porcine model. J Am Coll Cardiol. 1992; 19:267–74.

51. Weinberger J, Amols H, Ennis RD, et al. Intracoronary irradiation: dose response fro prevention of restenosis in swine. Int J Radiat Oncol Biol Phys 1996;36:767–75.

52. Sabaté M, Costa MA, Kozuma K, et al. Geographic miss: a cause of treatment failure in radio-oncology applied to intra-coronary radiation therapy. Circulation 2000;101:2467–71.

53. Paterson R. The Treatment of Malignant Disease by Radiotherapy. London: Edward Arnold, 1963.

54. Kay IP, Wardeh AJ, Kozuma K, et al. The pattern of restenosis and vascular remodelling after cold-end radioactive stent implantation. Eur Heart J 2001;22:1311–17.

55. Serruys PW, Kay IP. I like the candy, I hate the wrapper. The ^{32}P radioactive stent. Circulation 2000;101:3–7.

56. Hall EJ, Miller RC, Brenner DJ. The basic radiobiology of intravascular irradiation. In: Vascular Brachytherapy, 2nd edn (Waksman R, ed). Armonk, NY: Futura, 1999: 63–72.

57. Teirstein PS, Massullo V, Jani S, et al. Three-year clinical and angiographic follow-up after intracoronary radiation. Results of a randomized clinical trial. Circulation 2000; 101:360–5.

58. Waksman R, White LR, Chan RC, et al. Intracoronary radia-tion therapy for patients with in-stent restenosis: 6 month follow up of a randomized clinical study. Circulation 1998;98(Suppl):I-651 (abst).

59. Waksman R, Ajani AE, White RL, et al. Two-year follow-up after beta and gamma intracoronary radiation therapy for patients with diffuse in-stent restenosis. Am J Cardiol 2001;88:425–8.

60. Carlier SG, Marijnissen JPA, Coen VLMA, et al. Comparison of brachytherapy strategies based on dose-volume histograms derived from quantitative intravascular ultrasound. Cardiovasc Radiat Med 1999;1:115–24.

61. Sabaté M, Marijnissen JPA, Carlier SG, et al. Residual plaque burden, delivered dose and tissue composition predict the 6-month outcome after balloon angioplasty and β-radiation therapy. Circulation 2000;101:2472–7.

62. Teirstein PS, Massullo V, Jani S, et al. A subgroup analysis of the Scripps Coronary Radiation to Inhibit Proliferation Poststenting Trial. Int J Radiat Oncol Biol Phys 1998; 42:1097–104.

63. Waksman R, Zimarino M, Mehran R, et al. Device influence on outcome in the treatment of in-stent restenosis with and without radiation. A sub-analysis from the WRIST study. J Am Coll Cardiol 2000;35(Suppl A):21^{a}A (abst).

64. Tripuraneni P. Coronary artery radiation therapy for the prevention of restenosis after precutaneous coronary angio-

plasty II: Outcomes of clinical trials. Semin Radiat Oncol 2002;12:17–30.

65. Waksman R, Ajani AE, White RL, et al. Intravascular gamma radiation for in-stent restenosis in saphenous-vein bypass grafts. N Engl J Med 2002;346:1194–9.

66. Leon MB, Teirstein PS, Moses JW, et al. Localized intra-coronary gamma-radiation therapy to inhibit the recurrence of restenosis after stenting. N Engl J Med 2001;344:250–6.

67. Gruberg L, Waksman R, Ajani AE, et al. The effect of intra-coronary radiation for the treatment of recurrent in-stent restenosis in patients with diabetes mellitus. J Am Coll Cardiol 2002;39:1930–6.

68. Meerkin D, Tardiff JC, Crocker IR, et al. Effects of intra-coronary beta-radiation therapy after coronary angioplasty: an intravascular ultrasound study. Circulation 1999;99:1660–5.

69. Waksman R, White LR, Chan RC, et al. Intracoronary beta-radiation therapy for patients with in-stent restensosis: the 6 months clinical and angiographic results. Circulation. 1999;100(Suppl I):I-75 (abst).

70. Popma JJ, Suntharalingam M, Lansky AJ, et al. START: ran-domized trial of ^{90}Sr/^{90}Y β-radiation versus placebo control for treatment of in-stent restenosis. Circulation 2002; 106:1090–6.

71. Suntharalingam M, Laskey W, Lanskey AJ, et al. Clinical and angiographic outcomes after use of ^{90}strontium/^{90}yttrium beta radiation for the treatment of in-stent restenosis: results from the Stents and Radiation Therapy 40 (START 40) registry. Int J Radiat Oncol Biol Phys. 2002;52:1075–82.

72. Waksman R, Raizner AE, Yeung AC, et al. Use of localised intracoronary beta radiation in treatment of in-stent restenosis: the INHIBIT randomised controlled trial. Lancet 2002;359:551–7.

73. Raizner AE, Oesterle SN, Waksman R, et al. Inhibition of restenosis with beta-emitting radiotherapy: report of the Proliferation Reduction with Vascular Energy Trial (PRE-VENT). Circulation 2000;102:951–8.

74. Tripuraneni P. Coronary artery radiation therapy for the prevention of restenosis after precutaneous coronary angioplasty II: Outcomes of clinical trials. Semin Radiat Oncol 2002;12:17–30.

75. Verin V, Popowski Y, de Bruyne B, et al. Endoluminal beta-radiation therapy for the prevention of coronary restenosis after balloon angioplasty. The Dose-Finding Study Group. N Engl J Med 2001;344:243–9.

18

Drug-eluting stents

Marco A Costa

Introduction

The number of percutaneous coronary interventions performed each year has expanded considerably since the introduction of coronary stents. Angioplasty procedures doubled in Europe from 1992 to 1996,[1] while an estimated 601 000 percutaneous coronary revascularizations were performed in the USA in 1997.[2] Stents, certainly a step forward since the invention of balloon angioplasty, effectively prevent the remodeling component of restenosis. Neointimal proliferation, however, is still not counteracted and poses the last hurdle in the percutaneous treatment of coronary artery disease, namely in-stent restenosis. Thus, the focus of the prevention of restenosis over the past two decades has been through the application of antiproliferative pharmacologic agents. As a result, drug-eluting stents have emerged as an ultimate solution for restenosis. Drug-eluting stents are coated stents capable of releasing single or multiple bioactive agents into the bloodstream and surrounding tissues. The development of drug-eluting stent technology and its introduction into clinical practice will be discussed in this chapter.

Rationale for drug-eluting stents

Antithrombotic stent coatings represented the first step towards loading medications onto stents. These devices were developed to decrease the inherent thrombogenicity of coronary metallic stents, which were facing skepticism due to an unacceptably high (20–25%) incidence of thrombotic complications.[3] There are three heparin-coated stents currently available for clinical use: the BX-Velocity Carmeda-coated stent (Johnson & Johnson, Warren, NJ), the Wiktor Hepamed-coated stent (Medtronic, Inc, Minneapolis, MN) and the Jostent Corline-coated stent (Jomed International AB, Helsingborg, Sweden). It is nevertheless important to note that heparin-coated stents differ from drug-eluting stents because the medication is covalently bonded to the device and hence may remain attached long after deployment.

The success and safety of coronary stenting has dramatically increased with high-pressure stent deployment and the use of antiplatelet agents. However, in-stent restenosis remains as a hindrance to stenting. The incidence of restenosis may vary from 8% to as high as 80% at 6 months, depending on both anatomic and clinical risk factors.[4] Metallic stent struts activate platelets and macrophages, and stimulate the release of cytokines and growth factors and upregulation of genes as well as metalloproteinases. The consequence is smooth muscle cell migration, cellular growth, and remodeling of extracellular matrix.[4] Each of these processes is a potential target for anti-restenosis therapy (Figure 18.1).

Mechanical approaches have proven ineffective in preventing in-stent restenosis. Interfering with molecular cell division appears to be a much more effective manner to alter the healing process after stenting. The potential toxicity of systemic pharmacologic therapy poses significant limitations on a systemic approach to restenosis. Local drug delivery systems have been developed to provide high concentrations of drug at the site of vascular injury with minimal systemic effect. However, catheter-based local drug delivery has been largely unsuccessful in humans due to a rapid washout of the drug downstream into the coronary circulation, and potential flow or pressure-mediated vessel wall injury.[5] Recently, the emergence of

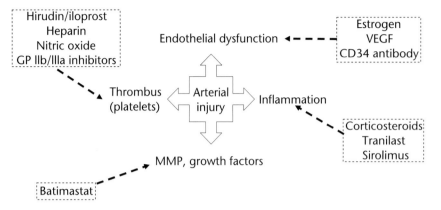

Figure 18.1
The leading processes of restenosis (arrows) and corresponding inhibitory (dashed lines) effects of different biologic agents.

drug-eluting stent technology has offered a new perspective for the pharmacologic prevention of restenosis.

The concept of using stents as vehicles for prolonged and sufficient intramural drug delivery is appealing. Stents represent an ideal platform for local drug delivery because of their permanent scaffolding properties, which prevent vessel recoil and negative remodeling. In addition, they represent drug reservoirs, as medications are released from various coatings at different time intervals. The achievement of a hospitable relationship between stent, coating matrix, drug, and vessel wall is extremely challenging. In general, drug-eluting stent technology faces many potential limitations[6–9] (Table 18.1). The scientific community, pharmaceutical and engineering industries, and clinicians have utilized a multidisciplinary approach to address these many issues in the formulation of a successful drug-eluting stent, which generally contains three basic components: stent, coating, and biologic agent.

Step I: the stent platform

Stents were initially designed as scaffolding structures, not to carry medications. Thus, stent designs have been altered to afford more flexibility, greater radial strength, and minimal metallic coverage. These properties are unfavorable for drug loading and elution. Compared with current stents, the ideal drug-delivery stent might have a much larger surface area, minimal gaps between cells, and minimal strut deformation after deployment. Ultimately, new drug-eluting stents still need to maintain a low profile, conformability, radial support, and flexibility to reach complex anatomies. Stent designs dedicated to drug delivery have been developed, and clinical investigations are currently ongoing.

Efforts are now being directed at coating stents with a sufficient amount of medication, which should be delivered uniformly to the underlying tissue. However, uniform drug distribution in diseased human coronary arteries is unrealistic. Besides stent geometry, other factors govern drug diffusion, such as vessel wall morphology, drug physicochemical characteristics, and the multifaceted milieu of the underlying atherosclerotic plaque.

So far, all clinical trials have tested conventional stent designs as drug carriers. The optimal results of these studies may obviate such design requirements for successful drug-eluting stents. However, compounds with narrow toxic–therapeutic window or different physicochemical properties may require a customized stent platform.

Table 18.1   Requirements for drug-eluting stents
<ul><li>Stent, drug and coating should be both blood- and tissue-compatible[6]</li><li>Current stents have limited surface area (usually <20%) to load large amounts of drugs</li><li>Adherence of the drug to the stent must not alter the biologic activities of the compound or the mechanical properties of the stent.</li><li>Local tissue properties and drug solubility affect the pharmacokinetics of the drug in vivo.[7,8]</li><li>The coating and drug must endure both sterilization and stent expansion</li><li>Coatings and biologic agents should not induce inflammation or other vascular proliferative responses[9,10]</li></ul>

Step II: stent coating – a crucial step

The coating material should act as a biologically inert barrier. However, only a few have satisfied this requirement.[11] The selection of a non-inflammatory, inert coating matrix has been a major obstacle for the development of drug-eluting stents. van der Giessen and co-workers[9] tested eight different polymers attached longitudinally across 90° of the circumferential surface of coil wire stents (Medtronic Inc, Minneapolis, MN). These coated stents were implanted in porcine coronary arteries, but none proved to be physiologically inert.

Coating materials must maintain their physicochemical characteristics after sterilization and after stent expansion

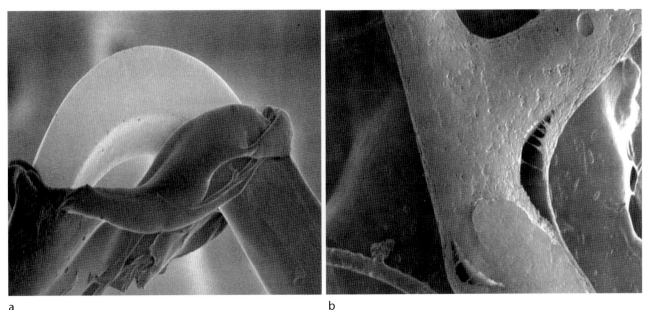

a   b

Figure 18.2
Potential alterations in stent surface after expansion (a) and sterilization (b) of a polymer-coated stent.

(Figure 18.2). The list of candidate substances for stent coatings is long and ever-expanding.[11] These substances may be categorized as organic, inorganic, bioerodable, non-bioerodable, synthetic, or naturally occurring substances.

Synthetic polymers

While problems have been observed with the use of synthetic polymers in the vascular bed, their ability to adhere, incorporate, degrade, and release pharmacologic agents still places these substances among the leading candidates for coating metallic stents. Polymers are long-chain molecules consisting of small repeating units. Polymer toxicity results in enhanced neointimal hyperplasia.[9] This type of response is influenced by the molecular weight and thickness of the coating layer. Slowly degrading coatings may elicit less inflammatory reaction. Metabolites of biodegradable polymers also play a role in inflammation.

Poly-L-lactic acid (PLLA) is a synthetic polymer completely degraded in vivo by enzymatic or nonenzymatic hydrolysis. Entirely biodegradable stents have been constructed with this polymer, while others have tested PLLA as a coating matrix for metallic prosthesis. Interestingly, different inflammatory reactions have been observed with PLLA, which illustrates the complexity of manufacturing inert polymer-coated stents.

The most successful drug-eluting stents tested clinically have been coated with synthetic polymers: poly-n-butyl methacrylate and polyethylene–vinyl acetate with sirolimus,[12] and a poly(lactide-co-ε-caprolactone) copolymer with a paclitaxel-eluting platform.[13]

Biological materials

Coating metallic surfaces with substances that mimic a biological vascular structure is highly appealing. Fibrin, cellulose, and albumin, all of which are naturally occurring, have been tested to improve the quality of stent surfaces with promising results from the animal studies. Phosphorylcholine (PC) is a neutral, zwitterionic naturally occurring phospholipid polymer. In vivo experiments have shown that PC does not interfere with stent re-endothelialization and elicits a similar amount of neointimal hyperplasia compared with uncoated stents. PC-coated BiodivYsio stents are currently available for clinical use and can be loaded with variety of compounds.

Inorganic coatings

Recently, pilot clinical investigations have been initiated with stents coated with inorganic substances. A nonporous ceramic layer of 300 μm containing tacrolimus has been used. In addition, other ongoing studies have tested stents with a deep reservoir for drug loading coated with a pyrolytic carbon thin layer (Carbofilm).

Drug loading and release kinetics

Some drugs can be loaded directly onto metallic surfaces (e.g. prostacyclin and paclitaxel), but a coating matrix is

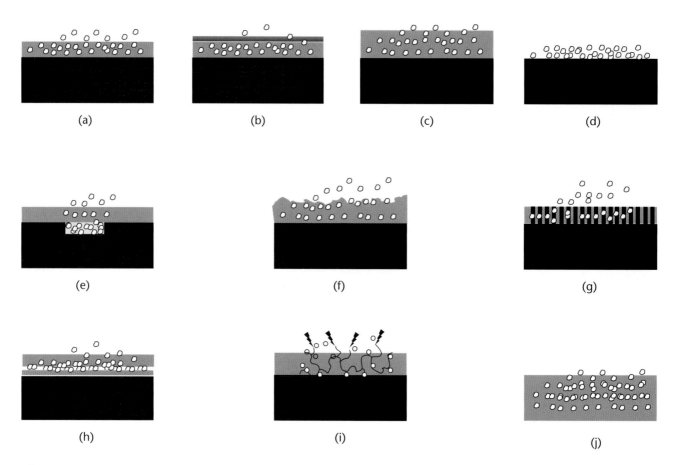

Figure 18.3
Schematic representation of different modalities of drug-eluting stent platforms (black, stent strut; gray, coating):
(a) drug–polymer blend, release by diffusion; (b) drug diffusion through an additional polymer coating; (c) drug release
by swelling of the coating; (d) nonpolymer-based drug release; (e) drug loaded in stent reservoir; (f) drug release by
erosion of coating; (g) drug loaded in nanoporous coating reservoirs; (h) drug loaded between coatings (coating
sandwich); (i) polymer–drug conjugate cleaved by hydrolysis or enzymatic action; (j) bioeradable polymeric stent.

required for most biologic agents (Figure 18.3) to ensure
drug retention during deployment and to modulate elution
kinetics. Drugs may be held by covalent bonds (C–C
bonds, sulfur bridges, etc.) or noncovalent bonds (ionic
and hydrogen bonds).[10] The blended matrix may then be
attached to the stent surface by dipping or spraying the
stent.

Drugs are released by particle dissolution or diffusion
when nonbioerodable matrices are used, or during polymer breakdown when absorbed into a biodegradable substance. Drug diffusion kinetics from coating matrices are
influenced by a variety of factors:

- coating thickness;
- physicochemical properties of the drug (soluble components diffuse faster than hydrophobic materials);
- physicochemical properties of the polymer;
- degree of crosslinking;
- porosity of the polymer;
- total amount of drug;
- local drug concentration (per unit area);
- underlying tissue characteristics.

Step III: the biological agent

Paradoxically, the ideal antirestenotic agent for local delivery should have potent antiproliferative effects, yet should
preserve vascular healing. Furthermore, such a compound
should contain hydrophobic elements to ensure high local
concentrations as well as hydrophilic properties to allow
homogeneous drug diffusion. In addition, the drug should
have a wide therapeutic-to-toxic ratio and should not provoke inflammation and thrombosis. Other factors, such as
molecular weight, charge, and degree of protein binding,[14]
may also affect drug kinetics and ultimately influence the
biologic success. The search for an effective biologic agent
to prevent restenosis has extended beyond the realm of
cardiology (Table 18.2). Anticancer and anti-transplant
rejection agents are now being considered in the fight
against restenosis. Only a few agents have demonstrated
clinical efficacy, but the search is still ongoing. Drugs that
interfere earlier in the cell cycle (G_1 phase) are generally
considered cytostatic, and potentially elicit less cellular

Table 18.2   Drug-eluting stent investigations

Drug	Stent	Coating	Manufacturer	Clinical trials	In-stent* late loss (mm)	In-stent* restenosis rate (%)
Sirolimus (rapamycin)	BX Velocity	Poly-n-butylmethacrylate/polyethylene–vinyl acetate (PBMA/PEVA)	Cordis, Jonhson & Johnson	FIM RAVEL SIRIUS ISR Registry SECURE, ARTS-2, FREEDOM, EC-SIRIUS, RESEARCH, e-CYPHER, STELLAR	0.16 (SR), −0.02 (FR) −0.01 0.14 0.36	0 0 2 4 (Brazil cohort)
Taxane	QuaDS	Polyacrylate sleeves	QUANAN QUANAN QUANAN/ Boston Scientific	SCORE Registry SCORE Randomized ISR Registry	0.35 0.47	0 6.4 13
Paclitaxel	NIR NIRx Comformer Express Express 2 Supra G V-Flex Plus/Logic Logic PTX Multi-Link Penta	Poly (lactide-co-ε-caprolactone) Surface modification	Boston Scientific Cook Guidant/Cook	TAXUS I TAXUS II TAXUS III TAXUS IV ASPECT ELUTES ELUTES-ISR PATENCY DELIVER, DELIVER II	0.36 0.31 (SR), 0.30 (MR) 0.44 0.39 0.29 (HD) 0.57 (LD) 0.1 (HD) 0.47–0.5 (ID) 0.7 (LD)	0 2.3 (SR), 4.7 (MR) 16 5.5 4 (HD) 12 (LD) 3.1 (HD) 11.8–13.5 (ID) 20 (LD) 38
Actinomycin D (dactinomycin)	Multi-Link Tetra	Proprietary	Guidant	ACTION		
Everolimus	S Stent	Proprietary	Biosensor/Guidant	FUTURE, FUTURE II		
Dexamethasone		Phosphorylcholine	Abbott/Biocompatibles	STRIDE DELIVER, Dose-Finding	0.45	13.3
Estrogen	BiodivYsio			EASTER EASTER-II	0.57	10
Batimastat				BRILLIANT	0.88	21
Angiopeptin				SWAN		

Table 18.2 Drug-eluting stent investigations (continued)

Drug	Stent	Coating	Manufacturer	Clinical trials	In-stent* late loss (mm)	In-stent* restenosis rate (%)
ABT-578				PREFER		
c-myc antisense	S7, S660, Driver		Medtronic Medtronic	ENDEAVOUR	0.33	2.1
Mycophenolic acid	Duraflex	Proprietary	Avantec Vascular Devices	IMPACT	1.04 (FR) 0.94 (SR)	12% (both formulations)
Tacrolimus	JoStent Graft JoStent	PTFE-covered Nanoporous ceramic	Jomed	EVIDENT PRESENT		
Tranilast	Igaki–Tamai stent	Biodegradable polymer stent	Igaki–Tamai			
Cyclosporine	R Stent	Proprietary	ORBUS MT	HEALING		
CD34 antibody						

* Follow-up period (≥4 month-follow up) varies considerably between trials SR, slow release; FR, fast release; LD, low dose; HD, high dose.

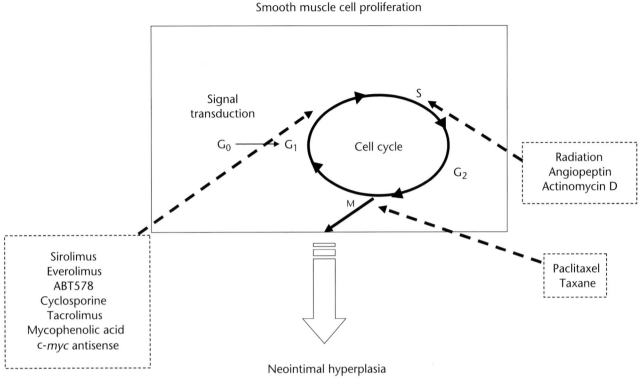

Figure 18.4
Mechanism of action of smooth muscle cell cycle inhibitors (dashed lines).

necrosis and inflammation compared with agents that affect the cell cycle in a later stage (beyond S phase)[15] (Figure 18.4). Based on the mechanism of action of the biologic compound and its target in the restenotic process, drug-eluting stents may be generally classified as antithrombotic, anti-inflammatory, immunosuppressive, antiproliferative, or pro-healing. Some agents, such as sirolimus, may affect multiple targets in the restenotic process.

Antithrombotic-eluting stents

Platelet aggregation and thrombus formation play a prominent role in the development of restenosis.[4] Antithrombotic pharmacologic approaches to inhibit restenosis, however, have proven ineffective. Nitric oxide (NO) and glycoprotein IIb/IIIa inhibitors have been used as stent coatings, but their efficacy has yet to be demonstrated.[16] Hirudin and iloprost were blended with a polylactic acid polymer and loaded onto a stent. Iloprost was slowly released by the breakdown of the polymer, but hirudin was mainly eluted in the first 24 hours.[17] Decreased neointimal formation was observed in sheep and pig injury models treated with this antithrombotic-eluting stent, but clinical data are still pending.

Anti-inflammatory-eluting stents

Inflammatory cells have been found early after vascular injury. Thus, these cells appeared to be an optimal target in the fight against restenosis. Corticosteroids have long been shown to reduce the influx of mononuclear cells, to inhibit monocyte and macrophage function, and to influence smooth muscle cell proliferation.[18] Nonetheless, clinical trials have failed to demonstrate any benefit of systemic steroid therapy.[19]

Corticosteroid-eluting stents

Experimental studies showed conflicting results of stents coated with steroid agents.[20,21] The STRIDE study was a phase II, multicenter registry conducted in Europe. Stents were immersed on-site in a solution of dexamethasone. Sixty patients with de novo lesions were treated with these dexamethasone-eluting BiodivYsio stents. At 6-month follow-up, angiographic binary restenosis (>50% diameter stenosis at follow-up) was 13.3% and late loss (the difference between the minimal luminal diameter (MLD) post procedure and the MLD at follow-up) was 0.45 mm (de Scheerder I, unpublished data, 2002). Another registry, the DELIVER study, will enroll 30 patients to test the feasibility of dexamethasone-eluting stents (average dose of 0.27 $\mu g/mm^2$ of stent) for the treatment of small coronary arteries. A dose-finding, multicenter study using the BiodivYsio stent preloaded with dexamethasone is currently ongoing in Germany.

Tranilast-eluting stent

Tranilast, N-(3,4-dimethoxycinnamoyl)anthranilic acid, has been shown to inhibit the proliferation and migration of vascular smooth muscle cells in experimental models. The systemic use of this agent for the prevention of restenosis was tested in a large multicenter trial, but the results were disappointing.[22] Initial experiments with the biodegradable Igaki–Tamai stent loaded with 184 μg of tranilast per stent have been initiated, but results are still pending.

Immunosuppressive-eluting stents

Encouraged by the early experience with ionizing radiation therapy, researchers have proposed sophisticated pharmacologic strategies interfering with cell cycle division.[15] Xenobiotic molecules (rapamycin, FK506, cyclosporine, and analogues) and antimetabolites (mycophenolate mofetil) have been utilized.

Sirolimus-eluting stents

Sirolimus is a macrolide antibiotic with potent antifungal, immunosuppressive, and antimitotic properties.[23] Sirolimus was discovered during an expedition to Easter Island in the South Pacific in 1975. The drug is produced by *Streptomyces hygroscopicus* in culture, and was initially named rapamycin after Rapa Mui, the native name of the island. Sirolimus (Rapamune) was approved by the US Food and Drug Administration (FDA) for the prophylaxis of renal transplant rejection in 1999. Shortly following this approval, the first sirolimus-eluting stents were implanted in human coronary arteries.[24]

The sirolimus-eluting stent is composed of a tubular stainless steel stent, the BX Velocity stent (Cordis, Warren, NJ), coated with a 5 μm thick layer of non-erodable polymer blended with sirolimus in a concentration of 140 μg sirolimus/cm^2 of stent.[12] The release kinetics can be modulated in such a way that both fast-release ($<$15-day drug release) and slow-release ($\geq$ 28-day drug release) formulations are obtained. Only slow-release formulations were tested in randomized studies and consequently became commercially available. In vivo studies demonstrated that sirolimus levels in whole blood peaked at 1 hour (0.9 $\pm$

0.2 ng/ml) after stent implantation and fell below the lower limit of quantification by 72 hours (0.4 ng/ml).[25]

Sirolimus binds to specific cytosolic proteins. The mechanism of action of sirolimus is distinct from that of other immunosuppressive agents, which act solely by inhibiting DNA synthesis. Upregulation of FK506-binding protein 12 (FKBP12) has been observed in human neointimal smooth muscle cells The sirolimus : FKBP complex binds to a specific cell cycle regulatory protein, mTOR (mammalian target of rapamycin) and inhibits its activation. Inhibition of mTOR ultimately induces cell cycle arrest in late G_1 phase,[15,23] and consequently arrests smooth muscle cell growth.

The first clinical experience with a sirolimus-eluting stent, the FIM ('First-In-Man') trial, was initiated in 1999 and involved 45 patients with native coronary artery disease and angina pectoris.[24,26] Thirty patients were treated in São Paulo, Brazil and 15 patients were treated in Rotterdam, the Netherlands. Two different formulations of sirolimus-eluting stents were used: slow release ($n = 30$) and fast release ($n = 15$). A virtual absence of neointimal proliferation was documented by serial intravascular ultrasound (IVUS) and angiography at all time points (4, 6, 12, and 24 months) in both groups. No stent malapposition, aneurysm formation, or edge effects were seen in this cohort of patients. One patient had target vessel thrombosis at 14 months. There was no in-stent restenosis up to 2 years and the overall major adverse cardiac event (MACE) rate was 11.1%, including procedural complications. No death occurred after hospital discharge.[27] Concerns about potential late complications such as late occlusion, thromboses, late restenosis, has not been confirmed after almost 4 years after stent implantation. This pioneering investigation provides unique long-term data on sirolimus-eluting stents (Figure 18.5), and allays some of the concerns about a potential late 'catch-up' of restenosis or late side-effects.

The RAVEL trial was the first randomized trial to compare slow-release sirolimus-eluting stents with bare BX Velocity stents for revascularization of single, de novo lesions in native coronary arteries.[28] The trial included 238 patients at 19 medical centers in Europe and Latin America. The primary end point was in-stent late luminal loss. Patients received clopidogrel or ticlopidine for 2 months. In-stent late loss was significantly lower in the sirolimus-stent group (–0.01 mm) than in the standard-stent group (0.80 mm, $p < 0.001$). None of the patients in the sirolimus-stent group had binary restenosis, and the incidence of MACE was 5.8% in the sirolimus-stent group after 1 year. Importantly, no episodes of stent thrombosis occurred. This study uniquely reported zero percent restenosis after coronary stenting, substantiating the striking results of the FIM study. The CYPHER stent, BX-Velocity sirolimus-eluting stent, is currently approved for clinical use in Europe.

Data have recently been presented from the SIRIUS trial, a US multicenter, randomized, double-blind study of a sirolimus-eluting stent in de novo native coronary

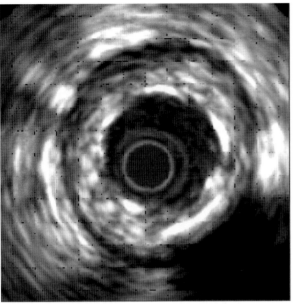

a

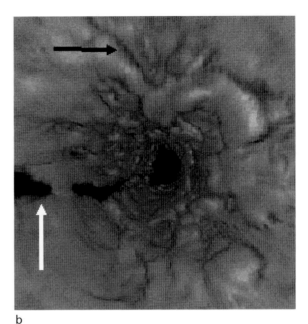

b

Figure 18.5

Intravascular ultrasound (IVUS) planar (a) and 'endoscopic' (reconstructed from 3D-IVUS) (b) visualization of a sirolimus-coated stent 1 year after implantation in a human coronary artery. Almost complete absence of neointimal hyperplasia is noted in both views. Black arrow indicates stent struts in black (negative image), and white arrow indicates the shadow of the metallic wire.

lesions.[29] Patients ($n = 1100$) with de novo coronary disease were randomized to receive slow-release sirolimus-eluting stents or bare BX Velocity stents at 53 sites. The inclusion criteria were more liberal than in the previous studies and allowed the implantation of more than one stent per lesion, which could vary from 15 to 30 mm in length. The primary endpoint was target vessel failure (TVF), which included cardiac death, myocardial infarction (MI), or target vessel revascularization (TVR) at 9-month follow-up. Multiple stents were implanted in 27.4% of patients (a mean of 1.4 stents per patient). In-stent late loss was 0.17 mm and in-lesion late loss was 0.25 mm. After 9 months, 10.5% of the patients receiving the Cypher stent reached the primary endpoint of TVF as compared with 19.5% in the control group. In the sirolimus group, the in-stent restenosis rate was 2.0% and the in-lesion restenosis rate was 9.1%. This large-scale randomized trial confirmed the potent anti-restenosis effects of Cypher stents. The FDA approved the clinical use of Cypher stent in April 2003.

The European–Canadian SIRIUS (EC-SIRIUS) trial randomized 350 patients with similar baseline characteristics to the US SIRIUS study. The 8-month angiographic results were similar to SIRIUS (Table 18.2).

In-stent restenosis studies

The In-Stent Restenosis Registry involved 41 patients treated in Brazil ($n = 25$) and the Netherlands ($n = 16$). This was an open-label safety study involving only patients with single vessel in-stent restenotic lesions. The protocol allowed the implantation of up to two Cypher stents. In the Brazilian cohort, all vessels were patent at the time of 12-month follow-up angiography.[30] Late loss averaged 0.36±0.46 mm in-stent and 0.16±0.42 mm in-lesion. One of the 25 patients developed in-stent restenosis at 1-year follow-up. There were no deaths, stent thromboses, or repeat revascularizations. The Rotterdam cohort included a more complex group of patients. In this group, 19% of the patients had previous brachytherapy failure, and one heart transplant patient was treated. There were two deaths, one late thrombosis, one vessel occlusion, and two in-lesion restenoses.

Complex scenarios

In the USA, the FDA approved the SECURE (compassionate use of sirolimus-eluting stents) protocol for patients with in-stent restenosis who have failed other approved therapies, such as radiation therapy and coronary artery bypass surgery (CABG). This registry is being conducted at five US sites and has enrolled 250 patients. SECURE data will provide unique information on the applicability of the Cypher stent in highly complex situations.

In ARTS-2 (Arterial Revascularization Therapies Study-2), sirolimus-eluting stent will be used to treat multivessel coronary disease. In the USA, another randomized trial comparing CABG and Cypher stents (the FREEDOM trial) in diabetic patients with multivessel coronary disease has been planned.

Sirolimus derivative-eluting stents

Everolimus (40-O-(2-hydroxyethyl)rapamycin) is also an inhibitor of mTOR. It has been shown to inhibit the proliferation of hematopoietic and nonhematopoietic cells. Although the immunosuppressive activity of everolimus is two- to threefold lower than sirolimus in vitro, animal studies have shown a potent anti-restenosis effect of everolimus given orally or via a drug-eluting stent.[31] The S-Stent (Biosensor) has been impregnated with a blend of everolimus and slowly biodegradable hydroxyacid polylactic acid polymer. Low-dose (186 μm per stent) and high-dose (360 μm per stent) everolimus-eluting stents were implanted in pig coronary arteries. Preliminary data showed a reduction of neointimal hyperplasia in the everolimus group as compared with control (Honda H, unpublished data, 2002).

The FUTURE (First Use To Underscore Reduction in Restenosis with Everolimus) study completed enrollment of 36 patients in July 2002. The study tested the safety of the Challenge stent, an everolimus-eluting stent, in de novo coronary lesions. There was no in-stent restenosis and only 0.10 mm late loss at 6-month follow-up, suggesting the potential of this new DES to prevent restenosis. The FUTURE II study has started in three German sites, and will randomize 90 patients with de novo lesions, treated either with eluting or bare stents.

ABT-578 (methylrapamycin) is another synthetic derivative of sirolimus. Preliminary animal studies have shown significant inhibition of intimal proliferation after stenting. The BiodivYsio stent has been loaded with ABT-578, and clinical studies have been initiated in Australia. A US multicenter randomized study (PREFER) will compare the ABT-578-eluting stent versus the standard BiodivYsio stent in 950 patients with de novo coronary lesions (Kuntz R, unpublished data, 2002). The ENDEAVOR trial tested the DRIVER, cobalt alloy stent coated with PC and ABT-578 in 100 patients in New Zealand and Australia. Initial 4-month data (Meredith I, unpublished data, 2003) showed 2.1% restenosis and 0.33 mm of late loss, which suggest the potential of this technology to prevent restenosis.

FK506 (tacrolimus)

Tacrolimus is a hydrophobic immunosuppressive agent that has been used clinically to prevent renal transplant rejection. It binds to the FKBP12 protein, but its mechanism of action differs from that of sirolimus.[32]

The EVIDENT registry will include 15 patients with saphenous vein graft disease treated with tacrolimus-eluting stent grafts.

In the PRESENT study, 30 patients with de novo lesions will be treated with a novel eluting stent design. In this study, nanoporous ceramic-coated stents (Jomed) loaded with tacrolimus will be utilized.

Cyclosporine-eluting stents

Cyclosporine is a calcineurin suppressor that has long been used as an immunosuppressive agent to prevent transplant rejection and to treat autoimmune diseases. Cyclosporine has inhibitory effects on T-cell activation, but its inhibitory effect on smooth muscle cells proliferation is controversial.[33,34] The R Stent, a stainless steel double-helix stent approved for clinical use in several countries, has been coated with a 7–12 μm slowly bioerodable polymer loaded with cyclosporine. These cyclosporine-eluting stents have been utilized in a porcine model. Preliminary data showed a 40% reduction in late loss but no significant reduction in neointimal thickness by morphometry (van der Giessen WJ, personal communication, 2002).

Mycophenolic acid-eluting stent

Mycophenolic acid (MPA) is the active metabolite of mycophenolate mofetil. It has been used clinically for prophylaxis of renal and heart transplant rejection. The Duraflex stent (Avantec Vascular Devices) is a tubular stainless steel stent that has been available in Europe since 2001. This stent, coated with a 5 μm layer of polyhydrocarbon polymer loaded with MPA, was tested in the IMPACT trial. This study included 150 patients with de novo coronary lesions. Slow-release (45 days) and fast-release (15 days) eluting stents coated with 4.5 μm of MPA per square millimeter were compared with bare Duraflex stents. Preliminary results suggest no differences in angiographic outcomes between groups, but final data are still pending.

Antiproliferative-eluting stents

A number of antineoplastic agents have been considered for the prevention of restenosis. Paclitaxel and its derivatives have been the most widely investigated compounds of this group.

Paclitaxel-eluting stents

Paclitaxel (Taxol) is a microtubule-stabilizing agent with potent antitumor activity,[35] which was originally isolated from the bark of the Pacific yew tree (Taxus brevifolia).

Many different platforms using polymer coating or surface modifications to adhere paclitaxel onto stents have been utilized over the past few years.

Unlike other antimitotic agents, paclitaxel shifts the cytoskeletal equilibrium towards assembly, leading to reduced vascular cell proliferation, migration, and signal transduction.[36] Paclitaxel is highly lipophilic, resulting in a rapid cellular uptake and a long-lasting effect in the cell.[8]

Paclitaxel-coated stents showed a marked reduction in neointimal and medial cell proliferation in pig coronary arteries at different time points (7, 28, 56, and 180 days).[13] However, arteries treated with paclitaxel showed incomplete healing, late persistence of a large number of macrophages, and fibrin deposition. Similar findings were observed with a stent platform coated with crosslinked biodegradable polymer (chondroitin sulfate and gelatin) and 42.0, 20.2, 8.6, or 1.5 μg of paclitaxel in rabbit iliac arteries.[37] Incomplete healing and increased inflammation were observed for the higher-dose paclitaxel-eluting stents.[37,38] These studies suggest the need for a more controlled drug release due to the narrow toxic–therapeutic window and high hydrophobic character of paclitaxel. The QuaDS drug-eluting stent (Quanam Medical Corp) is a slotted 316-L stainless steel tube with 50% of its surface area covered by multiple nonbiodegradable polyacrylate sleeves that release 7-hexanoylpaclitaxel (QP2 or taxane). Taxane is a less hydrophobic paclitaxel derivative. Approximately 800 μg of the drug was loaded per 2.4 mm of sleeve length, such that 13 mm-long stents have a total drug dose of 2400 μg and 17 mm-long stents contain 3200 μg of taxane.[39] These were the first drug-eluting stents implanted in human coronary arteries. This registry enrolled 26 patients randomly assigned to receive drug-loaded stents (n = 13; 14 stents) or bare stents (n = 13; 18 stents). At 18-month follow-up, there was no binary restenosis in the drug-eluting group. A fivefold decrease in neointimal proliferation was detected by IVUS in the paclitaxel group. None of the patients treated with QP2-eluting stents had any cardiac events.

The SCORE trial was a randomized study conducted in 15 sites in Europe to test the effectiveness of the QuaDs-QP2 stent.[40] The trial was interrupted prematurely after the enrollment of 266 patients because of a high incidence of stent thrombosis (9.4%) and myocardial infarction (14.5%) in the eluting-stent group. These clinical events were probably related to poor stent design and extremely high concentrations of taxane. The QuaDS-QP2 stent was further evaluated in 15 consecutive patients with in-stent restenosis Combined antiplatelet therapy with aspirin (at least 100 mg/day) and ticlopidine 500 mg/day (or clopidogrel 75 mg/day) was continued for at least 6 months.[41] Restenosis occurred in two lesions (13.3%) at 6 months and eight lesions (61.5%) at 12 months, suggesting a late catch-up of restenosis.[38]

A series of clinical trials (TAXUS I–VII) have been designed to test the feasibility and effectiveness of polymer-based paclitaxel-eluting stents in a variety of clinical settings.

The TAXUS I study evaluated the safety of the slow-release polymer-coated NIRx Conformer stent loaded with 85 μg of paclitaxel (1.0 μg/mm²). About 80% of the drug is released within the first 1–3 days. Sixty-one patients with short (<15 mm) de novo coronary lesions were randomized to either drug-eluting or bare stents. The 6-month MACE rate was 0% in the treatment arm compared with 7% in the control group. The in-stent late loss was 0.36 mm in the drug-eluting stent group versus 0.71 mm in control group (Grube E, unpublished data, 2001). At 1 year, the MACE rate was 3% in the eluting-stent group versus 10% in the uncoated-stent group (Silber S, unpublished data, 2002). There were no reports of death, stent thrombosis, target lesion revascularization (TLR), or binary restenosis in the drug-eluting group.

TAXUS II, a randomized multicenter trial, tested the efficacy of two formulations of the paclitaxel-eluting NIRx Conformer stent to treat patients with short de novo coronary lesions. The study included 536 patients divided into four groups: 267 treated with either bare (n = 136) or slow-release (n = 131) eluting stents, and 269 treated with bare (n = 134) or moderate-release eluting stents (n = 135). All cohorts were treated with a 15 mm NIRx Conformer stent. All eluting stents were coated with the Translute polymer loaded with 1 μg of paclitaxel per square millimeter. Clopidogrel (75 mg qid) was administered for 6 months. The primary endpoint was percentage in-stent volume neointimal hyperplasia (by IVUS) at 6 months. The binary in-stent restenosis rates were 2.3% for slow release and 4.7% for moderate release, versus 17.9% and 20.2% in the control groups, respectively. The late loss was 0.31 mm for slow release and 0.30 mm for moderate release in the eluting-stent groups. The percentage neointimal hyperplasia volume was markedly reduced in the eluting groups (7.85% for slow release and 7.84% for moderate release) versus control (23.17% and 20.54%, respectively). There were no late stent thromboses or aneurysms. This randomized study established the 6-month safety and efficacy of both formulations of polymer-based paclitaxel in patients with de novo lesions.[42]

TAXUS IV and TAXUS V are large randomized US trials testing the efficacy of moderate-release paclitaxel-eluting Express stents in patients with de novo lesions. TAXUS IV included 1326 patients with de novo coronary lesions varying from 10 or 28 mm in length, treated with a single stent. Stones et al presented the 1-year data of the TAXUS IV trial at the American Heart Association meeting in Orlando, 2003. The data show a sustained benefit of paclitaxel-eluting stents up to 1 year. No further deaths or MI events were observed in paclitaxel-treated patients between 9 and 12 months, while 1 patient died and 7 had a myocardial infarction in the bare stent group. After 1 year of follow-up, patients treated with paclitaxel stents had significantly less target vessel revascularization (6.8% vs 16.7%; p < 0.01) and combined event rates (10.6% vs 19.8%; p < 0.01. TAXUS V will include a more complex population with longer lesions (up to 40 mm) and will allow the implantation of multiple moderate-release stents. TAXUS VI is the European counterpart of the TAXUS V trial. Results are expected in 2003.

TAXUS III was a feasibility study utilizing a short-release paclitaxel-eluting NIRx Conformer platform for the treatment of patients with in-stent restenosis, and was conducted at two sites in Europe, enrolling 30 patients. The protocol allowed the implantation of up to two (15 mm) eluting stents. The in-stent late loss averaged 0.44 mm after 6 months. The overall binary restenosis rate was 16% (4/25), but two restenoses occurred at the gap between eluting stents and another within a bare stent implanted adjacent to the eluting-stent. There were no deaths, and repeat revascularizations occurred in 21.4% of the patients (Tanabe K, unpublished data, 2002).

The European ELUTES study compared the V-Flex stent loaded with four different doses of paclitaxel (0.2, 0.7, 1.4, and 2.7 μg/mm^2) versus bare metal stents for the treatment of de novo coronary lesions. Stents were directly impregnated with paclitaxel without a polymer. Patients ($n = 180$) were randomized evenly among the five groups. A dose-dependent effect on in-stent late loss was observed: 0.1 mm in the high-dose group, 0.47 and 0.5 mm in the intermediate-dose groups, and 0.7 mm in both low-dose and control groups. The binary restenosis rate was 3.1% in the high-dose group. The 1-year MACE rates were similar between groups. Thee were no reports of deaths or stent thromboses (de Scheerder I, unpublished data, 2002).

The In-Stent ELUTES study is a European trial comparing two doses of paclitaxel-eluting V-Flex Plus PTX stent with conventional non-radiation treatment for in-stent restenosis. A total of 600 patients will be enrolled in the study, starting in 20 European sites.

The Asian Paclitaxel-Eluting Clinical Trial (ASPECT) is a randomized study compared Supra-G stents directly impregnated with two different doses of paclitaxel (1.3 and 3.1 μg/mm^2) versus bare metal stents. Patients ($n = 180$) with de novo coronary lesions were treated with single stents. Antiplatelet therapy was administered for 6 months. In 37 patients, cilostazol was used in place of clopidogrel or ticlopidine. The neointimal hyperplasia volumes were 12, 18, and 31 mm^3, and restenosis rates were 4%, 12%, and 27% for the high-dose, low-dose, and control groups, respectively. Overall, the 1-year MACE and target lesion revascularization rates were similar among all groups. However, 4 of the 12 patients receiving the high-dose eluting stents, who were also receiving cilostazol, had stent thromboses (Park SJ, unpublished data, 2002).

The PATENCY study compared Logic PTX paclitaxel-eluting stents (2.0 μg/mm^2) with bare stents in de novo coronary lesions. A total of 50 patients were enrolled in two US sites. Clopidogrel was administered for 3 months. There were no stent thromboses up to 9 months, but restenosis rates were similar in the two groups (38% in the eluting-stent group and 35% in the control arm) (Heldman A, unpublished data, 2002).

The DELIVER randomized study compared Multilink Penta stents directly impregnated with 3 μg/mm^2 of paclitaxel using surface modification with bare stents. Patients with de novo coronary lesions ($n = 1043$) were enrolled in 50 US sites. The primary endpoint is TVF at 9 months. This study demonstrated the lack of anti-restenosis effect of non-polymeric paclitaxel eluting stents. Late loss was 0.81 mm and 15% of patients had restenosis.

DELIVER-2 will evaluate the Achieve stent, a paclitaxel-eluting Multilink Penta, in a higher-risk subset, including patients with bifurcation and in-stent restenotic lesions. The study will enroll 1500 patients at 83 sites.

Angiopeptin-eluting stents

Somatostatin, an angiopeptin analogue, has been shown to reduce tissue response to several growth factors, including platelet-derived growth factor (PDGF), basic fibroblast growth factor (bFGF), and insulin-like growth factors (IGF). In humans, systemic administration of angiopeptin has improved the clinical outcome after angioplasty, but showed no effect on restenosis.[43] Angiopeptin-loaded PC-coated BiodivYsio stents decreased neointimal proliferation compared with bare stents in pig coronary models.[42]

SWAN, an open-label registry, tested the feasibility and safety of angiopeptin-eluting BiodivYsio stents in 13 patients with coronary de novo lesions. Thirteen stents were loaded with 22 μg of angiopeptin, and 1 stent was loaded with 126 μg of the drug. There were no in-hospital or 30-day MACE (Kwok OH, unpublished data, 2002). Long-term follow-up data are pending.

Tyrosine kinase inhibitor-eluting stents

Tyrosine kinases are both transmembrane and intracellular protein kinases that are fundamental to a number of extracellular signals that regulate proliferation, differentiation, and specific functions of differentiated cells.[43] PLLA (185 kDa) biodegradable stents loaded with ST638 (0.8 mg), a specific tyrosine kinase inhibitor, were implanted in pig coronary arteries. After 3 weeks, the amount of neointimal proliferation was significantly decreased in the ST638 stents compared with its inactive metabolite (ST494).[44] Clinical studies are still pending.

Actinomycin D-eluting stents

Actinomycin D (dactinomycin) is an anticancer drug that selectively inhibits RNA synthesis. Little information regarding the use of actinomycin D for the prevention of smooth muscle cell proliferation and restenosis is available. The ACTION study was a large randomized trial designed to test the safety, feasibility, and effectiveness of two different doses of actinomycin D-eluting Tetra stents for the treatment of de novo coronary lesions. The study was interrupted prematurely because of a high incidence of repeat revascularization in the treated arms.

c-myc *antisense-eluting stents*

Upregulation of genes such as c-*myc*, which regulates cell division, leads to cellular proliferation. Antisense oligonucleotides have the ability to block critical phases of the smooth muscle cell growth cycle. c-*myc* antisense oligonucleotides have also been shown to inhibit inflammation and extracellular matrix production.[45] However, the first clinical experience using catheter-based local delivery of c-*myc* antisense oligonucleotides was disappointing.[46] In a porcine coronary model, AVI-4126, a specific c-*myc* antisense sequence eluted from a PC-coated stent, prevented c-*myc* expression and decreased neointimal hyperplasia as compared with control.

Extracellular matrix modulators

The extracellular matrix (ECM) constitutes a major component of the restenotic lesion and therefore represents a potential target for anti-restenosis therapy. Matrix metalloproteinases (MMPs), particularly MMP-2 (a 72 kDa type IV collagenase) and MMP-9 (a 92 kDa type IV collagenase), have the ability to digest collagen and facilitate smooth muscle cell migration. Batimastat, a nonspecific MMP inhibitor, and other MMP inhibitors have been shown to inhibit neointimal hyperplasia in animal models.[47,48] BRILLIANT-I was a multicenter registry designed to test the feasibility of a batimastat-eluting BiodivYiso stent to treat de novo coronary lesions in 173 patients. While safety was demonstrated, late loss was 0.88 mm and 21% of the patients developed binary restenosis (de Scheerder I, unpublished data, 2002). Further clinical studies have not yet been planned.

Pro-healing-eluting stents

The promotion of vascular healing seems a more natural and consequently safer approach to the prevention of restenosis. Endothelial denudation and dysfunction is common at the site of endovascular interventions and has been

associated with vessel thrombosis and restenosis.[49] In addition, delayed re-endothelialization has been associated with late side-effects of potent antiproliferative therapies, such as with radiation therapy.[50,51] Endothelial cell seeding has been proposed as the ultimate method to assure immediate stent endothelialization,[52] but cell viability has been a limitation. Stents may be used to attract circulating endothelial cells (CEC). R stents coated with antibodies to CD34 receptors on progenitor CEC have been implanted in pig coronary arteries. Preliminary results suggested the feasibility of capturing endothelial cells in-situ (Kutryk M, unpublished data, 2002). These non-drug-based stents should ultimately promote elution of biologically active substances through a functioning endothelium monolayer. The effects of these ingenious stents on restenosis remains to be demonstrated.

Nitric oxide, vascular endothelial growth factor (VEGF), and 17β-estradiol have all been tested as pro-healing, anti-restenotic agents as well. Local delivery of VEGF to prevent restenosis has been evaluated in animal models,[53] but the results were conflicting.

Estradiol-eluting stents

Estradiol may improve vascular healing, reduce smooth muscle cell migration and proliferation, and promote local angiogenesis.[54] Recently, estradiol-eluting PC-coated stents (Abbott/Biocompatibles) implanted in porcine coronary arteries have reduced neointimal hyperplasia by 40% compared with control stents.[55]

EASTER (Estrogen and Stent to Eliminate Restenosis) was a single-center feasibility study testing 17β-estradiol-eluting BiodivYsio stents in 30 patients with de novo coronary lesions. Stents were loaded on-site by immersion in a solution of estradiol. The average concentration was 2.54 μg/mm² of stent. The late loss was 0.32 mm in-lesion and 0.57 mm in-stent. The IVUS-detected neointimal hyperplasia rate was 23.5%. There were no deaths or stent thromboses, and only one patient underwent repeat revascularization. A second phase of the EASTER study is ongoing in Italy. Patients with de novo coronary lesion are randomized to estradiol-eluting BiodivYsio stents or unloaded stents. Results are still pending.

General clinical considerations

As expected, some drug-eluting stents were effective in animal models but produced disappointing clinical data. Clinical studies investigating paclitaxel-eluting stents provided relevant information on the importance of correct drug dosing and stent design in order to produce a successful drug-eluting stent. In these studies, minimal variations in pharmacologic properties, drug concentration, and stent-coating technologies elicited different vascular reactions and clinical outcomes.

The first wave of drug-eluting stent studies have demonstrated that *not all stents are equal*. Currently, only two drug-eluting stent platforms have proven effective in large randomized trials: sirolimus-eluting stents and polymer-based paclitaxel-eluting stents. A concern about potential late complications, such as late thrombosis and aneurysm formation, associated with drug-eluting stents is a legacy from our previous experience with intracoronary radiation therapy. A high incidence of incomplete stent

apposition was indeed observed in the sirolimus-eluting stent arm of the RAVEL study. Although intriguing, these IVUS findings were not associated with any clinical event up to 1-year follow-up. Late thrombosis and aneurysm formation have not been associated with the use of sirolimus-eluting stents so far. The high incidences of stent thrombosis observed in the early paclitaxel[51] studies have been associated with extremely high drug concentrations, poor stent design (SCORE), and inadequate antiplatelet therapy (ASPECT). No late thrombosis has been reported in the randomized TAXUS-II trial, but patients were taking clopidogrel up to 6-month follow-up.

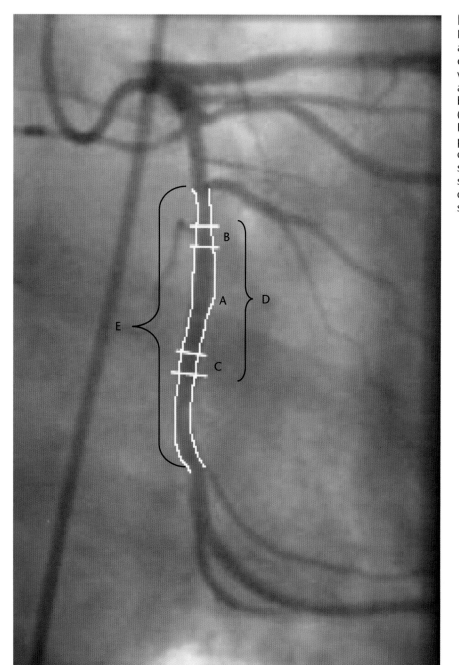

Figure 18.6
Proposed quantitative coronary angiographic methodology for drug-eluting stent trials. A, in-stent, which better describes the antiproliferative effect of the biological agent; B, proximal edge (5 mm); C, distal edge (5 mm); D, in-lesion, which determines potential paradoxical effects of low drug concentrations at traumatized stent edges ('edge effect'); E, in-segment, which is the ultimate determinant of angiographic success from a patient's perspective.

Methodologic considerations

There has been no standard format to analyze and report drug-eluting study findings. Angiographic and clinical data have been compiled at different time points (4, 6, 8, 9, or 12 months). The classical binary restenosis rate is not an appropriate endpoint to determine whether a device had restraining or inhibitory effects on neointimal proliferation, particularly in small clinical studies. Rather, angiographic late lumen loss and neointimal hyperplasia volume detected by IVUS seem to be the best available parameters to evaluate the performance of drug-eluting stents. Especially when testing a novel device, IVUS imaging should become an integral component of clinical investigations, in order to identify arterial wall reactions that would be unappreciated by conventional angiography. IVUS and angiographic analysis should involve both stented and edge segments, commonly defined as the stent plus at least 5 mm proximal and distal to the stent borders (Figure 18.6). Finally, the incidence of late thrombosis (>30 days) and repeat target *vessel* revascularization should be reported among traditional endpoints, given the clinical implications of these events.

Patient selection

Patient selection for drug-eluting stents is an evolving issue. Today, available data from randomized studies

(a)

(b)

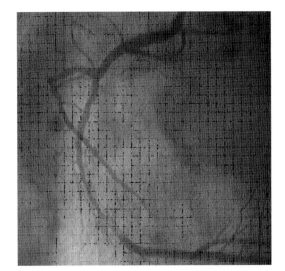

(c)

(d)

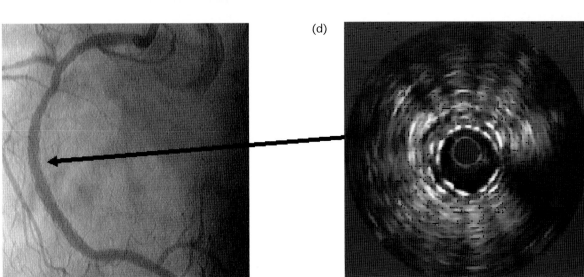

Figure 18.7
Potential future indications for drug-eluting stents. Sequential coronary angiography pre (a), post (b), and at 4-month follow-up (c), and IVUS cross-sectional image (d) showing the absence of intimal hyperplasia at 4 months after implantation of two overlapping Cypher stents for the treatment of diffuse in-stent restenosis.

Table 18.3   Drug-eluting stenting technique

Potential problems	Solutions
Coating disruption	• Careful device handling
	• Perform pre-dilation in tight, calcified stenosis
'Geographic miss' and secondary in lesion restenosis	• Always use a balloon shorter than the stent length for pre- or postdilatation (if required)
	• Complete lesion coverage
	• Avoid mechanical trauma outside the stented segment
	• Avoid gap between stents
	• Appropriate stent size (IVUS guidance), particularly in small vessels and long lesions
	• Appropriate patient selection
Non-target-lesion revascularization	• Appropriate patient selection
Restenosis in adjacent bare metal stents	• If a second stent is required, use another drug-eluting stent[a]

[a] Overlapping may not be safe for all drug-eluting stents.

demonstrate that drug-eluting stents are effective in patients with de novo coronary lesions. Complex anatomy such as diffuse disease, ostial location, bifurcation lesions, and chronic total occlusions have not been included in these randomized studies. However, indications for drug-eluting stents are expected to expand considerably in the near future, while future studies may further broaden clinical indications (Figure 18.7). The financial burden of drug-eluting stents will have a major impact on patient selection. Substantial costs may limit utilization of such devices to patients at high risk for restenosis, in spite of the positive results of clinical trials involving low-risk patients.

The sirolimus experience further illustrates the importance of patient selection. High-risk anatomic features such as diffuse disease, in-stent restenosis, and failed brachytherapy also impact the clinical outcomes of patients treated with drug-eluting stents. Differences in angiographic outcomes between RAVEL and SIRIUS have been attributed to the treatment of a higher-risk population in the US trial. Subanalyses of these studies, however, demonstrated a greater benefit in terms of absolute reduction in restenosis among high-risk patients.

Drug-eluting stent technique

The implantation of drug-eluting stents does not require vast changes in current stenting techniques (Table 18.3). However, diligent stent placement in various plaque morphologies may be more important than ever. The new drug-eluting stents abolish neointimal proliferation within the stent, and any tissue growth in segments adjacent to the stents become unmasked. Thus, operator-related factors such as incomplete lesion coverage, arterial trauma outside the stented segment, and gaps between stents rep-

resent the new face of 'geographic miss' in the drug-eluting stent era, and have been linked to treatment failures.

Overlapping sirolimus-eluting stents appear to be safe, but it is unclear if doubling the drug concentration at the overlapping zone with other drug-eluting stents will have similar profiles. Careful handling of the stent prior to stent deployment should be undertaken to avoid potential disruption of the coating surface. Operator- and technique-related factors will become the ultimate determinants of clinical outcomes. The STELLAR trial investigators will enroll 1500 patients, treated with Cypher stent in 50 US clinical sites. All operators will follow specific criteria for stent deployment, particularly stent sizing, angiographic data acquisition and documentation throughout the procedure. Angiographic data will be transmitted 'on line' to an independent core laboratory, which will prospectively scrutinize whether there was axial or longitudinal geographical miss. Quantitative measurements of the actual size of the largest balloon at maximal inflation pressure will be performed to define proper balloon artery ratio in DES era. Patients will be followed for 12 months in order to define whether SES deployment technique has an impact on acute and late clinical outcomes. Until then, we should follow the Instruction for Use in the stent packages.

References

1. Maier W, Windecker S, Boersma E, et al. Evolution of percutaneous transluminal coronary angioplasty in Europe from 1992–1996. Eur Heart J 2001;22:1733–40.
2. American Heart Association. 2002 Heart and Stroke Statistical Update. Dallas, TX: American Heart Association, 2001.
3. Serruys PW, Strauss BH, van Beusekom HM, et al. Stenting of coronary arteries: Has a modern Pandora's box been opened? J Am Coll Cardiol 1991;17:143B–54B.

4. Costa MA, Foley DP, Serruys PW. Restenosis: The problem and how to deal with it. In: (Grech ED, Ramsdale DR, eds) Practical Interventional Cardiology, 2nd edn. London: Martin Dunitz, 2002:279–94.

5. Lincoff AM, Topol EJ, Ellis SG. Local drug delivery for the prevention of restenosis. Fact, fancy, and future. Circulation 1994;90:2070–84.

6. Ratner BD. The blood compatibility catastrophe. J Biomed Mater Res 1993;27:283–7.

7. Hwang CW, Edelman ER. Arterial ultrastructure influences transport of locally delivered drugs. Circ Res 2002; 90:826–32.

8. Hwang CW, Wu D, Edelman ER. Physiological transport forces govern drug distribution for stent-based delivery. Circulation 2001;104:600–5.

9. van der Giessen WJ, Lincoff AM, Schwartz RS, et al. Marked inflammatory sequelae to implantation of biodegradable and nonbiodegradable polymers in porcine coronary arteries. Circulation 1996;94:1690–7.

10. Whelan DM, van Beusekom HM, van der Giessen WJ. Mechanisms of drug loading and release kinetics. Semin Interv Cardiol 1998;3:127–31.

11. Costa MA. Drug-coated Stents for restenosis. In: Restenosis: A Therapeutic Guide (Faxon DP, ed). London: Martin Dunitz, 2001:113–29.

12. Suzuki T, Kopia G, Hayashi S, et al. Stent-based delivery of sirolimus reduces neointimal formation in a porcine coronary model. Circulation 2001;104:1188–93.

13. Drachman DE, Edelman ER, Seifert P, et al. Neointimal thickening after stent delivery of paclitaxel: change in composition and arrest of growth over six months. J Am Coll Cardiol 2000;36:2325–32.

14. Lovich MA, Creel C, Hong K, et al. Carrier proteins determine local pharmacokinetics and arterial distribution of paclitaxel. J Pharm Sci 2001;90:1324–35.

15. Braun-Dullaeus RC, Mann MJ, Dzau VJ. Cell cycle progression: new therapeutic target for vascular proliferative disease. Circulation 1998;98:82–9.

16. Aggarwal RK, Ireland DC, Azrin MA, et al. Antithrombotic potential of polymer-coated stents eluting platelet glycoprotein IIb/IIIa receptor antibody. Circulation 1996; 94:3311–17.

17. Alt E, Haehnel I, Beilharz C, et al. Inhibition of neointima formation after experimental coronary artery stenting: a new biodegradable stent coating releasing hirudin and the prostacyclin analogue iloprost. Circulation 2000;101:1453–8.

18. Berk BC, Gordon JB, Alexander RW. Pharmacologic roles of heparin and glucocorticoids to prevent restenosis after coronary angioplasty. J Am Coll Cardiol 1991;17:111B–17B.

19. Pepine CJ, Hirshfeld JW, Macdonald RG, et al. A controlled trial of corticosteroids to prevent restenosis after coronary angioplasty. M-HEART Group. Circulation 1990; 81:1753–61.

20. de Scheerder I, Wang K, Wilczek K, et al. Local methylprednisolone inhibition of foreign body response to coated intracoronary stents. Coron Artery Dis 1996;7:161–6.

21. Lincoff AM, Furst JG, Ellis SG, et al. Sustained local delivery of dexamethasone by a novel intravascular eluting stent to prevent restenosis in the porcine coronary injury model. J Am Coll Cardiol 1997;29:808–16.

22. Holmes DR, Jr., Savage M, LaBlanche JM, et al. Results of Prevention of REStenosis with Tranilast and its Outcomes (PRESTO) trial. Circulation 2002;106:1243–50.

23. Marx SO, Marks AR. Bench to bedside: the development of rapamycin and its application to stent restenosis. Circulation 2001;104:852–5.

24. Sousa JE, Costa MA, Abizaid A, et al. Lack of neointimal proliferation after implantation of sirolimus-coated stents in human coronary arteries: a quantitative coronary angiography and three-dimensional intravascular ultrasound study. Circulation 2001;103:192–5.

25. Klugherz BD, Llanos G, Lieuallen W, et al. Twenty-eight-day efficacy and phamacokinetics of the sirolimus-eluting stent. Coron Artery Dis 2002;13:183–8.

26. Sousa JE, Costa MA, Abizaid AC, et al. Sustained suppression of neointimal proliferation by sirolimus-eluting stents: one-year angiographic and intravascular ultrasound followup. Circulation 2001;104:2007–11.

27. Sousa JE, Costa MA, Abizaid A, et al. Two-year angiographic and intravascular ultrasound follow-up after implantation of sirolimus-eluting stents in human coronary arteries. Circulation 2003;107:381–3.

28. Morice MC, Serruys PW, Sousa JE, et al. A randomized comparison of a sirolimus-eluting stent with a standard stent for coronary revascularization. N Engl J Med 2002; 346:1773–80.

29. Moses JW, Leon MB, Popma JJ, et al. Sirolimus-eluting stents versus standard stents in patients with stenosis in a native coronary artery. N Engl J Med 2003;349:1315–23.

30. Sousa JE, Costa MA, Abizaid A, et al. Sirolimus-eluting stent for the treatment of in-stent restenosis. A quantitative coronary angiography and three-dimensional intravascular ultrasound study. Circulation 2003;107:24–7.

31. Farb A, John M, Acampado E, et al. Oral everolimus inhibits in-stent neointimal growth. Circulation 2002;106:2379–84.

32. Marx SO, Jayaraman T, Go LO, et al. Rapamycin-FKBP inhibits cell cycle regulators of proliferation in vascular smooth muscle cells. Circ Res 1995;76:412–17.

33. Jonasson L, Holm J, Hansson GK. Cyclosporin A inhibits smooth muscle proliferation in the vascular response to injury. Proc Natl Acad Sci USA 1988;85:2303–6.

34. Gregory CR, Pratt RE, Huie P, et al. Effects of treatment with cyclosporine, FK 506, rapamycin, mycophenolic acid, or deoxyspergualin on vascular muscle proliferation in vitro and in vivo. Transplant Proc 1993;25:770–1.

35. Rowinsky EK, Donehower RC. Paclitaxel (Taxol). N Engl J Med 1995;332:1004–14.

36. Sollott SJ, Cheng L, Pauly RR, et al. Taxol inhibits neointimal smooth muscle cell accumulation after angioplasty in the rat. J Clin Invest 1995;95:1869–76.

37. Farb A, Heller PF, Shroff S, et al. Pathological analysis of local delivery of paclitaxel via a polymer-coated stent. Circulation 2001;104:473–9.

38. Virmani R, Liistro F, Stankovic G, et al. Mechanism of late instent restenosis after implantation of a paclitaxel derivateeluting polymer stent system in humans. Circulation 2002;106:2649–51.

39. Honda Y, Grube E, de La Fuente LM, et al. Novel drugdelivery stent: intravascular ultrasound observations from the first human experience with the QP2-eluting polymer stent system. Circulation 2001;104:380–3.

40. Kataoka T, Grube E, Honda Y, et al. 7-Hexanoyltaxol-eluting stent for prevention of neointimal growth: an intravascular ultrasound analysis from the Study to COmpare REstenosis rate between QueST and QuaDS-QP2 (SCORE). Circulation 2002;106:1788–93.

41. Liistro F, Stankovic G, Di Mario C, et al. First clinical experience with a paclitaxel derivate-eluting polymer stent system implantation for in-stent restenosis: immediate and long-term clinical and angiographic outcome. Circulation 2002;105:1883–6.

42. Colombo A, Drzewiecki J, Banning A, et al. Randomized study to assess the effectiveness of slow- and moderate-release polymer-based paclitaxel-eluting stents for coronary artery lesions. Circulation 2003;108:788–94.

43. Serruys PW. Long-term effects of angiopeptin treatment in coronary angioplasty: reduction of clinical events but not angiographic restenosis. Circulation 1995;92:2759–60.

44. Armstrong J, Gunn J, Arnold N, et al. Angiopeptin-eluting stents: observations in human vessels and pig coronary arteries. J Invasive Cardiol 2002;14:230–8.

45. Bilder G, Wentz T, Leadley R, et al. Restenosis following angioplasty in the swine coronary artery is inhibited by an orally active PDGF-receptor tyrosine kinase inhibitor, RPR101511A. Circulation 1999;99:3292–9.

46. Yamawaki T, Shimokawa H, Kozai T, et al. Intramural delivery of a specific tyrosine kinase inhibitor with biodegradable stent suppresses the restenotic changes of the coronary artery in pigs in vivo. J Am Coll Cardiol 1998;32:780–6.

47. Kipshidze NN, Kim HS, Iversen P, et al. Intramural coronary delivery of advanced antisense oligonucleotides reduces neointimal formation in the porcine stent restenosis model. J Am Coll Cardiol 2002;39:1686–91.

48. Kutryk MJ, Foley DP, van den Brand M, et al. Local intracoronary administration of antisense oligonucleotide against c-myc for the prevention of in-stent restenosis: results of the randomized investigation by the Thoraxcenter of antisense DNA using local delivery and IVUS after coronary stenting (ITALICS) trial. J Am Coll Cardiol 2002;39:281–7.

49. Li C, Cantor WJ, Nili N, et al. Arterial repair after stenting and the effects of GM6001, a matrix metalloproteinase inhibitor. J Am Coll Cardiol 2002;39:1852–8.

50. Lovdahl C, Thyberg J, Hultgardh-Nilsson A. The synthetic metalloproteinase inhibitor batimastat suppresses injury-induced phosphorylation of MAP kinase ERK1/ERK2 and phenotypic modification of arterial smooth muscle cells in vitro. J Vasc Res 2000;37:345–54.

51. Van Belle E, Tio FO, Couffinhal T, et al. Stent endothelialization. Time course, impact of local catheter delivery, feasibility of recombinant protein administration, and response to cytokine expedition. Circulation 1997;95:438–48.

52. Costa MA, Sabate M, van der Giessen WJ, et al. Late coronary occlusion after intracoronary brachytherapy. Circulation 1999;100:789–92.

53. Liistro F, Colombo A. Late acute thrombosis after paclitaxel eluting stent implantation. Heart 2001;86:262–4.

54. Rogers C, Parikh S, Seifert P, et al. Endogenous cell seeding. Remnant endothelium after stenting enhances vascular repair. Circulation 1996;94:2909–14.

55. Van Belle E, Perie M, Braune D, et al. Effects of coronary stenting on vessel patency and long-term clinical outcome after percutaneous coronary revascularization in diabetic patients. J Am Coll Cardiol 2002;40:410–17.

56. Geraldes P, Sirois MG, Bernatchez PN, et al. Estrogen regulation of endothelial and smooth muscle cell migration and proliferation: role of p38 and p42/44 mitogen-activated protein kinase. Arterioscler Thromb Vasc Biol 2002; 22:1585–90.

57. New G, Moses JW, Roubin GS, et al. Estrogen-eluting, phosphorylcholine-coated stent implantation is associated with reduced neointimal formation but no delay in vascular repair in a porcine coronary model. Cathet Cardiovasc Interv 2002;57:266–71.

19

Intravascular ultrasound

Dominick J Angiolillo, Fernando Alfonso

Introduction

Intravascular ultrasound (IVUS) is a tomographic technique with the ability to provide a direct and comprehensive visualization of atherosclerotic plaque and residual coronary lumen in vivo.[1-4] In addition, the echogenic characteristics of the plaque may be used as a surrogate to determine its underlying histology.[3] This information has represented a major advancement in our understanding of coronary artery disease, a disease of the vessel wall.[1-4] Until very recently, selective coronary angiography was the only available technique to study coronary anatomy in patients. Lumen stenoses are readily detected by angiography, a technique well suited for depicting the coronary lumen silhouette as a shadowgram image.[1-5] Comparing the minimal lumen diameter of the target lesion with the adjacent angiographically normal reference segment provides a valid measurement of relative lumen narrowing. This, in turn, has been classically considered a valid surrogate of stenosis severity. Angiography provides a rough estimation of the physiologic implications of coronary lesions, but fails to provide critical anatomic insights to predict lesion-related flow limitations.[5-8] However, nowadays the limitations of conventional angiography are well known.[5-7] In addition, despite complete and exhaustive angiographic examination, we often encounter lesions that elude accurate characterization. The paradigm of considering coronary angiography as the 'gold standard' for the diagnosis of coronary artery disease has been critically challenged.[1-7] This is relevant because our previous preoccupation with 'coronary luminology'[5] has recently turned into concerns on how to gauge precise physiologic insights, a critical issue in decisions concerning coronary interventions.[8]

IVUS studies have confirmed previous anatomopathologic observations suggesting that angiography underestimates the extent and severity of coronary artery disease.[1-4] The angiographically normal reference segment is universally involved in the atheromatous process and most lesions exhibit positive remodeling, explaining the underestimation of lesion severity by angiography.[1-4]

In this chapter, we will review the basic physical and technical principles of IVUS, the rationale for use of IVUS, the interpretation and measurements of images, diagnostic applications, and applications during coronary interventions.

Physical and technical principles of intravascular ultrasound

Physical principles

Medical ultrasound images are produced by passing an electrical current through a piezoelectric (pressure–electric) crystal that expands and contracts to produce sound waves when electrically excited.[9] Sound waves are reflected by tissue, with part of the ultrasound energy returning to the transducer, which produces an electrical impulse that is converted into an image. After leaving the transducer, the beam remains parallel for a short distance ('near field') and then begins to diverge ('far field'). Ultrasound images are of greater quality in the near field because the beam is narrower and more parallel, the resolution greater, and the characteristic backscatter (reflection of ultrasound energy) from a given tissue more accurate. The length of the near field is expressed by the equation $L = r^2/\lambda$, where L is the length of the near field, r is the radius of the transducer, and λ is the wavelength. Therefore, larger transducers with lower frequencies (longer wavelength) are used for examination of large vessels.

Image quality can be described by two important factors: spatial resolution and contrast resolution. Spatial resolution is defined as the ability to discriminate small objects within the ultrasound image and presents two principal directions: axial (parallel to the beam, primarily a function of wavelength) and lateral (perpendicular to the beam, a function of wavelength and transducer size, or aperture). For a 20–40 MHz IVUS transducer, the typical resolution is 80 μm axially and 200–250 μm laterally. Contrast resolution is the distribution of the gray scale of the reflected signal and is often referred to as dynamic range. An image of low dynamic range appears as black and white with a few in-between gray scale levels; images at high dynamic range are often softer, with preserved subtleties in the image presentation.

As an ultrasound pulse encounters a boundary between two tissues (e.g. fat and muscle), the beam will be partially reflected and partially transmitted. The degree of reflection depends on the difference between the mechanical impedances of the two materials. For instance, imaging of highly calcified structures is associated with acoustic shadowing: nearly complete reflection of the signal at the soft tissue–calcium interface. As the wave passes through many tissue interfaces, the energy is reduced (attenuation). Attenuation is a function of the tissue characteristics, the scattering of energy by small objects, and the absorption by tissue. Thus, only a small percentage of the emitted signal returns to the transducer. The received signal is converted to electrical energy and sent to an external signal processing system for amplification, filtering, scan-conversion, user-controlled modification, and, finally, graphic presentation.

Equipment and technique for IVUS imaging

Ultrasound catheters

The equipment required to perform IVUS consists of two major components: (1) a catheter incorporating a miniaturized transducer and (2) a console containing the electronics necessary to reconstruct the image.[10] High ultrasound frequencies are used, typically centered at 20–40 MHz and able to provide excellent resolution. At 30 MHz, the wavelength is 50 μm, yielding a practical axial resolution of approximately 150 μm. Determinants of

lateral resolution are more complicated and depend on imaging depth, which averages 250 μm at typical coronary diameters. Current catheters range from 2.6 to 3.5 French (1 Fr = 0.33 mm) and can be placed through conventional 6 Fr guiding catheters. Currently, two different approaches to transducer design exist: mechanically rotated devices and multielement electronic arrays (phase-array systems). Mechanical probes use a drive cable to rotate a single piezoelectric transducer at 1800 rpm, yielding 30 images per second. Alternatively, in electronic systems, multiple transducer elements (currently up to 64) in an annular array are activated sequentially to generate the image.[10] Multielement designs typically result in catheters that are easier to set up and use, whereas mechanical probes have traditionally offered superior image quality. Videotape or digital recording of imaging studies may be performed.

Examination technique

Standard techniques for IVUS imaging are usually applied. Intracoronary nitroglycerin (200 μg) and heparin (5000 IU) should be administered before advancing the IVUS catheter. Afterwards, the operator advances or retracts the imaging device over the guidewire. Our protocol includes advancement of the IVUS catheter 1 cm distal to the region of interest. A motorized pullback device is then used to withdraw the catheter at a constant speed (most frequently at 0.5 mm/s) until the guiding catheter (or aortic coronary junction) is visualized. Side branches visualized by angiography or ultrasound are useful landmarks to facilitate interpretation and comparisons in sequential examinations. Audio recording of relevant angiographic data together with online description of the finding is also systematically performed.

Rationale for ultrasound imaging

Limitations of angiography

Angiography has endured for over 40 years as the predominant method used to define coronary anatomy. It depicts arteries as a planar silhouette of the contrast-filled lumen, and any arbitrary angiographic projection can misrepresent the true extent of luminal narrowing. Visual assessment of coronary stenosis is convenient and rapid, but it is associated with large inter- and intraobserver variability. Therefore, quantitative coronary angiography (QCA) has been used during the last decade whenever accurate measurements of lumen diameters and stenosis severity have been needed.[11] In fact, multicenter clinical trials have systematically required this technique, which has eventually become a standard for clinical research.[11] In the clinical setting, however, many limitations of conventional angiography also apply to QCA.[11,12] Unrecognized disease at the reference segments remain a common limitation of any angiographic technique, potentially leading to underestimation of lesion severity.[1–4,9,10,13] Vessel foreshortening and overlapping side branches also remain practical limitations of QCA.[5–8,12] In addition, despite the use of multiple views, angiography may misrepresent the extent of luminal narrowing in eccentric lesions. Ostial lesions and bifurcated lesions are particulary challenging.[9,10,13]

Advantages of ultrasound

Several characteristics inherent to ultrasound imaging offer potential advantages in the evaluation of coronary disease. The tomographic orientation of ultrasound enables a visualization of the full circumference of the vessel wall, not just two surfaces, and is the method of choice to accurately determine coronary lumen area.[1–4,8–10,13] IVUS-derived minimal luminal area correlates better with the physiologic significance of coronary lesions than quantitative angiography does.[14,15]

Measurement of lumen diameters also remain an important diagnostic application.[9,10,13] Furthermore, the tomographic perspective of ultrasound enables an assessment of ambiguous lesions that are difficult to image by angiography. Angiographically ambiguous lesions[13] typically include: (1) intermediate lesions of uncertain severity; (2) aneurysmal lesions; (3) ostial stenoses; (4) disease at branching sites; (5) tortuous vessels; (6) left main stem lesions; (7) sites with complex lesions such as those with plaque rupture; (8) intraluminal filling defects and angiographically hazy lesions; (9) dissection after coronary angioplasty and assessment of the results of interventions. IVUS is frequently employed to examine lesions with these characteristics, in some cases providing additional evidence useful in determining whether the stenosis is clinically significant; however, it must be emphasized that IVUS does not provide physiologic information per se. Moreover, other factors, such as the mechanical characteristics of the vessel wall (e.g. coronary vessel compliance, including coronary distensibility), may be also studied by IVUS.[16,17] Finally, the penetrating nature of ultrasound provides unique images of the atherosclerotic plaque, not merely the lumen. IVUS has been fundamental in obtaining an understanding of the mechanism of action of some interventional devices, as well as of restenosis mechanisms, introducing some new concepts such as the negative remodeling. It was also due to IVUS that correct deployment of stents was developed and the burden of anticoagulation was taken away, improving results and decreasing costs – the ultimate goal of any new technology.

Limitations of IVUS

Although IVUS currently provides the most precise tool for measuring vessel lumen area and atherosclerotic plaque burden, this technique also has some specific problems and inherent limitations.[9,10,12,13] Nonuniform rotational distortion (NURD) artifact, typical from mechanical catheters, arises from friction preventing even rotation of the transducer, and generates an image distortion that affects the determination of lumen and plaque size. Transducer oscillations generate a ring-down artifact that obscures the near field. In fact, although the physical size of currently available catheters has improved to a large extent, this still represents a problem when measuring severe stenoses.[18,19] Off-axis positioning of the IVUS catheter may produce geometric distortion and elliptical vessel shapes, leading to overestimation of lumen area.[20] Careful interrogation to identify the image slide with the smallest lumen may be challenging, especially in focal stenosis or when only a manual pullback has been performed. Poor image quality may cause relevant information to be missed.[9,10,12,13] Finally, it should also be kept in mind that lumen area changes during the cardiac cycle and the maximal lumen area occurs in mid-systole.[9,10,13] Although in normal segments this lumen pulsatility accounts for a significant change in lumen area (up to 20%), this phenomenon is nearly absent at sites with severe stenosis.[16,17]

Although contemporary IVUS devices produce remarkably detailed views of the vessel wall, interpretation must rely on simple visual inspection of acoustic reflections to determine plaque composition. Different tissue components may have comparable echogenicities and textures, and therefore appear quite similar. A sonolucent luminal mass of tissue may represent intracoronary thrombus, while a nearly identical appearance may result from an atheroma with a high lipid content. Thus, IVUS is accurate in determining the thickness and echogenicity of vessel wall structures, but it is not consistently able to provide actual histology.

Finally, it should be emphasized that with IVUS only specific areas of interest can be studied, and not the entire coronary anatomy, while with angiography a more complete anatomic estimate (including small vessels, not assessed by IVUS) of the epicardial coronary artery vessels is obtained. Furthermore, coronary angiography is mandatory for subsequent IVUS study. In fact, coronary angiography represents a 'road map' for intravascular imaging.

IVUS is a relatively safe technique, having complication rates varying from 1% to 3%.[21,22] The complication most frequently reported is transient spasm, which responds rapidly to intracoronary nitroglycerin. Major complications (dissection or vessel closure) occur in less than 0.5%. Nearly all major complications occur in patients undergoing intervention rather than diagnostic procedures. Despite the favorable safety profile, subselective coronary instrumentation always carries a potential risk of vessel injury. IVUS should be performed only by operators experienced in intracoronary catheter manipulation.

Image interpretation and measurements

Image interpretation

Lumen appearance

Flowing blood exhibits a characteristic pattern of echogenicity, observed as finely textured echoes moving in a swirling pattern, at frequencies > 20–25 MHz.[10] The pattern of blood echogenicity depends on blood flow velocity, showing increased intensity with a coarser texture when flow is reduced.[23] At higher imaging frequencies, blood speckle is also more prominent; this may interfere with delineation of the blood–tissue interface. This phenomenon has so far limited IVUS imaging devices to frequencies < 40–45 MHz. Blood 'speckle' may be useful in image interpretation (e.g. it can help confirm the communication between a dissection plane and the

lumen). Assessment of luminal dimensions represents an important application for IVUS.[23] Lumen area is determined by planimetry of the leading edge of the blood–intima acoustic interface. Because of the speckled nature of ultrasound, individual video frames may not contain a continuous intimal leading edge. Therefore, a review of moving images is generally performed to assist edge detection by 'filling-in' a discontinuous border. Comparisons of ultrasound luminal measurements with angiography usually show a close correlation for vessels without atherosclerosis, while for diseased arteries only a moderate correlation exists.[23–25] The greatest disparities between angiography and ultrasound are observed after mechanical interventions, in which the shape of the lumen may be extremely complex (plaque fissures, wall dissections, etc.).[26,27] The reduced correlation between IVUS and angiography is probably explained by an irregular, noncircular cross-sectional profile, which cannot be adequately depicted by angiography.[28]

Normal arterial appearance

An ultrasound reflection is generated at a tissue interface if there is an abrupt change in acoustic impedance.[23] In muscular arteries, such as the coronary arteries, there are frequently three layers (Figure 19.1).[29–31] The innermost

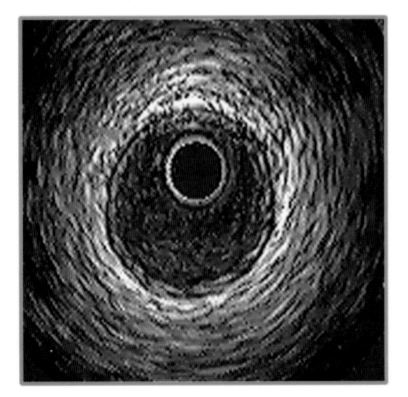

a

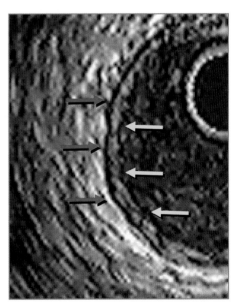

b

Figure 19.1
(A) Three-layered appearance of the coronary vessel wall by IVUS. (B) Magnified image. The intimal leading edge is highlighted by yellow arrows and the media–adventitia border (EEM) by red arrows.

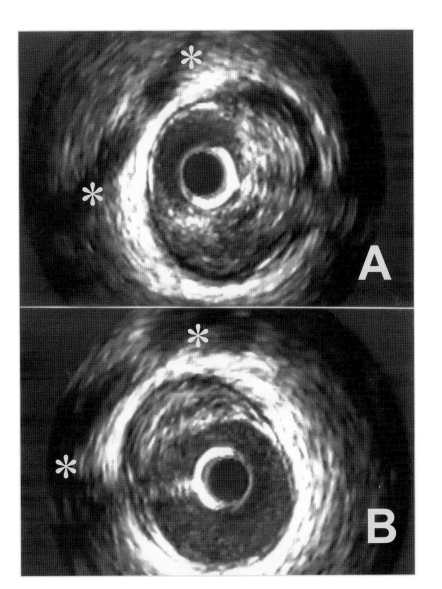

Figure 19.2
Plaque location. Pericardium (*) may be used as a landmark to describe plaque location. (A) Plaque located within the vessel wall not adjacent to the pericardium. (B) Plaque located within the vessel wall adjacent to the pericardium.

layer consists of a complex of two elements: intima and internal elastic membrane. This innermost layer is relatively echogenic compared with the lumen and media. In 30–50% of normal coronary arteries, the thin intima reflects ultrasound poorly, so it is not visualized as a separate layer. This finding has led some observers to propose that a trilaminar wall represents evidence of early atherosclerosis.[29] The reported normal value for intimal thickness in young subjects is typically 0.15 ± 0.07 mm.[23,30] Moving outward from the lumen, the second layer is the media, which is typically less echogenic than the intima. In some cases, the media may appear artifactually thin because of blooming – an intense reflection from the intima or external elastic membrane (EEM). In other cases, the media can appear artifactually thick because of signal attenuation and the weak reflectivity of the internal elastic membrane. In elastic arteries such as the carotid artery, the media is more echo-reflective because of its higher elastin content. The third and outer layer consists of the adventitia and periadventitial tissues.

The IVUS beam penetrates beyond the artery, providing images of perivascular structures, including the cardiac veins, the myocardium, and the pericardium. These structures have a characteristic appearance when viewed from different positions within the arterial tree, so they provide useful landmarks regarding the position of the imaging plane (Figure 19.2).

Characterization of atherosclerosis

Standards for acquisition, measurement, and reporting of IVUS have been overviewed in the American College of Cardiology Clinical Expert Consensus Document on IVUS.[9] In the following subsections, we briefly describe qualitative assessment and quantitative measurements of atheroma according to this consensus document.

Atheroma morphology   Ultrasound provides a unique method for studying the morphology of atherosclerosis in vivo.[9,10,13] Studies have compared the ultrasound appearance of plaques with histology in freshly explanted human

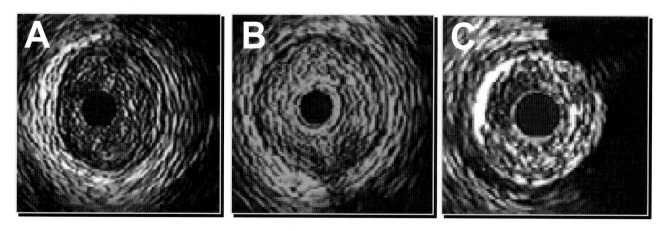

Figure 19.3
Plaque characteristics by IVUS: (A) hypoechogenic (soft); (B) fibrotic; (C) calcified atheromas.

arteries.[31–33] However, ultrasound images are fundamentally different from histology, and IVUS cannot be used to detect and quantify specific histologic contents. The following definitions may be used to describe plaque morphology (Figure 19.3):

- *Soft (echolucent) plaques*: these are generally due to high lipid content in a mostly cellular lesion.[9,10] It should be emphasized that the term 'soft' refers not to the plaque's structural characteristics, but rather to the acoustic signal (low echogenicity). However, a zone of reduced echogenicity may also be attributable to a necrotic zone within the plaque, an intramural hemorrhage, or a thrombus. Most soft plaques contain minimal collagen and elastin.
- *Fibrous plaques*: these have an echogenicity intermediate between that of soft (echolucent) atheromas and that of highly echogenic calcific plaques.[9,10] Fibrous plaques represent the majority of atherosclerotic lesions. In general, the greater the fibrous tissue content, the greater the echogenicity of the tissue. Very dense fibrous plaques may produce sufficient attenuation or acoustic shadowing to be misclassified as calcified.
- *Calcific plaques*: calcific deposits appear as bright echoes that obstruct the penetration of ultrasound (acoustic shadowing).[9,10] Because high-frequency ultrasound does not penetrate the calcium, IVUS can detect only the leading edge and cannot determine the thickness of the calcium. Therefore, measurements of calcified areas are not possible. Calcium can also produce reverberations or multiple reflections that result from the oscillation of ultrasound between transducer and calcium and cause concentric arcs in the image at reproducible distances. The angle subtended by the calcified arc is often used to quantify the severity of calcification. IVUS has shown significantly higher sensitivity than fluoroscopy in the detection of coronary calcification.[34,35] Target lesion calcification is detected

by ultrasound in 70–80% of patients undergoing intervention, whereas fluoroscopy detects calcium in 10–35%. The presence, depth, and circumferential distribution of calcification are very important factors for selecting the type of interventional device (e.g. rotational atherectomy when extense superficial calcium is present) and for estimating the risk of complications (i.e. disections post-PTCA, usually occuring at the border between calcium and soft tissue).[36–38] Calcium deposits should be described qualitatively according to their location (e.g. lesion versus reference) and distribution: superficial (the leading edge of the acoustic shadowing appears within the shallowest 50% of the plaque plus media thickness) or deep (the leading edge of the acoustic shadowing appears within the deepest 50% of the plaque plus media thickness).

- *Mixed*: plaques frequently contain more than one acoustic subtype.
- *Thrombus*: a thrombus is usually recognized as an intraluminal mass, often with a layered, lobulated, or pedunculated appearance.[9,39,40] The differential diagnosis should be done with flow turbulence (Figure 19.4), air, eccentric calcified plaques, Ventouri effect distal to a severe stenosis, among others. Thrombi may appear relatively echolucent or have a more variable gray scale with speckling or scintillation. Blood flow in 'microchannels' may also be apparent within some thrombi. Stagnant blood flow can simulate a thrombus with a grayish-white accumulation of specular echoes within the vascular lumen. Injection of contrast or saline may disperse the stagnant flow, clear the lumen, and allow differentiation of stasis from thrombosis. However, none of these features is a hallmark for thrombus, and the diagnosis of thrombus by IVUS should always be considered presumptive.
- *Intimal hyperplasia*: this is characteristic of early in-stent restenosis, and it appears as tissue with very low echogenicity, at times less echogenic than the blood speckle in the lumen. The intimal hyperplasia of late

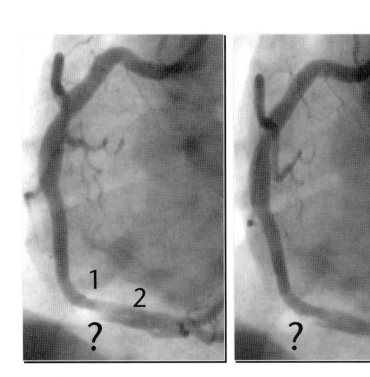

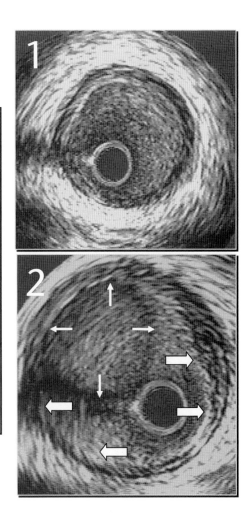

Flow streaming

Figure 19.4
Ambiguous lesion: angiographic image of an ectasic right coronary artery (RCA) of a patient with unstable angina. Flow streaming was observed in the distal segment of the RCA, raising the suspicion of intracoronary thrombus. IVUS imaging proved that this was due to vessel ectasia in the distal RCA generating blood flow with different velocities (2) not observed at the proximal reference (1).

in-stent restenosis often appears more echogenic (Figure 19.5).

Arterial remodeling   The term 'arterial remodeling' refers to changes in vascular dimensions during the development of atherosclerosis. Glagov et al[41] initially described this phenomenon from necropsy specimens, in which a positive correlation between EEM and atheroma area was observed. For lesions with a cross-sectional area less than 40%, an increase in arterial size compensated for plaque accumulation, resulting in a preserved lumen area. For advanced lesions, remodeling failed to maintain lumen size, and therefore lumen narrowing was present.

IVUS provides cross-sectional areas of the lumen, atheroma, and EEM, allowing the study of arterial remodeling in vivo. If the EEM area increases during atheroma development, the process is termed 'positive remodeling'. If the EEM area decreases, the process is termed 'nega-

tive' or 'constrictive remodeling'. In fact, in positive remodeling, the increase in EEM area may overcompensate for increasing plaque area, resulting in a net increase in lumen size. Alternatively, remodeling can either exactly compensate for increasing plaque area, resulting in no change in lumen size, or undercompensate for increasing plaque area, often termed 'inadequate' remodeling (Figure 19.6).

An index that describes the magnitude and direction of remodeling is expressed in terms of cross-sectional area (CSA) as (lesion EEM CSA)/(reference EEM CSA).[9] If the lesion EEM area is greater than the reference EEM area, then positive remodeling has occurred, and the index will be greater than unity; if the lesion EEM area is smaller than the reference EEM area, then negative remodeling has occurred, and the index will be less than unity. Direct evidence of remodeling can be derived only from serial changes in the EEM CSA that have been determined by two or more measurements obtained at different times,

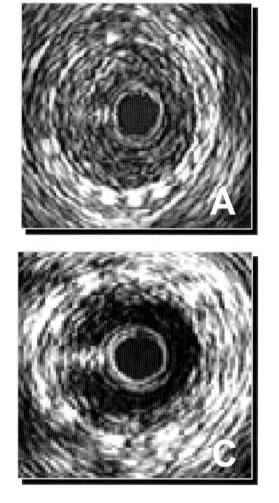
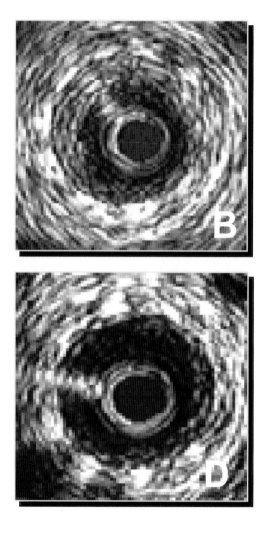

Figure 19.5
In-stent restenosis as assessed by IVUS: extensive (A), eccentric moderate (B), mild (C), and absence (D) of neointimal proliferation.

since remodeling may also be encountered at the 'normal' reference site.

Recent and intriguing IVUS studies have examined the relationship between remodeling and clinical presentation in patients with coronary artery disease.[42] In unstable patients, both EEM and plaque areas were significantly larger than the corresponding measurements in stable patients. Positive remodeling seems to be significantly more prevalent in the unstable group and negative remodeling more prevalent in the stable group.

Unstable lesions and ruptured plaque   No definitive IVUS features define a plaque as vulnerable.[39,40] However, necropsy studies demonstrated that unstable coronary lesions are usually lipid-rich with a thin fibrous cap, and hypoechoic plaques without a well-formed fibrous cap are presumed to represent potentially vulnerable atherosclerotic lesions (Figure 19.7).

Ruptured plaques have a highly variable appearance on IVUS. In patients studied after an acute coronary syndrome, IVUS may reveal an ulceration, often with remnants of the ruptured fibrous cap evident at the edges of the ulcer. A variety of other appearances are common, including fissuring or erosion of the plaque surface. The following definitions are recommended:[9]

- *Plaque ulceration*: a recess in the plaque beginning at the luminal–intimal border.
- *Plaque rupture*: a plaque ulceration with a tear detected in a fibrous cap. Contrast injections may be used to prove and define the communication point.

The presence of thrombi may obscure IVUS detection of plaque fissuring or ulceration.

Unusual lesion morphology (definitions)
- *True aneurysm*: a lesion that includes all layers of the vessel wall with an EEM and lumen area more than 50% larger than the proximal reference segment.
- *Pseudoaneurysm*: disruption of the EEM, usually observed after intervention.[9]
- A *true lumen* is surrounded by all three layers of the vessel: intima, media, and adventitia. Side branches communicate with the true, but not with the false lumen.

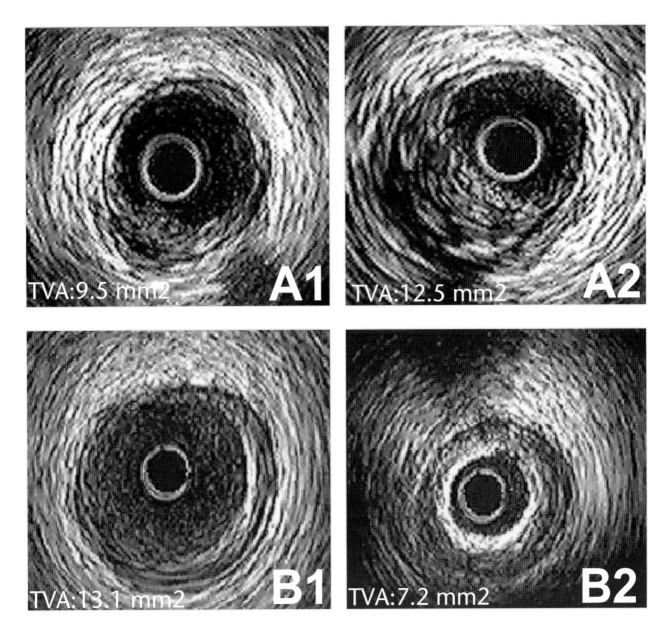

Figure 19.6
Remodeling. (A) Example of positive remodeling: despite a large increase in plaque burden (A2), the lumen size is similar to that observed at the proximal reference (A1) due to a compensatory increase in total vessel area (TVA). (B) Example of negative remodeling: the increase in plaque burden (B2) is not accompanied by an increase in TVA, which leads to 'shrinkage' of the vessel as compared with the proximal reference (B1), determining a reduction in lumen area.

- A *false lumen* is a channel, usually parallel to the true lumen, that does not communicate with the true lumen over a portion of its length.[9]

Measurements

Border identification

Measurements should be performed at the leading edge of boundaries.[9,10] With few exceptions, the location of the leading edge is accurate and reproducible regardless of system settings or the image-processing characteristics of different ultrasound scanners.[43] Measurements at the trailing edge are inconsistent and frequently yield erroneous results.

Lumen measurements

Lumen measurements are performed using the interface between the lumen and the leading edge of the intima.[9,10] The following lumen measurements can be derived:[9]

- *Lumen cross-sectional area (CSA)*: the area bounded by the luminal border.

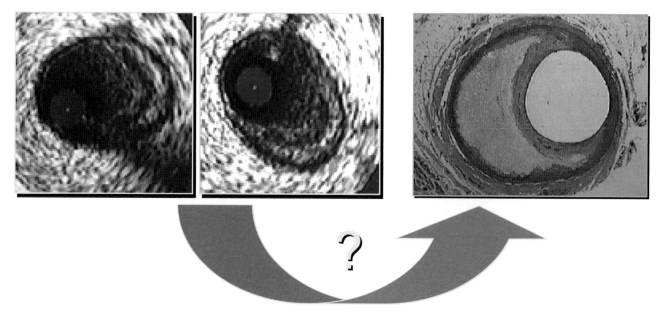

Figure 19.7
Vulnerable plaque: IVUS images (thin fibrous cap and large lipid core) resembling the histologic feature of the vulnerable plaque.

- *Minimal lumen diameter (MLD)*: the shortest diameter through the center point of the lumen.
- *Lumen eccentricity*: (maximal lumen diameter – minimal lumen diameter)/(maximal lumen diameter).
- *Lumen area stenosis*: (reference lumen CSA – minimal lumen CSA)/(reference lumen CSA). The reference segment used should be specified (proximal, distal, largest, or average).

EEM measurements

A discrete interface at the border between the media and the adventitia is almost invariably present within IVUS images and corresponds closely to the location of the EEM.[9,10] The recommended term for this measurement is 'EEM CSA', rather than alternative terms such as 'vessel area' or 'total vessel area'.[9]

EEM CSA cannot be measured reliably at sites where large side branches originate or in the setting of extensive calcification, because of acoustic shadowing. In addition, some stent designs may obscure the EEM border and render measurements unreliable.

Disease-free coronary arteries are circular, but atherosclerotic arteries may remodel into a noncircular configuration. If maximal and minimal EEM diameters are reported, measurements should bisect the geometric center of the vessel rather than the center of the IVUS catheter.

Atheroma measurements

Because the leading edge of the media (the internal elastic membrane) is not well delineated, IVUS measurements cannot determine the true histological atheroma area (the area bounded by the internal elastic membrane).[43] Accordingly, IVUS studies use the EEM and lumen CSA measurements to calculate a surrogate for the true atheroma area, the 'plaque plus media' area. In practice, the inclusion of the media in the atheroma area does not constitute a major limitation of IVUS, because the media represents only a very small fraction of the atheroma CSA. It has been suggested that the term 'plaque plus media' (or atheroma) be used and that the following measurements be performed:[9]

- *Plaque plus media (or atheroma) CSA*: EEM CSA – lumen CSA.
- *Plaque plus media (or atheroma) eccentricity*: (maximal plaque plus media thickness – minimal plaque plus media thickness)/(maximal plaque plus media thickness).
- *Plaque (or atheroma) burden*: (plaque plus media CSA)/(EEM CSA). The atheroma burden is distinct from the luminal area stenosis. The former represents the area within the EEM occupied by atheroma regardless of lumen compromise. The latter is a measure of luminal compromise relative to a reference lumen analogous to the angiographic diameter stenosis.

Calcium assessment

The arc of calcium can be measured (in degrees) by using an electronic protractor centered on the lumen.[9,10] Semiquantitative grading has also been described, which classifies calcium as absent or subtending 1, 2, 3, or 4 quadrants. The length of the calcific deposit can be measured using motorized transducer pullback.

Length measurements

Length measurements using IVUS can be performed using motorized transducer pullback (number of seconds × pullback speed). This approach can be used to determine the length of a lesion, stenosis, calcium, or any other longitudinal feature.[9]

Diagnostic applications

Angiographically normal coronary vessels

Angiographically normal coronary arteries are encountered in 10–15% of patients undergoing cardiac catheterization for suspected coronary disease. If any luminal irregularity is present by angiography, ultrasound will usually demonstrate disease at most other examined sites.[28,30] The prevalence of disease at angiographically normal sites confirms the finding, previously reported from necropsy studies, that coronary disease is usually diffuse, not focal, and that angiography frequently underestimates disease burden (Figure 19.8).[44] Although IVUS commonly detects occult disease in patients with a 'true normal' angiography, its impact on prognosis remains uncertain.[28,45,46]

Angiographically indeterminate lesions

Intermediate stenoses (angiographic severity ranging from 40% to 75%) are particularly problematic in patients whose symptomatic status is difficult to assess. In

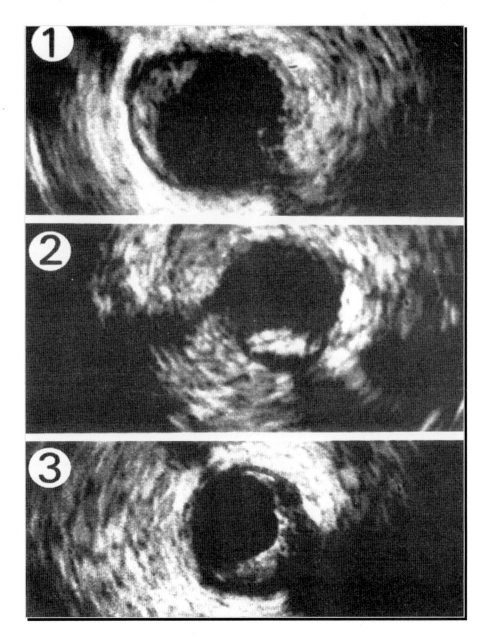

Figure 19.8
Assessment of the vessel wall: evidence of plaque burden by IVUS in an angiographically normal vessel. On IVUS (20 MHz), 80% of angiographically normal segments, proximal to the target lesion, had plaque; (1,3) semilunar appearance; (1,2,3) lumen shape preserved; (1,2,3) heterogeneous features. (Reproduced from Alfonso F et al. Am Heart J 1994;127:536–44[4] with permission from Elsevier.)

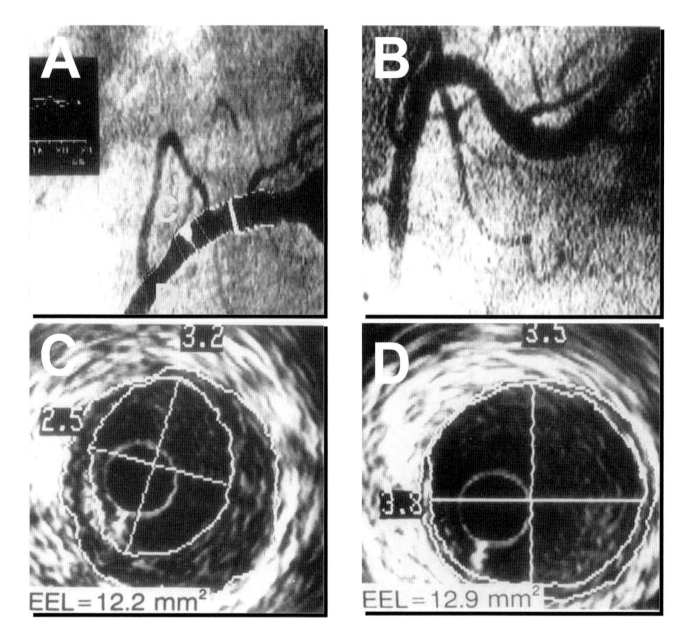

Figure 19.9
Coronary pseudostenosis induced by a stiff guidewire during PTCA (A) resolved after wire removal (B). IVUS image at site of pseudostenosis (C) and at distal reference (D).

ambiguous lesions, IVUS provides a tomographic perspective, independent of the radiographic projection, that often permits lesion quantification. Several studies have used IVUS to perform or defer a coronary intervention. Abizaid et al[47] studied with IVUS 300 patients with 357 intermediate ('uncertain') coronary stenosis (< 70% diameter stenosis on visual assessment). In this study, no angiographic measurement was predictive of events (death, myocardial infarction, or target vessel revascularization) at 13-month follow-up. It is noteworthy that the only independent predictors of events (after adjusting for clinical and angiographic variables) were IVUS minimal lumen area and percentage area stenosis as detected by

IVUS. In addition, the only independent predictors of target lesion revascularization were diabetes mellitus, IVUS minimal lumen area, and IVUS percentage area stenosis. In 248 lesions with a minimal lumen area of 4 mm² or more, the requirement for revascularization at follow-up was only 2.8% and the event rate 4.4%. Therefore, IVUS imaging was a valuable alternative to physiologic assessment in patients with intermediate coronary lesions on angiography. In addition, the long-term follow-up after IVUS-guided deferred interventions was similar to that previously reported after direct physiologic lesion assessment.[48,49] Therefore the clinical usefulness of this cut-off value (≥ 4 mm²) appears well validated for IVUS-based deferred interventions. A potential limitation of this parameter is the assessment of lesions in small or secondary vessels. Few of these vessels were included in previous studies, so one may speculate that percentage area stenosis may be more useful in this subset of patients.

Another indication for IVUS is the evaluation of coronary 'pseudostenosis'.[50] In some patients, the use of stiff guidewires induces an artificial straightening of the vessels that in angled coronary segments facilitates the appearance of intimal wrinkles or coronary intussusceptions that create functional stenosis. Physiologic study of these 'pseudoestenoses' reveals that they are indeed able to cause an obstruction to flow.[51] However, this phenomenon (also called the 'accordion effect' or a 'crumpled coronary artery') is benign, spontaneously resolving after the procedure, but requires appropriate diagnosis and management. IVUS is able to readily detect the asymmetric lumen associated with the typical image of intussusception and to exclude significant atheroma burden or residual dissections at sites with misleading angiographic images (Figure 19.9).[50]

Left main coronary disease

Assessment of left main coronary disease by angiography represents a particularly difficult clinical problem (Figure 19.10).[52] Ultrasound may help overcome the three major anatomic factors that impair angiographic left main evaluation: (1) aortic cusp opacification or 'streaming' of contrast may obscure the ostium; (2) the short length of the vessel may leave no normal segment for comparison; (3) the distal left main artery may be concealed by bifurcation or trifurcation.[53] There is no consensus regarding the cross-sectional area at which the left main obstruction is considered critical. In the study by Abizaid et al,[54] patients with moderate left main disease and ambiguous angiograms were evaluated with IVUS and subsequently did not undergo coronary revascularization. At 1-year clinical follow-up, there was a 14% total event rate; diabetes mellitus, an untreated vessel and IVUS-derived MLD were independent predictors of cardiac events. In particular, MLD was the most important predictor of cardiac events, whereas patients with MLD less than 3 mm present an increased risk. A stenosis area greater

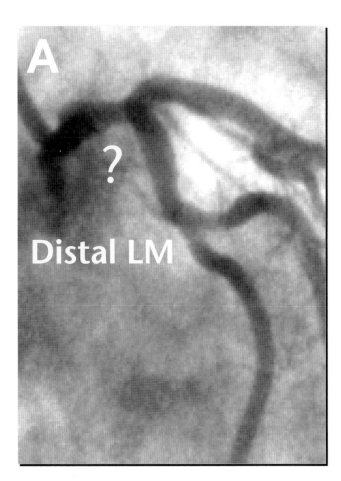

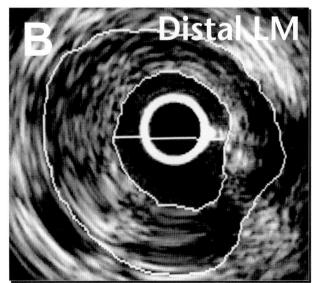

Figure 19.10
(A) Angiographically borderline stenosis in the distal segment of the left main stem. (B) An IVUS image demonstrates that this stenosis is severe. Minimal lumen diameter 2.3 mm; minimal lumen area 5.3 mm².

than 50% or an absolute area less than 9 mm² have also been proposed as criteria for left main stenosis severity requiring revascularization.[9]

Transplant coronary artery disease

Coronary disease represents the major cause of death in the first year after transplantation.[10] This disease is often clinically silent, because the heart is denervated and ischemia by functional testing does not usually occur until the disease is advanced.[55–57] Although angiography has been performed annually for surveillance, the diffuse nature of the disease often impairs detection.[58] IVUS has emerged as the optimal method for early detection.[59] Disease by angiography is present in 10–20% of patients at 1 year and in 40–50% by 5 years,[60,61] while the prevalence of arteriopathy detected by ultrasound is much higher.[60–62]

IVUS studies have demonstrated an association between the severity of disease by ultrasound and clinical outcome, with an increased incidence of death, myocardial infarction, or retransplantation in those with more severe disease.[63,64] Rapidly progressive intimal thickening (≥ 0.5 mm increase) in the first year after transplantation has major negative prognostic significance (Figures 19.11 and 19.12).[64]

Interventional applications

IVUS examination offers advantages over angiography for deciding which specific treatment modality is most appropriate for a given lesion. The main limitation of IVUS assessment before treatment is that, despite the extreme miniaturization of IVUS catheters, the probe occludes the lesion in most cases, precluding a prolonged assessment because of development of myocardial ischemia and disturbance of the image interpretation due to blood stagnation.

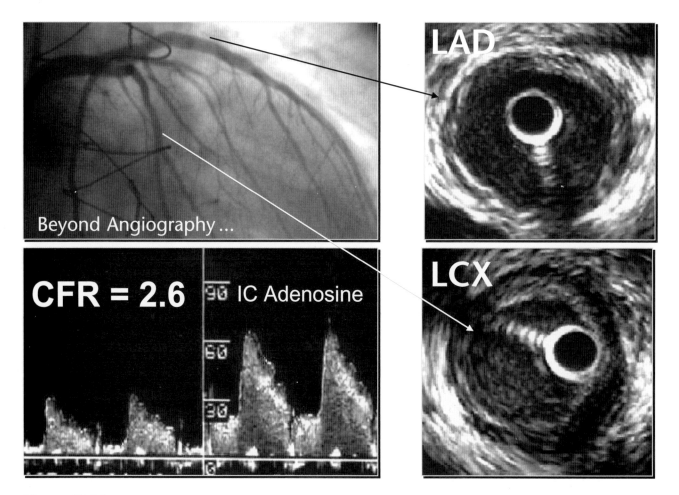

Figure 19.11
Intimal thickening observed by IVUS in angiographically normal vessels of a transplanted heart. Despite such echographic evidence, coronary flow reserve (CFR), following adenosine-induced hyperemia, is preserved.

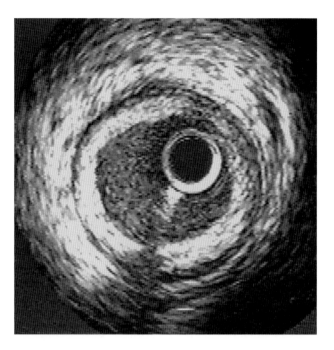

Figure 19.12
Intimal thickening with fibrotic component observed by IVUS in an epicardial vessel of a transplanted heart.

Lee et al[65] evaluated the effect of IVUS imaging on decision making in the performance of coronary interventions; angiographically acceptable results were deemed inadequate by IVUS in 29% of angioplasties and 30% of stent deployments, and planned procedures were subsequently altered. The additional information provided by IVUS on lesion composition, eccentricity, and length accounted for modification of treatment in almost 20% of the cases of the Washington Heart Center experience.[66] The presence, depth, and circumferential distribution of calcification are very important factors for selecting the type of interventional device (e.g. rotational atherectomy when extensive superficial calcium is present) and for estimating the risk of complications (e.g. dissections post PTCA, usually occuring at the border between calcium and soft tissue) (Figure 19.13).[36–38] The presence of highly eccentric bulky plaques, without significant subendothelial calcification, could be an indication to use directional atherectomy. The origin of side branches from the diseased part of the vessel wall with an eccentric plaque is a predictor of occlusion after PTCA or stent deployment. IVUS can also clarify unusual lesion morphologies, such as aneurysm versus pseudoaneurysm. The ability to serially assess interventioned lesions and thereby determine the mechanism of vessel remodeling (restenosis) is also an important advantage of IVUS.[38] The importance of IVUS in different interventional strategies is reviewed in the following subsections.

IVUS during balloon angioplasty

IVUS has helped to understand the mechanism of balloon angioplasty.[67] Modifications of the dilatation strategy based on IVUS results include changes in balloon size and inflation pressure. The most important information obtained with IVUS concerns the results of the procedure: after angioplasty, IVUS can detect circumferential and longitudinal extension of plaque fracture or dissection, which may require immediate treatment. In the setting of acute coronary syndromes, IVUS showed that plaque area reduction is the major cause of luminal gain, suggesting that compression, redistribution, or dislodgement of mural thrombus occurs in these syndromes.[68]

With IVUS, the selection of balloon size can be based on measurements of total vessel diameter. The Clinical Outcomes with Ultrasound Trial (CLOUT) reported that the IVUS reference segment midwall dimensions could be used to safely upsize percutaneous transluminal coronary angioplasty (PTCA) balloons.[69] In CLOUT, PTCA was first performed using conventional angiographic balloon sizing; then PTCA was repeated using IVUS balloon sizing. This study showed that on the basis of the vessel size and extent of plaque burden in the reference segment evaluated with IVUS, 73% of the lesions needed larger balloons even after achieving an optimal angiographic result. The success rate of IVUS-guided PTCA was 99.0%. IVUS-guided oversized balloon angioplasty resulted in a greater final MLD and a decrease in stenosis diameter without increased rates of dissection or ischemic complications. These findings have been confirmed in other studies.[70–72]

IVUS studies to define predictors of restenosis have also been performed. Despite some contradictory results, there is currently some evidence that residual plaque burden is an important predictor of restenosis. The Post-Intracoronary Treatment Ultrasound Evaluation (PICTURE), however, did not show any predictors of outcome.[73] Single-center studies, though, identified residual plaque burden as an independent predictor of outcome in multivariable analysis.[74] The GUIDE II trial examined this issue more completely and observed that ultrasound-derived residual percentage plaque burden was the most powerful predictor of clinical outcome.[74,75] In this trial, in addition to residual plaque burden, MLD measured by IVUS was also a predictor of restenosis.[75] However, the long-term clinical impact of differences in angiographic result has not been completely established.

IVUS is commonly employed to detect and direct the treatment of dissections and other complications after intervention (Figure 19.13).[67] Dissections may be classified into five categories: (1) intimal; (2) medial; (3) adventitial; (4) intramural hematoma (an accumulation of blood within the medial space, displacing the internal elastic membrane inward and the EEM outward); (5) intrastent.[9] The severity of a dissection can be quantified according to (i) depth; (ii) circumferential extent (in degrees of arc) using a

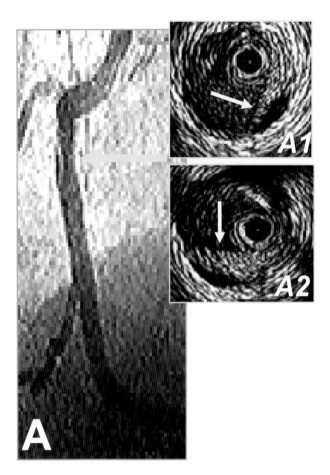
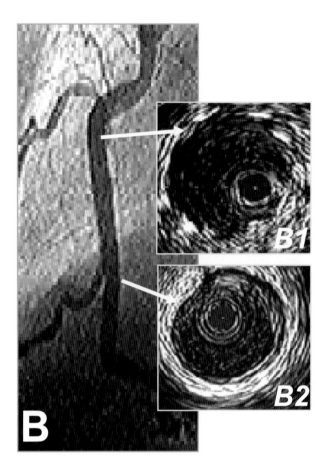

Figure 19.13
(A) Angiographic image of edge dissection following balloon angioplasty. (A1, A2) IVUS images with evidence of dissection and intimal flap (arrows). (B) Angiographic result following stent implantation. (B1) IVUS image at site of dissection (note the stent struts). (B2) Distal reference.

protractor centered on the lumen; (iii) length using motorized transducer pullback; (iv) size of residual lumen (CSA); (v) CSA of the luminal dissection.[9] Additional descriptors of a dissection may include the presence of a false lumen, the identification of mobile flap(s), the presence of calcium at the dissection border, and dissections in close proximity to stent edges. In a minority of patients, the dissection may not be apparent by IVUS, because of the scaffolding by the imaging catheter or because the dissection is located behind calcium.

For the first 15 years of interventional cardiology, investigators believed that the predominant mechanism of restenosis after angioplasty and atherectomy was intimal proliferation. Ultrasound studies in the peripheral vessels by Pasterkamp et al[76] presented the first indication that negative remodeling, or localized shrinkage of the vessel, was a major mechanism of late lumen loss. Mintz et al[77] studied 212 native coronary arteries in patients undergoing repeat catheterization for recurrent symptoms or research protocols after coronary interventions. At follow-up, there was a decrease in EEM area and an increase in plaque area at the target lesion. Interestingly, over 70%

of lumen loss was attributable to the decrease in EEM area, whereas the neointimal area accounted for only 23% of the loss. Moreover, the change in lumen area correlated more strongly with the change in EEM area than with the change in plaque area, and lesions with an increase in EEM area at follow-up were associated with a significant reduction in angiographic restenosis.[77]

IVUS during stenting

Intracoronary stenting currently represents the standard method of percutaneous catheter intervention. IVUS has provided important insights into the anatomy of stented coronary segments, not achievable by angiographic techniques alone. By depicting stent expansion patterns in a cross-sectional view, it could be shown by IVUS that most stents were underexpanded and that some of them had no full vessel wall apposition (Figures 19.14 and 19.15).[78,79] These insights led to a change in implantation techniques and the development of so-called 'high-pressure stent

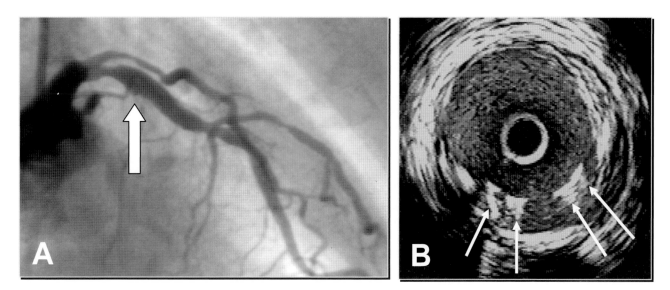

Figure 19.14
Stent malapposition. (A) Angiographic image of ectasia in the left anterior descending coronary artery (arrow) observed following coronary stent implantation. This corresponded to the proximal portion of the stent, which showed (B) an incomplete apposition (arrows) to the vessel wall, despite full stent expansion.

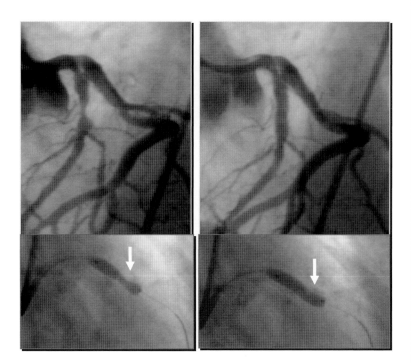

Balloon indentation

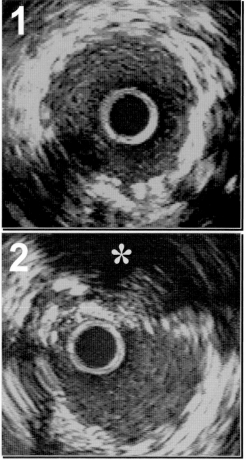

Figure 19.15
Severe calcified lesion in the proximal segment of the left anterior descending coronary artery treated by percutaneous transluminal coronary angioplasty. The severity of calcium is observed by balloon indentation despite the use of high-balloon-pressure inflation. Following stent implantation, IVUS showed a fully deployed stent (1) except for in its distal portion (2) due to the severe calcium deposit beyond the stent (*), observed as shadowing.

implantation'. This new implantation strategy, together with the routine use of combined antiplatelet treatment with aspirin and thienopyridines (ticlopidine and clopidogrel), decreased the rate of stent malapposition and subacute stent thrombosis.[80,81] However, despite these improvements, in-stent restenosis has emerged as a new disease, difficult to treat and involving between 10% and 40% of patients, depending on their risk profile.[82]

Another important issue with IVUS in coronary stenting concerns the degree of stent expansion to be reached, yielding what is called 'optimal stent expansion'. Following the concept of 'the bigger the better' introduced in coronary intervention for different treatment modalities by Kuntz and colleagues in 1991,[83] the impact of optimal stent expansion on the rate of restenosis came into the focus of scientific interest and was supported by observational clinical studies.[84,85] However, in balloon angioplasty models, after excessive overdilatation, an exaggerated neointimal proliferation occurs.[86,87] Therefore, IVUS could potentially lead to an optimal compromise between stent expansion relative to the true coronary vessel dimension, plaque volume and composition on one site, and minimal vessel overstretch or trauma on the other site.

The guidelines of the Milano group modified by the MUSIC investigators[80] represent useful criteria for optimal coronary stenting. These guidelines are based on a comparison between the lumen inside the stent and the lumens of the proximal and distal reference segments. The MUSIC criteria for optimal coronary stent deployment are: (1)

1. Complete apposition of the stent over its complete length.
2. In-stent minimal lumen area greater than or equal to 90% of the average reference area or greater than or equal to 100% of the lumen area of the reference segment with the smallest lumen area. This criterion is modified (80% of the average reference area and 90% of the lumen area of the reference segment with smallest area) if the minimal lumen area inside the stent is 9 mm^2 or greater.
3. Symmetric stent expansion defined by a ratio of minimal to maximal lumen diameter of 7 or more.

Since a variety of observational single- and multicenter observational studies demonstrated very favorable angiographic and clinical restenosis rates, even below 10%,[84] some multicenter randomized trials were performed to further assess the effect of IVUS on clinical outcome. The single-center randomized Strategy for Intracoronary Ultrasound-Guided PTCA and Stenting (SIPS) trial tested the concept of provisional stenting, with around 50% of the randomized patients receiving a stent and the others balloon angioplasty.[88] The CRUISE ('Can Routine Ultrasound Influence Stent Expansion?') study represents an observational study as a substudy of a randomized multicenter trial that addressed different antithrombotic regimens.[89] In this substudy, patients were assigned to

angiographic or ultrasound guidance on a center-by-center basis. The CRUISE and SIPS studies, however, were positive in their endpoints: target vessel revascularization after 9 months and clinically driven target vessel revascularization after 24 months, respectively.[88,89] There are only four randomized multicenter stent trials dealing with the effect of IVUS on outcome: RESIST, OPTICUS, AVID, and TULIP.[90–93] Restensosis was the primary endpoint in the RESIST, OPTICUS, and TULIP trials, and target vessel revascularization in the AVID trial. Only the TULIP trial, in which long lesions (< 20 mm) were included, reached the primary endpoint (restenosis). There was just a trend in favor for the ultrasound-guided group in the RESIST and AVID studies with respect to restenosis rate and target vessel revascularization, respectively, while the OPTICUS study was a negative study.

IVUS studies have provided a key insight into the reduction of restenosis observed with stenting. Unlike the restenotic response to angioplasty or atherectomy, which is a mixture of arterial remodeling and neointimal growth, in-stent restenosis is primarily due to neointimal proliferation. In serial ultrasound studies, late lumen loss correlated strongly with the degree of in-stent neointimal growth.[77,94] The amount of intimal proliferation has been shown to correlate with the pre-stent plaque burden[95,96] and with the residual plaque burden.[97] In a serial study of stented coronary segments using IVUS, although the arterial remodeling process occurred, no significant change was observed in the area bounded by stent struts, indicating that stents can resist the arterial remodeling process.[94] This phenomenon, combined with the greater initial lumen expansion accomplished with stenting, results in a lower net restenosis rate than that with angioplasty or atherectomy.

Results from clinical studies on IVUS during coronary stenting led to the development of combined ultrasound–stent devices for clinical use. This system allows one to assess lesion morphology before treatment and to check whether the stent was deployed correctly (and to optimize the result if it was not), using a single catheter on which balloon, stent, and probe are mounted.

IVUS studies have been useful in providing a more detailed morphologic analysis of the local biological effects of the implantation of drug-eluting stents. An IVUS substudy was performed in a subset of patients of the RAVEL trial.[98] Neointimal hyperplasia and percentage of volume obstruction at 6 months were significantly lower in patients randomized to receive a sirolimus-eluting stent compared with an uncoated stent, emphasizing the nearly complete abolition of the proliferative process inside the drug-eluting stent. Analysis of the distal edge volumes showed no significant difference between the two groups in EEM or lumen and plaque volume at the stent edges. The SIRIUS trial also compared a sirolimus-eluting stent with an uncoated stent in more complex patients (longer lesions, higher number of diabetics, multivessel disease, overlapping stents).[99] The IVUS substudy showed 93% and 92% reductions in neointimal hyperplasia and percentage of volume obstruction at 8 months. These were significantly reduced (although to a lesser extent) also at the distal edges, suggesting a lower antiproliferative effect at the stent edges; this is in accordance with the pattern of restenosis at the site of the proximal margin with sirolimus-eluting stents. New late incomplete apposition was seen only with sirolimus-eluting stents; however, this has not yet been associated with clinical events.

IVUS during atherectomy

Directional coronary atherectomy (DCA)

Direct visualization of the quadrants of maximal plaque accumulation has great potential for guidance of interventions directed at selective plaque removal. However, combined ultrasound–atherectomy devices are not available for clinical use. During atherectomy, serial ultrasound examinations are generally performed:

- before intervention, to confirm the indication (absent or deep calcification, short stenosis, ideally soft plaques);
- between subsequent atherectomy passes, to assess the completeness of plaque removal and avoid deep cuts in the periadvential tissue;
- after atherectomy, to determine the degree of adjunctive balloon dilatation or stent implantation to be used to tackle the flaps and smooth the irregular wall contours often induced by the atherectomy cuts.

Usually the use of IVUS during atherectomy results in a more aggressive strategy and leads to greater plaque removal and a larger lumen diameter.[100] Therefore, the use of IVUS may help to overcome some of the limitations of angiographically guided directional atherectomy, such as its inability to provide a clinically relevant reduction in restenosis as documented in randomized multicenter comparisons with balloon dilatation.[101,102] Two randomized trials, CAVEAT[101] and CCAT,[102] comparing DCA with conventional balloon angioplasty for the treatment of de novo native coronary lesions failed to show a significant benefit of DCA over angioplasty. However, these trials did not take advantage of the potential of this approach. Concern that deep-tissue resection might cause perforation or increased tissue proliferation biased the technique toward the use of relatively small cutter sizes and limited tissue resection. The results of the Optimal Atherectomy Restenosis Study (OARS),[103] however, demonstrated the possibility of achieving an improved immediate result and a high procedural success with aggressive ultrasound-guided atherectomy; however, the angiographic restenosis rate was high. More encouraging results arise from the Adjunctive Balloon Angioplasty following Coronary Atherectomy Study (ABACAS),[104] in which a more complete plaque removal than in the OARS trial was achieved,

resulting in a reduction of the angiographic restenosis rate. The Balloon vs Optimal Atherectomy Trial (BOAT)[105] showed that acute lumen results and late angiographic restenosis could be significantly improved by DCA over PTCA. As studies suggest that residual plaque burden after stenting is predictive of late restenosis, the role of DCA in conjunction with coronary stents has also been evaluated. The Stenting after Optimal Lesion Debulking (SOLD) registry[106] demonstrated that DCA followed by coronary stenting could be performed with excellent angiographic results. This represented the rationale to perform the AMIGO trial.[107] This randomized trial, however, failed to show a benefit in terms of angiographic restenosis of DCA followed by coronary stenting compared to coronary stenting alone.

Rotational atherectomy

Rotational atherectomy has been suggested in patients with moderate to severe coronary lesion calcification.[13] Since IVUS is superior to angiography in the evaluation of calcium, this has been a useful tool to evaluate the results of rotational atherectomy. In fact, IVUS is able to demonstrate the effectiveness of rotational atherectomy to 'debulk' calcified plaques; in addition, IVUS allows to assess the results of additional balloon dilatation or stent implantation. On the other hand, data from single-center studies demonstrated the feasibility and safety of rotational atherectomy in in-stent restenosis and its effectiveness in debulking neointima.[108–110] However, data from nonrandomized trials indicate a wide range of clinical or angiographic restenosis.[109,110] The Angioplasty versus Rotational Atherectomy for Treatment of Diffuse In-Stent Restenosis Trial (ARTIST)[111] was a multicenter, randomized, prospective trial comparing rotational atherectomy followed by low-pressure balloon angioplasty with high-pressure balloon angioplasty, in which balloon angioplasty alone was shown to be a better strategy (with higher mean net gains in MLD and in stenosis diameter, and lower restenosis and event rates). IVUS was performed in a substudy of this trial, which demonstrated a significant decrease of the neointima after rotational atherectomy, indicating effective debulking but no stent overexpansion. In contrast, balloon angioplasty with higher pressures resulted in a significant increase in stent area. Neointimal tissue growth between intervention and follow-up did not differ between groups. IVUS results suggest that if rotational atherectomy is used to treat patients with in-stent restenosis, adjunctive balloon PTCA should be performed at relatively high pressures.

IVUS during brachytherapy

The occurrence of restenosis after stent implantation remains unresolved, especially in small vessels and long lesions, where it may exceed 30% of cases.[112] It is primarily caused by neointimal hyperplasia, which occurs due to trauma of the arterial wall by the stent struts. The treatment of in-stent restenosis with conventional techniques (balloon angioplasty or debulking) is rather disappointing, with high reccurrent restenosis rates.[108,113,114] Radiation therapy can be delivered to the coronary arteries by external radiation or by brachytherapy methods, using either catheter-based systems or radioactive stents.[115] Catheter-based systems can handle both β- or γ-emitters, which can deliver the prescribed dose at either high or low dose rates.

IVUS imaging studies have been helpful to determine the morphologic effect of brachytherapy on the vessel wall, as well as the nature of the complications and limitations of this technique. Further, a more accurate way to calculate radiation dose delivered at a certain point into the vessel wall has been possible from IVUS analysis.

Mechanism of action of intracoronary brachytherapy to prevent restenosis as assessed by IVUS

Enhancement of positive remodeling   The effect of intracoronary radiation therapy on vascular remodeling has been clinically demonstrated in the Beta Energy Restenosis Trial (BERT).[116] In a careful volumetric IVUS analysis of the irradiated coronary segment following successful balloon angioplasty, vessel size (i.e. the volume encompassed by the EEM) appeared to increase significantly during the 6-month follow-up. This vessel enlargement (positive remodeling) was able to accommodate a parallel increase in plaque volume. As a result, the luminal volume remained unchanged at follow-up.[117] The same phenomenon has been observed in patients treated because of diffuse in-stent restenosis (Figure 19.16).

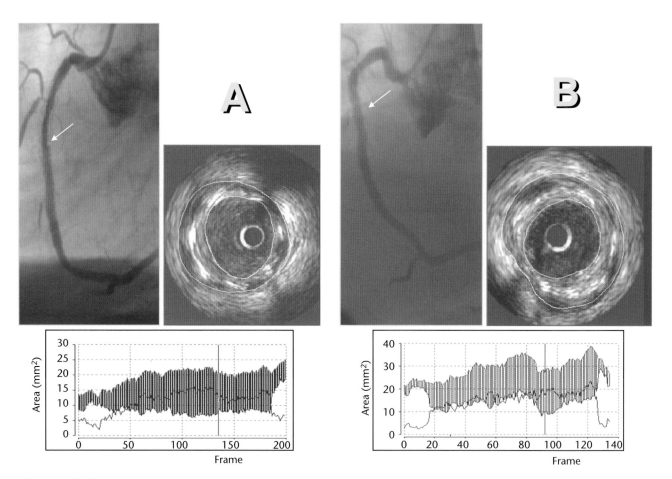

Figure 19.16
Example of positive remodeling following intracoronary brachytherapy. (A) Angiographic (left) and echographic (right) images following balloon dilatation in a patient with in-stent restenosis; the bottom plot is a 3D reconstruction of the analyzed segment: the green line delimits the vessel area (20.4 mm²), the red line delimits lumen area (9.1 mm²), the area between green and red lines or delimited by the blue line represents the plaque area (11.3 mm²). (B) Six-month angiographic and echographic results: despite an increase in plaque area (16.6 mm²), the lumen area does not vary (10.2 mm²) due to an increase in vessel area (26.8 mm²).

Inhibition of neointimal hyperplasia   The efficacy of γ-radiation therapy to prevent recurrence of in-stent restenotic lesions was serially assessed by IVUS. Data derived from IVUS analysis of various randomized trials[118–120] demonstrated that irradiated coronary arteries had significantly less increase in in-stent neointimal hyperplasia during the follow-up as compared with placebo.

IVUS and limitations of intracoronary brachytherapy

Aneurysm formation   Theoretically, the early beneficial effect of intravascular brachytherapy on arterial remodeling could lead to undesired aneurysm formation. The incidence of aneurysm formation after radiation therapy is low, probably less than 1% using current dosimetric guidelines.

Edge effect (the 'candy wrapper' effect)   A potential limitation of intracoronary brachytherapy is the development of a new stenotic lesion at both edges of the irradiated segments. This so-called 'edge effect' or 'candy wrapper' effect was originally described after high-activity radioactive stent implantation.[121] However, this phenomenon is not exclusive to radioactive stents but may also affect coronary segments treated by means of a catheter-based system.[117] Vessel wall injury concomitant with low-dose radiation at the edge of the irradiated segment may be involved in the pathophysiology of this phenomenon ('geographic miss').[122] Volumetric IVUS studies demonstrated that lack of positive remodeling together with plaque increase were the contributors to the lumen shrinkage at both edges of the irradiated segment after catheter-based brachytherapy.[117] To minimize this harmful edge effect, the use of longer sources to allow enough margin to fully cover the injured segment has been advocated when catheter-based brachytherapy is applied.[123]

Late thrombosis   Late thrombosis became apparent in the first series of patients treated with brachytherapy worldwide.[124] Delay in stent re-endothelialization has been considered as a trigger mechanism of this event. Besides, the possibility that brachytherapy may induce late stent malapposition, easily recognized by IVUS, by not being able to follow the vessel enlargement promoted by radiotherapy, has been advocated in this process.[125,126] Moreover, the implantation of a conventional stent within the irradiated segment has been considered a main contributor to this phenomenon. To overcome this late thrombosis, long-term use (> 6 months) of double antiplatelet therapy (aspirin and ticlopidine or clopidogrel) is clearly advocated when intracoronary radiation therapy is performed.

Black hole   This term stands for an echo-lucent area within the lumen of the coronary artery, noted uniquely by the use of IVUS.[127] By definition, this type of lesion should have a homogeneous black appearance without backscatter. This characteristic allows one to distinguish it from images with ring-down or other causes of relatively echo-lucency, such as contrast, thrombus, or a lipid lake. This phenomenon is associated more commonly with radioactive stent implantation in areas adjacent to the stent struts, with radiation fall-off, and may causes of restenosis.[127]

IVUS and radiation dose calculation

Dose delivered to the vessel wall may be calculated by means of so-called dose–volume histograms.[128] This method condenses into a plot the information on the dose distribution data derived from IVUS analysis. In brief, radial distances (24 pie slices, 15° for instance) from the center of the lumen (for centered systems) or from the IVUS probe (for noncentered systems) to the lumen–intima and media–adventitia boundaries may be obtained from several equidistant cross-sectional areas within the irradiated coronary segment (e.g. every 0.2 mm). Given the prescribed dose, the type of the isotope used and its activity at the time of the procedure, the dose received in those boundaries may be calculated and depicted as a cumulative dose distribution over a specific volume.

Conclusions

IVUS represents the most precise diagnostic tool for analysis of coronary artery anatomy. Atherosclerosis is a disease of the vessel wall, and currently IVUS constitutes the technique of choice to recognize atheroma and the resultant compromise of the coronary lumen. IVUS has several diagnostic applications and is useful in choosing the most adequate interventional strategy and optimizing its results. Its application during interventional techniques has also given important pathophysiologic insights into what is still considered the Achilles heel of interventional cardiology, namely restenosis. A better understanding of the mechanisms involved in this phenomenom has been the rationale for the development of new therapeutic approaches (e.g. drug-eluting stents), and therefore should always be considered when new interventional strategies are applied.

References

1. Nissen SE, Gurley JC, Grines CL, et al. Intravascular ultrasound assessment of lumen size and wall morphology in normal subjects and patients with coronary artery disease. Circulation 1991;84:1087–99.
2. Tobis JM, Mallery J, Mahon D, et al. Intravascular ultrasound imaging of human coronary arteries in vivo. Analysis of tissue characterizations with comparison to in vitro histological specimens. Circulation 1991;83:913–26
3. Mintz GS, Kent KM, Pichard AD, et al. Contribution of inadequate arterial remodeling to the development of

focal coronary artery stenoses. An intravascular ultrasound study. Circulation 1997;95:1791–8.

4. Alfonso F, Macaya C, Goicolea J, et al. Intravascular ultrasound imaging of angiographically normal coronary segments in patients with coronary artery disease. Am Heart J 1994;127:536–44.

5. Topol TJ, Nissen SE. Our preoccupation with coronary lumenology: the dissociation between clinical and angiographic findings in ischemic heart disease. Circulation 1995;92:2333–42.

6. Grondin CM, Dyrda I, Pasternac A, et al. Discrepancies between cineangiographic and postmortem findings in patients with coronary artery disease and recent coronary revascularization. Circulation 1974;49:703–8.

7. Arnett EN, Isner JN, Redwood DR, et al. Coronary artery narrowing in coronary heart disease: comparison of cineangiographic and necropsy findings. Ann Intern Med 1979;91:350–6.

8. Kern MJ. Coronary physiology revisited. Practical insights from the cardiac catheterization laboratory. Circulation 2000;101:1344–51.

9. Mintz GS, Nissen SE, Anderson WD, et al. American College of Cardiology Clinical Expert Consensus Document on Standards for Acquisition, Measurement and Reporting of Intravascular Ultrasound Studies (IVUS). A report of the American College of Cardiology Task Force on Clinical Expert Consensus Documents. J Am Coll Cardiol 2001;37:1478–92.

10. Nissen SE, Yock P. Intravascular ultrasound: novel pathophysiological insights and current clinical applications. Circulation 2001;103:604–16.

11. Mancini GBJ. Quantitative coronary arteriographic methods in the interventional catheterization laboratory: an update and perspective. J Am Coll Cardiol 1991;17:23B–33B.

12. Alfonso F. Videodensitometric versus edge-detection quantitative angiography. Insights from intravascular ultrasound imaging. Eur Heart J 2000;21:604–7.

13. Di Mario C, Görge R, Peters R, et al, on behalf of the Working Group of Echocardiography of the European Society of Cardiology. Clinical application and image interpretation in intracoronary ultrasound. Eur Heart J 1998; 19:207–29.

14. Takagi A, Tsurumi Y, Ishii Y, et al. Clinical potential of intravascular ultrasound for physiological assessment of coronary stenosis. Relationship between quantitative ultrasound tomography and pressure-derived fractional flow reserve. Circulation 1999;100:250–5.

15. Hanekamp CEE, Koolen JJ, Pijls NHJ, et al. Comparison of quantitative angiography, intravascular ultrasound and coronary pressure measurement to assess optimun stent deployment. Circulation 1999;99:1015–21.

16. Alfonso F, Macaya C, Goicolea J, et al. Determinants of coronary compliance in patients with coronary artery disease: an intravascular ultrasound study. J Am Coll Cardiol 1994;23:879–84.

17. Nakatani S, Yamagishi M, Tamai J, et al. Assessment of coronary artery distensibility by intravascular ultrasound. Application of simultaneous measurements of luminal area and pressure. Circulation 1995;91:2904–10.

18. Alfonso F, Macaya C, Goicolea J, et al. Angiographic changes (Dotter effect) produced by intravascular ultrasound imaging before coronary angioplasty. Am Heart J 1994;128:244–51.

19. Alfonso F, Goicolea J, Perez.Vizcaíno MJ, et al. Intracoronary ultrasound before coronary interventions: a prospective comparison of two different catheters. Cathet Cardiovasc Diagn 1997;40:33–9.

20. Di Mario C, Madretsma S, Linker D, et al. The angle of incidence of ultrasonic bean: a critical factor for image quality in intravascular ultrasonography. Am Heart J 1993;125:442–8.

21. Hausmann D, Erbel R, Alibelli-Chemarin MJ, et al. The safety of intracoronary ultrasound: a multicenter survey of 2207 examinations. Circulation 1995;91:623–30.

22. Batkoff BW, Linker DT. Safety of intracoronary ultrasound: data from a Multicenter European Registry. Cathet Cardiovasc Diagn 1996;38:238–41.

23. Nissen SE, Gurley JC, Grines CL, et al. Intravascular ultrasound assessment of lumen size and wall morphology in normal subjects and patients with coronary artery disease. Circulation 1991;84:1087–99.

24. Nissen SE, Grines CL, Gurley JC, et al. Application of a new phased-array ultrasound imaging catheter in the assessment of vascular dimensions: in vivo comparison to cineangiography. Circulation 1990;81:660–6.

25. Tobis JM, Mallery JA, Gessert J, et al. Intravascular ultrasound cross-sectional arterial imaging before and after balloon angioplasty in vitro. Circulation 1989; 80:873–82.

26. Honye J, Mahon DJ, Jain A, et al. Morphological effects of coronary balloon angioplasty in vivo assessed by intravascular ultrasound imaging. Circulation 1992;85: 1012–25.

27. Waller BF. 'Crackers, breakers, stretchers, drillers, scrapers, shavers, burners, welders, and melters': the future treatment of atherosclerotic coronary artery disease? A clinical–morphologic assessment. J Am Coll Cardiol 1989;13:969–87.

28. Topol EJ, Nissen SE. Our preoccupation with coronary luminology: the dissociation between clinical and angiographic findings in ischemic heart disease. Circulation 1995;92:2333–42.

29. Fitzgerald PJ, St. Goar FG, Connolly AJ, et al. Intravascular ultrasound imaging of coronary arteries. Is three layers the norm? Circulation 1992;86:154–8.

30. St Goar FG, Pinto FJ, Alderman EL, et al. Intravascular ultrasound imaging of angiographically normal coronary arteries: an in vivo comparison with quantitative angiography. J Am Coll Cardiol. 1991;18:952–8.

31. Gussenhoven EJ, Essed CE, Lancee CT, et al. Arterial wall characteristics determined by intravascular ultrasound imaging: an in vitro study. J Am Coll Cardiol 1989; 14:947–52.

32. Potkin BN, Bartorelli AL, Gessert JM, et al. Coronary artery imaging with intravascular high-frequency ultrasound. Circulation 1990;81:1575–85.

33. Nishimura RA, Edwards WD, Warnes CA, et al. Intravascular ultrasound imaging: in vitro validation and pathologic correlation. J Am Coll Cardiol 1990;16:145–54.

34. Mintz GS, Douek P, Pichard AD, et al. Target lesion calcification in coronary artery disease: an intravascular ultrasound study. J Am Coll Cardiol 1992;20:1149–55.

35. Tuzcu EM, Berkalp B, De Franco AC, et al. The dilemma of diagnosing coronary calcification: angiography versus intravascular ultrasound. J Am Coll Cardiol 1996; 27:832–8.

36. Baptista J, Di Mario C, Osaki Y, et al. Impact of plaque morphology and composition on the mechanisms of lumen enlargement using intracoronary ultrasound and quantitative angiography after balloon angioplasty. Am J Cardiol 1996;77:115–21.

37. Mintz JS, Pichard AD, Poppma JJ, et al. Preliminary experience with adjunct directional coronary atherectomy in the treatment of calcific coronary artery disease. Am J Cardiol 1994;73:423–30.

38. Fitzgerald PJ, Ports TA, Yock PG. Contribution of localized calcium deposits to dissection after angioplasty in vivo assessed by intravascular ultrasound imaging. Circulation 1992;86:64–70.

39. Siegel RJ, Ariani M, Fishbein MC, et al. Histopathologic validation of angioscopy and intravascular ultrasound. Circulation 1991;84:109–17.

40. Kearney P, Erbel R, Rupprecht HJ, et al. Differences in the morphology of unstable and stable coronary lesions and their impact on the mechanisms of angioplasty. An in vivo study with intravascular ultrasound. Eur Heart J 1996; 17:721–30.

41. Glagov S, Weisenberg E, Zarins C, et al. Compensatory enlargement of human atherosclerotic coronary arteries. N Engl J Med 1987;316:1371–5.

42. Shoenhagen P, Ziada K, Kapadia SR, et al. Extent and direction of arterial remodeling in stable versus unstable coronary syndromes: an intravascular ultrasound study. Circulation 2000;101:598–603.

43. Wong M, Edelstein J, Wollman J, et al. Ultrasonic–pathological comparison of the human arterial wall. Verification of intima–media thickness. Arterioscler Thromb 1993; 13:482–6.

44. Roberts WC, Jones AA. Quantitation of coronary arterial narrowing at necropsy in sudden coronary death. Am J Cardiol 1979;44:39–44.

45. Erbel R, Ge J, Bockisch A, et al. Value of intracoronary ultrasound and Doppler in the differentiation of angiographically normal coronary arteries: a prospective study in patients with angina pectoris. Eur Heart J 1996;17:880–9.

46. Mintz GS, Painter JA, Pichard AD, et al. Atherosclerosis in angiographically 'normal' coronary artery reference segments: an intravascular ultrasound study with clinical correlations. J Am Coll Cardiol 1995;25:1479–85.

47. Abizaid AS, Mintz GS, Mehran R, et al. Long-term follow-up after precutaneous transluminal coronary angioplasty was not performed based on intravascular ultrasound findings. Importance of lumen dimensions. Circulation 1999;100:256–61.

48. Kern MJ, Donohue TJ, Aguirre FV, et al. Clinical outcome of deferring angioplasty in patients with normal translesional pressure–flow velocity measurements. J Am Coll Cardiol 1995;25:178–87.

49. Bech GJ, De Bruyne B, Bonnier HJ, et al. Long-term follow-up after deferral of percutaneous transluminal coronary angioplasty of intermediate stenosis on the basis of coronary pressure measurement. J Am Coll Cardiol 1998;31:841–7.

50. Alfonso F, Delgado A, Magalhaes D, et al. Value of intravascular ultrasound in the assessment of coronary pseudostenosis during coronary interventions. Cathet Cardiovasc Diagn 1999;46:327–32.

51. Escaned J, Flores A, García P, et al. Guidewire-induced coronary pseudostenosis as a source of error during physiological guidance of stent deployment. Cathet Cardiovasc Interv 2000;51:91–4.

52. Isner JM, Kishel J, Kent KM. Accuracy of angiographic determination of left main coronary arterial narrowing. Circulationsa 1981;63:1056–61.

53. Hermiller JB, Buller CE, Tenaglia AN, et al. Unrecognized left main coronary artery disease in patients undergoing interventional procedures. Am J Cardiol 1993;71:173–6.

54. Abizaid AS, Mintz GS, Abizaid A, et al. One-year follow-up after intravascular ultrasound assessment of moderate left main coronary artery disease in patients with ambiguous angiograms. J Am Coll Cardiol 1999;34:707–15.

55. Stark RP, McGinn AL, Wilson RF. Chest pain in cardiac-transplant recipients: evidence of sensory reinnervation after cardiac transplantation. N Engl J Med 1991; 324:1791–4.

56. Mairesse GH, Marwick TH, Melin JA, et al. Use of exercise electrocardiography, technetium-99m-MIBI perfusion tomography, and two-dimensional echocardiography for coronary disease surveillance in a low-prevalence population of heart transplant recipients. J Heart Lung Transplant 1995;14:222–9.

57. Smart FW, Ballantyne CM, Cocanougher B, et al. Insensitivity of noninvasive tests to detect coronary artery vasculopathy after heart transplant. Am J Cardiol 1991; 67:243–7.

58. Dressler FA, Miller LW. Necropsy versus angiography: How accurate is angiography? J Heart Lung Transplant 1992;11:S56–9.

59. Pinto FJ, Chenzbraun A, Botas J, et al. Feasibility of serial intracoronary ultrasound imaging for assessment of progression of intimal proliferation in cardiac transplant recipients. Circulation 1994;90:2348–55.

60. Uretsky BF, Murali S, Reddy PS, et al. Development of coronary artery disease in cardiac transplant patients receiving immunosuppressive therapy with cyclosporine and prednisone. Circulation 1987;76:827–34.

61. Gao SZ, Alderman EL, Schroeder JS, et al. Accelerated coronary vascular disease in the heart transplant patient: coronary arteriographic findings. J Am Coll Cardiol 1988;12:334–40.

62. Yeung AC, Davis SF, Hauptman PJ, et al. Incidence and progression of transplant coronary artery disease over 1 year: results of a multicenter trial with use of intravascular ultrasound: Multicenter Intravascular Ultrasound Transplant Study Group. J Heart Lung Transplant 1995; 14:S215–20.

63. Tuzcu EM, Hobbs RE, Rincon G, et al. Occult and frequent transmission of atherosclerotic coronary disease with cardiac transplantation: insights from intravascular ultrasound. Circulation 1995;91:1706–13.

64. Mehra MR, Ventura HO, Stapleton DD, et al. Presence of severe intimal thickening by intravascular ultrasonography predicts cardiac events in cardiac allograft vasculopathy. J Heart Lung Transplant 1995;14:632–39.

65. Lee DY, Nishioka T, Tabak SW, et al. Effect of intracoronary imaging on clinical decision making. Am Heart J 1995;129:1084–93.

66. Mintz GS, Pichard AD, Kovach JA, et al. Impact of preintervention intravascular ultrasound imaging on transcatheter treatment strategies in coronary artery disease. Am J Cardiol 1994;73:423–30.

67. Honye J, Mahon DJ, Jain A, et al. Morphological effects of coronary balloon angioplasty in vivo assessed by intravascular ultrasound imaging. Circulation 1992;85:1012–25.

68. Kearney P, Koch L, Ge J, et al. Differences in morphology of stable and unstable coronary lesions after impact on the mechanism of angioplasty. An in vivo study with IVUS. Eur Heart J 1996;17:721–30.

69. Stone GW, Hodgson JM, St. Goar FG, et al., for the Clinical Outcomes with Ultrasound Trial (CLOUT) Investigators. Improved procedural results of coronary angioplasty with intravascular ultrasound guided balloon sizing. Circulation 1997;95:2044–52.

70. Abizaid A, Pichard AD, Mintz GS, et al. Acute and long-term results of an IVUS-guided PTCA/provisional stent implantation strategy. Am J Cardiol 1999;84:1381–4.

71. Schroeder S, Baumbach A, Haase KK, et al. Reduction of restenosis by vessel size adapted percutaneous transluminal coronary angioplasty using intravascular ultrasound. Am J Cardiol 1999;83:875–9.

72. Haase KK, Athanasiadis A, Mahrholdt H, et al. Acute and one year follow-up results after vessel size adapted PTCA using intracoronary ultrasound. Eur Heart J 1998;19:263–72.

73. Peters RJ, Kok WE, Di Mario C, et al. Prediction of restenosis after coronary balloon angioplasty: Results of PICTURE (Post-IntraCoronary Treatment Ultrasound Result Evaluation), a prospective multicenter intracoronary ultrasound imaging study. Circulation 1997;95:2254–61.

74. Fitzgerald PJ, Yock PG. Mechanisms and outcomes of angioplasty and atherectomy assessed by intravascular ultrasound imaging. J Clin Ultrasound 1993;21:579–88.

75. The GUIDE Trial Investigators. IVUS-determined predictors of restenosis in PTCA and DCA: an interim report from the GUIDE trial, Phase II. Circulation 1994;90:4;2:I-23.

76. Pasterkamp G, Wensing PJ, Post MJ, et al. Paradoxical arterial wall shrinkage may contribute to luminal narrowing of human atherosclerotic femoral arteries. Circulation 1995;91:1444–9.

77. Mintz GS, Kent KM, Pichard AD, et al. Contribution of inadequate arterial remodeling to the development of focal coronary artery stenoses: an intravascular ultrasound study. Circulation 1997;95:1791–8.

78. Nakamura S, Colombo A, Gaglione A, et al. Intracoronary ultrasound observations during stent implantation. Circulation 1994;89:2026–34.

79. Mudra H, Klauss V, Blasini R, et al. Ultrasound guidance of Palmatz–Schatz intracoronary stenting with a combined intravascular ultrasound balloon catheter. Circulation 1994;90:1252–61.

80. Colombo A, Hall P, Nakamura S, et al. Intracoronary stenting without anticoagulation accomplished with intravascular ultrasound guidance. Circulation 1995;91:1676–88.

81. Moussa I, Di Mario C, Di Francesco L, et al. Subacute stent thrombosis and the anticoagulation controversy: changes in drug therapy, operator technique, and the impact of intravascular ultrasound. Am J Cardiol 1997;78(Suppl 3A):13–17.

82. de Feyter PJ, Kay P, Disco C, et al. Reference chart derived from post-stent-implantation intravascular ultrasound predictors of 6-month expected restenosis on quantitative coronary angiography. Circulation 1999;100:1777–83.

83. Kuntz RE, Baim DS. Defining coronary restenosis: newer clinical and angiographic paradigms. Circulation 1993;88:1310–23.

84. DeJaegere P, Mudra H, Figulla H, et al. Intravascular ultrasound-guided optimized stent deployment: Immediate and 6 months clinical and angiographic results from the multicenter ultrasound stenting in coronaries study (MUSIC study). Eur Heart J 1998;19:1214–23.

85. Serruys PW, van der Giessen W, Garcia E, et al. Clinical and angiographic results with the Multi-Link stent implanted under ultrasound guidance (WEST-2 study). J Invasive Cardiol 1998;10:20B–7B.

86. Schwartz RS, Huber KC, Murphy JG, et al. Restenosis and the proportional neointimal response to coronary artery injury: results in a porcine model. J Am Coll Cardiol 1992;19:267–74.

87. Staab ME, Srivatsa SS, Lerman A, et al. Arterial remodeling after experimental injury is highly dependent on adventitial injury and histopathology. Int J Cardiol 1997;58:31–40.

88. Frey AW, Hodgson JM, Müller C, et al. Ultrasound-guided strategy for provisional stenting with focal balloon combination catheter. Results from the randomized Strategy for Intracoronary Ultrasound-Guided PTCA and Stenting (SIPS) trial. Circulation 2000;102:2497–502.

89. Fitzgerald PJ, Oshima A, Hayase M, et al. Final results of the Can Routine Ultrasound Influence Stent Expansion (CRUISE) study. Circulation 2000; 102:523–530.

90. Mudra H, di Mario C, de Jaegere P, et al. Randomized comparison of coronary stent implantation under ultrasound or angiographic guidance to reduce stent restenosis (OPTICUS study). Circulation 2001;104:1343–9.

91. Russo RJ, Attubato MJ, Davidson CJ, et al. Angiography versus intravascular ultrasound-directed stent placement: final results from AVID. Circulation 1999;100:I-N234(abst).

92. Schiele F, Meneveau N, Vuillemenot A, et al. Impact of intravascular ultrasound guidance in stent deployment on 6-month restenosis rate: a multicenter, randomized study comparing two strategies – with and without intravascular ultrasound guidance (RESIST study). J Am Coll Cardiol 1998;32:320–8.

93. Oemrawsingh PV, Mintz GS, Schalij MJ, et al. Intravascular ultrasound guidance improves angiographic and clinical outcome of stent implantation for long coronary artery stenoses: final results of a randomized comparison with angiographic guidance (TULIP study). Circulation 2003;107:62–7.

94. Painter JA, Mintz GS, Wong SC, et al. Serial intravascular ultrasound studies fail to show evidence of chronic Palmaz–Schatz stent recoil. Am J Cardiol 1995;75:398–400.

95. Hoffmann R, Mintz GS, Mehran R, et al. Intravascular ultrasound predictors of angiographic restenosis in lesions treated with Palmaz–Schatz stents. J Am Coll Cardiol 1998;31:43–9.

96. Prati F, Di Mario C, Moussa I, et al. In-stent neointimal proliferation correlates with the amount of residual plaque burden outside the stent: an intravascular ultrasound study. Circulation 1999;99:1011–14.

97. Alfonso F, Garcia P, Pimentel G, et al. Predictors and implications of residual plaque burden after coronary stenting. An intravascular ultrasound study. Am Heart J 2003;152:248–53.

98. Serruys PW, Degertekin M, Tanabe K, et al. Intravascular ultrasound findings in the multicenter, randomized, double-blind RAVEL (RAndomized study with the sirolimus-eluting VElocity balloon-expandable stent in the treatment of patients with de novo native coronary artery Lesions) trial. Circulation 2002;106:798–803.

99. Moses JW, Leon MB, Popma JJ, et al. for the SIRIUS Investigators. Sirolimus-eluting stents versus standard stents in patients with stenosis in a native coronary artery. N Engl J Med 2003;349:1315–23.

100. Umans VA, Baptista J, Di Mario C, et al. Angiographic, ultrasonic, and angioscopic assessment of the coronary artery wall and lumen area configuration after directional atherectomy: the mechanism revisited. Am Heart J 1995;130:217–27.

101. Topol EJ, Leya F, Pinkerton CA, et al. A comparison of directional atherectomy with coronary angioplasty in patients with coronary artery disease. N Engl J Med 1993;329:221–7.

102. Adelman AG, Cohen M, Kimball BP, et al. Canadian coronary atherectomy trial. A randomized comparison of directional atherectomy and percutaneous transluminal coronary angioplasty for lesions of the proximal left anterior descending artery. N Engl J Med 1993;329:228–34.

103. Simonton CA, Leon MB, Kuntz RE, et al. Acute and late clinical angiographic results of directional atherectomy in the Optimal Atherectomy Restenosis Study (OARS). Circulation 1995;92:I-545.

104. Sumitsuji T, Suzuki T, Katoh O, et al. for the ABACAS investigators. Restenosis mechanism after aggressive directional coronary atherectomy assessed by intravascular ultrasound in Adjunctive Balloon Angioplasty following Coronary Atherectomy Study (ABACAS). J Am Coll Cardiol 1997;129A(abst).

105. Baim DS, Cutlip DE, Sharma SK, et al. Final results of the Balloon vs Optimal Atherectomy Trial (BOAT). Circulation 1998;97:322–31.

106. Moussa I, Moses J, Di Mario C, et al. Stenting after Optimal Lesion Debulking (SOLD) registry. Angiographic and clinical outcome. Circulation 1998;98:1604–9.

107. Colombo A. AMIGO study. Proceedings from TCT-2002.

108. Sharma SK, Duvuri S, Dangas G, et al. Rotational atherectomy for in-stent restenosis: acute and long-term results of first 100 cases. J Am Coll Cardiol 1998;32:1358–65.

109. vom Dahl J, Radke P, Haager P, et al. Clinical and angiographic predictors of recurrent restenosis after percutaneous transluminal rotational atherectomy for treatment of diffuse in-stent restenosis. Am J Cardiol 1999;83:862–7.

110. Mehran R, Dangas G, Mintz G, et al. Treatment of in-stent restenosis with excimer laser coronary angioplasty versus rotational atherectomy: comparative mechanisms and results. Circulation 2000;101:2484–9.

111. vom Dahl J, Dietz U, Haager PK, et al. Rotational atherectomy does not reduce recurrent in-stent restenosis: results of the Angioplasty versus Rotational Atherectomy for Treatment of Diffuse In-Stent Restenosis Trial (ARTIST). Circulation 2002;105:583–8.

112. Dussaillant GR, Mintz GS, Pichard AD, et al. Small stent size and intimal hyperplasia contribute to restenosis: a volumetric intravascular ultrasound analysis. J Am Coll Cardiol 1995;26:720–4.

113. Eltchaninoff H, Koning R, Tron C, et al. Balloon angioplasty for the treatment of coronary in-stent restenosis: immediate results and 6-month angiographic recurrent restenosis rate. J Am Coll Cardiol 1998;32:980–4.

114. Bauters C, Banos JL, Van Belle E, et al. Six-month angiographic outcome after successful repeat percutaneous intervention for in-stent restenosis. Circulation 1998; 97:318–21.

115. Waksman R (ed). Vascular Brachytherapy, 2nd edn. Armonk, NY: Futura, 1999.

116. King SB III, Williams DO, Chogule P, et al. Endovascular beta-radiation to reduce restenosis after coronary balloon angioplasty. Results of the Beta Energy Restenosis Trial (BERT). Circulation 1998;97:2025–30.

117. Sabaté M, Serruys PW, van der Giessen WJ, et al. Geometric vascular remodeling after balloon angioplasty and beta-radiation therapy: a three-dimensional intravascular ultrasound study. Circulation 1999;100:1182–8.

118. Teirstein PS, Massullo V, Jani S, et al. Catheter-based radiotherapy to inhibit restenosis after coronary stenting. N Engl J Med 1997;336:1697–703

119. Ahmed JM, Mintz GS, Waksman R, et al. Serial intravascular ultrasound assessment of the efficacy of intracoronary gamma-radiation therapy for preventing recurrence in very long, diffuse, in-stent restenosis lesions. Circulation 2001;104:856–9.

120. Mintz GS, Weissman NJ, Teirstein PS et al. Effect of intracoronary gamma radiation therapy on in-stent restenosis: an intravascular ultrasound analysis from the Gamma-1 study. Circulation 2000;102:2915–18.

121. Albiero R, Adamian M, Kobayashi N, et al. Short- and intermediate-term results of ^{32}P radioactive beta-emitting stent implantation in patients with coronary artery disease. The Milan Dose–Response study. Circulation 2000;101:18–26.

122. Sabaté M, Costa MA, Kozuma K, et al. Geographic miss: a cause of treatment failure in radio-oncology applied to intracoronary radiation therapy. Circulation 2000; 101:2467–71.

123. Pötter R, van Limbergen E, Dries W, et al. Recommendations of the EVA GEC ESTRO Working Group: prescribing, recording, and reporting in endovascular brachytherapy. Quality assurance, equipment, personnel and education. Radiother Oncol 2001;59:339–60.

124. Costa M, Sabaté M, van der Giessen WJ, et al. Late coronary occlusion after intracoronary brachytherapy. Circulation 1999;100:789–92.

125. Sabaté M, van der Giessen WJ, Deshpande NV, et al. Late thrombotic occlusion of a malapposed stent 10 months after intracoronary brachytherapy. Int J Cardiovasc Interv 1999;2:55–9.

126. Kozuma K, Costa MA, Sabaté M, et al. Late stent malapposition occurring after intracoronary beta-irradiation detected by intravascular ultrasound. J Invasive Cardiol 1999; 11:651–5.

127. Kay IP, Wardeh AJ, Kozuma K, et al. The pattern of restenosis and vascular remodelling after cold-end radioactive stent implantation. Eur Heart J 2001;22:1311–17.

128. Drzymala RE, Mohan R, Brewster L, et al. Dose-volume histograms. Int J Radiat Oncol Biol Phys 1991;21:71–8.

20

Physiological assessment of coronary circulation using pressure and Doppler guidewires

Javier Escaned

Introduction

As stated elsewhere in this book, soon after its introduction as a diagnostic technique, the limitations of coronary angiography in assessing the underlying atherosclerotic involvement of the studied vessel became evident.[1-5] Cardiologists have focused on coronary lumenology, despite the dissociation between coronary angiography and clinical manifestations.[2] This approach, when allied to facilitated coronary intervention, may lead to the use of the feared 'oculostenotic reflex'. The implications of using 'lumenology' for the grading of coronary disease according to the number of vessels with angiographic stenoses has also been questioned. As remarked by Plotnick,[3] clinical decisions based only on the number of vessels exemplify a unidimensional approach to a multidimensional problem, which could be amended if 'less anatomy and more physiology' were used in the assessment of ischemic heart disease. It was against this background that intracoronary guidewires fitted with flow velocity Doppler and pressure sensors were developed during the late 1980s and through the 1990s.[6,7]

How can pressure and Doppler guidewires complement the information obtained during angiography? By far the most common question raised during the review of a coronary angiogram is whether a given stenosis is hemodynamically significant and therefore is a cause of myocardial ischemia. On other occasions, the physician or investigator would like to assess the status of the coronary microcirculation, which can be affected by many conditions and which not only can constitute a cause of cardiopathy but also may interfere with some techniques used for assessment of coronary stenoses. And in which way should these new technologies help the clinician? An

ideal physiological assessment of the discussed aspects of coronary circulation should (1) provide information that incorporates different aspects of coronary physiology, (2) be accurate, (3) be independent of changing hemodynamic conditions, (4) be easy to perform, (5) be safe, and (6) be easy to interpret.

In this chapter, we will focus on the use of intracoronary guidewires fitted with pressure or flow velocity microsensors for physiological assessment of coronary circulation in the catheterization laboratory. We shall review, firstly, the basic concepts of coronary physiology that are required for an adequate understanding of intracoronary physiological techniques. Then we shall move to a review of the technological and practical principles of intracoronary guidewires with pressure and flow velocity sensors. This will be followed by a separate discussion of the different indices for assessment of coronary circulation that can be obtained either with one type of guidewire or by combining the information obtained with both. Finally, we shall review the degrees of evidence supporting the use of intracoronary physiology for diagnostic purposes or for guidance of revascularization procedures.

Some relevant physiological aspects of coronary circulation

An understanding of the principles underlying intracoronary physiological techniques is essential for its adequate use and for a correct interpretation of the results obtained. It is customary to describe the coronary circulation in terms of analogies with simple electrical or hydraulic circuits. However, these analogies are far from capable of integrating the complexity of the phenomena that occur during the cardiac cycle. For this reason, we will combine this approach with specific comments about aspects that require an alternative description to those provided by that model.

Heart function is highly dependent on the maintenance and modulation of coronary blood flow

The myocardium, particularly the subendocardium, is the tissue with the highest baseline aerobic demands in the body (8–10 ml O_2/min/100 g versus 0.15 ml O_2/min/100 g in the skeletal muscle). The three main determinants of this demand are wall stress, inotropic state, and heart rate.[8–10]

Coronary blood flow is influenced by extravascular compression

Throughout the cardiac cycle, variations in intramyocardial and intracavitary pressure modify coronary vascular resistance drastically.[11] Coronary blood flow is modulated by variations in the resistance of the vascular bed. Whereas blood flow is predominantly diastolic in the left coronary artery, in the right coronary artery there is also systolic blood flow due to the low extravascular compression exerted by the right ventricle and atrium.[11,12] As a result, the phasic characteristics of the transtenotic gradient are also different, paralleling the blood flow pattern through the stenosis. If the microcirculation presents significant obliteration (e.g. by microvascular embolization or myocardial damage), then systolic extravascular compression is not followed by the normally expected antegrade flow towards capillaries and veins, but is translated into retrograde flow in the epicardial vessels.[13] Extravascular compression of epicardial vessels by a myocardial bridge may also cause systolic backflow in the coronary segments proximal to the bridge.[14]

Under baseline circumstances, the relation between blood pressure and flow in the coronary arteries is not linear

If the only situation considered from now on is mid end-diastole, that is to say, a situation in which extravascular compression is minimal and constant and there are no variations in coronary conductance, then coronary blood flow remains stable over a broad range of pressures. This phenomenon is termed coronary self-regulation and is the result of intrinsic myogenic tone, a response by the smooth muscle cells of the coronary arterioles to pressure

variations[4,15,16] (Figure 20.1). Coronary self-regulation is only effective within a certain range of pressures indicated: when the perfusion pressure falls below this pressure, coronary blood flow decreases.

During maximum coronary hyperemia, the relation between coronary blood pressure and flow is linear

In contrast to the situation just described, during complete vasodilation of resistance vessels induced by a maximum physiological or pharmacological hyperemic stimulus (increased myocardial metabolism), a fixed relation between coronary perfusion pressure and blood flow can be observed (Figure 20.1). The slope of this relation (which is the coronary conductance) is influenced by the resistance of the system: the lower this slope is, the greater the resistance of the system will be.[17,18] The pressure–flow relation during maximum hyperemia constitutes a ceiling of expected coronary flow values for different perfusion pressures.[19]

The increase in blood flow from self-regulation to the maximum hyperemia situation is an indicator of the functional state of the coronary system

This concept constitutes the coronary flow reserve, a functional indicator of the state of coronary circulation that is widely used in diagnostic techniques.[5,19,20] In Figure 20.1, this principle is illustrated schematically. It is important to remember that under normal conditions, the coronary reserve is transmurally heterogeneous: in the subendocardium, the coronary reserve is smaller because there is a greater baseline degree of arteriolar vasodilation as a result of greater subendocardial metabolic requirements.

The presence of epicardial stenosis causes a loss of energy associated with blood flow that is expressed as a fall in effective perfusion pressure

The hydraulic resistance of a stenosis has two distinct components: one related to friction (f) and the other related to flow turbulence at the exit site of the stenosis (s) (Figure 20.2). The transtenotic pressure gradient, ΔP, has a nonlinear relation with the f and s components and flow Q, in accordance with the expression $\Delta P = fQ + sQ^2$. The resistive components of friction and turbulence are

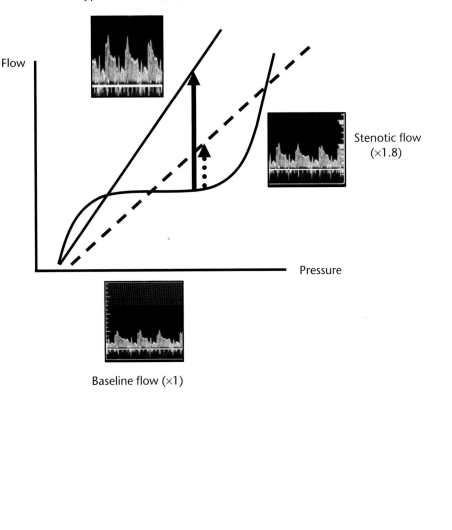

Hyperemic flow (×3)

Flow

Stenotic flow (×1.8)

Pressure

Baseline flow (×1)

Figure 20.1
Application of the relation between intracoronary pressure and flow to the diagnostic study of coronary circulation. The basic concept of coronary reserve is shown. Under baseline conditions, the relation between pressure and flow is not linear, but is characterized by a broad plateau of pressures for which coronary flow remains constant – a phenomenon modulated by arteriolar resistance. Nevertheless, during maximum hyperemia induced by myocardial oxygen demand or the administration of vasodilator drugs, this relation is linear (solid lines). The slope of this relation expresses coronary resistance (R). A situation is considered physiological when resistance is normal (small R). The induction of hyperemia means that, for a given pressure, coronary flow increases 3 times over baseline values (arrow). Nevertheless, an increase in resistance (large R) resulting from epicardial stenosis or microcirculatory dysfunction, and manifested as a less pronounced slope in the pressure–flow relation, is associated with a smaller increase in flow in relation to baseline values for the same pressure (1.8 times the baseline flow value). The intracoronary velocity tracings obtained with a Doppler guidewire make it possible to obtain, in accordance with this principle, the coronary flow velocity reserve (CFVR).

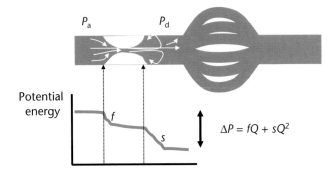

P_a P_d

Potential energy

f

s

$\Delta P = fQ + sQ^2$

Figure 20.2
The development of an intracoronary gradient results from the loss of energy of coronary flow due to friction (f) across the stenosis and to the development of turbulence (s) during the separation of flow lines at the distal aspect of the stenosis. Since coronary flow is also modulated by the status of the microcirculation, it is possible to infer from the formula that transstenotic gradient is also influenced by microcirculatory status.

influenced by characteristics of the blood (viscosity and density) and the geometry of the stenosis (reduction of luminal area, length, and the inflow and outflow angles).[16,19,20] The complex interrelation between these factors contrasts with the simplicity of the indices of angiographic severity commonly used in clinical practice (e.g. the percentage of luminal diameter), and illustrates the limitations of angiography for evaluating the functional repercussions of stenosis.

Coronary self-regulation compensates for the fall in blood pressure caused by stenosis in order to maintain constant coronary blood flow

The mechanism of self-regulation, which under physiological conditions adjusts microcirculatory resistance to myocardial blood flow requirements, has a chronic compensatory function in response to the fall in intracoronary pressure secondary to stenosis. As the stenosis increases in severity, sustained arteriolar vasodilation increasingly compromises the self-regulatory function to maintain an adequate myocardial blood flow. In other words, the compensatory function of coronary self-regulation in a stenotic vessel is at the expense of reducing coronary reserve. The compromised coronary reserve is first evident in the subendocardium, where baseline arteriolar vasodilation is greater due to higher energy demands.

The hemodynamic effect of a stenosis is manifested in the smaller slope of the pressure–flow relation

The diagnostic utility of the coronary reserve concept derives from this finding. The potential increase in coronary blood flow from a given pressure at baseline to maximum hyperemia (i.e. the coronary reserve) decreases in the presence of stenosis. This effect is quantifiable if measurements obtained at baseline and in hyperemia are obtained (Figure 20.1). In addition, because adjacent vascular beds have a preserved coronary reserve, the induction of maximum hyperemia tends to increase the heterogeneity of myocardial perfusion, a phenomenon that constitutes the basis for some noninvasive imaging diagnostic techniques. In this sense, pure arterial vasodilators (adenosine, papaverine, and dipyridamole), administered systemically, enhance the heterogeneity of regional and transmural myocardial perfusion (inducing a steal phenomenon when the vessel of the epicardial layers dilate). Dobutamine exhausts the coronary reserve in the stenotic vessel as a result of metabolically increasing myocardial demand (it increases contractility and myocardial oxygen consumption more than physical exercise) and specifically inducing vasodilation of the microcirculation (doses of 30–40 μg/kg/min produce overall coronary vasodilation similar to that of adenosine administered systemically).[21] Finally, physical exercise is the most physiological stimulus, since it combines metabolic stimuli with neural modulation of the coronary circulation.

Microcirculatory dysfunction is also manifested as a smaller slope of the pressure–flow relation

This is important for a correct interpretation of diagnostic techniques based on coronary reserve, and explains the development of techniques for the specific assessment of epicardial and microcirculatory resistance.[6,7,22] Many clinical entities that cause remodeling of the coronary microcirculation also participate in the development of epicardial stenoses, such as diabetes mellitus, systemic

arterial hypertension, smoking, and hypercholesterolemia, as well as heart transplant vasculopathy.[22] Likewise, microcirculatory resistance can increase in relation to α-adrenergic stimulation (e.g. in relation to physical exercise or mental stress),[23] during acute myocardial ischemia,[24] or as a result of microembolization (platelet or thrombotic aggregates, or particles resulting from rotational atherectomy).[13] Another important observation for diagnostic techniques and, particularly fractional flow reserve, is that microcirculatory dysfunction reduces the gradient of transstenotic pressure in an epicardial stenosis that, as discussed above, is dependent on coronary blood flow.[7] This phenomenon can lead to an incorrect interpretation of diagnostic tests that are based on the Bernouilli formula or measurement of the translesional gradient.[6,25] This again explains the importance of tests that allow independent assessment of the severity of an epicardial stenosis and the state of microcirculation.

Technical aspects of pressure and Doppler guidewires

Although various invasive techniques have been used for the physiological assessment of coronary circulation in the cardiac catheterization suite,[26] the instruments most used at present are very small-caliber guidewires equipped with speed or pressure sensors[6,7] (Figure 20.3). Two solid 0.014 inch pressure guidewires are currently available: the PressureWire (Radi Medical Systems, Uppsala, Sweden) and the WaveWire (Endosonics, Rancho Cordoba, CA). In both guidewires, the pressure transducer is located at the transition between the radiopaque guidewire tip and the non-radiopaque stem, thus allowing accurate positioning of the pressure transducer under fluoroscopy. The interface consoles for the two guidewires are, however, different. The WaveWire console (WaveMap) displays the aortic, intracoronary pressures and fractional flow reserve (FFR) in a digital format, the latter being calculated automatically either following intracoronary administration of adenosine or during continuous intravenous administration. It therefore requires an external polygraph for visualization and recording of pressure tracings. The RadiAnalyzer is a self-contained unit that allows visualization of aortic and intracoronary pressure, as well as instantaneous FFR, on a screen. The complete pressure tracing obtained during the induction of hyperemia is digitally recorded and can be postprocessed to overcome artifacts that might have led to an erroneous estimation of FFR in the automatic mode. Recording of mean pressures can also be performed on paper using a conventional polygraph. A word of caution must be added regarding the way in which mean pressures is calculated in this case by the polygraph, since those in which averaging of pressures

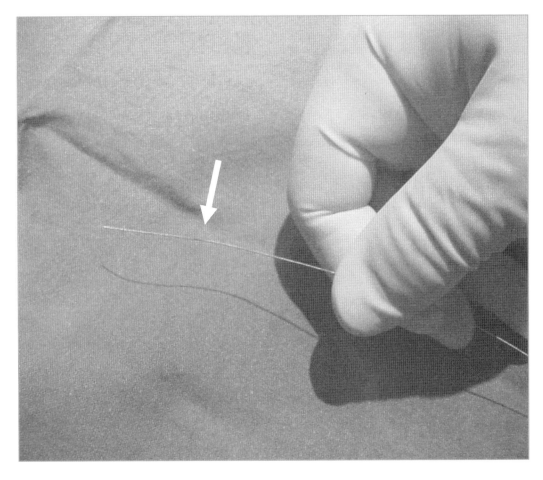

Figure 20.3
Pressure guidewire, showing the location of the pressure microsensor.

takes place over a long period of time (e.g. 10 s) may yield serious errors if a short-acting hyperemic stimulus (e.g. intracoronary adenosine) is used. The operator should be aware about this problem, which can be solved by adjusting the pressure-averaging settings in many polygraphs, or which may make mandatory the use of a sustained hyperemic stimulus for FFR measurements.

The only commercially available 0.014 inch Doppler guidewire to our knowledge is the FlowWire (Endosonics), which is used in combination with the FloMap console. A 12 MHz Doppler sensor is located at the guidewire tip. The console performs a spectral analysis of the radiofrequency signal, defining a sample volume at 5.2 mm from the tip, which is beyond the area of distortion of flow profile induced by the guidewire. Since the guidewire tip is curved to form a 14° angle, it is possible to obtain information on coronary flow velocity in the central area of the arterial lumen in a coronary artery of standard dimensions. The FloMap console provides information on average and peak flow velocities. Combining flow and electrocardiographic information, it calculates systolic and diastolic components of flow velocity and yields a diastolic/systolic velocity ratio. The system stores information on a baseline situation and, following induction of hyperemia, automati-

cally identifies the point of maximal flow velocity and calculates the coronary flow velocity reserve. It also provides a graphical representation of the flow velocity trend during recent minutes.

Practical aspects of intracoronary instrumentation with sensor-fitted guidewires

It is advisable that pressure guidewires be used in conjunction with coronary guiding catheters. This recommendation stems mainly from the potential need to perform an interventional procedure should a complication due to guidewire manipulation occur. Furthermore, diagnostic coronary catheters have a smaller lumen and less smooth inner coating, which may interfere with guidewire manipulation. The guiding catheter should not have side holes, since these may not only lead to spillage of hyperemic agents from the coronary ostium if given through them, but also may interfere with accurate pressure measurement.[27] During hyperemia, the increase in coronary blood flow can actually cause engagement of the guiding catheter in the coronary ostium, causing damping of pressure and decrease in flow. To avoid this phenomenon, it is advisable to monitor the phasic characteristics of aortic pressure at the catheter tip during hyperemia. The available 0.014 inch pressure guidewires are compatible with regular interventional devices, such as balloon catheters, intravascular ultrasound (IVUS) catheters, etc., but, as with other guidewires with floppy tips, pressure guidewires should be used with caution in those single operator exchange (SOE) devices with a short monorail segment, like some IVUS catheters, since kinking and entanglement of the wire by the device may occur.[28] In contrast to pressure guidewires, the increase in blood flow with the induction of hyperemia can cause a signal loss from Doppler guidewires, necessitating reorientation of the angled tip towards the center of the lumen. Guidewire manipulation in the coronary vessels is only performed following administration of heparin, either after administration of a minimum of 5000 units or by adjusting the heparin dose to achieve an activated clotting time (ACT) above 250 s.

Induction of hyperemia

Calculation of many of the indices that will be described below requires pharmacological induction of maximum coronary hyperemia. The agents most often used are adenosine (or adenosine triphosphate) and papaverine. Adenosine can be administered by the intracoronary (20–40 μg bolus) or intravenous (140–160 μg/kg/min) routes. It must be used with caution in patients with bronchial hyperreactivity, cardiac conduction disorders, or severe kidney failure. Its effect can be antagonized by concomitant xanthine treatment. Papaverine administered as an intracoronary bolus (12 mg in the left coronary and 8 mg in the right) provides a stable maximum hyperemia lasting approximately 1 minute. Finally (although it is not generally used in calculations of coronary reserve), the administration of maximal doses of dobutamine (30–40 μg/kg/min) is also associated with maximal coronary hyperemia.[21]

From a practical point of view, and taking adenosine as the hyperemic agent more frequently used, we can make several remarks. For practical reasons, many centers preferentially use the intracoronary route for administration of the agent, but this approach is more prone to pitfalls that might lead to erroneous results. Firstly, the operator should be aware that part of the dose of hyperemic agent given intracoronarily may be spilled out through the guidewire introducer and hemostatic valve, or may not reach the coronary microcirculation of the target vessel due to inappropriate canulation of the vessel, distribution of the drug preferentially to other coronary branches, etc.

(as discussed above, catheters with side holes cannot be used in this situation). It is recommended, in addition to adequate sealing of the angiography system and proper canulation of the vessel, to perform multiple measurements with increasing doses of intracoronary adenosine to ensure that the plateau of the dose–response curve of adenosine has been reached. Secondly, the operator should be aware that the peak effect of intracoronary adenosine is very short (Figure 20.4). The settings of the polygraph should therefore be adjusted for calculation of mean pressure over a very short period (1–3 beats). Otherwise, the obtained pressure reading may not represent the true values during the peak effect of adenosine. It is also critical that flushing of the catheter following administration of the adenosine bolus be performed as rapidly as possible. Thirdly, it should be noted that some validation studies, particularly those used to establish its optimal cutoff value for fractional flow reserve,[29] have been performed using intravenous adenosine infusion. In a study on this subject performed by our group,[30] FFR values obtained with incremental doses of intracoronary adenosine and intravenous adenosine infusion were compared in a cohort of selected patients. The results demonstrated that intracoronary doses of 20, 40, and 80 μg were associated with a percentage of false negatives of 21%, 13%, and 10%, taking the FFR measured with intravenous adenosine as a reference. In spite of performing the study following all the above recommendations, this appears to be an unacceptably high number of false-negative FFR values using the intracoronary administration route. Similar concerns have been raised with regard to the measurement of coronary flow velocity reserve.[31]

Coronary flow velocity reserve

The most direct use of Doppler guidewires is for the calculation of coronary flow velocity reserve (CFVR), an index equivalent to classic, or volumetric, coronary reserve.[26] CFVR is the ratio between intracoronary mean velocity in baseline conditions and following pharmacological induction of maximum hyperemia. This index does not discriminate between the effect on coronary reserve of epicardial stenoses or microcirculatory disorders. Its usefulness in the hemodynamic assessment of epicardial stenoses has been studied widely. The most relevant studies in this field are listed in Table 20.1, with the type of test used to detect ischemia used as a reference.[32–40] The cut-off point for determining the hemodynamic relevance of these studies varies, with CFVR < 2 generally being accepted as indicative of abnormal coronary reserve. The main limitation of the concept of CFVR is its dependence on values obtained with respect to the baseline flow velocity, which can be modified by many factors, including sex, blood pressure, and heart rate.[6,26,41–43] CFVR also is

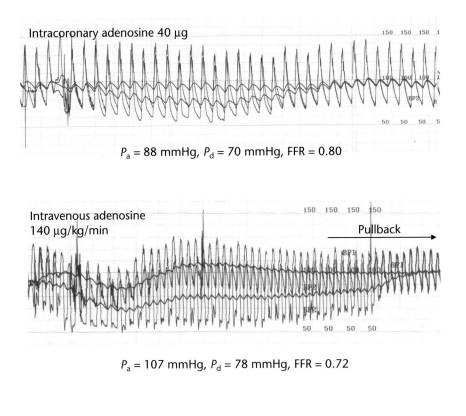

Intracoronary adenosine 40 µg

$P_a = 88$ mmHg, $P_d = 70$ mmHg, FFR = 0.80

Intravenous adenosine
140 µg/kg/min

Pullback

$P_a = 107$ mmHg, $P_d = 78$ mmHg, FFR = 0.72

Figure 20.4
Pressure tracings obtained during induction of coronary hyperemia with either intracoronary bolus or intravenous infusion of adenosine. Intracoronary adenosine induces a short period of hyperemia that can be missed if the average pressure is calculated by the polygraph using a long time constant, or if a long delay occurs between bolus administration and flushing of the guiding catheter. In contrast, intravenous adenosine infusion induces a long, sustained period of hyperemia that facilitates adequate measurements. Note the typical increase in blood pressure preceding the hyperemic period. An additional advantage of intravenous infusion is that a pullback can be performed during hyperemia to perform an 'FFR mapping' of the segment and to facilitate corrections if a pressure shift has occurred. In this case, a brisk change in pressure gradient occurs when crossing back through the stenosis, and a perfect matching of pressures denotes the persistence of pressure calibration during the study. The two tracings were obtained in different patients. The recording speed is different in the two cases (slower for the intravenous adenosine infusion).

influenced by age.[44] For this reason, a model has been proposed to adjust CFVR measurements to the baseline speed and age of the patient, a concept designated corrected coronary flow velocity reserve ($CFVR_{corrected}$),[44] expressed by the formula

$$CFVR_{corrected} = 2.85(CFVR_{measured}$$
$$\times 10^{0.48 \log(APV\ baseline) + 0.0025age - 1.16}),$$

where APV is the averaged peak flow velocity. The fact that $CFVR_{corrected}$ standardizes CFVR for basal flow velocity and age makes it possible to assess more accurately those patients in whom microcirculatory dysfunction is expected, such as diabetics.

Relative coronary flow velocity reserve

As mentioned, coronary reserve and therefore CFVR provide combined information on the epicardial (stenosis) and microcirculatory components of the vessel studied. The potential coexistence of both anomalies can lead to problems in clinical decision-making.[6,7,25] The concept of relative coronary flow velocity reserve (CFVR-r) provides a solution to this problem.[45–47] CFVR-r is the ratio between the CFVR obtained in a stenotic vessel and CFVR in a nonstenotic reference vessel (Figure 20.5). CFVR-r can have a maximum value of 1, corresponding to the complete absence of hemodynamic relevance in the problem stenosis. Below 0.60–0.65 (Table 20.1), the problem stenosis would be considered hemodynamically significant regardless of the presence of microvascular dysfunction. This technique therefore offers the theoretical advantage of providing simultaneous information on the state of the microcirculation (CFVR < 2 in the reference vessel indicates that the subject has microcirculatory dysfunction). The limitations of the method are the assumption that microcirculation presents a similar degree of impairment in the two territories in which CFVR measurements are made – an assumption that has been challenged by recent observations[48] – and by need for a nonstenotic reference vessel, which might be absent in patients with multivessel disease.

Table 20.1   Validation studies on coronary physiology indices

Study	n	Reference standard	OCV	Sensitivity (%)	Specificity (%)
CFVR					
Miller et al[32]	33	SPECT	2.0	82	100
Joye et al[33]	30	SPECT	2.0	94	95
Deychak et al[34]	17	SPECT	1.8	94	94
Heller et al[35]	55	SPECT	1.7	81	87
Danzi et al[36]	30	Stress echo	2.0	91	84
Verberne et al[37]	37	SPECT	1.9	67	86
Abe et al[38]	46	SPECT	2.0	88	95
Chamuleau et al[39]	127	SPECT	1.7	50	90
El-Shafei et al[40]	48	SPECT	1.9	63	88
CFVR-r					
Verberne et al[37]	37	SPECT	0.65	78	89
Chamuleau et al[39]	127	SPECT	0.60	48	91
El-Shafei et al[40]	48	SPECT	0.75	71	83
FFR					
Pijls et al[55]	45	ETT + SPECT + stress echo	0.75	88	100
Abe et al[38]	46	SPECT	0.75	83	100
Rieber et al[83]	148	SPECT	0.75	91	63
Chamuleau et al[39]	127	MIBI-SPECT	0.74	65	85
Diastolic FFR					
Abe et al[38]	46	SPECT	0.76	96	100
Hyperemic stenosis resistance index					
Meuwissen et al[75]	151	SPECT	0.80	79	90
Pulse transmission coefficient					
Brosh et al[78]	56	FFR	0.60	100	98

OCV, optimal cutoff value; CFVR, coronary flow velocity reserve; CFVR-r, relative CFVR; FFR, fractional flow reserve; SPECT, single-photon emission computed tomography; stress echo, stress echocardiography; ETT, excercise tolerance test.

Diastolic/systolic flow velocity ratio

Another index derived from Doppler guidewires is the ratio between the systolic and diastolic components of flow velocity (DSVR), which is automatically calculated by the FloMap console. In assessing the hemodynamic significance of a coronary stenosis, the rationale for this index is that, as discussed in the introduction to coronary physiology above, subendocardial flow is abolished during systole to a much higher degree than subepicardial flow. The ratio between the two might therefore reflect the impact of stenosis severity on transmural flow distribution and subendocardial flow.[34,36,49,50] However, the DSVR does not constitute an index for this purpose, particularly in the right coronary artery, since, as discussed previously, the phasic characteristics of flow in that vessel reflect the differences in extramural compression of vessels in the left and right ventricles.[50] More recently, observations on phasic characteristics of coronary blood flow in the context of acute myocardial infarction with Doppler guidewires have

created a renewed interest in this index. This aspect will be discussed in the following section.

Deceleration time of diastolic flow velocity

In the context of acute myocardial infarction, several investigators[51–53] have demonstrated that coronary flow may follow two distinct patterns. The type I pattern is characterized by diastolic flow with long diastolic deceleration time and normal antegrade systolic flow. The type II pattern has a decreased diastolic deceleration time and retrograde systolic flow. The rationale behind type II is the occurrence of retrograde displacement of blood in a plugged or obliterated microvasculature when squeezed by systolic extravascular compression. The rapid deceleration of diastolic flow is related to the absence of antegrade flow through the myocardial bed, since antegrade diastolic blood flow only occurs as a result of the capacitance of the

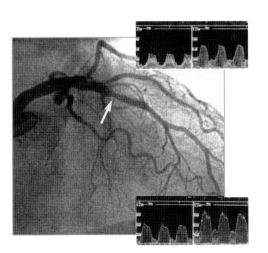

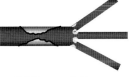

CFVR $_{LAD}$ = 1.9

Relative CFVR =
1.9/2.0 = 0.95

CFVR $_{LCX}$ = 2.0

Figure 20.5
Usefulness of the coronary flow velocity reserve (CFVR) in a diabetic patient with angiographically mild restenosis (arrow) in a stent previously implanted in the anterior descending branch and persistent angina. Noninvasive tests to detect ischemia detection were inconclusive. The CFVR in the problem vessel is abnormal (1.9), which can lead to the conclusion that the restenosis is hemodynamically significant. Nevertheless, CFVR in the circumflex branch, without angiographically evident stenosis, demonstrates a borderline value with normality that suggests the presence of microvascular dysfunction. The ratio between the two CFVR vales (relative CFVR) permits normalization of the results of the stenotic vessel for the documented microcirculatory substrate in the reference vessel, and demonstrates a normal value (>0.65). In the context of the patient's microvascular impairment, revascularization of the restenosis indicated would contribute, in the best of cases, only 5% more flow in the anterior descending branch, and for that reason should not be performed.

vascular bed up to the level of microvascular obstruction. As a result of this, a decreased and even negative DSVR is observed in type II flow (in recent work by Akasaka et al,[51] the DSVR in type I and II flows were 1.3 ± 0.6 and -2.1 ± 1.4, respectively). The relevance of these findings is that type I and II flows constitute a reflection of the extent of myocardial damage in the infarct territory, and predict not only the potential recovery of myocardial function but also the additional benefit of stenting to balloon angioplasty, information which is not provided by TIMI flow grade alone.[51,52] Future studies will confirm these potential advantages, at a time when assessment of microvascular damage in myocardial infarction is an area of active investigation and clinical interest.

the possibility of calculating volumetric coronary flow reserve on the grounds of the thermodilution principle. The technique is based on calculation of the mean transit times of an indicator (normal saline at room temperature) from the coronary ostium to the location of the intracoronary temperature sensor, both at rest and following induction of coronary hyperemia with adenosine. Validation of this technique in humans[55] demonstrated that the measurements obtained correlated fairly well with CFVR measurements ($r = 0.80$), although individual differences of more than 20% were seen in a quarter of all arteries. Among other factors, the presence of major side branches, bradycardia, and displacement of the transducer within the artery between measurements may influence the accuracy of this method.

Coronary flow reserve calculated from intracoronary thermodilution

Using a combined pressure/temperature sensor fitted in an intracoronary guidewire, De Bruyne et al[54] investigated

Absolute intracoronary pressure gradients

From a historical point of view, coronary pressure measurements were used to assess the severity of coronary stenoses or the result of percutaneous interventions,[56,57] and even to predict the development of cardiac events.[58,59]

However, this approach was unsuccessful for several reasons. Firstly, the relatively large diameters of the intracoronary or balloon catheters used in these studies interfered with the measurements performed, to the point that significant gradients could be documented in coronary arteries without stenoses.[60] Secondly, the theoretical framework in which translesional pressure gradients were used to estimate stenosis severity was incorrect. The transstenotic pressure gradient is influenced by translesional blood flow, which is modulated by the degree of distal microvascular resistance, which is highly variable.[25,48] Even when complete hyperemia is achieved, or when the vasodilatory reserve of the distal microvascular bed is exhausted by a severe stenosis, the absolute value of the transstenotic pressure gradient varies with aortic pressure. For these reasons, the reliability of intracoronary pressure measurements for assessment of coronary stenoses was poor, and they were never widely used in clinical practice. A major breakthrough in the use of intracoronary pressure gradients for functional assessment of coronary stenoses came from the introduction of a different theoretical framework, namely fractional flow reserve, which will be discussed next.

Myocardial fractional flow reserve

FFR constitutes a link between intracoronary pressure gradient measurements and the assessment of stenosis severity in terms of flow impairment.[29,42,61-63] The cornerstone principle underlying this technique is that the pressure–flow relation in the coronary tree becomes linear during hyperemia. When such linearity is achieved, the ratio between two intracoronary pressures is identical to the ratio between the coronary flows corresponding to these pressures (Figure 20.6). If this concept is applied to pressures proximal (P_a) and distal (P_d) to a stenosis, we will be able to calculate the percentage fall in coronary flow caused by the stenosis: for example, $P_d/P_a = 0.5$ will be interpreted as a 50% reduction in blood flow in the dependant myocardial territory caused by the stenosis in relation to a non-stenotic situation (in which case, there would be no difference between P_a and P_d, and $P_d/P_a = 1$). This P_d/P_a ratio obtained during maximum hyperemia constitutes the myocardial fractional flow reserve (FFRmyo). The term 'myocardial' here refers to the fact that the reduction in blood flow is estimated as that occurring in the myocardial territory vascularized by that vessel, and which therefore takes into consideration other sources of blood flow such as collateral support. In recent years, the terms FFR and FFRmyo have become synonymous, although in the original work by Pijls and co-workers[61,63] a distinction between myocardial (FFRmyo) and coronary (FFRcor) fractional flow reserve was made, the latter being calculated by subtracting from FFRmyo the collateral contribution to myocardial blood flow.

To its credit, FFR has created unprecedented expectations among interventional cardiologists,[64,65] and has boosted interest in intracoronary physiology among

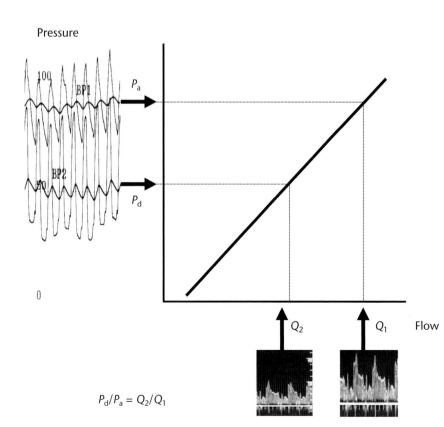

Pressure

P_a

P_d

Q_2 Q_1 Flow

$P_d/P_a = Q_2/Q_1$

Figure 20.6
Physiological principles of fractional flow reserve (FFR). During maximal hyperemia, there is a linear relationship between pressure and flow. Let us consider two pressure measurements P_a and P_d with their corresponding coronary flows Q_1 and Q_2. Since P_d results from the effect of a coronary stenosis, it is possible to infer that the relative loss of intracoronary pressure is proportional to the loss in coronary flow induced by the same stenosis. See text for details.

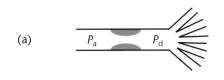
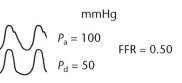
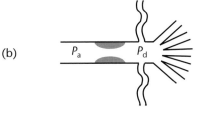
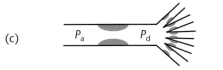

mmHg

(a) P_a P_d $P_a = 100$ $P_d = 50$ FFR = 0.50

(b) P_a P_d $P_a = 100$ $P_d = 75$ FFR = 0.75

(c) P_a P_d $P_a = 100$ $P_d = 85$ FFR = 0.85

(d) P_a P_d $P_a = 100$ $P_d = 95$ FFR = 0.95

(e) S_1 S_2 P_{d1} P_{d2}

S_1 $P_a = 100$ $P_{d1} = 85$ FFR = 0.85

$S_1 + S_2$ $P_a = 100$ $P_{d2} = 50$ FFR = 0.50

Figure 20.7

Fractional flow reserve (FFR) is an index of stenosis that incorporates different variables with a net effect on coronary circulation. This figure deals with some of these factors. (a) Effect of coronary stenosis on the hyperemic pressure gradient in the presence of a normal microcirculation. (b) The same stenosis under the circumstances of having good collateral support. As a consequence of collateral supply, P_d and consequently FFR are higher than in (a). (c) Effect of microcirculatory dysfunction on FFR. Since the increase in microvascular resistance decreases coronary blood flow, and since the hyperemic gradient is a function of trans-stenotic blood flow, P_a and FFR are higher. This does not in itself constitute a problem for clinical applications of FFR, which, from a pragmatic point of view, produces valid information to judge whether revascularization is needed in that vessel. (d) Expected result if coronary stenting is performed in that situation. From a hemodynamic point of view, a small increase in FFR would be noticed but, more importantly, no significant net benefit would be obtained, since treatment would be limited to the epicardial vessel but would not improve the underlying problem in the microcirculation. (e) Effect of serial stenoses on FFR measurements. Even when the severity of the stenosis located upstream, S_1, is similar to that in (a), FFR measurements obtained when the pressure transducer is left between both stenosis (P_{d1}) would show a lower value, since the stenosis located downstream is limiting trans-stenotic flow. If FFR is performed across the two serial stenoses (P_{d2}), one would assess the combined effect of them, but might underestimate the severity of S_1. The issue of serial stenoses is treated in detail elsewhere in this book.

interventional and non-interventional cardiologists alike. Two aspects that are critical to the success of FFR are its ease of performance and interpretation. For the former, only two mean pressures (obtained from the guiding catheter and the pressure guidewire) recorded during maximal hyperemia induced pharmacologically are required. The latter is facilitated by a clear cut-off value of 0.75 for identification of significant coronary stenoses (that

is, those which are associated with inducible myocardial ischemia in noninvasive tests).

The interpretation of FFR relies critically, however, on a number of specific features of this technique that stem from the previously described physiological characteristics of coronary circulation (Figure 20.7). First, FFR is a specific technique for the hemodynamic assessment of stenoses. In contrast to intracoronary Doppler, its use in coronary arteries without epicardial stenosis will not provide information on coronary microcirculation, and will only show that coronary conductance is maximal (a FFR=1 would be documented). Secondly, FFR performs an assessment of the stenosis that is relative to a theoretical hemodynamic situation in which that stenosis would be absent. This characteristic makes FFR an especially useful index for assessing the need for percutaneous revascularization. It is also in marked contrast with CFVR, in which the reference element is flow velocity before induction of hyperemia. Thirdly, as anticipated above, the information provided by FFR refers to blood flow in the myocardial area of distribution of the studied vessel, and incorporates not only anterograde flow through the stenosis but also collateral circulation provided from other vessels. In vessels with important collateral support, the relative effect of stenosis on the perfusion of the territory is smaller, and consequently higher FFR values would be expected. Fourthly, the status of coronary microcirculation is also incorporated in the assessment of a stenosis with FFR. Since the transstenotic pressure gradient is a function of coronary flow, attenuation of the hyperemic response by microcirculatory impairment will be associated with higher FFR values than those obtained in cases of normal microcirculation. From a practical viewpoint, this may not constitute a limitation of the technique: the finding of a normal FFR value in a stenosis with important underlying microcirculatory involvement would make it possible to anticipate a small percentage increment in myocardial blood flow if this vessel is revascularized. And fifthly, an important aspect of FFR is its applicability under variable hemodynamic conditions, since it is relatively unaffected by them.[42]

Assessment of a coronary stenosis in the presence of additional distal stenoses constitutes a major problem. As elegantly demonstrated by De Bruyne et al,[66] distal stenoses decrease the maximal transstenotic pressure gradient across those located upstream, causing underestimation of their hemodynamic severity with FFR. Although on experimental grounds it is possible to ascertain the individual contributions of two stenoses in series, the clinical application of this is hampered by the fact that wedge pressure – which is normally obtained during balloon dilatation – is one of the terms in the calculation. For the purpose of this introduction to the practice of FFR, it is enough to warn the operator about this potentially misleading setting.

Pressure-pullback FFR for the assessment of diffuse disease

As demonstrated by De Bruyne et al,[67] the additive effect of multiple coronary irregularities in diffuse disease may lead to the development of a significant drop in pressure along the vessel, which may cause myocardial ischemia, as demonstrated with positron emission tomography (PET).[68] This phenomenon can be studied with intracoronary pressure wires by performing a so-called pressure pullback curve, a pressure tracing obtained during sustained maximal hyperemia and continuous slow withdrawal of the pressure guidewire along a complete coronary segment or vessel. This technique allows assessment not only of a single stenosis but also of serial lesions or of multiple irregularities resulting from diffuse atherosclerotic narrowing. Since the complete sequence is obtained during maximal hyperemia, this technique also makes it possible to introduce corrections for unforeseen drift of the intracoronary pressure signal.

Diastolic fractional flow reserve

Diastolic FFR is characterized by using the ratio of pressures obtained only during diastole.[38] This technique, aside from demonstrating a higher sensitivity for the detection of inducible ischemia than conventional FFR, can potentially avoid the interference of systolic phenomena that affect calculations based on mean pressures, such as those resulting from differences in flow patterns in the right and left coronary arteries[69] or from the systolic compression of epicardial vessels by myocardial bridges.[70] None of the systems currently available commercially, however, allows the measurement of diastolic FFR.

Instantaneous hyperemic diastolic pressure–flow slope index (coronary conductance)

In introducing the elementary principles of coronary physiology, we described the importance of the relation between coronary blood pressure and flow as a method of characterizing coronary function. This principle was developed by Mancini et al[18] to be used as a diagnostic application, and was designated as the instantaneous hyperemic diastolic pressure–flow slope index (i-HDPFS). The slope is calculated only from measurements obtained in mid end-diastole, since during protodiastole there is no relation between pressure and flow due to the capacitance of intramyocardial vessels and microcirculation (Figure 20.8). Experimental studies have shown a good correlation between the severity of epicardial stenoses and the degree of subendocardial conductance measured with radiospheres.[18] Di Mario et al[71] have adapted the method for

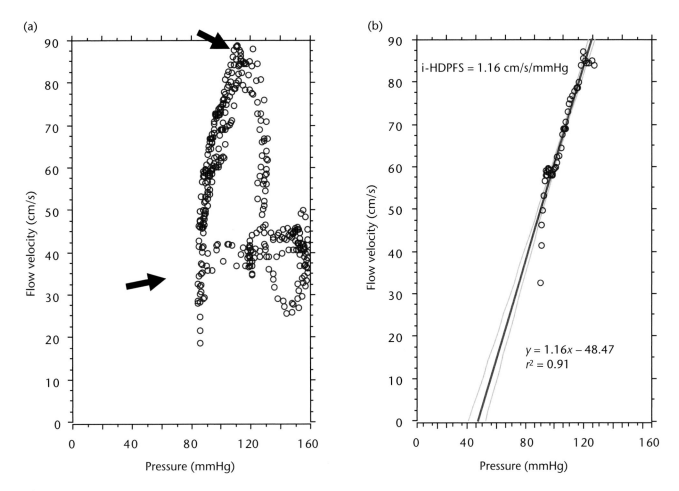

Figure 20.8
The slope of the pressure–flow relation in hyperemia, an index of coronary resistance, can be estimated directly from intracoronary pressure and flow data. To do so, it is necessary to have instantaneous information on intracoronary pressure and flow. (a) The complete cycle of pressure–flow relationship during several consecutive beats. Using only data collected in mid end-diastole (the interval between the arrows), regression analysis can be used to establish the slope of this relation (b). This index is termed the instantaneous hyperemic diastolic pressure–flow slope (i-HDPFS), which in this particular case performed at our institution was 1.16 cm/s/mmHg.

clinical use by combining pressure and Doppler guide-wires. The principle of i-HDPFS is similar to that of the hemipressure time used in the assessment of mitral stenosis with Doppler echocardiography. It has the advantage of not needing baseline reference measurements, because data are collected only during maximum hyperemia. The main limitation of i-HDPFS is the technical difficulty of obtaining the measurement: there are no commercial systems for the measurement of this variable, and, in clinical studies, the poor quality of the Doppler signal has made it impossible to perform this calculation in 20% of cases. Controversy exists regarding its dependence on changes in preload, heart rate, and cardiac contractility.[42,72]

With regard to the application of i-HDPFPS to the assessment of coronary microcirculation, our group has found in patients with cardiac allografts in whom endomyocardial biopsies were obtained at the time of physiological assessment that it is closely correlated with structural changes in the microvasculature, namely arteriolar obliter-

ation and capillary rarefaction.[73] Using the same model, i-HDPFS demonstrated a better correlation with histological findings than other indices such as coronary flow velocity reserve, coronary resistance, and coronary resistance reserve.[74]

Coronary resistance and hyperemic stenosis resistance index

The resistance of an epicardial stenosis has also been calculated on the basis of the translesional pressure gradient (obtained with a pressure guidewire) and flow (measured simultaneously with a Doppler guidewire). Meuwissen et al[75] have recently reported the superiority of this hyperemic stenosis resistance index over CFVR or FFR for the identification of stenosis associated with inducible myocardial ischemia documented with SPECT. Interestingly, in the subset of patients with conflicting results of FFR and CFVR, the hyperemic stenosis resistance index demonstrated better agreement with SPECT than either of the other two techniques.[75] Coronary resistance has also been used to assess the status of coronary microcirculation, expressed either in absolute terms[24] or as a ratio between resistance in baseline conditions and hyperemia.[76] This approach has demonstrated the potential of coronary resistance and she hyperemic stenosis resistance index for identifying structural histological changes in microcirculation[70] and for observations about their role in different coronary syndromes.[24,77]

Pulse transmission coefficient

A non-hyperemic index of stenosis severity based on the analysis of pressure wave transmission across the stenosis has been proposed and compared with FFR in a recent work by Brosh et al.[78] The cornerstone of this method is the impairment in the transmission of pressure waves across a stenosis, which behaves in this regard as a low-pass filter. Using a specific digital console (SmartFlow, Florence Medical Inc., Wellesley, MA) and computational flow dynamics, the transmission of high-frequency components of the pressure signal through the stenosis is analyzed using as the region of interest the dichrotic notch in the aortic waveform. The derived index, the pulse transmission coefficient, has only been compared with FFR measurements, and not with noninvasive tests for the detection of ischemia (Table 20.1).

Safety of clinical decisions based on intracoronary physiological techniques

A growing amount of information is available not only on the safety of intracoronary maneuvers with pressure and flow guidewires[79] but also on decision-making about revascularization based on intracoronary physiological data obtained with these techniques.[79–86] The first study on the safety of deferring percutaneous treatment on the basis of physiological evidence was published by Kern et al.[80] In that work, the cardiac event rate during follow-up of 88 patients with revascularization treatment deferred on the grounds of pressure or flow measurements was found to be similar to that of a control group of 45 patients treated with percutaneous transluminal coronary angioplasty (PTCA). Following a similar study design, Ferrari et al[81] documented a lower event rate during follow-up in those patients in whom PTCA was deferred for having a normal CFVR – although apparently at the cost of having more symptoms in the long term than a control group treated with PTCA. Two major trials have been conducted on the same issue. Based upon nonrandomized evidence supporting the safety of clinical decision-making based on FFR measurements,[82] the DEFER study enrolled 300 patients in a randomized, multicenter study design.[84] The enrolled patients presented one stenosis judged suitable for PTCA but without conclusive documentation of associated myocardial ischemia. After performing FFR, the 181 patients with FFR > 0.75 were randomly assigned either to a performance (n = 90) or to a deferral group (n = 91), while all patients with FFR < 0.75 underwent PTCA (reference group, n = 144). Clinical follow-up after 2 years demonstrated that the cardiac event rate and symptomatic status were not superior in the treatment group than in the deferral group, while both groups presented fewer events and fewer symptoms than those in the reference group. A second multicenter trial, the ILIAS study,[85] explored the usefulness of characterizing the severity of an intermediate stenosis for clinical decision-making with either CFVR or SPECT in 191 patients with multivessel disease. All patients presented a severe stenosis treated electively with PTCA and a stenosis with intermediate angiographic severity in a different vessel. Treatment of the intermediate stenosis was deferred in 182 patients on the grounds of having a negative SPECT or CFVR > 2.0. At 1-year follow-up, the distribution of cardiac events in groups defined by the result of SPECT and CFVR demonstrated thet the latter was a more accurate predictor of events (relative risk 3.9) than SPECT (relative risk 0.5). Statistical adjustment with multivariate analysis demonstrated that CFVR was the only significant predictor for the development of cardiac events. These results suggest that selective evaluation of stenosis severity with a Doppler guidewire allows more accurate risk stratification than does SPECT, and improves clinical decision-making.

The validity of physiological decision-making has also been extended to intermediate stenoses in the left main coronary artery. Bech et al[86] followed a strategy of deferring coronary revascularization in 24 patients in whom FFR > 0.75. Freedom from death, myocardial infarction, or revascularization was compared at a mean follow-up time of 29 months with that of 30 patients who underwent coronary surgery on the grounds of FFR < 0.75 (angiographic severity was virtually identical in both groups). The survival rates of the patients were 100% and 97% in the deferral and surgical groups respectively. The event-free survival rates were 76% and 83%, resulting from the crossover of some patients to the surgical strategy during follow-up. These data suggest that FFR can also be applied for clinical decision-making in this subset of patients.

Use of intracoronary physiological measurements to guide the performance of percutaneous coronary interventions

One of the advantages of the compatibility of pressure and flow velocity guidewires is that they can be used to monitor the result of percutaneous coronary interventions (PCI). The first large multicenter trial investigating this issue was DEBATE (Doppler Endpoints Balloon Angioplasty Trial Europe),[87] which demonstrated that PTCA procedures resulting in a CFVR greater than 2.5 and a residual stenosis rate of 35% or less presented an excellent clinical course with a low restenosis rate at follow-up. These results, published at the time of the generalization of the use of coronary stents, encouraged many investigators to test the so-called provisional stenting strategy, which aimed to optimize balloon angioplasty with intracoronary physiological techniques to reduce as much as possible the implantation of coronary stents. The multicenter studies DEBATE II,[88] DESTINI,[89] and FROST[90] demonstrated that provisional stenting is a safe strategy, with similar results to those obtained with elective stenting. The design of DEBATE II, however, suggested that in spite of achieving optimal physiological results, patients do still benefit in the long term from stent implantation. Although stents currently constitute currently the most widely used modality of PCI, the information provided by these studies is still useful under circumstances in which avoidance of stent implantation is recommended due to the anatomical location of the lesion, etc. In that regard, measurement of FFR following balloon angioplasty has been found to predict the likelihood of cardiac events in the long term.[91]

Optimization of stent implantation has also been an issue for measurements performed with pressure guidewires. In an initial work, Hanekamp et al[92] found an FFR greater than 0.94 in all cases in which the IVUS MUSIC criteria were fulfilled. Although this issue was contested by other groups,[93] recently published data from an international multicenter registry on stent implantation and FFR including 900 patients have demonstrated a clear relationship between the final FFR after stenting and the development of cardiac events during follow-up.[94] Other groups have focused their work in assessing optimal stent deployment using Doppler guidewires.[95]

Conclusions

The introduction of intracoronary guidewires fitted with sensors of pressure, flow velocity, and temperature has opened new possibilities of applying concepts of coronary physiology in living humans that were previously only applied in the experimental domain. These instruments are based on different theoretical frameworks. Some of them (e.g. FFR and CFVR) have facilitated the technique and have thus contributed to a growing expansion of the use of physiological assessment of coronary circulation. Others are still under evaluation, but may become equally important for clinical purposes. The fact that measurements are performed selectively on a vessel or even a stenosis basis gives an unprecedented spatial resolution to such measurements, which is likely to complement the more limited information in this regard provided by noninvasive imaging techniques. Furthermore, the compatibility of these tools with percutaneous revascularization devices allows the guidance of procedures or their ad hoc performance if judged adequate. The interpretation and performance of intracoronary functional assessment requires a good understanding of the physiological principles of the technique; otherwise, major mistakes in diagnosis can occur when applying these techniques under clinical circumstances in which they have not been validated or when the prerequisites for their performance (e.g. maximal hyperemia) are not fulfilled.

References

1. White CW, Wright CB, Doty DB, et al. Does visual interpretation of the coronary arteriogram predict physiologic importance of a coronary stenosis? N Engl J Med 1984; 310:819–24.
2. Topol EJ, Nissen SE. Our preoccupation with coronary luminology. The dissociation between clinical and angiographic findings in ischemic heart disease. Circulation 1995; 92:2333–42.
3. Plotnick GD. Coronary artery bypass surgery to prolong life? Less anatomy/more physiology. Am J Cardiol 1986; 8:749–51.
4. Klocke FJ. Measurements of coronary blood flow and degree of stenosis; current clinical implications and continuing uncertainties. J Am Coll Cardiol 1983;1:131–41.
5. Klocke FJ. Measurements of coronary flow reserve: Defining pathophysiology versus making decisions about patient care. Circulation 1987;76:1183.
6. Serruys PW, Di Mario C, Meneveau N, et al. Intracoronary pressure and flow velocity with sensor-tipped guidewires: a new methodologic approach for assessment of coronary hemodynamics before and after coronary interventions. Am J Cardiol 1993;71:41D–53D.
7. Kern MJ. Coronary physiology revisited. Practical insights from the cardiac catheterization laboratory. Circulation 2000;101:1344–51.
8. Opie LH. The Heart: Physiology, from Cell to Circulation. Philadelphia: Lippincott-Raven, 1998: 267–94.
9. Marcus ML. Metabolic regulation of coronary blood flow. In: The Coronary Circulation in Health and Disease (Marcus ML, ed). New York: McGraw-Hill, 1983: 65–92.

10. Marcus ML. Differences in the regulation of coronary perfusion to the right and left ventricles. In: The Coronary Circulation in Health and Disease (Marcus ML, ed). New York: McGraw-Hill, 1983: 337–47.

11. Akasaka T, Yoshikawa J, Yoshida K, et al. Comparison of relation of systolic flow of the right coronary artery to pulmonary artery pressure in patients with and without pulmonary hypertension. Am J Cardiol 1996;76:240–4.

12. Eeckhout E, Kern MJ. The coronary non-reflow phenomenon: a review of mechanisms and therapies. Eur Heart J 2001;22:729–39.

13. Ge J, Jeremias A, Rupp A, et al. New signs characteristic of myocardial bridging demonstrated by intracoronary ultrasound and Doppler. Eur Heart J 1999;20:1707–16.

14. Gould KL. Pressure–flow characteristics of coronary stenoses in unsedated dogs at rest and during coronary vasodilation. Circ Res 1978;43:242–3.

15. Gould K. Coronary artery stenosis and reversing atherosclerosis. London: Arnold, 1999: 3–29.

16. Klocke FJ. Measurements of coronary blood flow and degree of stenosis; current clinical implications and continuing uncertainties. J Am Coll Cardiol 1983;1:131–41.

17. Hoffman J, Spaan JAE. Pressure–flow relations in coronary circulation. Physiol Rev 1990;70:331–90.

18. Mancini GBJ, McGillem MJ, DeBoe SF, Gallagher KP. The diastolic hyperemic flow vs pressure relation: a new index of coronary stenosis severity and flow reserve. Circulation 1989;80:941–50.

19. Gould KL, Lipscomb K, Hamilton GW. Physiological basis for assessing critical coronary stenosis: instantaneous flow response and regional redistribution during coronary hyperemia as measures of coronary flow reserve. Am J Cardiol 1974;33:87–94.

20. Kirkeeide RL, Gould KL, Parsel L. Assessment of coronary stenosis by myocardial perfusion imaging during pharmacologic coronary vasodilatation. VII. Validation of coronary flow reserve as a single integrated functional measure of stenosis severity reflecting all its geometric dimensions. J Am Coll Cardiol 1986;7:103–13.

21. Bartunek J, Wijns W, Heyndrickx GR, de Bruyne B. Effects of dobutamine on coronary stenosis physiology and morphology. Comparison with intracoronary adenosine. Circulation 1999;100:243–9.

22. L'Abatte A, Sambuceti G, Haunsø S, Schneider-Eicke. Methods for evaluating coronary microvasculature in humans. Eur Heart J 1999;200:1300–13.

23. Baumgart D, Haude M, Görge G, et al. Augmented alpha-adrenergic constriction of atherosclerotic human coronary arteries. Circulation 1999;99:2090–7.

24. Marzilli M, Sambuceti G, Fedele S, L'Abbate A. Coronary microcirculatory vasoconstriction during ischemia in patients with unstable angina. J Am Coll Cardiol 2000;35:327–34.

25. Meuwissen M, Chamuleau SAJ, Siebes M, et al. Role of variability in microvascular resistance on fractional flow reserve and coronary blood flow velocity reserve in intermediate coronary lesions. Circulation 2001;103:184–7.

26. Nitenberg A, Anyony I. Coronary vascular reserve in humans: a critical review of methods of evaluation and of interpretation of the results. Eur Heart J 1995;16(Suppl I): 7–21.

27. Pijls NHJ, Kern MJ, Yock PG, De Bruyne B. Practice and potential pitfalls of coronary pressure measurement. Cathet Cardiovasc Interv 2000;49:1–16.

28. Alfonso F, Flores A, Escaned J, et al. Pressure wire kinking, entanglement, and entrapment during intravascular ultrasound studies: a potentially dangerous complication. Cathet Cardiovasc Intervent 2000;50:221–5.

29. Pijls NHJ, de Bruyne B, Peels K, et al. Measurement of myocardial fractional flow reserve to assess the functional severity of coronary-artery stenoses. N Engl J Med 1996;334:1703–8.

30. Camacho D, Escaned J, Garcia J, et al. Intracoronary or intravenous adenosine during fractional flow reserve: influence of stenosis severity, collateral steal and branch order. Eur Heart J 2002;23:13.

31. Di Segni E, Higano ST, Rihal CS, et al. Incremental doses of intracoronary adenosine for the assessment of coronary velocity reserve for clinical decision making. Cathet Cardiovasc Interv 2001;54:34–40

32. Miller DD, Donouhue TJ, Younis LT, et al. Correlation of pharmacological ^{99m}Tc-sestamibi myocardial perfusion imaging with poststenotic coronary flow reserve in patients with angiographically intermediate artery stenoses. Circulation 1994;89:2150–60.

33. Joye ID, Schulman DS, Lasorda D, et al. Intracoronary Doppler guide wire versus stress single photon emission computed tomographic thallium-201 imaging in assessment of intermediate coronary stenoses. J Am Coll Cardiol 1994;24:940–7.

34. Deychak YA, Segal J, Reiner JS, et al. Doppler guide wire flow-velocity indexes measured distal coronary stenoses associated with reversible thallium perfusion defects. Am Heart J 1995;129:219–27.

35. Heller LI, Cates C, Popma J, et al. Intracoronary Doppler assessment of moderate coronary artery disease: comparison with ^{201}Tl imaging and coronary angiography. FACTS Study Group. Circulation 1997;96:484–90.

36. Danzi GB, Pirelli S, Mauri L, et al. Which variable of stenosis severity best describes the significance of an isolated left anterior descending coronary artery lesion? Correlation between quantitative angiography, intracoronary Doppler measurements and high dose dipyridamole echocardiography. J Am Coll Cardiol 1998;31:526–33.

37. Verberne HJ, Piek JJ, van Liebergen RAM, et al. Functional assessment of coronary artery stenosis by Doppler derived absolute and relative coronary blood flow velocity reserve in comparison with ^{99m}Tc MIBI SPECT. Heart 1999;82:509–14.

38. Abe M, Tomiyama H, Yoshida H, Doba N. Diastolic fractional flow reserve to assess the functional severity of moderate coronary stenoses. Comparison with fractional flow reserve and coronary flow velocity reserve. Circulation 2000;102:2365–70.

39. Chamuleau SAJ, Meuwissen M, van Eck-Smit BLF, et al. Fractional flow reserve, absolute and relative coronary blood flow velocity reserve in relation to the results of technetium-99m sestamibi single-photon emission computed tomography in patients with two-vessel coronary artery disease. J Am Coll Cardiol 2001;37:1316–22.

40. El-Shafei A, Chiravuri R, Stikovac MM, et al. Comparison of relative coronary Doppler flow velocity reserve to stress myocardial perfusion imaging in patients with coronary artery disease. Cathet Cardiovasc Interv 2001;53:193–201.

41. Serruys PW, Murphy ES, Pijls NHJ. Application of coronary flow measurements to decision making in angioplasty. In: Quantitative Coronary Angiography in Clinical Practice. (Serruys PW, Foley DP, de Feyter PJ, eds). Dordrecht: Kluwer, 1994: 181–230.

42. De Bruyne B, Bartunek J, Sys SU, et al. Simultaneous coronary pressure and flow velocity measurements in humans: feasibility, reproducibility and hemodynamic dependence of coronary flow velocity reserve, hyperemic flow versus pressure slope index, and fractional flow reserve. Circulation 1996;94:1842–9.

43. Anderson HV, Stokes MJ, Leon M, et al. Coronary artery flow velocity is related to lumen area and regional left ventricular mass. Circulation 2000;102:48–54.

44. Wieneke H, Haude M, Ge J, et al. Corrected coronary flow velocity reserve: a new concept for assessing coronary perfusion. J Am Coll Cardiol 2000;35:1713–20.

45. Baumgart D, Haude M, Gorge G, et al. Improved assessment of coronary stenosis severity using the relative coronary flow reserve. Circulation 1998;98:40–6.

46. Verberne HJ, Piek JJ, van Liebergen RAM, et al. Functional assessment of coronary artery stenosis by Doppler derived absolute and relative coronary blood flow velocity reserve in comparison with ^{99m}Tc MIBI SPECT. Heart 1999;82:509–14.

47. Chamuleau SAJ, Meuwissen M, van Eck-Smit BLF, et al. Fractional flow reserve, absolute and relative coronary blood flow velocity reserve in relation to the results of technetium-99m sestamibi single-photon emission computed tomography in patients with two-vessel coronary artery disease. J Am Coll Cardiol 2001;37:1316–22.

48. Wieneke H, Schmermund A, Ge J, et al. Increased heterogeneity of coronary perfusion in patients with early coronary atherosclerosis. Am Heart J 2001;142:691–7.

49. Ofili EO, Kern MJ, St Vrain JA, et al. Differential characterization of blood flow, velocity, and vascular resistance between proximal and distal normal epicardial human coronary arteries: analysis by intracoronary Doppler spectral flow velocity. Am Heart J 1995;130:37–46.

50. Segal J, Kern MJ, Scott NA, et al. Alterations of phasic coronary artery flow velocity in humans during percutaneous coronary angioplasty. J Am Coll Cardiol 1992; 20:276–86.

51. Akasaka T, Yoshida K, Kawamoto T, et al. Relation of phasic coronary flow velocity characteristics with TIMI perfusion grade and myocardial recovery after primary percutaneous transluminal coronary angioplasty and rescue stenting. Circulation 2000;101:2361–7.

52. Kawamoto T, Yoshida K, Akasaka T, et al. Can coronary blood flow velocity pattern after primary percutaneous transluminal coronary angioplasty predict recovery of regional left ventricular function in patients with acute myocardial infarction? Circulation 1999;100:339–45.

53. Iwakura K, Ito H, Takiuchi S, et al. Alternation in the coronary blood flow velocity pattern in patients with no reflow and reperfused acute myocardial infarction. Circulation 1996;94:1269–75.

54. De Bruyne B, Pijls NH, Smith L, et al. Coronary thermodilution to assess flow reserve: experimental validation. Circulation 2001;104:2003–6.

55. Pijls NH, De Bruyne B, Smith L, et al. Coronary thermodilution to assess flow reserve: validation in humans. Circulation 2002;105:2482–6.

56. Aueron H, Gruentzig A. Percutaneous transluminal coronary angioplasty: indication and current status. Prim Cardiol 1984;10:97–107.

57. Anderson H, Roubin G, Leimburger P, et al. Measurements of transtenotic pressure gradient during percutaneous transluminal coronary angioplasty. Circulation 1986; 73:1223–30.

58. Ellis S, Gallison L, Grines C, et al. Incidence and predictors of early recurrent ischemia after successful percutaneous transluminal coronary angioplasty for acute myocardial infarction. Am J Cardiol 1989;63:263–8.

59. Urban P, Meier B, Finci L, et al. Coronary wedge pressure: a predictor of restenosis after balloon angioplasty. J Am Coll Cardiol 1987;10:504–9.

60. De Bruyne B, Sys S, Heyndrickx G. Percutaneous transluminal coronary angioplasty catheters versus fluid-filled pressure monitoring guidewires for coronary pressure measurements and correlations with quantitative coronary angiography. Am J Cardiol 1993;72:1101–6.

61. Pijls NHJ, van Gelder B, van der Voort P, et al. Fractional flow reserve. A useful index to evaluate the influence of an epicardial coronary stenosis on myocardial blood flow. Circulation 1995;92:3183–93.

62. Bartunek J, van Schuerberbeeck E, De Bruyne B. Comparison of exercise electrocardiography and dobutamine echocardiography with invasively assessed myocardial fractional flow reserve in evaluation of severity of coronary arterial narrowing. Am J Cardiol 1997;79:478–81.

63. Pijls NHJ, De Bruyne B (eds). Coronary Pressure. Dordrecht: Kluwer, 1997:60–8.

64. Hodgson JMcB. FFR for all. Cathet Cardiovasc Interv 2001;54:435–6.

65. Wilson RF. Looks aren't everything. Circulation 2001;103:2873–5.

66. De Bruyne B, Pijls NHJ, Heyndrickx GR, et al. Pressure-derived fractional flow reserve to assess serial epicardial stenoses: theoretical basis and validation. Circulation 2000;101:1840–7.

67. De Bruyne B, Hersbach F, Pijls NH, et al. Abnormal epicardial coronary resistance in patients with diffuse atherosclerosis but 'normal' coronary angiography. Circulation 2001;104:2401–6.

68. Gould KL, Nakagawa Y, Nakagawa K, et al. Frequency and clinical implications of fluid dynamically significant diffuse coronary artery disease manifest as graded, longitudinal, base-to-apex myocardial perfusion abnormalities by noninvasive positron emission tomography. Circulation 2000;101:1931–9.

69. Escaned J, Cortés J, Goicolea J, et al. Angiographic and intracoronary physiological assessment of myocardial bridging during dobutamine challenge. Circulation 1999;100(Suppl I): 731.

70. Escaned J, Flores A, Cortés J, et al. Influence of flow characteristics of the right and left coronary arteries on fractional flow reserve measurements. Circulation 2000;102 (Suppl II):639.

71. Di Mario C, Krams R, Gil R, Serruys PW. Slope of the hyperemic diastolic coronary flow velocity-pressure relation. A new index for assessment of the physiological significance of coronary stenosis in humans. Circulation 1994;90:1215–24.

72. Cleary RM, Ayon D, Moore NB, et al. Tachycardia, contractility and volume loading alter conventional indexes of coronary flow reserve, but not the instantaneous hyperemic flow versus pressure slope index. J Am Coll Cardiol 1992;20:1261–9.

73. Escaned J, Flores A, Segovia J, et al. Assessment of coronary microcirculation in cardiac allografts. A comparison of intracoronary physiology, intravascular ultrasound and histological morphometry. J Heart Lung Transplant 2001;20(Suppl.):204–5 (abst).

74. Garcia J, Escaned J, Segovia J, et al. A comparison of four intracoronary physiology indices of coronary microcirculation.

Validation with histomorphometry in endomyocardial biopsies. Eur Heart J 2002;4:250.

75. Meuwissen M, Siebes M, Chamuleau SA, et al. Hyperemic stenosis resistance index for evaluation of functional coronary lesion severity. Circulation 2002;106:441–6.

76. Krams R, Kofflard MJM, Duncker DJ, et al. Decreased coronary flow reserve in hypertrophic cardiomyopathy is related to remodeling of the coronary microcirculation. Circulation 1998;97:230–3.

77. Sambuceti G, Marzilli M, Marraccini P, et al. Coronary vasoconstriction during myocardial ischemia induced by rises in metabolic demand in patients with coronary artery disease. Circulation 1997;95:2652–9.

78. Brosh D, Higano ST, Slepian MJ, et al. Pulse transmission coefficient: a novel nonhyperemic parameter for assessing the physiological significance of coronary artery stenoses. J Am Coll Cardiol 2002;39:1012–19.

79. Quian J, Ge J, Baumgart D, et al. Safety of intracoronary Doppler flow measurement. Am Heart J 2000;140:502–10.

80. Kern MJ, Donohue TJ, Aguirre FV, et al. Clinical outcome of deferring angioplasty in patients with normal translesional pressure–flow velocity measurements. J Am Coll Cardiol 1995;25:178–87.

81. Ferrari M, Schnell B, Werner GS, Figulla HR. Safety of deferring angioplasty in patients with normal coronary flow velocity reserve. J Am Coll Cardiol 1999;33:82–7.

82. Bech GJW, de Bruyne B, Bonnier HJRM, et al. Long-term follow-up after deferral of percutaneous transluminal coronary angioplasty of intermediate stenosis on the basis of coronary pressure measurement. J Am Coll Cardiol 1998;31:841–7.

83. Rieber J, Stemplfle HU, Jung P, et al. Safety of deferring patients with coronary multivessel disease and normal fractional flow reserve. Circulation 2000;102:II-478.

84. Bech GJ, De Bruyne B, Pijls NH, et al. Fractional flow reserve to determine the appropriateness of angioplasty in moderate coronary stenosis: a randomized trial. Circulation 2001;103:2928–34.

85. Chamuleau SA, Tio RA, de Cock CC, et al. Prognostic value of coronary blood flow velocity and myocardial perfusion in intermediate coronary narrowings and multivessel disease. J Am Coll Cardiol 2002;39:852–8.

86. Bech GJ, Droste H, Pijls NH, et al. Value of fractional flow reserve in making decisions about bypass surgery for equivocal left main coronary artery disease. Heart 2001;86:547–52.

87. Serruys PW, Di Mario C, Piek J, et al. Prognostic value of intracoronary flow velocity and diameter stenosis in assessing the short- and long-term outcomes of coronary balloon angioplasty: the DEBATE study (Doppler Endpoints Balloon Angioplasty Trial Europe). Circulation 1997;96:3369–77.

88. Serruys PW, de Bruyne B, Carlier S, et al. Randomized comparison of primary stenting and provisional balloon angioplasty guided by flow velocity measurement. Circulation 2000;102:2930–7.

89. Di Mario C, Moses JW, Anderson TJ, et al. Randomized comparison of elective stent implantation and coronary balloon angioplasty guided by online quantitative angiography and intracoronary Doppler. Circulation 2000;102:2938–44.

90. Lafont A, Dubuis-Randé JL, Steg PG, et al. The French Randomized Optimal Stenting Trial: a prospective evaluation of provisional stenting guided by coronary velocity reserve and quantitative angiography. J Am Coll Cardiol 2000; 36:404–9.

91. Bech GJW, Pijls NHJ, De Bruyne B, et al. Usefulness of fractional flow reserve to predict clinical outcome after balloon angioplasty. Circulation 1999;99:883–8.

92. Hanekamp CEE, Koolen JJ, Pijls NHJ, et al. Comparison of quantitative coronary angiography, intravascular ultrasound and coronary pressure measurement to assess optimal stent deployment. Circulation 1999;99:1015–21.

93. Fearon WF, Luna J, Samady H, et al. Fractional flow reserve compared with intravascular ultrasound guidance for optimizing stent deployment. Circulation 2001;104:1917–22.

94. Pijls NH, Klauss V, Siebert U, et al. Coronary pressure measurement after stenting predicts adverse events at follow-up: a multicenter registry. Circulation 2002;105:2950–4.

95. Haude M, Baumgart D, Verna E, et al. Intracoronary Doppler- and quantitative coronary angiography-derived predictors of major adverse cardiac events after stent implantation. Circulation 2001;103:1212–17.

21

Invasive imaging of vulnerable plaque

Glenn Van Langenhove, Johannes Schaar, Stefan Verheye

Introduction

Cardiovascular disease remains the single most important cause of death, with close to 1 million people dying annually in the USA alone (1998 figures). Amongst those, 220 000 people a year die of coronary heart disease without being hospitalized. According to the American Heart Association, most of these are sudden deaths.[1] Also, autopsy studies have shown that 68% of all myocardial infarctions are associated with lesions of less than 50% severity on angiographic assessment.[2-5] It is therefore clear that non-obstructive and hemodynamically insignificant atherosclerotic plaques can be responsible for sudden death due to myocardial infarction. These potentially high-risk plaques are still left untreated, as it is unknown which of them are harmful (leading to rupture). Also, it is still unclear whether all harmful plaques show an equally high risk of rupture. The main reason for the absence of an accepted therapeutic strategy is the fact that no diagnostic tool has yet become widely available. Unfortunately, current standard technology such as coronary angiography is unable to predict the likelihood of rupture of such plaques.

Because of the increased death rate and rate of acute coronary events, early recognition of other parameters (functional parameters, in addition to anatomical parameters) of angiographically nonsignificant plaques is essential. We therefore need not only to better understand the pathogenesis of plaque rupture, but also to improve current imaging techniques. Today, angiography and intravascular ultrasound as sole techniques do not have a resolution high enough to differentiate between benign and potentially hazardous plaques.

Currently, invasive and noninvasive techniques are being developed in a quest to detect plaque that is at increased risk for rupture. The purpose of the overview in this chapter is to describe evolving techniques for invasive imaging of vulnerable plaques.

Pathophysiology of vulnerable plaque

Plaque that is at increased risk of rupture, also called 'vulnerable' plaque, is defined as plaque that is often not stenotic but has a high likelihood of becoming disrupted, thereby forming a thrombogenic focus after exposure to an acute risk factor.[6] Several factors may play a role in the propensity for rupture, but plaque composition is undoubtedly a key player. The histopathological correlate of vulnerable plaque is plaque with a lipid pool and a necrotic core, with a thin fibrous cap (between 65 and 150 μm), infiltrated by macrophages. Although any plaque may rupture, rupture-prone plaques have been associated with a high tensile mechanical stress within such a thin fibrous cap and a large lipid and necrotic core. Nonetheless, not only cap thickness and mechanical forces help determine the potential to withstand the stress but also the composition of the cap: mechanical stress at the start of fracture of a fibrous cap is decreased when the cap contains macrophages.[7] This finding was underscored in a report by van der Wal et al,[8] who demonstrated that the underlying morphology of complex atherosclerotic lesions leading to acute coronary syndromes and acute myocardial infarction is heterogeneous with respect to both plaque architecture and cellular composition. At sites of rupture, they found a huge inflammatory response with an increased number of macrophages.

The presence of macrophages suggests an inflammatory reaction. Indeed, atherosclerosis is an inflammatory disease, and numerous factors may play a role in the induction and promotion of inflammation, involving several cells (including endothelial cells, monocytes, and T cells) and their chemical end-products, as well as flow variations (shear stress).[5,9–12] The production of matrix metalloproteinases, tissue factor, and other substances released by apoptotic macrophages is found to be associated with plaque rupture and thrombosis.[13] Since rupture of a hemodynamically nonsignificant plaque may result in a cardiac event, it is important that newer 'imaging' techniques, based on recent insights into 'vulnerable' plaques, are being developed. These imaging modalities should be designed to prospectively assess the potential of rupturing of the plaque at an early stage prior to the occurrence of a coronary event.

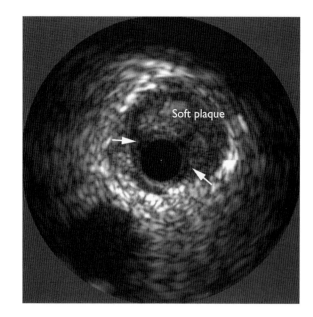

Figure 21.1
Intravascular ultrasound (IVUS) image of a soft plaque (from 9 to 5 o'clock – arrows) in a circumflex artery. Using this technique, it remains difficult to identify plaques that have a high likelihood of rupture.

New invasive techniques

Intravascular ultrasound (IVUS)

This is a well-known technique and is currently considered as the only one capable of addressing the amount of plaque burden.[14] IVUS images allow discrimination between plaques with high echodensity (more fibrous composition) and plaques with low echodensity (more lipid or less fibrous). Despite improvements in imaging quality, the resolution of IVUS (around 200 μm, depending on wavelength) remains too low to measure cap thickness and thus to discriminate between stable plaques and plaques at risk. As shown in Figure 21.1, recent improvements in IVUS imaging technology have made some operators believe that ruptured plaques can be detected – albeit at a stage where prevention is no longer possible and therefore the clinical utility may be questioned.

Derivatives of IVUS such as virtual histology, developed by the Cleveland Clinic group, or plaque characterization, originating from the Thoraxcenter in Rotterdam, have yet to prove their added value in defining plaque vulnerability.

Optical coherence tomography (OCT)

This is analogous to IVUS except that it uses light rather than sound.[15] OCT is a new class of ultrahigh-resolution imaging technology that utilizes high-bandwidth light sources, fiberoptics, and advanced signal processing. OCT has an axial resolution of 20 μm, allowing the determination of small structural details such as cap thickness and extent of lipid collections. This invasive but promising technique provides reliable anatomical information, but is

hampered by lack of functional plaque assessment. Another limitation is interference from blood between the probe and the vascular wall, which results in decreased image quality. Intracoronary saline infusions may alleviate this problem. Further improvements of this technique are eagerly awaited. Figure 21.2 provides an example of the potential of this technique in assessing vascular wall anatomical properties.

Intravascular elastography/palpography

This is a recently developed invasive technique based on IVUS. However, as opposed to IVUS, elastography takes into account the mechanical properties of the plaque, and may thus provide details of functional characteristics of the plaque.[16] Images obtained by elastography are based on radial strain, determined by means of the ultrasound signal. This imaging modality is therefore able to discriminate soft from hard material, allowing detection of regions with elevated strain due to increased stress. The inventors found different strain values between fibrous, fibrofatty, and fatty plaque components; this technique was recently validated in vivo.[17] A current limitation is that it is a time-consuming process due to the complex data acquisition. Figure 21.3 provides an example of a palpogram of part of a right coronary artery, with clear delineation of regions with high versus low strain.

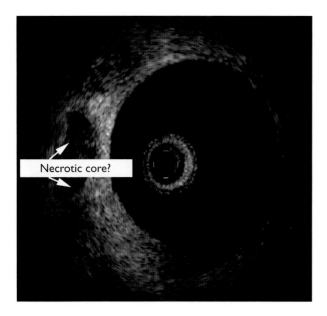

Figure 21.2
Optical coherence tomography (OCT) image of a right coronary artery, showing an area suggestive of the presence of fatty material. The zone of decreased density is possibly an area with fibrofatty tissue and a necrotic core. Opposite the plaque, normal vascular wall is seen.

Spectroscopic techniques

Raman and infrared spectroscopy can yield information on the chemical composition of atherosclerotic tissue. These techniques can be combined with other more established imaging techniques such as IVUS. Recently, this technique has been able to identify plaque composition and features associated with plaque vulnerability in postmortem human aortic specimen.[18,19] Limitations are background fluorescence, long acquisition time, and absorption of laser light by blood.

Thermography catheters

Currently, thermography catheters seem to be closest to becoming clinically applicable and valuable for the diagnosis of plaque instability. Indeed, the first thermography catheter has recently received CE mark approval (Thermosense thermography catheter, Thermocore Medical Systems NV, Merelbeke, Belgium), and is currently being used in several cathlabs in Europe. With this in mind, we would like to focus on these devices.

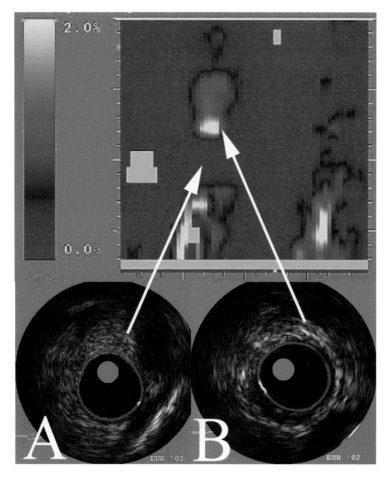

Figure 21.3
Palpogram of a right coronary artery. The upper part shows color coding of the strain of the vessel wall surface, ranging from 0% to 2%. To the right is an outlaid color map of an interrogated vessel segment. A and B show palpography data collated upon IVUS images, revealing the absence of high-strain spots in part of the vessel, and the presence of potentially dangerous high-strain spots in other parts, respectively.

Temperature

Inflammation

The link between inflammation or disease and temperature is as old as medicine itself, and since atherosclerosis is an inflammatory process, local temperature is expected to be elevated. 'Thermography' has been used in cardiology since the mid 1960s. Initially, the term indicated the use of a thermographic camera to monitor and record temperature changes in the human heart during coronary surgery and to use the data obtained to draw conclusions applicable to regional blood supply and to blood flow during coronary artery bypass graft (CABG) surgery.[20] Changes in temperature have been associated with inverse changes in death rates in vascular diseases. For myocardial infarctions, the temperature 1–2 days before death was found to be the most relevant to death rate.[21]

However, it is only fairly recently that a relation between atherosclerotic plaques (more specifically macrophages) and local temperature increase has been described.[22] Using a thermistor needle-tip (24-gauge), temperature differences were measured in human carotid plaques. It was found that in atherosclerotic plaques retrieved during surgical atherectomy of carotid artery lesions, the ex vivo temperature derived by a microprobe immediately after retrieval correlated positively with cell density (most cells were macrophages) and inversely with the distance from the dense cell clusters to the vessel's internal surface. Surface temperature differences within one plaque were measured up to 2.2°C.

Neovascularization within an atherosclerotic plaque could have been a confounding factor due to its partial contribution to temperature heterogeneity. However, since plaque neovascularization correlates with inflammation and both processes are considered to be risk factors for plaque rupture, the authors feel that temperature still may be predictive. Another interesting finding is that the temperature was highest when cells were closest to the probe and thus just below the surface of the plaque. However, it is not clear whether macrophages in the deeper regions of a plaque may also contribute to temperature heterogeneity due to heat release and eventually leading to plaque rupture. The conduction of heat produced by cells located in the deeper layers of the plaque through the superficial layer towards the probe remains unknown. Another unknown factor is the phenotypic appearance of a macrophage: the heat production of an 'active' macrophage may be different from that produced by macrophages influenced by lipid-lowering medication or macrophages undergoing apoptosis.

Recently, we described for the first time that in vivo temperature heterogeneity is determined by plaque composition and more specifically by the total macrophage mass.[23] In a hypercholesterolemic rabbit model, we found that there was marked temperature heterogeneity (up to >1 °C) at sites of thick plaques with a high macrophage content. Temperature heterogeneity was not present in thick plaques with low macrophage content. In addition, this animal study suggested that changes in the macrophage content in the plaque can be detected by in vivo thermography, since the temperature heterogeneity disappeared when the animals received a lipid-lowering diet during 3 months, which is histopathologically characterized by a marked decrease in macrophage content despite unchanged plaque thickness. This also indicates that the effect of cholesterol lowering on at least one parameter of plaque vulnerability (i.e. the number of macrophages) can be evaluated in vivo. This study further illustrated that the beneficial effect of cholesterol lowering would have been missed if the results were only based on measurements by IVUS or angiography – illustrating the shortcomings of these techniques with respect to mild atherosclerotic plaques. Furthermore, using this simplified model, a confounding factor such as neovascularization could be excluded, since this is not present in this model.

The obvious question that arises is why cells produce heat – or is the increased temperature (i.e. temperature heterogeneity) just an epiphenomenon. Inflammatory cells such as macrophages are metabolically very active, with a higher turnover rate of adenosine triphosphate (ATP) than other cells, at least in vitro.[24] Previous observations have shown that an increased metabolic rate found at sites of macrophage accumulation may result in increased heat production as opposed to cellular areas lacking inflammatory cells.[25] The reason for the increased temperature is unknown, but mitochondrial uncoupling proteins (UCP) may be involved. These molecules are homologues of thermogenin, also known as UCP-1, which is involved in the thermogenesis of brown fat tissue.[26,27] We have previously shown that human atherosclerotic plaques are associated with an increased and focal accumulation of UCP-2-positive macrophages, which could explain the temperature heterogeneity. The increased UCP–2 expression could reflect a response to the increased oxidative stress and fatty acid accumulation in plaques, finally resulting in cell death by ATP depletion.[28] It is probably still too early to say whether this may have therapeutic implications, and this needs further investigation.

An important step in translating the ex vivo findings into the clinic was taken by a group of Greek researchers, who reported the safety and feasibility of intracoronary temperature measurement using a single-thermistor catheter in humans.[29] They showed that atherosclerotic plaques of human coronary arteries demonstrated temperature heterogeneity of up to 2°C. In addition, the degree of heterogeneity was associated with the severity of the clinical presentation of the patient. The temperature heterogeneity was higher in lesions from patients with unstable angina/infarction than in those measured in patients with stable angina and patients without visible atherosclerosis (minimal to absent temperature differences), suggesting that temperature heterogeneity may be related to the pathogenesis or plaque rupture. Indeed, the same group found a good correlation between acute phase proteins such as C-reactive protein (CRP) as well as serum amyloid A and temperature.[30] Furthermore, the authors found increased local temperature heterogeneity in such atherosclerotic plaques to be a strong predictor of an unfavorable clinical outcome in patients undergoing percutaneous revascularization.[31]

Temperature-measuring devices

The thermography catheter used by Stefanadis et al[29] was a rapid-exchange modified balloon catheter incorporating a thermistor probe at the distal end embedded in a polyurethane shaft. By wedging the catheter into the lesion under investigation, measurement of surface temperature at a specific point of the vessel was possible. The thermistor guaranteed a temperature accuracy of 0.05°C, a time constant of 300 ms, a spatial resolution of 0.5 mm, and a linear correlation between resistance and temperature over the range of 33–43°C.

It is not clear, however, that the thermistor, based on its design, was in continuous contact with the surface of the vessel wall, since the diameter of a coronary artery lumen may vary along the analyzed segment. This may have resulted in incorrect values due to the cooling effect of circulating coronary blood. In addition, this catheter measured only at a single point along the circumference of the vessel wall and possibly did not take into account other diseased segments of the wall. Because of the shortcomings of this device, other catheters have been designed. One of these is a 4 French (Fr) side-viewing infrared thermography catheter capable of imaging the temperature of the vessel wall with a 180° scope.[32] The catheter is constructed from fiberoptic material with a 1 mm wide wedge-shaped mirror assembly made of zinc selenide at its tip. It is transparent to infrared radiation and is placed in such a way that it reflects temperature only from the side of the catheter. The fibreoptic catheter is connected to a focal plane array-cooled infrared camera. The system has a thermal resolution of 0.01°C, and real-time image reconstruction software continuously records the linear images obtained through the 1 mm window and processes them into two-dimensional and virtual longitudinal color-coded thermographic images of the lumen. In vitro tests with this device seemed to provide reliable images of thermal information. So for, no in vivo experiments have been reported. Another device developed by the same group is a thermography basket, existing of a 4 Fr catheter with an expandable and externally controllable basket with nine built-in thermosensors.[33] The expandable basket at the end of the catheter is made of six highly flexible hollow wires with built-in thermocouples. Each wire has two sensors located at the maximum curve, 0.5 mm apart, allowing monitoring of

temperature between and within plaques. The catheter also has a central wire with a thermal sensor to monitor blood temperature simultaneously. The real-time data acquisition software supports digital transmitters for each channel with a thermal resolution of 0.0025°C and a sampling rate of 20 readings per second. It can also display a circumferential and longitudinal thermal map of the vessel wall. Although still in the investigational phase, this system has been tested in five inbred atherosclerotic dogs and ten Watanabe rabbits, in all of which temperature heterogeneity has been found.

The findings of the in vivo study described by our group were obtained using an over-the-wire thermography catheter (Thermocore Medical Ltd, Guildford, UK) consisting of a functional end that can be engaged by retracting a covering sheath.[23] The distal part has four dedicated thermistors at the distal ends of four flexible nitinol strips (evenly distributed along a 360° circumference) that after engagement, with an expansion width of 9 mm, ensure endoluminal surface contact of the vascular wall. The thermistors are made of 5k7 bare chips (5 kohm resistance, curve 7 material), with gold metallization and 40 awg wires soldered onto the metallization; they can perform up to 25 measurements per second, and are delivered with a certified accuracy of 0.01°C. Results derived from animal studies have been shown to be reliable and reproducible; recent data derived from clinical trials investigating safety, feasibility, and reproducibility show that this catheter system is safe for use in humans, and that indeed important temperature heterogeneity can be appreciated along coronary artery systems of different patient populations. Figure 21.4 shows the absence of coronary temperature heterogeneity in anatomically perfectly normal coronary arteries, in patients without clinical signs of coronary lesion instability. Figure 21.5 shows an example of a thermographic assessment, revealing the presence of temperature heterogeneity in another patient. Figure 21.6 reveals that it is often not the hemodynamically most significant lesion that experiences the highest thermographic burden.

Our group has repeatedly found that temperature differences did not reach the 1–2°C (and even higher) difference found in the initial experience published previously. Indeed, patients who exhibit an unstable clinical syndrome, and in whom unstable plaques are expected, reveal temperature heterogeneities in the region of 0.10–0.25°C. Although clinical syndromes are not necessarily correlated with the presence/absence of unstable plaques and thus temperature heterogeneity, these data appear suggestive of unstable plaques revealing temperature heterogeneity in these regions. Potential reasons for these lower-than-originally envisaged temperature ranges are the presence of flow (with blood having a cooling effect), the fact that the patients included in this first trial potentially did not have truly unstable plaques, and that heat dissipation from metabolic activity of the vascular wall was not taken into account.

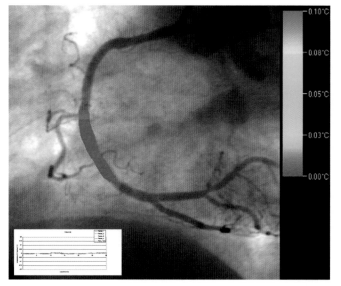

Figure 21.4
Result of an online collation of thermographic data upon an angiographic image. Immediately after performing an automated pullback, the temperature data are collated upon the stored angiographic image, and an online combination picture is provided, so that the cardiologist can immediately assess the hotter regions or the extent of temperature heterogeneity. This image reveals the absence of temperature heterogeneity, also shown by the raw data in the lower left corner, in this perfectly healthy vessel.

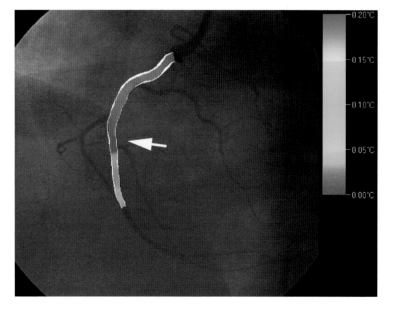

Figure 21.5
Thermography of a desobstructed right coronary artery (RCA). This 27-year-old patient presented with symptoms of an acute inferior myocardial infarction. After passing a wire through the obstructed RCA, flow was restored, and a thermography was performed. The assessment of the region where a plaque had just ruptured (with the acute myocardial infarction as a consequence) revealed temperature heterogeneity of up to 0.18°C (white arrow).

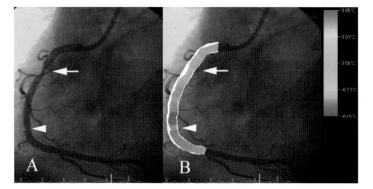

Figure 21.6
(A) Angiogram of a right coronary artery with a significant stenosis (arrow) and a small, nonsignificant eccentric plaque (arrowhead). (B) Collation of temperature data upon the angiographic image, revealing the absence of any temperature increase at the site of the significant stenosis, and the presence of a 'hot spot' at the site where the plaque proved to be angiographically insignificant. These images suggest that these so-called unimportant plaques may prove to be hazardous and prone to rupture.

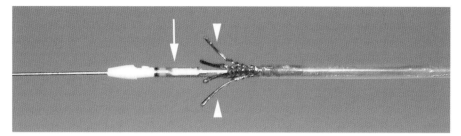

Figure 21.7
The Thermosound catheter, the first intracoronary plaque anatomy/functionality-testing combination catheter. The arrow shows the IVUS probe located distally from the dedicated thermistor-holding nitinol arms (arrowheads).

Combination thermography/ultrasound/IVUS flow/palpography catheter

Recently, Thermocore Medical Ltd (Guildford, UK) produced the first ever combination catheter, the Thermosound. The catheter is shown in Figure 21.7. This catheter is the first that can provide combined data from thermography, ultrasound, IVUS flow, and palpography. Using this catheter, it will be possible to assess anatomy (through IVUS), and in the same session record data providing details about the functionality of the vessel wall and plaques that are present (through thermography and palpography). Concurrently, quantification of flow through the vessel that is investigated can be assessed. Figure 21.8 shows an example of data that can be acquired using this combination catheter.

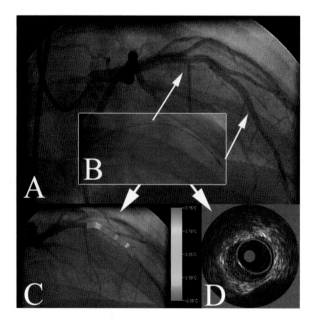

Figure 21.8
Angiogram of a mid left anterior descending segment (A) with a thermography catheter (B) present. Combined data from angiography/thermography (C) and IVUS/palpography (D), showing the type of data that can be generated using a combined catheter. The data reveal the presence of a hot lesion with high strain, strongly suggestive of a vulnerable plaque.

Conclusions

For thermography to be accepted by the clinical community, several hurdles need to be taken. First, the proof of principle needs to be irrevocably established in humans. Indeed, although previously mentioned trials have provided indications that thermal heterogeneity within coronary arteries exists, controlled, reproducible evidence is still lacking. Second, if plaque instability is indeed linked to temperature variances, and these plaques can be visualized using a thermography system, the cardiology community still has to investigate how to treat them. Also, the health-economic benefit of using a thermography system needs to be established. The likelihood of an invasive thermography system's gaining widespread acceptance will depend on the proof that it is indeed important to visualize unstable plaques, and that by treating them, lives can be saved and a beneficial effect on healthcare expenditure can be obtained. Researchers will then in the future possibly have a reliable method to detect unstable plaque in vivo and will further investigate the pathophysiological basis of the occurrence of temperature generation.

Nevertheless, we feel that intracoronary thermography is well on its way to becoming of the major players in the quest for the diagnosis of hot, vulnerable plaque in human coronary arteries. Early clinical data are being generated, and are necessary to prove a complex principle: by diagnosing and subsequently treating unstable coronary plaques, detrimental events such as myocardial infarctions and sudden death will be prevented, with an ensuing benefit both for the individual and for the healthcare system.

The recently constructed thermography/IVUS combination device may prove to be a giant step forward in this ingoing quest.

References

1. National Health and Nutrition Examination Survey III (NHANES III), 1988–1994. CDC/NCHS and the American Heart Association, 2002.
2. Ambrose JA, Tannenbaum MA, Alexopoulos D, et al. Angiographic progression of coronary artery disease and the development of myocardial infarction. J Am Coll Cardiol 1988;12:56–62.
3. Haft JI, Haik BJ, Goldstein JE, Brodyn NE. Development of significant coronary artery lesions in areas of minimal disease.

A common mechanism for coronary disease progression. Chest 1988;94:731–6.

4. Little WC, Constantinescu M, Applegate RJ, et al. Can coronary angiography predict the site of a subsequent myocardial infarction in patients with mild-to-moderate coronary artery disease? Circulation 1988;78:1157–66.

5. Falk E, Shah PK, Fuster V. Coronary plaque disruption. Circulation 1995;92:657–71.

6. Muller JE, Abela GS, Nesto RW, Tofler GH. Triggers, acute risk factors and vulnerable plaques: the lexicon of a new frontier. J Am Coll Cardiol 1994;23:809–13.

7. Lendon CL, Davies MJ, Born GV, Richardson PD. Atherosclerotic plaque caps are locally weakened when macrophages density is increased. Atherosclerosis 1991;87:87–90.

8. van der Wal AC, Becker AE, van der Loos CM, Das PK. Site of intimal rupture or erosion of thrombosed coronary atherosclerotic plaques is characterized by an inflammatory process irrespective of the dominant plaque morphology. Circulation 1994;89:36–44.

9. Ross R, Glomset JA. Atherosclerosis and the arterial smooth muscle cell: proliferation of smooth muscle is a key event in the genesis of the lesions of atherosclerosis. Science 1973;180:1332–9.

10. Ross R. Atherosclerosis is an inflammatory disease. Am Heart J 1999;138:S419–20.

11. Ross R. Atherosclerosis – an inflammatory disease. N Engl J Med 1999;340:115–26.

12. Libby P. Coronary artery injury and the biology of atherosclerosis: inflammation, thrombosis, and stabilization. Am J Cardiol 2000;86:3J–8J.

13. Aikawa M, Rabkin E, Okada Y, et al. Lipid lowering by diet reduces matrix metalloproteinase activity and increases collagen content of rabbit atheroma: a potential mechanism of lesion stabilization. Circulation 1998;97:2433–44.

14. Nissen SE, Yock P. Intravascular ultrasound: novel pathophysiological insights and current clinical applications. Circulation 2001;103:604–16.

15. Brezinski ME, Tearney GJ, Weissman NJ, et al. Assessing atherosclerotic plaque morphology: comparison of optical coherence tomography and high frequency intravascular ultrasound. Heart 1997;77:397–403.

16. de Korte CL, Pasterkamp G, van der Steen AF, et al. Characterization of plaque components with intravascular ultrasound elastography in human femoral and coronary arteries in vitro. Circulation 2000;102:617–23.

17. de Korte CL, Sierevogel MJ, Mastik F, et al. Identification of atherosclerotic plaque components with intravascular ultrasound elastography in vivo; a yucatan pig study. Circulation 2002;105:1627–30.

18. Moreno PR, Lodder RA, Purushothaman R, et al. Detection of lipid pool, thin fibrous cap, and inflammatory cells in human aortic atherosclerotic plaques by near-infrared spectroscopy Circulation 2002;105:927.

19. Fayad ZA, Fuster V. Clinical imaging of the high-risk or vulnerable atherosclerotic plaque. Circ Res 2001;89:305–16.

20. Robicsek F, Masters TN, Svenson RH, et al. The application of thermography in the study of coronary blood flow. Surgery 1978;84:858–64.

21. Bull GM, Morton J. Relationships of temperature with death rates from all causes and from certain respiratory and arteriosclerotic diseases in different age groups Age Ageing 1975;4:232–46.

22. Casscells W, Hathorn B, David M, et al. Thermal detection of cellular infiltrates in living atherosclerotic plaques: possible implications for plaque rupture and thrombosis. Lancet 1996;347:1447–51.

23. Verheye S, De Meyer GR, Van Langenhove G, et al. In vivo temperature heterogeneity of atherosclerotic plaques is determined by plaque composition. Circulation 2002;105:1601.

24. Newsholme P, Newsholme EA. Rates of utilization of glucose, glutamine and oleate and formation of end-products by mouse peritoneal macrophages in culture. Biochem J 1989;261:211–18.

25. Bjornheden T, Bondjers G. Oxygen consumption in aortic tissue from rabbits with diet-induced atherosclerosis. Arteriosclerosis 1987;7:238–47.

26. Palou A, Pico C, Bonet ML, Oliver P. The uncoupling protein, thermogenin. Int J Biochem Cell Biol 1998;30:7–11.

27. Ricquier D, Bouillaud F. The uncoupling protein homologues: UCP1, UCP2, UCP3, StUCP and AtUCP. Biochem J 2000;345:161–79.

28. Kockx MM, Knaapen MW, Martinet W, et al. Expression of the uncoupling protein UCP-2 in macrophages of unstable human atherosclerotic plaques. Circulation 2000;102:18A.

29. Stefanadis C, Diamantopoulos L, Vlachopoulos C, et al. Thermal heterogeneity within human atherosclerotic coronary arteries detected in vivo: a new method of detection by application of a special thermography catheter. Circulation 1999;99:1965–71.

30. Stefanadis C, Diamantopoulos L, Dernellis J, et al. Heat production of atherosclerotic plaques and inflammation assessed by the acute phase proteins in acute coronary syndromes. J Mol Cell Cardiol 2000;32:43–52.

31. Stefanadis C, Toutouzas K, Tsiamis E, et al. Increased local temperature in human coronary atherosclerotic plaques: an independent predictor of clinical outcome in patients undergoing a percutaneous coronary intervention. J Am Coll Cardiol 2001;37:1277–83.

32. Naghavi M, Melling M, Gul K, et al. First prototype of a 4 French 180 degree side-viewing infrared fiber optic catheter for thermal imaging of atherosclerotic plaque. J Am Coll Cardiol 2001;37:3A.

33. Gul K, O'Brien T, Siadaty S, et al. Coronary thermosensor basket catheter with thermographic imaging software for thermal detection of vulnerable atherosclerotic plaques. J Am Coll Cardiol 2001:37:18A.

22

Noninvasive coronary imaging with multislice spiral computed tomography

Pedro A Lemos, Koen Nieman

Introduction

Since its introduction in the late 1950s, invasive coronary angiography has been utilized as the gold standard method to evaluate coronary anatomy and detect coronary luminal stenosis. In clinical practice, however, invasive coronary angiograms are generally not utilized as a first-line diagnostic tool. A variety of noninvasive ischemia detection tests are currently available and are usually performed as an initial risk-stratification approach. Indeed, in recently issued clinical guidelines, invasive coronary angiography has been considered not to be useful for most patients without clear evidence of myocardial ischemia.[1] Nevertheless, although routinely performed, noninvasive testing does not preclude the need for coronary angiography. Indeed, more liberal early coronary angiography has been increasingly advocated for high-risk patients, such as those with acute coronary syndromes. In this context, a noninvasive test capable of direct visualization of the coronary tree would be desirable.

In the last few years, several reports have shown that magnetic resonance imaging (MRI), electron-beam computed tomography (CT), and early-generation (4-slice) multislice computed tomography (MSCT) have the potential to delineate the lumen of proximal coronary branches.[2–10] However, diagnostic accuracy has been insufficient to provide an alternative to invasive angiography. Recently, significant improvements in MSCT technology have markedly improved image quality, introducing into the clinical scenario a noninvasive method that is capable of reliably defining luminal integrity even for smaller coronary branches.[11,12] This chapter reviews the main technical aspects of the latest (16-slice) MSCT technology and describes the potential role of MSCT in clinical practice.

Requirements for an ideal coronary imaging method

The ideal coronary imaging for the detection and quantification of luminal stenosis should represent a true three-dimentional dataset that can be acquired on an operator- and patient-independent basis. To quantify a 50% diameter stenosis in an average-sized coronary artery (e.g. 2.0–3.0 mm), a spatial resolution in all three dimensions of at least 1–1.5 mm is needed – perhaps better in smaller branches. In fact, to monitor stenosis progression or regression, variations in diameter as small as 0.4 mm have been utilized in previous studies with conventional coronary angiography.[13]

High temporal resolution is mandatory to take account of cardiac motion.[14] Obviously, temporal resolution requirements are higher for imaging during the phases of the cardiac cycle where motion is more rapid (e.g. midsystole) than for phases with relatively decreased motion (e.g. telediastole). Although difficult to estimate, it is expected that artifacts should be largely minimized at a temporal resolution of 100 ms for 'slow' phases and 50 ms or less for 'rapid' phases, at normal heart rates (<100 bpm).[15]

Scan time should be short. Acquisition of all data within a single breath hold is mandatory in contrast-enhanced CT angiography, in order to avoid repetitive contrast injection, radiation exposure, and artifacts due to breathing. Ideally, all data should be collected during a single cardiac cycle (or less) and available for immediate analysis, which should be quick, quantitative, operator-independent, and well presented. Finally, the diagnostic tool should be noninvasive, harmless (e.g. radiation- and contrast-free), and costless. Unfortunately, these prerequisites are not achievable by any noninvasive method currently in use, and should not be expected within the foreseeable future.

Multislice spiral CT imaging

Image acquisition

In contrast to conventional sequential CT, spiral CT requires continuous movement of the table, while data from up to 16 detector rows, each with submillimeter slice width, acquire data simultaneously and continuously (Figure 22.1). During table (patient) movement through the scanner, the tube current can be altered according to the ECG. At systole, radiation is lowered to 20%, while nominal exposure is used during diastole. The change in tube current is triggered at a predefined time point coincident with 50% of the estimated RR interval, when nominal exposure begins and is maintained for 400 ms to acquire high-quality images (Figure 22.1). In this way, the total dose can be reduced by 50%. Importantly, image data are gathered continuously during the whole cardiac cycle and, although not appropriate for coronary anatomy, systolic images can be used for evaluation of contractile function. From the acquired data, ECG-gated cross-sectional images are retrospectively reconstructed (in contrast) to prospective ECG-synchronized data acquisition as in conventional and electron-beam CT scanners). By varying the position of the reconstruction window within the relatively motion-sparse diastolic phase (e.g. at 350 ms, 400 ms, or 450 ms prior to the R wave), selection of the most optimal imaging results is permitted for further analysis (Figure 22.1).

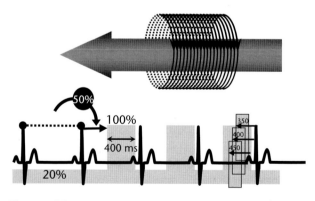

Figure 22.1
Data are acquired by 16 parallel detector rows, while the patient moves continuously through the scanner. Triggered by the patient's ECG, nominal radiation exposure is limited to the diastolic phase (400 ms). Retrospectively, a number of reconstructions are performed, during slightly different intervals within the diastolic phase images, gated at predefined position relative to the next R wave.

Practical considerations and image quality

The cranio-caudal size of the heart averages 10–12 cm, although it can be significantly larger in patients with coronary heart disease. In most instances, however, the entire length of the heart can be comfortably imaged during one breath hold with current 16-slice MSCT scanners,[11] which provides a scan range of nearly 1 cm/s (a breath hold of under 20 s is enough to scan the entire heart).

The previous generation of 4-slice scanners had an individual detector width of 1.0 mm with a reconstructed slice width of 1.3 mm. Current 16-slice MSCT provides a reconstructed slice width of 0.75–1.0 mm and an in-plane spatial resolution of up to 0.5 mm × 0.5 mm. This resolution allows assessment of almost the entire coronary tree, including intermediate to small epicardial branches.

The duration of the diastolic phase, the most motion-sparse period in the cardiac cycle, is directly related to heart rate, being markedly reduced in patients with tachycardia. Because CT requires a defined period of time to acquire its data per heart cycle, the heart rate plays an important role in image quality with respect to motion artifacts.[16] Sixteen-slice MSCT requires 210 ms for heart rates below 70 bpm, and between 105 and 210 ms for heart rates above 70 bpm (based on adaptive algorithms). It has been shown that MCST provides better diagnostic accuracy in patients with heart rates below 65 bpm. Pharmacological heart rate control for patients with rates above 65 bpm (metoprolol 100 mg 1 hour before the examination) has been defined as an important step to enhance the final quality of MSCT imaging.[11] The reliability of CT in patients with irregular cardiac rhythm, such as those with atrial fibrillation, is limited. The consequent variable filling conditions between consecutive heartbeats and the reconstruction of slices at different cycle phases may lead to interslice discontinuity, potentially resulting in the false appearance of coronary obstructions (Figure 22.2).

The differences in X-ray attenuation between non-enhanced blood, the vessel wall, and the perivascular fat are not sufficient to distinguish them by CT. Iodine contrast media are necessary to increase the opacification of the coronary lumen and make it distinguishable from the surrounding tissues. A bolus of 100–140 ml of intravenous contrast is usually utilized (4–5 ml/s). After injection, the signal density level in the ascending aorta is monitored until a predefined threshold of 100 Hounsfield units is reached. The patient is then instructed to maintain an inspiratory breath hold (usually around 20 s) while CT data are acquired.

The presence of calcification represents a true limitation of MSCT. The beam hardening and partial volume effects can completely obscure the coronary lumen, precluding reliable evaluation of the coronary anatomy. Similarly, metal objects, such as stents, surgical clips, sternal wires, and pacemaker wires, can also reduce the inter-

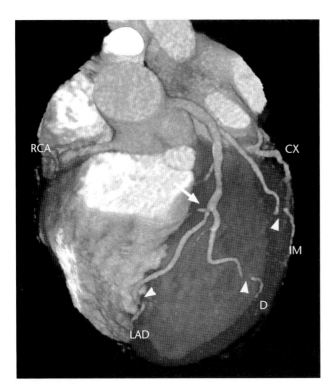

Figure 22.2
Volume-rendered reconstruction of an MSCT angiogram. The left anterior descending coronary artery (LAD), at the level of the second septal branch, is mildly narrowed (arrow). The distal segments of the LAD and the diagonal and intermediate branches show interruptions (arrowheads) that are caused by an irregular heartbeat. CX, left circumflex branch; D, diagonal branch; RCA, right coronary artery.

pretability of MSCT. In addition to dedicated filtering algorithms, use of the thinnest slice possible reduces partial volume artifacts and may enhance image quality in calcified vessel segments.[17]

The X-ray dose ultimately determines the final image quality. Increased doses are required to maintain a good contrast-to-noise ratio in large patients as well as acquisition with thin slices. Despite a thin slice width, the contrast-to-signal ratio in MSCT is high, which is crucial to the discrimination of non-enhanced structures.

Image interpretation and diagnostic accuracy
Postprocessing techniques

The coronary lumen can be assessed through different postprocessing techniques (Figure 22.3). Maximum-intensity projections of thin slabs and multiplanar reformations are used in addition to the axial source images. Maximum-intensity projections provide smooth high-contrast images, with the advantage that longer vessel sections can be visualized in the same plane. However, the presence of calcifications or stents can markedly reduce the interpretability of the lumen contours, in which case multiplanar reformations or the axial source images are more suitable. Although not used as the initial means for image interpretation, advanced postprocessing techniques

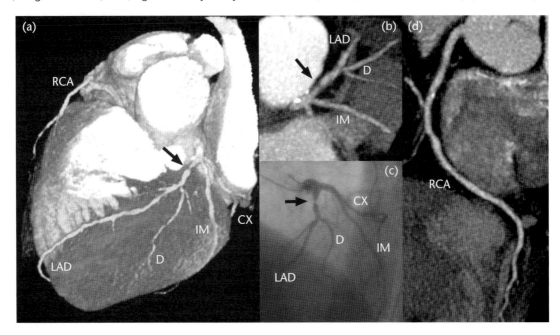

Figure 22.3
Three-dimensional volume-rendered reconstruction (a), maximum-intensity projection (b), conventional angiogram (c) of a left coronary artery with a short and significant lesion (arrow) in the most proximal segment, and curved multiplanar reformation of the right coronary artery (d). LAD, left anterior descending coronary artery; D, diagonal branch; IM, intermediate branch; CX, left circumflex branch; RCA, right coronary artery.

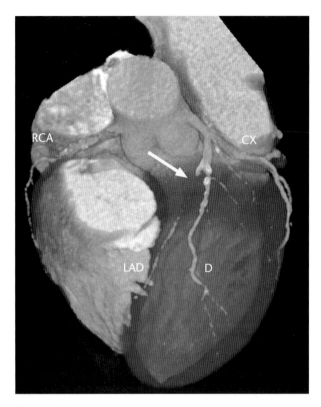

Figure 22.4
Occlusion (arrow) of a small left anterior descending
coronary artery (LAD) with collateral filling of the distal
segment. CX, left circumflex branch; D, diagonal branch;
RCA, right coronary artery.

such as curved multiplanar reformations, volume render-
ing, and virtual angioscopy may add important information
with regard to three-dimensional orientation for the referring physician (Figures 22.3 and 22.4).

Data analysis and clinical results

The 16-slice spiral MSCT scanners have provided major
improvements in image quality and robustness of noninvasive coronary imaging, compared with the previous
generation (4-slice) of MSCT and electron-bean CT
scanners.[2–6,9,11,12,16,18–23] The assessability of the entire
coronary tree has significantly increased to more than
90% of all branches of 'clinical interest', including smaller
branches and distal segments (Figures 22.2–22.4). Oblique
and multiplanar reconstructions have been made possible
by the submillimeter resolution, permitting the display of
longer stretches of vessels, which facilitates data analysis
with improved vessel sharpness.

In a recent study by Nieman et al,[11] the sensitivity to
identify significantly stenosed coronary arteries was
reported as 95%, with a specificity of 86%. These results
were obtained without exclusion of any segments due to

suboptimal quality. In another study, Roper et al[12] excluded 12% of the segments and found a similar sensitivity
(92%) with a higher specificity (93%). These figures compare favorably with results obtained with electron-beam
CT and 4-slice MSCT scanners. In previous studies utilizing these modalities, analysis was often restricted to the
proximal and middle coronary segments. Exclusion rates
ranged from 6% to 32%, while the sensitivity and
specificity to detect significant stenosis in the evaluable
coronary arteries ranged from 75% to 95% and from
79% to 97%, respectively.[2–6,9,16,18–23]

Coronary wall and plaque imaging

Initially, the major application of cardiac CT scanning was
quantification of coronary calcium. However, the current
generation of 16-slice MSCT scanners permit the identification of non-obstructive atherosclerotic plaques.
Furthermore, plaque components such as fat, fibrous tissue, and calcium have distinct X-ray attenuation characteristics, resulting in differences in CT density values
expressed in Houndsfield units. Thus, differentiation
among 'soft' (fat, thrombus, necrotic), 'hard' (fibrous),
and calcific plaques is theoretically possible and has been
reported in preliminary studies comparing 4-slice MSCT
imaging with intravascular ultrasound.[24] It is worth noting, however, that identification of plaque composition
with MSCT is currently rather crude and requires further confirmation by clinical and histological studies.
Nevertheless, these first results highlight that MSCT may
become a future technique for the noninvasive
identification of rupture-prone coronary plaques and
may be used as a valuable tool for risk stratification
(Figure 22.5).

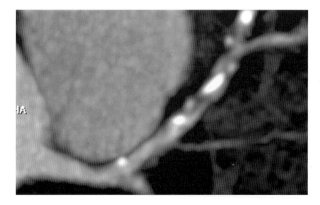

Figure 22.5
Diffusely diseased left anterior descending coronary artery.
The atherosclerotic material consists of high-density
(bright) calcified tissue to low-density (dark) noncalcified
tissue.

Conclusions

The new generation of MSCT scanners have been demonstrated to provide reliable information concerning coronary anatomy and the presence of coronary stenosis, thereby representing a potential noninvasive alternative to conventional catheter-based coronary angiography. Currently, MSCT imaging does not provide enough clinical reliability to replace diagnostic conventional angiography. However, the noninvasive nature of the method, and the possibility to evaluate plaque constitution, as well as cardiac function, may increase the clinical applicability of MSCT in daily practice.

References

1. Scanlon PJ, Faxon DP, Audet AM, et al. ACC/AHA Guidelines for Coronary Angiography. A report of the American College of Cardiology/American Heart Association Task Force on Practice Guidelines (Committee on Coronary Angiography). Developed in collaboration with the Society for Cardiac Angiography and Interventions. J Am Coll Cardiol 1999;33:1756–824.
2. Nakanishi T, Ito K, Imazu M, et al. Evaluation of coronary artery stenoses using electron-beam CT and multiplanar reformation. J Comput Assist Tomogr 1997;21:121–7.
3. Reddy GP, Chernoff DM, Adams JR, et al. Coronary artery stenoses: assessment with contrast-enhanced electron-beam CT and axial reconstructions. Radiology 1998; 208:167–72.
4. Schmermund A, Rensing BJ, Sheedy PF, et al. Intravenous electron-beam computed tomographic coronary angiography for segmental analysis of coronary artery stenoses. J Am Coll Cardiol 1998;31:1547–54.
5. Rensing BJ, Bongaerts A, van Geuns RJ, et al. Intravenous coronary angiography by electron beam computed tomography: a clinical evaluation. Circulation 1998;98:2509–12.
6. Achenbach S, Moshage W, Ropers D, et al. Value of electron-beam computed tomography for the noninvasive detection of high-grade coronary-artery stenoses and occlusions. N Engl J Med 1998;339:1964–71.
7. Achenbach S, Ropers D, Regenfus M, et al. Contrast enhanced electron beam computed tomography to analyse the coronary arteries in patients after acute myocardial infarction. Heart 2000;84:489–93.
8. Achenbach S, Ropers D, Regenfus M, et al. Noninvasive coronary angiography by magnetic resonance imaging, electron-beam computed tomography, and multislice computed tomography. Am J Cardiol 2001;88:70E–3E.
9. Nieman K, Oudkerk M, Rensing BJ, et al. Coronary angiography with multi-slice computed tomography. Lancet 2001;357:599–603.
10. Nieman K, van Geuns RJ, Wielopolski P, et al. Noninvasive coronary imaging in the new millennium: a comparison of computed tomography and magnetic resonance techniques. Rev Cardiovasc Med 2002;3:77–84.
11. Nieman K, Cademartiri F, Lemos PA, et al. Reliable noninvasive coronary angiography with fast submillimeter multislice spiral computed tomography. Circulation 2002;106:2051–4.
12. Ropers D, Baum U, Pohle K, et al. Detection of coronary artery stenoses with thin-slice multi-detector row spiral computed tomography and multiplanar reconstruction. Circulation 2003;107:664–6.
13. White CW, Gobel FL, Campeau L, et al. Effect of an aggressive lipid-lowering strategy on progression of atherosclerosis in the left main coronary artery from patients in the post coronary artery bypass graft trial. Circulation 2001; 104:2660–5.
14. Nieman K, Rensing BJ, van Geuns RJ, et al. Non-invasive coronary angiography with multislice spiral computed tomography: impact of heart rate. Heart 2002;88:470–4.
15. Wang Y, Watts R, Mitchell I, et al. Coronary MR angiography: selection of acquisition window of minimal cardiac motion with electrocardiography-triggered navigator cardiac motion prescanning – initial results. Radiology 2001; 218:580–5.
16. Giesler T, Baum U, Ropers D, et al. Noninvasive visualization of coronary arteries using contrast-enhanced multidetector CT: influence of heart rate on image quality and stenosis detection. AJR 2002;179:911–16.
17. Nieman K, Cademartiri F, Raaijmakers R, et al. Noninvasive angiographic evaluation of coronary stents with multi-slice spiral computed tomography. Herz 2003;28:136–42.
18. Budoff MJ, Oudiz RJ, Zalace CP, et al. Intravenous three-dimensional coronary angiography using contrast enhanced electron beam computed tomography. Am J Cardiol 1999;83:840–5.
19. Achenbach S, Giesler T, Ropers D, et al. Detection of coronary artery stenoses by contrast-enhanced, retrospectively electrocardiographically-gated, multislice spiral computed tomography. Circulation 2001;103:2535–8.
20. Knez A, Becker CR, Leber A, et al. Usefulness of multislice spiral computed tomography angiography for determination of coronary artery stenoses. Am J Cardiol 2001;88:1191–4.
21. Vogl TJ, Abolmaali ND, Diebold T, et al. Techniques for the detection of coronary atherosclerosis: multi-detector row CT coronary angiography. Radiology 2002;223:212–20.
22. Kopp AF, Schroeder S, Kuettner A, et al. Non-invasive coronary angiography with high resolution multidetector-row computed tomography. Results in 102 patients. Eur Heart J 2002;23:1714–25.
23. Nieman K, Rensing BJ, van Geuns RJ, et al. Usefulness of multislice computed tomography for detecting obstructive coronary artery disease. Am J Cardiol 2002;89:913–18.
24. Schroeder S, Kopp AF, Baumbach A, et al. Noninvasive detection and evaluation of atherosclerotic coronary plaques with multislice computed tomography. J Am Coll Cardiol 2001;37:1430–5.

23

Myogenesis: an update on muscle regeneration

Chi Hang Lee, Pieter C Smits

Introduction

It is a traditional belief that adult myocardium is incapable of self-repair after infarction[1] and that the damaged area is replaced by noncontracting fibrous scar tissue. Initially, ventricular remodeling helps to preserve overall myocardial function. However, this compensatory mechanism fails and clinical heart failure ensues when the infarcted area is large. Medical treatment and alternative therapies, including biventricular pacing, surgical cardiomyoplasty and left ventricular assist devices, have only limited success. Currently, heart transplantation is the last option for patients with end-stage heart failure.[2] However, side-effects from lifelong immunosuppressive therapy, limitations in the availability of donor organs, and strict eligibility criteria remain critical issues. These constraints mandate a continuing search for alternative treatments for patients with irreversibly damaged myocardium.

Myogenesis, the transplantation of contractile cells to the failing heart in order to replenish the number of functioning cardiomyocytes and improve cardiac function, has recently emerged as a novel strategy for the treatment of heart failure. It represents a paradigm shift in our therapeutic approach, from substitution to regeneration of irreversibly damaged cardiac tissues and structures. In the past decade, encouraging progress has been made in myogenesis research. Survival, differentiation, and engraftment of the transplanted cells, as well as improvements in myocardial contractility, have been demonstrated in animal studies. Currently, several phase I/II clinical trials are in progress.

Different routes of cell delivery

There are a number of different methods of delivering cells to the host myocardium. Among these, direct intramyocardial injection under open thoracotomy and intravenous infusion have been the common routes employed in animal studies. However, due to their invasive nature and suboptimal efficiency, respectively, these two methods are less favored for clinical trials. Instead, the feasibility of using an intracoronary approach for delivery of cells has been established. The development of nonfluoroscopic electromechanical mapping guidance has facilitated direct intramyocardial injection using a percutaneous transcatheter approach.

Intramyocardial injection

Direct myocardial injection via thoracotomy (transepicardial approach)

There is a theoretical advantage to direct intramyocardial injection of cells into the myocardium. The most precise and accurate delivery can be achieved by direct visualization during thoracotomy. In fact, the initial experiments on myogenesis in animal models were performed using an open- or mini-thoracotomy approach.[3,4] Therefore, this delivery method has been well validated and established. When used in patients, the myocardial injection can be performed either as an adjunct to coronary artery bypass grafting (CABG) or, theoretically, as sole therapy. However, the thoracotomy approach is invasive. General anaesthesia is required during the procedure and there follows a prolonged postoperative recovery course. These are associated with substantial morbidity and/or mortality. For the same reasons, repeated administration of cells to the same patient is less possible. Apart from being an adjunct to CABG, thoracotomy for sole injection of cells into patient myocardium does not seem justified at present.

Endomyocardial injection via transcatheter (transendomyocardial approach)

Compared with thoracotomy, the percutaneous approach to cell delivery using an injection catheter is relatively less invasive. During the procedure, the catheter traverses the femoral artery and enters the left ventricular cavity by the retro-aortic approach. Often, there is a radiopaque tip at the distal end of the catheter for fluoroscopic navigation. Positioning of the catheter and injection is done under fluoroscopic guidance. Once the injection site has been confirmed, the injection needle can be protruded and cells can be injected directly into the myocardium.

A novel transcatheter approach using the electromagnetic navigation and injection catheter NOGA system (Biosense-Webster, Waterloo, Belgium)[5] has achieved promising results. This system allows nonfluoroscopic in vivo navigation and three-dimensional mapping of the left ventricle. There are several advantages to using this system. Radiation exposure of the patient and operator is minimized. This system is designed to acquire, analyze, and display three-dimensional electro-anatomical maps of the heart by integrating information obtained from intracardiac electrograms and kinesia acquired at multiple endocardial locations. These help to demarcate the normal, hibernating, and infarcted myocardium, and serve as a platform for positioning the injection catheter.[6,7] The accuracy of this system has been validated in both in vivo and in vitro settings.[8] The feasibility and safety of transcatheter delivery of skeletal myoblasts in a porcine model of myocardial infarction under electromagnetic guidance have recently been reported.[9]

Intramyocardial injection via the coronary vein (transvenous)

The transvascular catheter is a newly designed catheter under investigation. There is an intravascular ultrasound (IVUS) probe attached to the catheter tip and a retractable injection needle is located proximal to the probe. Under fluoroscopic guidance, the injection catheter goes through the inferior vena cava and right heart, enters the coronary sinus and cardiac vein, running parallel to the infarct-related artery. The spatial orientation of the injection needle within the cardiac vein is determined by IVUS. Under IVUS guidance, the needle is directed towards the myocardium. After penetration of the vein with the extendable needle, a microcatheter is then advanced intramyocardially. Cells or drugs can be injected through this microcatheter. The safety and feasibility of this new catheter approach still need to be investigated.

Intracoronary administration

Intracoronary administration of cells to the infarcted region of the myocardium is technically simple. Without direct contact of the catheter with endomyocardium, this method avoids mechanical injury and induction of an inflammatory response in the myocardium. This can be performed as an adjunct to percutaneous coronary intervention in the same setting. The main disadvantage is the need for a patent infarct-related vessel and the potential disadvantage of blocking capillaries with the injected cells.

Intravenous administration

Intravenous administration is the simplest and least invasive delivery route. It is associated with minimal morbidity and almost nil mortality. The procedure can easily be repeated if necessary. However, the problems of poor selectivity and efficiency make this approach less favorable, although it has been suggested that injected cells can home to the ischemic or infarcted region. The clinical significance and reliability of this homing mechanism have still to be demonstrated.

Different cell types used in myogenesis

Different cell types have been used in myogenesis research in animal models. These include skeletal myoblasts, fetal cardiomyocytes, embryonic stem cells, and bone marrow-derived stromal cells. Each cell type has its own merits and limitations. Skeletal myoblast transplantation has accumulated the most information and clinical experience (Table 23.1).

Autologous skeletal myoblasts

Characteristics features

Skeletal muscle is the most abundant muscle in the human body. There are more than 600 skeletal muscles in the

Table 23.1　Different cell types and concerns in clinical applications of cell transplantation

	Availability	Immunogenicity	Ethical issues	Potential oncogenicity	Experience
Skeletal myoblasts	***	***	***	***	**
Fetal cardiomycytes	*	*	*	***	*
Embryonic stem cells	**	*	*	*	*
Bone marrow stromal cells	***	***	***	**	*

*** More favorable. ** Moderately favorable. * Less favorable.

human body and these make up about 40% of the tissue of the whole body. Skeletal muscle is composed of different myofibers. In contrast to myocardium, skeletal muscle retains a population of myogenic cells (myoblasts) that offer a proliferative and regenerative capacity to repair damaged skeletal muscle fibers. Skeletal myoblasts (or satellite cells) are precursor cells of skeletal muscle. They normally lie in a quiescent state under the basal membrane of muscular fibers. Under normal conditions, skeletal myoblasts make up 4–8% of the total number of muscle cells in adult mammal skeletal muscles; this percentage decreases with age.[10] An injury or stress inflicted on myofibers activates dormant myoblasts through a chemotactic pathway; these then proliferate and migrate toward the damaged site, where they enter the mitotic cycle and later fuse with each other to form new myotubes and also fuse with the ends of damaged myofibers. The role of skeletal myoblasts in the regenerative capacity of skeletal muscle is well established.[11]

There are several theoretical advantages to using autologous skeletal myoblasts for myogenesis:

1. *Ease of availability*. Skeletal muscle is abundant throughout the human body, negating the problem of organ shortage. For the purpose of myoblast culture and expansion, only a limited amount (around 5–10 g) of skeletal muscle has to be removed through a small (10 cm) surgical incision. The procedure itself is only mildly invasive, and patients can be discharged on the same day.
2. *Autologous transplantation*. Although successful myogenesis has been demonstrated in animal models using heterogeneous cells, immunosuppressive therapy is required to prevent rejection. The regimen and duration of the immunosuppressive therapy that is required remain unknown. Moreover, the side-effects related to immunosuppressive agents can adversely affect patients. In contrast, skeletal myoblasts can be obtained from patients themselves; thus, the transplantation is autologous and so no immunosuppressive therapy is necessary.
3. *Ischemic resistance*. Fewer capillaries are found in skeletal muscle compared with myocardium. Accordingly, skeletal muscle is relatively more resistant to ischemia and has been shown to have increased survival in regions of reduced coronary perfusion.[12,13] This

feature favors the survival and engraftment of transplanted skeletal myoblasts within the infarcted myocardium.
4. *Low risk of tumor development*. Unlike multipotential noncommitted stem cells, skeletal myoblasts are committed to muscle development and have less chance of developing into tumor or other tissues after transplantation into myocardium.
5. *Continued replenishment of satellite cells*. Although most engrafted myoblasts differentiate into mature fibers after transplantation, some of them remain quiescent satellite cells. Theoretically, this provides a continuous source of precursor cells that can participate in tissue repair in subsequent ischemic episodes.[14]
6. *Absence of ethical controversy*. Unlike embryonic stem cells and fetal cardiomyocytes, the use of autologous skeletal myoblasts for myogenesis does not give rise in any ethical controversy.

Preclinical trials

Transplantation of skeletal myoblasts into normal as well as injured myocardium has been successfully demonstrated in several different animal models (Table 23.2). In early studies, the transplanted skeletal myoblasts formed striated muscle fibers with histological evidence of centrally located nuclei and intercalated discs in the host myocardium, suggesting their survival and differentiation into cardiomyocytes.[15,16] However, these findings were not reproduced in subsequent studies.[14] Moreover, staining for cardiac-specific α-myosin heavy chain and connexin-43 (a marker of cardiac-specific gap junctions between the grafted skeletal myoblasts and the surrounding host cardiomyocytes) remained negative in most studies.[14,17,18] Nowadays, it is generally believed that transplanted skeletal myoblasts will not differentiate into cardiomyocytes. Nevertheless, studies have shown improvement in functional performance of ischemic[19–21] and nonischemic[22] injured myocardium after skeletal myoblast transplantation. In one recent study, long-term (up to 1 year) survival of the graft and improvement of myocardial function has been reported.[23] This study also suggested that the degree of improvement is greater in the group with a worse baseline ejection fraction.[24] In one study, diastolic performance was found to improve before systolic performance.[21] This

Table 23.2   Studies of skeletal myoblast transplantation in animal models

Authors	Year	Animal	Injury induction	Delivery	Main results
Marelli et al[3]	1992	Dogs	Cryoinjury	Thoracotomy	Patch of muscle fibers formed
Chiu et al[15]	1995	Canines	Cryoinjury	Thoracotomy	Milieu-influenced differentiation of myoblasts into cardiac-like muscle cells
Murry et al[14]	1996	Rats	Cryoinjury	Thoracotomy	Myoblasts proliferated and differentiated into myofibers; contracted when stimulated
Robinson et al[16]	1996	Murine	Nil	Transventricular	Engraftment of myoblasts; cardiomyocyte phenotype
Taylor et al[20]	1998	Rabbits	Cryoinjury	Thoracotomy	Engraftment of striated muscle cells; improved cardiac function
Atkins et al[21]	1999	Rabbits	Cryoinjury	Thoracotomy	Improved diastolic prior to systolic function
Jain et al[19]	2001	Rats	Coronary ligation	Thoracotomy	Viable graft; enhanced exercise capacity; contractile function and attenuated ventricular dilatation
Suzuki et al[22]	2001	Rats	Doxorubicin	Intracoronary	Globally disseminated myoblasts survived and formed myotubes; improved cardiac function
Pouzet et al[24]	2001	Rats	Coronary ligation	Thoracotomy	LVEF <40% and number of cells injected predicted improvement in cardiac function
Suzuki et al[28]	2001	Rats	Coronary ligation	Thoracotomy	Infarct size reduced and cardiac function improved with VEGF-expressing myoblasts
Dib et al[9]	2002	Pigs	Coil placement	Endomyocardial	Multinucleated myotube found in infarcted region
Ghostine et al[23]	2002	Sheep	Embolization	Thoracotomy	Graft survival and improved myocardial function at 1 year

is an important observation, as diastolic dysfunction often occurs sooner and more insidiously than systolic dysfunction in myocardial ischemia and is the primary etiology for heart failure in up to 40% of patients with chronic ischemia.[25–27] Treatment options for diastolic heart failure are also more limited.

The mechanism of improved myocardial function after myogenesis remains unclear, and a number of hypotheses have been postulated.[24] The first hypothesis is that the transplanted myoblasts may limit infarct expansion owing to their elastic properties, thereby preventing adverse ventricular remodeling. Secondly, the grafted myoblasts may contribute directly to contractility by synchronously contracting with the host cardiomyocytes. The absence of gap junctions and hence electromechanical coupling between the graft and host cardiomyocytes has cast doubt on this hypothesis. Nevertheless, this may not exclude an inotropic involvement of the grafted cells if one assumes that they can be mechanically stimulated by the surrounding cardiomyocytes, through a stretch–contract mechanism. Another mechanism whereby transplanted myoblasts could improve function is through stimulation of angiogenesis by locally released growth factors.

Recently, a novel approach has been developed combining cell transplantation with gene therapy. Skeletal myoblasts transfected with a human angiogenic factor (vascular endothelial growth factor, $VEGF_{165}$) gene were injected into an infarction rat model.[28] It was hypothe-

sized that the increase in microcirculation due to the additional angiogenic factor could provide the grafted cells with enhanced blood supply. Compared with control-transfected myoblasts, $VEGF_{165}$ gene-transfected myoblasts transplantation demonstrated increased myocardial VEGF level, enhanced angiogenesis, superior reduction in infarct size, and better improvement in cardiac function.

In view of the limited availability of myoblasts in the elderly, attempts have been made to transform the more readily available fibroblasts into myogenic cells by genetic manipulation. MyoD is a transcription factor functioning as unique master gene that is able to prompt myogenesis in a variety of cells, including fibroblasts. An adenoviral vector encoding MyoD was transfected into cultured cardiac fibroblasts in an ex vivo experiment. Myogenic transformation of the fibroblasts was observed, and subsequent transplantation of the transformed myogenic cells into infarcted rat myocardium showed formation of viable graft.[29]

Clinical trials

Following the success of animal models, nonrandomized clinical trials with autologous skeletal myoblasts are being conducted (Tables 23.3 and 23.4). In France, ten post-myocardial infarction patients with direct intramyocardial injection of autologous skeletal myoblasts via a

Table 23.3 Ongoing surgical trials with skeletal myoblasts for myogenesis: clinical experience (November 2002)

Location(s)	Investigators	No. of patients	Context
Hôpital Bichot, Paris, France	Menasché et al[74]	10	Adjunct to CABG
Arizona Heart, UCLA, Temple University, USA	Dib et al[75]	6	Adjunct to LVAD
		12	Adjunct to CABG
University of Navarra, Spain	Herreros et al[76]		Adjunct to CABG
China	Kao et al	2	Adjunct to CABG
Hôpital Pompidou, Paris, France	Chachques et al[77]	5	Adjunct to CABG

CABG, coronary artery bypass grafting; LVAD, left ventricular assist device.

Table 23.4 Ongoing percutaneous trials with skeletal myoblasts for myogenesis: Clinical experience (November 2002)

Location	Investigators	No. of patients	Approach
Erasmus Medical Center, Rotterdam, Netherlands	Smits et al[78]	11	Transendocardial (Myostar)
		3	Transvenous (Transvascular)
Centre Cuore, Milan, Italy	Colombo et al	3	Transendocardial (Myocath)
Rostock, Germany	Nienaber et al	6	Transendocardial (Myocath)
Poznan, Poland	Siminiak et al	10	Transvenous

thoracotomy approach as an adjunct to bypass surgery by a team led by Philippe Menasché. There was one early postoperative death. Implantable cardioverter defibrillators (ICDs) were implanted in four of the nine surviving patients after the procedure due to ventricular arrhythmia. Only one patient experienced two shocks, while others have remained arrhythmia-free. At a mean follow-up of 10.9 months, there was significant improvement in functional status and myocardial contractility (Figure 23.1 and 23.2). One patient died from a stroke 18 months after treatment.

A phase I/II pilot study of catheter-based autologous skeletal myoblast transplantation for myogenesis was initiated at the Thoraxcenter in Rotterdam in 2001. The primary objectives of this pilot study were feasibility and safety. The secondary objective was to assess the postprocedural change in left ventricular (LV) function. Only symptomatic patients with New York Heart Association (NYHA) functional class II or III on optimal medical therapy were recruited. All patients had a history of previous anterior myocardial infarction more than 4 weeks old at the time of procedure and an impaired LV function (LV ejection fraction (LVEF) of

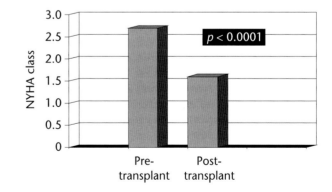

Figure 23.1
Change in New York Heart Association (NYHA) function class after skeletal myoblast transplantation by thoracotomy. Mean follow-up 10.9 months (range 5–17.5 months).

20–45% by radionuclide radiography). In total, five patients were recruited to this study.

Before the procedure, myocardial scar was defined as an area of akinesia on dobutamine stress echocardiography

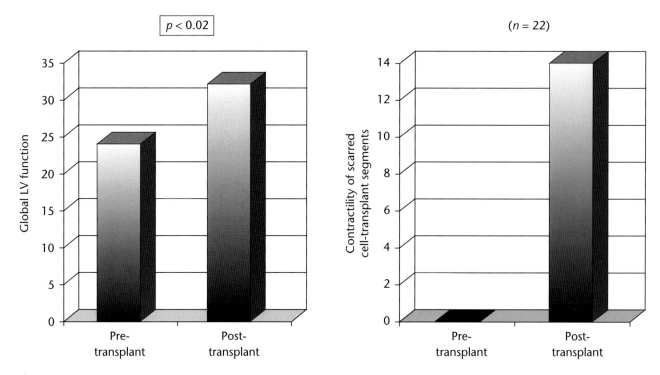

Figure 23.2
Change in cardiac function after skeletal myoblast transplantation by thoracotomy. Mean follow-up 10.9 months (range 5–17.5 months).

(DSE), LV angiography, and magnetic resonance imaging (MRI). Target regional wall thickness had to be greater than 5 mm. History of syncope or malignant ventricular arrhythmia were considered exclusion criteria.

Biopsy of the quadriceps muscle was done under local anesthesia. On average, 8.4 g (range 5–13 g) of muscle was excised through a 10 cm-long surgical incision (Figure 23.3). All five biopsy procedures were uneventful and were done on an outpatient basis. Biopsies were placed in bottles containing a proprietary solution designed to preserve the cell during controlled shipment and were then sent for culture and expansion. A rebiopsy was required in three patients, due to the desmin-staining results falling below the lot release criteria. In these patients, a prestimulation procedure was performed using multiple needle punctures of the muscle 3 days prior to the biopsy procedure, in order to activate myoblast proliferation.

After a culture period of 17 days (range 14–19 days), the cell transplantation procedure was performed in the cardiac catheterization laboratory under local anesthesia. Access was obtained through the femoral artery and 100 IU/kg heparin was given. The target activated clotting time (ACT) was 250–300 s. After a coronary and biplane LV angiogram with orthogonal views had been obtained, an outline of the LV chamber was drawn on transparent tabloids that were taped to the fluoroscopy monitors. An electromechanical NOGA map of the LV was then obtained using a 7 French (Fr) NOGASTAR catheter (F-curve) connected to the NOGA console. Areas exhibiting low voltages and linear local shortening (UV < 6 mV and LLS < 2%) on

the NOGA map were considered as the target area of treatment if these areas were geographically concordant with the scar areas assessed by the preprocedural DSE, MRI, and LV angiogram. With an 8 Fr MYOSTAR injection catheter, 16±4 (mean ± SD, range 9–19) transendocardial injections were made under the NOGA map guidance.

No procedural complication has occurred. Only in one patient were minor elevations of creatine kinase (CK) and CK-MB (less than twice the upper level) and troponin T (0.16 μg/l) noted after the procedure. In all five patients, the in-hospital stay was uneventful and the patients were discharged within 24 hours after the procedure. During follow-up, patient number 3 was rehospitalized due to decompensated heart failure and nonsustained ventricular tachycardia (NSVT) on Holter monitoring. He eventually received intracoronary device implantation 2 months after the procedure. At 6-month follow-up, all five patients had a moderate increase in LV function as shown by LV angiography (Figure 23.4), although this change was not observed by nuclear LVEF measurement. However, regional analysis by MRI showed a significant increase in wall thickening at the target areas.

Fetal cardiomyocytes

The fetal cardiomyocyte is different from the adult cardiomyocyte in that it can still enter the cell cycle and there-

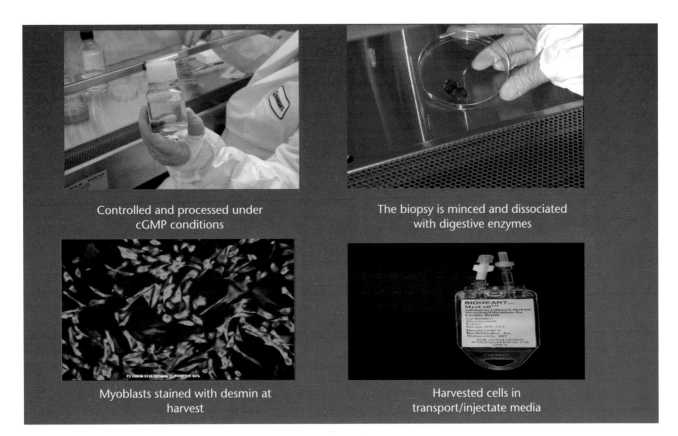

Controlled and processed under
cGMP conditions

The biopsy is minced and dissociated
with digestive enzymes

Myoblasts stained with desmin at
harvest

Harvested cells in
transport/injectate media

Figure 23.3
Myoblast selection and cell expansion.

fore can be expanded in culture. Due to their possessing the same inherent structural and functional properties as adult cardiomyocytes, fetal cardiomyocytes are theoretically ideal candidates for myogenesis. Survival of transplanted fetal cardiomyocytes was initially demonstrated in the rat hindlimb and myocardium.[30,31] After transplantation, the tissue derived from the transplanted cardiomyocytes increased in size and contracted spontaneously.[30] Electron microscopy revealed the presence of nascent intercalated discs connecting the fetal cardiomyocytes with the host myocardium, suggesting successful engraftment.[31] In a study investigating the functional significance of transplanted fetal cardiomyocytes, myocardial injury was incurred by cryoinjury in rats.[32] Fetal rat cardiomyocytes or culture medium were injected into the scar tissue 4 weeks after injury. At 8 weeks, scar size was significantly smaller in the transplantation group than in the control group. Myocardial function measured using a Langendorff preparation was also better in the transplantation group. In agreement with the results from small animals, successful myocardial regeneration using fetal cardiomyocytes in adult pigs and dogs was also demonstrated.[33,34] New vessels were formed in and around the cell graft area, which may enhance cell survival by transporting nutrients and growth factors to the grafted cells. In addition, similar efficacy of fetal cardiomyocyte and skeletal myoblast transplantation in augmenting ventricular func-

tion has been demonstrated in the ischemic rat model.[35] These experiments show that myogenesis using fetal cardiomyocyte transplantation is possible and clinically relevant.

However, one limitation to the use of fetal cardiomyocytes is that lifelong immunosuppressive therapy is necessary to prevent rejection. Besides this, the regime and dose of immunosuppressive agents for cell transplantation is still unknown. This is reflected by a study investigating the natural history of transplanted fetal cardiomyocytes into the adult rat heart.[36] Despite the administration of cyclosporine after the procedure, lymphocytic infiltration persisted around the region of transplantation, and the newly formed cardiac tissue decreased in size secondary to rejection. In addition, there are still ethical questions concerning the use of human fetal tissue that need to be addressed. It is virtually certain that human fetal donor cardiomyocytes cannot be obtained in sufficient quantities for use in a clinical setting.

Embryonic stem cells

Embryonic stem cells (ESC) are continuously growing stem cell lines of embryonic origin. They are found in the inner cell mass of the human blastocyst, an early stage of the

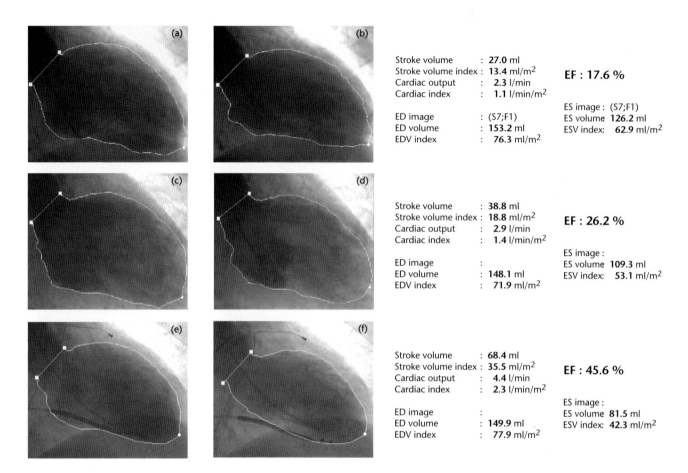

Stroke volume   : 27.0 ml
Stroke volume index : 13.4 ml/m^2 **EF : 17.6 %**
Cardiac output   : 2.3 l/min
Cardiac index   : 1.1 l/min/m^2

                                             ES image : (S7;F1)
ED image   : (S7;F1)   ES volume 126.2 ml
ED volume   : 153.2 ml   ESV index: 62.9 ml/m^2
EDV index   : 76.3 ml/m^2

Stroke volume   : 38.8 ml
Stroke volume index : 18.8 ml/m^2 **EF : 26.2 %**
Cardiac output   : 2.9 l/min
Cardiac index   : 1.4 l/min/m^2

                                             ES image :
ED image   :   ES volume 109.3 ml
ED volume   : 148.1 ml   ESV index: 53.1 ml/m^2
EDV index   : 71.9 ml/m^2

Stroke volume   : 68.4 ml
Stroke volume index : 35.5 ml/m^2 **EF : 45.6 %**
Cardiac output   : 4.4 l/min
Cardiac index   : 2.3 l/min/m^2

                                             ES image :
ED image   :   ES volume 81.5 ml
ED volume   : 149.9 ml   ESV index: 42.3 ml/m^2
EDV index   : 77.9 ml/m^2

Figure 23.4
Baseline left ventricular dimensions end diastolic (a) and end systolic (b) and quantitative measurements (ab). Changes in left ventricular dimensions and quantitative measurements at 3 (c,d,cd) and 6 months (e,f,ef) follow-up after autologous skeletal muscle cell transplantation. EDV, end diastolic volume; ESV, end systolic volume; EF, left ventricular ejection fraction.

developing embryo lasting from the fourth to the seventh day after fertilization. ESC extracted from the inner cell mass during the blastocyst stage, however, can be cultured in the laboratory, and under the right conditions will proliferate indefinitely. ESC growing in this undifferentiated state retain the potential to differentiate into cells of all three embryonic tissue layers.[37,38] ESC can be harvested from three sources: aborted fetuses (cadaveric stem cells), embryos left over from in vitro fertilization efforts (discarded embryos), and embryos created in the laboratory solely for the purpose of producing stem cells (research embryos). In recent years, there has been active discussion on the prospects of the medical application of ESC transplantation. Infinite opportunities have been predicted for human ESC as a source of 'spare parts' for the human body.

ESC transplantation for the treatment of a number of disorders that were previously incurable has been demonstrated. Since human fetal cardiomyocytes cannot be obtained in sufficient numbers for clinical purposes, the use of the human ESC line as a novel source of human cardiomyocytes may become an attractive option. In vitro differentiation of human ESC into cardiomyocytes has been demonstrated.[39] Successful selection of cardiomyocytes

from an ESC line and subsequent transplantation of the selected cardiomyocytes into mice has been reported.[40] More recently, intramyocardial injection of ESC into ischemic injured rat myocardium has been reported.[41] Compared with the control group injected with an equivalent volume of cell-free medium, cardiac function in ESC-implanted rats was significantly improved 6 weeks after cell transplantation. The characteristic phenotype of engrafted ESC was identified in implanted myocardium by strong positive staining of sarcomeric α-actin, cardiac α-myosin heavy chain, and troponin I. If ESC transplantation proves to be of therapeutic value in patients, the generation of cardiogenic human embryonic stem cell lines would preclude the requirement for either human fetal or xenotrophic tissue.

However, harvesting human ESC requires the destruction of an embryo – a potential human life. Opposition to the use of ESC comes mainly from those who believe human life begins at conception and that destroying an embryo at any stage of development is equal to infanticide. Protagonists of ESC research believe that while embryos certainly deserve respect, they are not yet fully human and that, furthermore, the profound therapeutic implications that may result from medical research justify their use. At present, European research programs do not and will not fund research on ESC that involves the creation of an embryo for research purposes only. In September 2001, the US government announced that they would permit Federal monies to be used for research on existing stem cell lines, but not to create new lines.

In addition, recipients of ESC must receive immunosuppressants because these cells are allogeneic. Transplanted ESC can potentially form teratomas if undifferentiated totipotent cells are still present. No experiments investigating the functional results after implantation of ESC-derived cardiomyocytes have yet been published. Thus, the transfer of ESC-derived cardiomyocytes is a relatively new technique with limited experience so far.

Bone marrow stromal cells

Bone marrow stromal cells have recently received much attention as an alternative cell type for transplantation. These are adult mesenchymal stem cells that show a high capacity for differentiation. Compared with totipotent ESC, there is a potentially lower inherent risk of tumor formation after transplantation. The cells can be obtained from patients themselves by simple bone marrow aspiration. With the use of autologous bone marrow stem cells, immunosuppression after transplantation becomes unnecessary. Studies suggest that bone marrow stromal cells have many characteristics of mesenchymal stem cells and possess greater functional plasticity than previously suspected.[42–44] Bone marrow stromal cells have been shown to have the potential of differentiating into cardiomyocytes in vitro,[45–47] and contract synchronously with native cardiomyocytes in a coculture system.[48] In the context of myocardial repair, it has been hypothesized that after transplantation, the myocardial microenvironment will supply the appropriate signals for cardiomyogenic differentiation of the transplanted bone marrow stem cells – a process known as milieu-dependent differentiation. The new cardiomyocytes thus achieve the purpose of replenishing the number of functioning cardiomyocytes.

Labeled bone marrow injection into normal myocardium of isogenic rats or mice has been shown to differentiate into cardiomycytes,[49,50] establishing proof of principle. In a preliminary but classic animal experiment, bone marrow stem cells from male mice were injected into the peri-infarction area of an ischemic female mouse model.[51,52] Nine days after the injection, newly formed myocardial tissue, comprising proliferating myocytes and neovascularization, was detected in the infarcted region, ameliorating the function of the infarcted heart. Cardiomyocyte-specific protein, connexin-43, and microscopic evidence of intercellular communication were detected at the injection sites. Similar results have recently been reported in a swine myocardial infarction model, which demonstrated success-

ful engraftment as well as attenuation of contractile dysfunction and pathological thinning of the left ventricle after injection of bone marrow stromal cells.[53] These preliminary in vivo findings demonstrated the capacity of adult bone marrow mesenchymal stem cells to integrate into host myocardium and regenerate into functional cardiomyocytes within the infarcted region. The exact in vivo signal or mechanism leading to cardiomyogenic differentiation, however, remains unknown.

The above strategy of bone marrow cell injection by surgical intervention was accompanied by high mortality in animal models. As a noninvasive alternative, researchers have attempted to maximize the number of circulating bone marrow stem cells by the administration of recombinant stem cell factor (SCF, steel factor) and granulocyte colony-stimulating factor (G-CSF) in an ischemic mouse model. This was associated with significant increase in the number of circulating stem cells and tissue regeneration, as well as improvement in hemodynamics and a reduction in mortality.[54] In a similar experiment presented at the 2002 Congress of the American Heart Association (AHA), while G-CSF was shown to improve myocardial function in a mouse infarction model, while granulocyte–macrophage colony-stimulating factor (GM-CSF) was found to have deleterious effects on myocardial function and to increase mortality.[55] This suggests that G-CSF and GM-CSF might have different effects on postinfarction heart failure.

Selective intracoronary transplantation of autologous bone marrow stem cells in patients with acute myocardial infarction in order to repair the infarcted myocardium has been reported.[56] This study involved 10 patients who received autologous bone marrow stem cells and coronary angioplasty in addition to standard therapy, and another 10 patients who received standard therapy alone. For the cell therapy group, stem cells were obtained by bone marrow aspiration around 1 week after infarction. After in vitro concentration, stem cells were injected into the infarct-related coronary artery, with concomitant angioplasty. After 3 months of follow-up, the infarct region was significantly decreased when compared with the standard therapy group. Imaging studies confirmed improvements in stroke volume index LV end-systolic volume, and contractility in the cell therapy group compared with the standard therapy group. Since percutaneous coronary intervention was also performed on these patients, it is unknown whether this hemodynamic effect was due to the cell transplantation, the coronary intervention, or simply the play of chance due to the small sample size.

Endothelial progenitor cells (EPCs)

Endothelial progenitor cells (EPCs) and hematopoietic stem cells (HSCs) share common cell surface antigens and thus are considered to be derived from a common precursor.[63] These cells play an important role in vasculogenesis by differentiating into vascular endothelial cells and blood cells, respectively. Several breakthrough experiments suggesting the potential role of transplanting EPCs to animals for the purpose of myocardial repair have been reported. This paradigm is now known as cell-mediated vascular regeneration. Instead of increasing the number of contracting muscle cells as demonstrated in skeletal myoblasts or fetal cardiomyocytes transplantation, EPC transplantation can potentially inhibit ventricular remodeling through improvement in myocardial blood flow. The TOP-CARE AMI[64] investigators have shown that injection of EPCs is safe and feasible and may attenuate the remodeling process in post-infarction patients (see below). EPCs can be identified in adult peripheral blood, bone marrow and human umbilical cord blood.

Peripheral blood. Experiments performed in various animal species have successfully isolated EPCs from peripheral blood.[65,66] Kalka and et al[66] successfully isolated, cultured and expanded adult human peripheral blood EPCs. The expanded cells were transplanted to the ischemic rat hind limb model for therapeutic neovascularization. Compared with controls, an improvement in neovascularization and a reduction in limb necrosis and auto-amputation were noted. Furthermore, ex vivo expanded human peripheral EPCs, when given intravenously, were associated with an improvement in left ventricular function.[67] Badorff et al recently reported that blood-derived human EPCs transdifferentiate into active cardiomyocytes when cultured with rat cardiomyocytes.[68] These studies demonstrated the feasibility of ex vivo culture and expansion of EPCs from peripheral blood and formed the basis for the early clinical trials of EPCs in therapeutic neovascularization.

Bone marrow. Since EPCs reside in the bone marrow, it is anticipated that bone marrow is a robust source of EPCs.[69] Direct intramyocardial injection of total bone marrow cells can enhance neovascularization.[70–73] After intravenous injection, Kocher et al[70] showed a six-fold reduction in myocyte apoptosis, a reduction in scar formation, and a significant restoration of cardiac function in an ischemic rat model. Compared with controls, there was a significant reduction in left ventricular dimensions and an improvement in systolic function. These studies suggest that adult bone marrow is a good source for isolating EPCs and that transplantation of EPCs can significantly augment postnatal neovascularization. The precise signal and homing mechanism of the EPCs require further elucidation. The advantage of using bone marrow derived or circulating EPCs is their autologous origin. However, the relatively low number of EPCs that can be obtained by this method may not be enough for therapeutic use. The clinical applications of either blood-derived or bone marrow-derived EPCs for myocardial angiogenesis has been demonstrated. The safety and efficacy of autologous implantation of bone marrow derived EPCs for thera-

peutic angiogenesis in patients with critical limb ischemia has been recently reported in a randomized clinical trial conducted in Japan.[79] However, the low numbers of identifiable EPCs in the bone marrow specimens used, curtailed the initial enthusiasm associated with this concept.

Umbilical cord blood. Human umbilical cord blood has been shown to contain a larger number of hematopoietic colony-forming cells.[80] Flow cytometric analysis revealed that cord blood contained a 10-fold excess of mononuclear cells (MNCs),[81] which are precursor of EPCs, compared to peripheral blood. Thus cord blood seems to be another rich source of EPCs. Moreover, isolation of EPCs from cord blood is less invasive than bone marrow aspiration. In fact, EPCs have been successfully isolated from human umbilical cord blood MNCs.[81] Kalka et al[82] reported that EPCs derived from human umbilical cord blood showed greater proliferative activity than EPCs derived from peripheral blood, suggesting that cord blood-derived EPCs may contribute more effectively to therapeutic vasculogenesis. Recently, Murohara et al[81,83] reported transplantation of human umbilical cord blood derived EPCs in a rat hind limb ischemic model. Serial laser Doppler blood flow analyses revealed significantly augmented blood flow in the EPC-transplanted group compared to the saline-treated control animals. However, as cryo-preserved cord blood derived EPCs are not generally available (although this may change in the future), cord blood derived EPCs transplantation is only allogeneic, thus subject to graft-versus host reactions and to rejection.

Controversies

Survival of transplanted cells in ischemic myocardium and improvements in contractility have been convincingly demonstrated in different animal models. In the short term, however, this new frontier contains many challenges, and several important questions remain to be answered before this novel strategy can be moved from bench to bedside.

1. What is the best cell type? Among the several cell types mentioned, skeletal myoblasts are the most extensively studied cells for myogenesis. On the other hand, the bone marrow stromal cell is another cell type that has shown promising results recently. Transdifferentiation of blood-derived endothelial progenitor cells into functionally active cardiomyocytes has also been demonstrated.[57]

2. There are different methods of cell delivery, and the best one is still unknown.

3. The optimal timing for the delivery of donor cells remains unknown. So far, there has been only one study investigating this issue. In a study using the cryo-injured adult rat heart model, embryonic rat cardiomyocytes were implanted at 0–8 weeks after creating the cryoinjury.[58] The success rate was highest (50%)

when donor cells were grafted 2 weeks post cryoinjury. It was postulated that the inflammation associated with myocardial damage during the acute phase limits efficiency during the initial period. This was supported by histological findings, which showed the presence of inflammatory cells up to 2 weeks after injury. On the other hand, established scar expansion also explains the suboptimal effect of delayed (>2 weeks) cell transplantation. However, humans with a different injury mechanism (atherosclerosis and/or thrombosis versus cryoinjury) may have a temporal inflammatory response different from that of the animal model. Therefore, the optimal time of cell delivery in patients remains to be determined.

4. Proof of concept in animal models is needed. Different methods of ischemic induction were used in animal models to simulate human myocardial ischemia. The most widely used methods were cryoinjury, coronary artery ligation, and embolization coils. The pathophysiological damage produced by these methods differs. Transmural scar produced by cryoinjury is more consistent in size, and myocardial dysfunction is less variable. On the other hand, coronary artery ligation produces a wide spectrum of necrosis, scar tissue, and ventricular dysfunction. The extent and homogeneity of the scar is dependent on the amount of collateral perfusion, which is variable.[31] In addition, little is known regarding the biological and physiological effects of the artificial ischemic induction in comparison with coronary ischemia secondary to atherosclerosis in patients.

5. Safety issues are always a major concern in novel technology. In each of two safety and feasibility studies on skeletal myoblast injection, one sudden death occurred within 8–9 days post procedure. These events were probably related to the occurrence of malignant arrhythmia. Whether these events are related to the cell transplantation procedure itself is difficult to determine, as these patients are high-risk and prone to malignant arrhythmia. Cardiomyocytes derived from ESC have also been shown to demonstrate electrophysiological features that facilitate arrhythmic potential,[59] suggesting the possibility of arrhythmia due to implanted cells. Therefore, stem cell engraftment in areas of injury is likely to promote any arrhythmic tendency. Furthermore, in vitro study of cultured skeletal myoblasts has shown a heterogeneicity in action potential under different conditions. This can potentially induce re-entry circuits and/or trigger activity, leading to arrhythmia.[59,60]

Conclusions

With the intrinsic limitations of cardiac transplantation, therapeutic myogenesis is definitely a potential novel treatment strategy for patients with heart failure. In principle, it aims to replenish the number of myocytes, and thus targets the pathophysiology of heart failure. Whether or not myogenesis will ever be successful in restoring the contractile function of the infarcted myocardium remains to be determined. Although preliminary, results of initial studies are promising. However, most of these early studies have been performed in small-animal models – some even without a control group. How far we can extrapolate these results to the clinical setting is still unknown. At present, the most intriguing issues are what is the best cell type and what is the best method of cell delivery. Apart from these, there are some other practical issues that need to be addressed (Table 23.5). Phase I clinical trials of cell transplantation for myocardial ischemia and myocardial scar repair in patients have suggested feasibility and safety from a procedural point of view. This sets the stage for more definitive experiments.

It will take a few years before we have a better idea from the results of randomized trials. In the future, perhaps the best outcome is the consignment to oblivion of organ transplantation with its waiting lists, together with the surgical risks and the side-effects of life-long immunosuppression. Future clinical trials are required to determine the best cell types and route and time of administration that provide effective and safe therapeutic myogenesis for patients with heart failure.

Recently, the traditional belief that adult myocardium is incapable of self-repair has been challenged. Mitotic figures have been detected within the myocytes of patients who died shortly after acute myocardial infarction.[61] In addition, there is evidence of cell migration from the recipient to the graft in patients who died of causes other than rejection.[62] These findings illustrate that regeneration exists in the adult human heart. At present, the clinical significance of this endogenous myogenesis process is very limited (with mitotic indices of 0.08% and 0.03% in zones adjacent to and distant from the infarct[61]), but should shown many promises once we have identified and expanded the source of these cells.

Table 23.5 Unresolved issues in cell transplantation for myocardial repair

- Best cell types
- Best delivery methods
- Immunogenicity
- Ethical considerations
- Number of cells required
- Efficacy
- Cell dissemination and associated side-effects
- Survival benefit versus symptomatic improvement
- Optimal timing of cell transplantation
- Arrhythmia

References

1. Rumyantsev PP (ed). Growth and Hyperplasia of Cardiac Muscle Cells. New York: Academic Press, 1991.

2. John R, Rajasinghe HA, Chen JM, et al. Long-term outcomes after cardiac transplantation: an experience based on different eras of immunosuppressive therapy. Ann Thorac Surg 2001;72:440–9.

3. Marelli D, Desrosiers C, el-Alfy M, et al. Cell transplantation for myocardial repair: an experimental approach. Cell Transplant 1992;1:383–90.

4. Soonpaa MH, Koh GY, Klug MG, et al. Formation of nascent intercalated disks between grafted fetal cardiomyocytes and host myocardium. Science 1994;264:98–101.

5. Ben-Haim SA, Osadchy D, Schuster I, et al. Nonfluoroscopic, in vivo navigation and mapping technology. Nat Med 1996; 2:1393–5.

6. Vale PR, Losordo DW, Tkebuchava T, et al. Catheter-based myocardial gene transfer utilizing nonfluoroscopic electro-mechanical left ventricular mapping. J Am Coll Cardiol 1999;34:246–54.

7. Kornowski R, Leon MB, Fuchs S, et al. Electromagnetic guidance for catheter-based transendocardial injection: a platform for intramyocardial angiogenesis therapy. J Am Coll Cardiol 2000;35:1031–9.

8. Gepsetin L, Hayam G, Ben-Haim SA. A novel method for nonfluoroscopic catheter based electroanatomical mapping of the heart. In vitro and in vivo accuracy results. Circulation 1997;95:1611–22.

9. Dib N, Diethrich EB, Campbell A, et al. Endoventricular trans-plantation of allogenic skeletal myoblasts in a porcine model of myocardial infarction. J Endovasc Ther 2002;9:313–19.

10. Campion DR. The muscle satellite cell: a review. Int Rev Cytol 1984;87:225–51.

11. Snow MH. An autoradiographic study of satellite cell differen-tiation into regenerating myotubes following transplantation of muscles in young rats. Cell Tissue Res 1978;186:535–40.

12. Leor J, Prentice H, Sartorelli V, et al. Gene transfer and cell transplant: an experimental approach to repair a 'broken heart'. Cardiovasc Res 1997;35:431–41.

13. Jennings RB, Reimer KA. Lethal myocardial ischemic injury. Am J Pathol 1981;102:241–55.

14. Murry CE, Wiseman RW, Schwartz SM, et al. Skeletal myoblast transplantation for repair of myocardial necrosis. J Clin Invest 1996;98:2512–23.

15. Chiu RC, Zibaitis A, Kao RL. Cellular cardiomyoplasty: myocardial regeneration with satellite cell implantation. Ann Thorac Surg 1995;60:12–18.

16. Robinson SW, Cho PW, Levitsky HI, et al. Arterial delivery of genetically labelled skeletal myoblasts to the murine heart: long-term survival and phenotypic modification of implanted myoblasts. Cell Transplant 1996;5:77–91.

17. Reinecke H, Murry CE. Transmural replacement of myocardium after skeletal myoblast grafting into the heart: too much of a good thing? Cardiovasc Pathol 2000; 9:377–44.

18. Scorsin M, Hagege A, Vilquin JT, et al. Comparison of the effects of fetal cardiomyocyte and skeletal myoblast trans-plantation on postinfarction left ventricular function. J Thorac Cardiovasc Surg 2000;119:1169–75.

19. Jain M, DerSimonian H, Brenner DA, et al. Cell therapy attenuates deleterious ventricular remodeling and improves cardiac performance after myocardial infarction. Circulation 2001;103:1920–7.

20. Taylor DA, Atkins BZ, Hungspreugs P, et al. Regenerating functional myocardium: improved performance after skeletal myoblast transplantation. Nat Med 1998;4:929–33.

21. Atkins BZ, Hueman TH, Meuchel JM, et al. Myogenic cell transplantation improves in vivo regional performance in infarcted rabbit myocardium. J Heart Lung Transplant 1999;18:1173–80.

22. Suzuki K, Murtuza B, Suzuki N, et al. Intracoronary infusion of skeletal myoblasts improves cardiac function in doxorubicin-induced heart failure. Circulation 2001;104(suppl I):213–17.

23. Ghostine S, Carrion C, Souza LC, et al. Long-term efficacy of myoblast transplantation on regional structure and function after myocardial infarction. Circulation 2002;106(12 Suppl I):I131–6.

24. Pouzet B, Vilquin JT, Hagege AA, et al. Factors affecting functional outcome after autologous skeletal myoblast transplantation. Ann Thorac Surg 2001;71:844–51.

25. Brogan WC 3rd, Hillis LD, Flores ED, et al. The natural history of isolated left ventricular diastolic dysfunction. Am J Med 1992;92:627–30.

26. Cohn JN, Johnson G. Heart failure with normal ejection frac-tion. The V-HeFT Study. Veterans Administration Cooperative Study Group. Circulation 1990;81(2 Suppl):III48–53.

27. Kessler KM. Heart failure with normal systolic function. Update of prevalence, differential diagnosis, prognosis, and therapy. Arch Intern Med 1988;148:2109–11.

28. Suzuki K, Murtuza B, Smolenski RT, et al. Cell transplantation for treatment of acute myocardial infarction using vascular endothelial growth factor-expressing skeletal myoblasts. Circulation 2001;104(Suppl I):207–12.

29. Etzion S, Barbash IM, Feinberg MS, et al. Cellular cardio-myoplasty of cardiac fibroblasts by adenoviral delivery of MyoD ex vivo: an unlimited source of cells for myocardial repair. Circulation 2002;106(12 Suppl I):I125–30.

30. Li RK, Mickle DA, Weisel RD, et al. In vivo survival and function of transplanted rat cardiomyocytes. Circ Res 1996;78:283–8.

31. Soonpaa MH, Koh GY, Klug MG, et al. Formation of nascent intercalated disks between grafted fetal cardiomyocytes and host myocardium. Science 1994;264:98–101.

32. Li RK, Jia ZQ, Weisel RD, et al. Cardiomyocyte transplantation improves heart function. Ann Thorac Surg 1996;62:654–60.

33. Watanabe E, Smith DM, Delcarpio JB, et al. Cardiomyocyte transplantation in a porcine myocardial infarction model. Cell Transplant 1998;7:239–46.

34. Koh GY, Soonpaa MH, Klug MG, et al. Stable fetal cardio-myocyte grafts in the hearts of dystrophic mice and dogs. J Clin Invest 1995;96:2034–42.

35. Scorsin M, Hagege A, Vilquin JT, et al. Comparison of the effects of fetal cardiomyocyte and skeletal myoblast trans-plantation on postinfarction left ventricular function. J Thorac Cardiovasc Surg 2000;119:1169–75.

36. Li RK, Mickle DA, Weisel RD, et al. Natural history of fetal rat cardiomyocytes transplanted into adult rat myocardial scar tissue. Circulation 1997;96(9 Suppl):II179–86.

37. Dinsmore J, Ratliff J, Deacon T, et al. Embryonic stem cells differentiated in vitro as a novel source of cells for trans-plantation. Cell Transplant 1996;5:131–43.

38. Maltsev VA, Wobus AM, Rohwedel J, et al. Cardiomyocytes differentiated in vitro from embryonic stem cells develop-

mentally express cardiac-specific genes and ionic currents. Circ Res 1994;75:233–44.

39. Kehat I, Kenyagin-Karsenti D, Snir M, et al. Human embryonic stem cells can differentiate into myocytes with structural and functional properties of cardiomyocytes. J Clin Invest 2001;108:407–14.

40. Klug MG, Soonpaa MH, Koh GY, et al. Genetically selected cardiomyocytes from differentiating embryonic stem cells form stable intracardiac grafts. J Clin Invest 1996;98:216–24.

41. Min JY, Yang Y, Converso KL, et al. Transplantation of embryonic stem cells improves cardiac function in postin-farcted rats. J Appl Physiol 2002;92:288–96.

42. Prockop DJ. Marrow stromal cells as stem cells for non-hematopoietic tissues. Science 1997;276:71–4.

43. Jackson KA, Majka SM, Wang H, et al. Regeneration of ischemic cardiac muscle and vascular endothelium by adult stem cells. J Clin Invest 2001;107:1395–402.

44. Goodell MA, Jackson KA, Majka SM, et al. Stem cell plasticity in muscle and bone marrow. Ann NY Acad Sci 2001;938:208–18.

45. Fukuda K. Development of regenerative cardiomyocytes from mesenchymal stem cells for cardiovascular tissue engineering. Artif Organs 2001;25:187–93.

46. Tomita S, Li RK, Weisel RD, et al. Autologous transplantation of bone marrow cells improves damaged heart function. Circulation 1999;100(19 Suppl II):II247–56.

47. Makino S, Fukuda K, Miyoshi S, et al. Cardiomyocytes can be generated from marrow stromal cells in vitro. J Clin Invest 1999;103:697–705.

48. Tomita S, Nakatani T, Fukuhara S, et al. Bone marrow stromal cells contract synchronously with cardiomyocytes in a co-culture system. Jpn J Cardiovasc Surg 2002;50:321–4.

49. Wang JS, Shum-Tim D, Galipeau J, et al. Marrow stromal cells for cellular cardiomyoplasty: feasibility and potential clinical advantages. J Thorac Cardiovasc Surg 2000;120:999–1006.

50. Toma C, Pittenger MF, Cahill KS, et al. Human mesenchymal stem cells differentiate to a cardiomyocyte phenotype in the adult murine heart. Circulation 2002;105:93–8.

51. Orlic D, Kajstura J, Chimenti S, et al. Bone marrow cells regenerate infarcted myocardium. Nature 2001;410:701–5.

52. Orlic D, Kajstura J, Chimenti S, et al. Transplanted adult bone marrow cells repair myocardial infarcts in mice. Ann NY Acad Sci 2001;938:221–9.

53. Shake JG, Gruber PJ, Baumgartner WA, et al. Mesenchymal stem cell implantation in a swine myocardial infarct model: engraftment and functional effects. Ann Thorac Surg 2002;73:1919–25.

54. Orlic D, Kajstura J, Chimenti S, et al. Mobilized bone marrow cells repair the infarcted heart, improving function and survival. Proc Natl Acad Sci USA 2001;98:10344–9.

55. Fujita J, Suzuki Y, Ando K, et al. G-CSF improves post-infarction heart failure by mobilizing bone marrow stem cells, but GM-CSF increases the mortality by deteriorating heart function in mice. Circulation 2002;106(Suppl II):II15 (abst).

56. Strauer BE, Brehm M, Zeus T, et al. Repair of infarcted myocardium by autologous intracoronary mononuclear bone marrow cell transplantation in humans. Circulation 2002;106:1913–18.

57. Badorff CM, Brandes RP, Popp R, et al. Transdifferentiation of blood-derived human adult endothelial progenitor cells into functionally active cardiomyocytes. Circulation 2002;106(Suppl II):II138 (abst).

58. Li RK, Mickle DA, Weisel RD, et al. Optimal time for cardio-myocyte transplantation to maximize myocardial function after left ventricular injury. Ann Thorac Surg 2001; 72:1957–63.

59. Zhang YM, Hartzell C, Narlow M, et al. Stem cell-derived cardiomyocytes demonstrate arrhythmic potential. Circulation 2002;106:1294–9.

60. Leobon B, Garcin I, Vilquin JT. Do engrafted skeletal skeletal myoblasts cntract in infarcted myocardium? Circulation 2002;106(Suppl II):II549 (abst).

61. Beltrami AP, Urbanek K, Kajstura J, et al. Evidence that human cardiac myocytes divides after myocardial infarction. N Engl J Med 2001;344:1750–7.

62. Quaini F, Urbanek K, Beltrami AP, et al. Chimerism of the transplanted heart. N Engl J Med 2002;346:5–15.

63. Weiss MJ, Orkin SH. In vitro differentiation of murine embryonic stem cells. New approaches to old problems. J Clin Invest 1996;97:591–5.

64. Assmus B, Schachinger V, Teupe C, et al. Transplantation of Progenitor Cells and Regeneration Enhancement in Acute Myocardial Infarction (TOPCARE-AMI). Circulation 2002; 106:3009–17.

65. Asahara T, Murohara T, Sullivan A, et al. Isolation of putative progenitor endothelial cells for angiogenesis. Science. 1997;275:964–7.

66. Kalka C, Masuda H, Takahashi T, et al. Transplantation of ex vivo expanded endothelial progenitor cells for therapeutic neovascularization. Proc Natl Acad Sci USA 2000; 97:3422–7.

67. Kawamoto A, Tkebuchava T, Yamaguchi J, et al. Intramyocardial transplantation of autologous endothelial progenitor cells for therapeutic neovascularization of myocardial ischemia. Circulation 2003;107:461–8.

67. Badorff C, Brandes RP, Popp R, et al. Transdifferentiation of blood-derived human adult endothelial progenitor cells into functionally active cardiomyocytes. Circulation 2003; 107:1024–32.

69. Takahashi T, Kalka C, Masuda H, et al. Ischemia- and cytokine-induced mobilization of bone marrow-derived endothelial progenitor cells for neovascularization. Nat Med 1999;5:434–8.

70. Kocher AA, Schuster MD, Szabolcs MJ, et al. Neovascularization of ischemic myocardium by human bone-marrow-derived angioblasts prevents cardiomyocyte apoptosis, reduces remodeling and improves cardiac function. Nat Med 2001;7:430–6.

71. Asahara T, Masuda H, Takahashi T, et al. Bone marrow origin of endothelial progenitor cells responsible for postnatal vas-culogenesis in physiological and pathological neovasculariza-tion. Circ Res 1999;85:221–8.

72. Tomita S, Li RK, Weisel RD, et al. Autologous transplantation of bone marrow cells improves damaged heart function. Circulation 1999;100:II247–56.

73. Kobayashi T, Hamano K, Li TS, et al. Enhancement of angio-genesis by the implantation of self bone marrow cells in a rat ischemic heart model. J Surg Res 2000;89:189–95.

74. Menasché P, Hagege AA, Vilquin JT, et al. Autologous skeletal myoblast transplantation for severe postinfarction left ven-tricular dysfunction. J Am Coll Cardiol 2003;41:1078–83.

75. Dib N, McCarthy P, Campbell A, et al. Two year follow-up of the safety and feasibility of autologous skeletal myoblast transplantation in patients with ischemic cardiomyopathy:

results from the United States Experience (abstract AHA 2003). Circulation 2003;108(Suppl II).

76. Herreros J, Prosper F, Perez A, et al. Autologous intramyocardial injection of cultured skeletal muscle-derived stem cells in patients with non-acute myocardial infarction. Eur Heart J 2003;24:2012–20.

77. Chachques JC, Cattadori B, Herreros J, et al. Treatment of heart failure with autologous skeletal myoblasts. Herz 2002;27:570–8.

78. Smits PC, Geuns R-J, Poldermans D, et al. Catheter-based intramyocardial injection of autologous skeletal myoblasts as a primary treatment of ischemic heart failure. J Am Coll Cardiol 2003;42:2063–9.

79. Tateishi-Yuyama E, Matsubara H, Murohara T, et al. Therapeutic angiogenesis for patients with limb ischaemia by autologous transplantation of bone-marrow cells: a pilot study and a randomised controlled trial. Lancet 2002; 360:427–35.

80. Nakahata T, Ogawa M. Hemopoietic colony-forming cells in umbilical cord blood with extensive capability to generate mono- and multipotential hemopoietic progenitors. J Clin Invest 1982;70:1324–8.

81. Murohara T, Ikeda H, Duan J, et al. Transplanted cord blood-derived endothelial precursor cells augment postnatal neovascularization. J Clin Invest 2000;105:1527–36.

82. Kalka C, Iwaguro H, Masuda H. Generation of differentiated endothelial cells from mononuclear cells of human umbilical cord blood. Circulation 1999;100(Suppl I):749.

83. Murohara T. Therapeutic vasculogenesis using human cord blood-derived endothelial progenitors. Trends Cardiovasc Med 2001;11:303–7.

24

Circulatory assist devices

Dominick J Angiolillo

Introduction

In the USA, more than 4000 patients are listed for heart transplantation; 30% of them will die before a suitable donor is found. Since the donor population is not expanding, there has been a need for the development and use of mechanical circulatory assist devices to prolong survival during the wait for definitive treatment. A large number of mechanical circulatory assist devices are available and can provide extended hemodynamic support for patients deteriorating acutely or chronically while waiting for a definitive treatment. In particular, implantable ventricular assist devices (VADs) have been shown to offer extended support, even for long periods of time, for patients hemodynamically deteriorating to a stage where it would be unlikely for them to survive until transplantation. In select individuals suffering from shock after acute myocardial infarction (MI) or myocarditis, insertion of mechanical support can allow recovery of the injured heart such that primary responsibility for hemodynamic support can ultimately once again be carried out by the heart: relieving pressure and stress-load burdens from the injured myocardium might be therapeutic in and of itself.

Many devices are available, with various ranges of circulatory support (Table 24.1). These range from the intraaortic balloon counterpulsation pump (IABP), univentricular and biventricular nonpulsatile and pulsatile devices, extracorporeal membrane oxygenation systems (ECMOs), and the total artificial heart.

Since a wide range of circulatory devices are available, an exhaustive description of all of them is impossible, for which we refer the reader to more specialized books. In this chapter, the circulatory assist devices that are commercially available for routine use are reviewed and more details are given on those most frequently used in clinical practice. First, the more widely used IABP is described and then VADs and future perspectives in this field are discussed.

Intraaortic balloon counterpulsation pump

The IABP is needed (1) to support hemodynamics in cardiogenic shock and (2) to relieve medically refractory

Table 24.1   Circulatory assist devices

- Intraaortic balloon counterpulsation (IABC)
- Extracorporeal membrane oxygenator (ECMO)
- Nonpulsatile extracorporeal centrifugal pumps
  - Biomedicus
  - Sarns/3M
- Nonpulsatile intracorporeal centrifugal pumps
  - Hemopump–Nimbus
  - De Bakey–NASA
- Extracorporeal pulsatile devices
  - Thoratec–Pierce/Donachy
  - Abiomed BVS 5000
- Intracorporeal pulsatile devices
  - Novacor
  - HeartMate
- Percutaneous transseptal ventricular assist
  - TandemHeart
- Total artificial heart
  - CardioWest
  - Penn State Pneumatic

ischemia in patients with severe coronary disease. Since multiple complications may occur in patients receiving circulatory assistance with this device, the duration of support with an IABP is short. Therefore, as for all circulatory assist devices, patient selection is of crucial importance and those patients who are selected to be treated require strict monitoring.

Indications

1. In patients with *cardiogenic shock*, the IABP may be considered as a bridge to revascularization. An IABP may provide temporary hemodynamic stabilization of patients with cardiogenic shock due to acute MI, allowing the physician to attempt revascularization in these patients. Early revascularization with percutaneous transluminal coronary angioplasty (PTCA) improves survival rates in cardiogenic shock caused by acute MI. In the GUSTO I (Global Utilization of Streptokinase and Tissue Plasminogen Activator for Occluded Coronary Arteries) trial, in which fibrinolytic regimens were compared for acute ST-elevation MI, PTCA was the only factor associated with a lower 30-day mortality rate in 2972 patients with cardiogenic shock.[1] Furthermore, early placement of an IABP in this cohort of patients was also associated with lower 30-day and 1-year mortality rates.[2] However, many hospitals do not have PTCA capabilities and it is known that in patients with cardiogenic shock, thrombolytic therapy alone is less successful than mechanical reperfusion. Therefore, the use of an IABP may be considered in patients with cardiogenic shock following acute MI treated with thrombolytic therapy to provide hemodynamic support and may be considered as a bridge to a tertiary center for revascularization.[3] While the use of an IABP followed by revascularization has a beneficial effect in this group of patients (acute MI and cardiogenic shock), an IABP alone (without revascularization) is associated with poor hospital survival rates (5–20%). Although the use of an IABP has shown to be beneficial in patients with acute MI and cardiogenic shock (when followed by revascularization), such beneficial effects remain uncertain in patients with acute MI but without cardiogenic shock treated with PTCA. In a randomized trial of 182 hemodynamically stable patients who underwent primary PTCA, the prophylactic use of an IABP for 2 days following the procedure reduced the incidence of recurrent ischemia and reocclusion of the infarct-related artery (IRA), but had no effect on survival or reinfarction.[4] In the PAMI II (Primary Angioplasty in Myocardial Infarction II) trial, 437 high-risk patients (age >70 years, multivessel coronary disease, reduced ejection fraction, vein graft disease, or persistent ventricular arrhythmias) treated with primary PTCA were randomized to 1–2 days of IABP or to no type of circulatory assistance, following the procedure.[5] Patients treated with an IABP had a slight reduction in recurrent ischemia but no reductions in mortality, reinfarction or reocclusion of the IRA. Therefore, this subset of patients with acute MI (hemodynamically stable) treated with PTCA are not likely to benefit from an IABP.

2. Patients with severe coronary disease having *refractory ischemia* or hemodynamic instability improve when an IABP is used prior to revascularization; therefore, in patients with medically refractory ischemia, IABP may be considered as a bridge to stabilize them before revascularization.[6]

3. There are no specific recommendations for using an IABP during *high-risk coronary interventions*. High-risk interventions include those with unprotected left main coronary disease, severe left ventricular (LV) dysfunction, target vessel supplying more than 40% of the myocardial territory, or severe congestive heart failure; these procedures have a two- to sixfold increase in periprocedural mortality.[7] The use of an IABP allows the operator a longer duration of ischemia during balloon inflation in these high-risk patients, postponing the development of hypotension and congestive heart failure. However, improved percutaneous revascularization techniques and adjunctive pharmacological treatments have reduced the need for prophylactic IABP placement in high-risk patients.[8,9]

4. Patients who develop *mechanical complications of acute MI*, such as ventricular septal defect and acute mitral regurgitation, frequently have hemodynamic deterioration progressing to cardiogenic shock. These patients may benefit from IABP placement prior to surgical repair.[10,11]

5. *Decompensated aortic stenosis* can be managed with temporary IABP support to reduce the transvalvular gradient and to improve stroke volume prior to aortic valve replacement. However, aortic insufficiency (see 'Contraindications' below) may be associated with aortic stenosis, and therefore monitoring of these patients to ensure that aortic insufficiency is not worsened by IABP is recommended.[12]

6. IABP support improves hemodynamics and facilitates *weaning from cardiopulmonary bypass*. In particular, patients with severe LV dysfunction or with prolonged runs on cardiopulmonary bypass can be difficult to wean from bypass after open heart surgery due to stunned myocardium resulting from prolonged cardioplegic arrest.[13]

7. Incessant ventricular tachycardia compromises LV filling, reduces stroke volume, and causes or worsens ischemia.[14] The use of an IABP improved hemodynamics, reduced ischemia, and controlled *refractory ventricular arrhythmias* in 86% of patients in a large case series.

8. High-risk patients (severe coronary artery disease, recent MI, or severe LV dysfunction) have a greater risk of cardiac complications when they undergo noncardiac surgery. Case reports have shown that prophylactic *IABP balloon support during and after noncardiac*

surgery hemodynamically stabilizes high-risk patients and improves postoperative outcome.[15]

9. An IABP improves cardiac output and lowers filling pressures in patients with end-stage cardiomyopathy and may be used as *bridge to cardiac transplantation*. However, the introduction into clinical practice of newly developed VADs, which may offer long-term support, has reduced IABP use in this subset of patients.[13]

Contraindications

IABP placement has a few contraindications.[16] Some of these are absolute – IABP placement may worsen patients' clinical status and therefore should be avoided. Others are relative, and IABP insertion should be carefully evaluated according to the necessity of circulatory support. Aortic dissection and abdominal/thoracic aneurysm are absolute contraindications; severe peripheral vascular disease and descending aortic and peripheral vascular grafts are relative contraindications.[17] During balloon inflation in diastole, blood is displaced in the proximal aorta and aortic insufficiency is worsened; however, there is no consensus as to the degree of aortic insufficiency at which use of an IABP is contraindicated, and therefore strict monitoring of patients with aortic insufficiency who absolutely require circulatory support with an IABP is strongly recommended for patients with severe coagulopathy or in whom anticoagulation is contraindicated for high bleeding risk, IABP use is discouraged and should be undertaken only for a short period of time. Patients with a contraindication to heparin (e.g. heparin-induced thrombocytopenia) can be anticoagulated with alternative agents such as low-molecular-weight heparins or hirudin.

Contraindications to IABP placement are summarized in Table 24.2.

Hemodynamics of IABP function

IABP hemodynamic effects are observed both in systole, when the balloon is deflated and afterload is decreased, and in diastole, when the balloon is inflated and diastolic pressure is increased (Figure 24.1).

As *systole* begins, the intraaortic balloon deflates rapidly, creating a negative pressure in the aorta; this causes a reduction in afterload (due to a reduction in aortic end-diastolic pressure) and therefore improves cardiac output (approximately 20% increase) and decreases mean pulmonary capillary wedge pressure (approximately 20% reduction). The overall hemodynamic benefit of IABP is a reduction in LV wall stress and myocardial oxygen consumption deriving from decreased filling pressures and decreased afterload, which in turn improves stroke volume and cardiac output.

In *diastole*, the intraaortic balloon inflates; this displaces blood to the proximal aorta, augmenting aortic diastolic pressure and therefore coronary perfusion. Augmentation of coronary perfusion is more pronounced when systemic hypertension is present. IABP support generally determines an increase in peak coronary flow velocity, as observed in Doppler flow studies; however, no improvement in coronary flow is observed distal to severe coronary stenosis. Collateral coronary flow does not even increase with IABP support. Therefore, in patients with severe coronary stenosis, IABP relieves ischemia through reduction of LV wall stress and of myocardial consumption of oxygen rather than through increasing coronary perfusion.

The optimal function of an IABP depends on correct balloon pump triggering and timing. Balloon pump inflation can be triggered by a surface ECG, the arterial pressure waveform, a paced rhythm, or an internal asynchronous mode. The surface ECG is preferably used to trigger IABP inflation. IABP inflation is delayed after the R wave, to begin at the time in the cardiac cycle when the aortic valve closes (the dicrotic notch). If the IABP fails to trigger properly from the surface ECG, the lead being evaluated should be changed, surface electrode placement checked, or ECG gain increased on the console monitor. For patients with poor surface ECG tracings, the balloon can be triggered from the arterial pressure waveform. Pacing spikes should be used to trigger the balloon in patients who are 100% paced. When patients are in cardiac arrest or when the other triggering mechanisms are not working correctly, an internal asynchronous mode can be used.

Ideal balloon pump timing takes place when the balloon inflates on the downslope of the systolic pressure waveform before the dicrotic notch and deflates prior to the onset of the next systolic pressure waveform (Figure 24.1). Timing can be adjusted manually or automatically by internal algorithms in the IABP console. Early inflation of the IABP (prior to aortic valve closure) causes premature closure of the aortic valve, with an increase in afterload, LV wall stress, and myocardial oxygen consumption; stroke volume and cardiac output are decreased. Late inflation of the IABP (well after the dicrotic notch) reduces diastolic pressure augmentation and leads to suboptimal coronary perfusion. Early deflation of the IABP (before isovolumetric LV contraction) results in suboptimal diastolic augmentation, coronary perfusion, and

Table 24.2	Contraindications to IABP placement

- Aortic dissection
- Abdominal or thoracic aneurysm
- Moderate to severe aortic insufficiency
- Severe peripheral vascular disease
- Descending aortic and peripheral vascular grafts
- Coagulopathy or contraindication to heparin

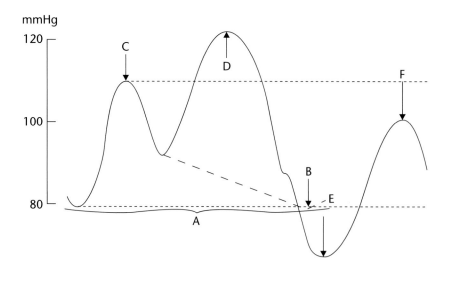

Figure 24.1
Correct timing of balloon function occurs when the balloon inflates on the downslope of the systolic pressure waveform and deflates before the onset of the next systolic waveform. The IABP inflation in diastole increases diastolic pressure to improve coronary artery perfusion and to increase mean arterial pressure. Additionally, aortic end-diastolic pressure is reduced when the balloon deflates in end-diastole to lower afterload and myocardial oxygen demand. 'A' represents one complete cardiac cycle, 'B' unassisted aortic end-diastolic pressure, 'C' unassisted systolic pressure, 'D' diastolic augmentation, 'E' assisted aortic end-diastolic pressure, and 'F' reduced systolic pressure. (Courtesy of Datascope Corp.)

afterload reduction, and thus increased myocardial oxygen demand. Late deflation of the IABP (after the onset of systole) leads to impaired LV emptying, increased afterload and preload, increased myocardial oxygen consumption, and reduced stroke volume. During tachyarrhythmias, adequate balloon pump function is difficult to achieve. With heart rates above 150 beats/min, there is insufficient time for the helium gas to move in and out of the balloon with each inflation. Adjusting balloon inflation to 1 : 2 can improve IABP function during tachyarrhythmias.

IABP insertion and removal techniques

Proximal and distal pulses are assessed in both legs, with the leg with the strongest pulses being chosen for access. This leg should be adequately prepared for sheath insertion (shaved and prepped with antiseptic solution). Following infiltration with a local anesthetic, the femoral artery is accessed using an 18-gauge introducer needle, and a 0.030 inch × 145 cm J-tipped guidewire is advanced through the needle to the aortic arch under fluoroscopy. The sheaths sizes are between 9 French (Fr) and 11 Fr and are 6–11 inches long; the balloon catheter is 0.5 Fr smaller than the sheath, ranging between 8.5 Fr and 10.5 Fr. A 10 Fr sheath and a 9.5 Fr balloon are most commonly used. Three common balloon sizes are available and are chosen according to the patient's height: 50 cm³ for patients over 6 ft (1.83 m), 40 cm³ for patients between 5 ft 4 in and 6 ft (1.63 m and 1.83 m), and 34 cm³ for patients under 5 ft 4 in (1.63 m). The balloon length and diameter increase with each larger size. The 40 cm³ balloon is the most commonly used. The prewrapped balloon is inserted

over the guidewire and is advanced until the proximal tip is positioned 1 cm below the left subclavian artery and 2 m below the carina. Afterwards, the guidewire is removed and the distal tip of the balloon should be visualized to ensure that it is out of the sheath. Although fluoroscopic guidance is recommended for IABP insertion, in some cases fluoroscopy is not available or the hemodynamic status of the patient requires immediate circulatory assistance without lost of time to reach fluoroscopy machinery. In these cases, the distance from the angle of Louis to the umbilicus and then to the common femoral artery insertion site is measured to determine the approximate distance the balloon must be advanced. An IABP may also be inserted surgically by directly exposing the common femoral artery or by suturing a 6–12 mm prosthetic graft end-to-side to the femoral artery to provide a conduit for the catheter. Surgical insertion of an IABP reduces the risk of limb ischemia but also requires surgical arterial repair; this type of approach may cause a loss of time, and generally the percutaneous approach is preferred.

Following insertion, the helium gas line of the balloon catheter is connected to the IABP console and the central lumen of the catheter is attached to an arterial pressure monitor device on the console. Balloon autoinflation is initiated from the console, the arterial line attached to the central lumen of the catheter is flushed, and the initial IABP inflation is at 1 : 2 per cardiac cycle while the timing is adjusted. Balloon inflation should be observed under fluoroscopy (Figure 24.2) to ensure that the balloon is completely out of the sheath and fully inflating. The sheath and balloon catheter should then be sutured in place and inflation changed to 1 : 1.

A chest X-ray should be taken immediately after IABP insertion to verify the catheter position (even if insertion was performed under fluoroscopic guidance) and repeated daily to ensure that the catheter position is ade-

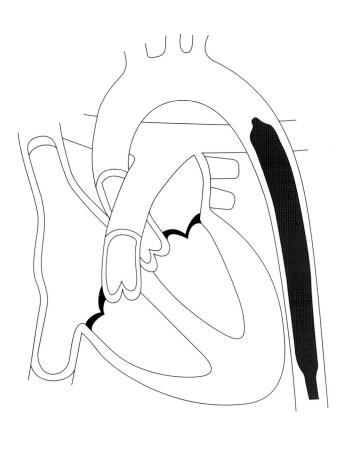

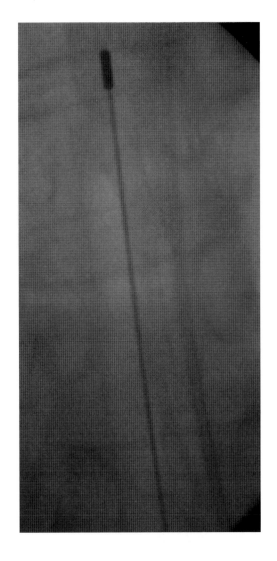

(a)

Figure 24.2
(a) Diagram and fluoroscopic image of inflated balloon: during diastole, the balloon inflates, with augmentation of diastolic pressure and increased coronary perfusion.

Figure 24.2 continued on next page

quately maintained. Daily hemoglobin, red blood cell, and platelet counts are recommended to detect hemolysis and thrombocytopenia. Infusion of intravenous heparin must be initiated immediately after IABP placement to maintain an activated partial thromboplastin time (aPTT) between 50 and 70 s.

Following IABP placement, the patient should be kept supine in bed and peripheral pulses and signs of limb ischemia periodically assessed. The accessed leg should be secured to prevent inadvertent patient movement. Blood samples should not be drawn from the central lumen of the IABP, because the risk of clotting the lumen is increased, and air or small thrombi can be injected through the small lumen during flushing of the tubing after blood withdrawal. Prophylactic antibiotic treatment is not recommended.

IABP support is usually short, since multiple complications may develop with prolonged circulatory assistance using this device. When IABP removal is planned, the usual practice is to change the IABP inflation rate to 1 : 2 for a few hours and then to 1 : 3. Monitoring the patient's hemodynamics is mandatory during weaning from an IABP. Afterwards, the timing and rate of reduction of balloon inflation depend on the hemodynamic status of the patient, LV function, and the duration of support. If weaning is hemodynamically tolerated, the balloon can then be removed. Drugs may be used during weaning to simulate hemodynamic effects of the IABP (e.g. dobutamine or milrinone to maintain cardiac output and stroke volume; sodium nitroprusside to replace the afterload reduction). Before beginning balloon catheter removal, the balloon is

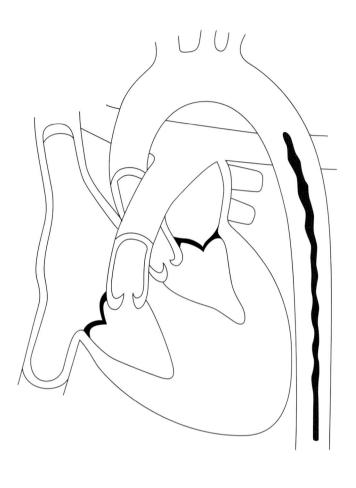

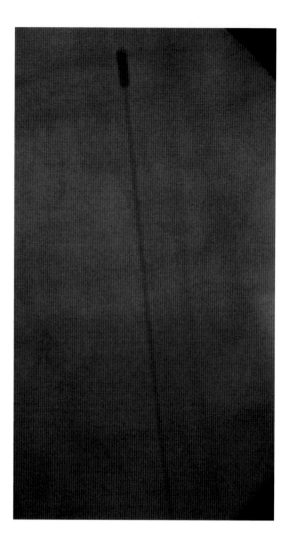

(b)

Figure 24.2 (Continued)
(b) Diagram and fluoroscopic image of deflated balloon: at the onset of systole, the balloon deflates, with decreased afterload, myocardial wall stress, cardiac work, and oxygen demand, and increased cardiac work.

changed to standby and the gas drive line disconnected; the balloon catheter is then pulled back until resistance is met, indicating that the catheter is in the sheath. Then the sheath and balloon catheter are removed together as a unit. Intravenous heparin should be discontinued for at least 4 hours prior to balloon catheter removal and the activated coagulation time (ACT) should be below 150 s. When the balloon catheter is placed percutaneously, it is removed manually, while surgically placed balloon catheters require surgical arterial repair. During manual pressure, to obtain hemostasis, and afterwards, following compressive dressing of the access site, the distal pulses of the leg and signs of limb ischemia should be periodically assessed. Strict bed rest is recommended for at least 12 hours following IABP withdrawal.

Complications

Vascular complications are the most frequent type with the use of an IABP.[18,19] These complications vary from 5% to 20% and include limb ischemia, hematoma at the access site, bleeding at the access site, and rarely pseudo-aneurysms. Female sex, peripheral vascular disease, diabetes, smoking habitus, and catheter size are independent risk factors associated with ischemic vascular complications from IABP use. In those cases in which ischemia develops, the balloon catheter and sheath should be removed and hemostasis obtained at the access site. If limb ischemia persists, vascular surgical consultation is required; surgical interventions for ischemic complications include thrombectomy, bypass grafts, and, rarely, amputations. Bleeding at the access site is usually controlled by manual pressure at the site, while hematomas and pseudoaneurysms may require surgical repair; in many of these complications, transfusion of blood products may be required. Other rare vascular complications include acute renal failure, mesenteric ischemia, and paraplegia caused by plaque embolization to or thrombosis of the renal, mesenteric, or spinal arteries. Extremely rare are dissections and perforations of the aorta, which usually occur during balloon catheter insertion.

Balloon rupture is another possible, although rare ($\leq 4\%$), complication, which should be taken into consideration when blood is detected in the gas drive line lumen or when balloon augmentation is interrupted.[20] Balloon damage and subsequent balloon leaks may be caused by rupture of the balloon surface against calcified plaques in the aorta during inflation. Incorrect selection of balloon size according to patient height has also been associated with a greater risk of balloon damage. Balloon leaks may lead to helium gas embolism. A damaged balloon may also allow blood to leak into the balloon, with clot formation within the balloon; this prevents adequate deflation and subsequent balloon entrapment. *Balloon entrapment* should be considered when resistance is encountered during balloon removal, and forceful removal should be avoided because of the high risk of causing serious vascular damage. In these cases, fluoroscopy should be carried out to assess the position of the balloon catheter and surgical extraction should be considered.

The shear forces of the balloon catheter may cause *hemolytic anemia* and *mild thrombocytopenia*.[21] Platelet and red blood cell counts are recommended daily. Severe thrombocytopenia (<50 000) is unlikely to be caused by the IABP, and therefore another cause should be sought.

Infectious complications are rare, and include infection at the access site, catheter infections, and bacteremia.[22]

Ventricular assist devices

VADs provide substantial advantages for extended support of patients awaiting cardiac transplantation. Although some devices remain extracorporeal, the intracorporeal pulsatile devices, such as the Novacor and HeartMate devices, allow patients to ambulate and enter cardiac rehabilitation programs. Potential recipients for a VAD must generally meet criteria for heart transplantation. These candidates usually have a cardiac index below 2 l/min/m^2, systolic blood pressure below 90 mmHg, pulmonary capillary wedge pressure above 15 mmHg, atrial pressures above 20 mmHg, systemic vascular resistance above 2100 dyn•s/cm^2, and oliguria with urine output below 20 ml/h despite aggressive medical therapy. Contraindications to VAD placement include any disease that precludes heart transplantation, including active malignant disease, infections, peripheral vascular disease, hepatic dysfunction, and chronic renal failure.[23]

The nonpulsatile intracorporeal centrifugal pumps are indicated for short-term use (several days) and are similar to an IABP, except that they completely unload the LV work rather than simply augmenting it. Inserted through the femoral artery, the system is based on a catheter that crosses the aortic valve into the LV. The catheter contains a flow pump that provides an output of 3.5–5.7 l/min. The system requires anticoagulation with heparin and has allowed a 38% survival rate at 30 days. The disadvantages of the system are the need for bed rest because of the femoral artery approach, prolonged supervision, and lack of right ventricular support, and it cannot be used in patients with aortic valve diseas.[24,25] The most common complications are hemolysis and ventricular arrhythmia caused by the catheter position.

Extracorporeal centrifugal pumps are commonly used for circulatory support in patients with postcardiotomy cardiogenic shock (inability to function without the cardiopulmonary bypass pump) and cardiogenic shock following MI, and provide biventricular support.[26,27] These devices are efficient, relatively simple, and reasonably inexpensive, but are feasible only for short-term support (several days). These pumps require venous and arterial cannulation, and the flow is a continuous nonpulsatile flow. Lines are typically left between an unclosed sternum, with only skin closure. Patients require systemic anticoagulation. The main complications with these devices are bleeding, consumptive coagulopathy, thromboembolism, renal dysfunction, systemic interstitial edema (due to mechanical difficulty with this preload-dependent device), and infections. Patients are restricted to prolonged supervision in an intensive care unit and are bedridden. Survival rates for the Biomedicus BioPump and the Sarns/3M devices are up to 40% and 50%, respectively, at 30 days. Survival is best if the systems are used for less than a week. These centrifugal devices may be used with an extracorporeal membrane oxygenation (ECMO) system. Current ECMO systems have a centrifugal pump to drive blood from the patient to a membrane for carbon dioxide and oxygen exchange similar to that provided by cardiopulmonary bypass systems in open heart surgery. The insertion is extrathoracic, however, with arterial and venous cannulation typically at the femoral vessels. These devices are particularly useful when respiratory failure accompanies circulatory collapse. They require systemic anticoagulation and may cause substantial trauma to blood components.[28]

Indications for use of external pulsatile (pneumatic drive) pumps are the same as for external centrifugal devices. These may provide left, right, or biventricular support. External pulsatile pumps have the advantage over centrifugal systems that subcostal lines allow sternal closure and there is a lower rate of thromboembolism,

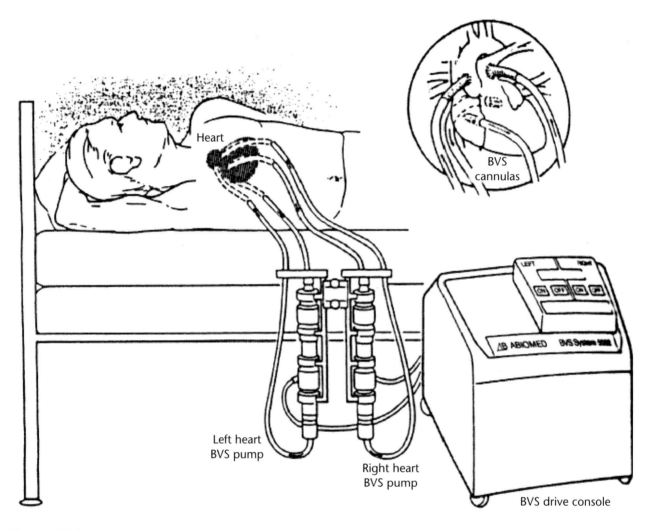

Heart

BVS
cannulas

Left heart
BVS pump

Right heart
BVS pump

BVS drive console

Figure 24.3
Diagram of the Abiomed BVS 5000 device for biventricular support. (Adapted from Topol EJ. Comprehensive
Cardiovascular Medicine. Philadelphia: Lipincott-Raven, 1998 with permission from Lippincott Williams & Wilkins.)

although systemic anticoagulation is still required. This type of device is not used in small patients (body surface area <1.3 m²), for whom an external centrifugal device is usually preferred. The lower interstitial edema with these devices is thought to be related to the pulsatile manner of the blood flow. The Abiomed BVS 5000 device (Figure 24.3) has been most successful when used for an average of 3.5 days; it can generate a stroke volume of 80 ml and a cardiac output of 5.5 l/min. Filling is determined by the venous return pressure, with gravity draining a cannula placed in the right or left atrium; outflow cannulas are inserted into the main pulmonary artery or aorta.[29] The Thoratec device (Figure 24.4) has been used for up to 75 days as a bridge to transplantation, and can generate stroke volumes of 65 ml and a cardiac output of 7.0 l/min.[30] Cardiovascular circuit cannulation is generally via the appropriate atria or ventricles, with outflow cannulas inserted into the pulmonary artery or aorta, depending on the ventricle being bypassed and supported.

If attempted removal of these VADs fails, causing irreversible ventricular dysfunction, longer-term management of the patients is required. Long-term management options include changing to a long-term VAD or cardiac transplantation. There is no implantable VAD without extracorporeal components. Important ideal parameters for long-term VAD use are effective pressure and flow support, small device size, potential for removal if the ventricle recovers, complete implantability, an efficient power source, absence of percutaneous connections, high reliability, long device lifetime, low risk of infection and thromboembolism, minimal blood component trauma, and lack of immunogenicity. The two implantable long-term VADs are the HeartMate and Novacor devices.[31,32] The HeartMate device (Figure 24.5) has an implanted pump that is pneumatically driven and electrically powered; it generates stroke volumes of 85 ml and a cardiac output of 11 l/min. The interior surfaces of the HeartMate are designed to allow pseudointimal layering, which reduces

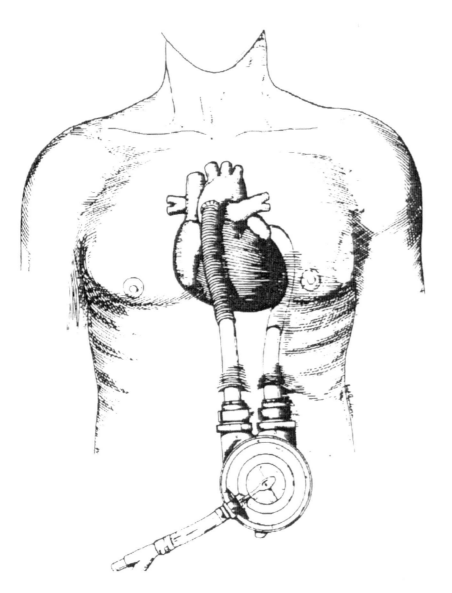

Figure 24.4
Diagram of the Thoratec ventricular assist device. (Adapted from Topol EJ. Comprehensive Cardiovascular Medicine. Philadelphia: Lipincott-Raven, 1998 with permission from Lippincott Williams & Wilkins.)

the risk of thromboembolism. In theory, no anticoagulation is required, but patients usually receive antiplatelet treatment. The Novacor device (Figure 24.6) has an electromagnetic converter and the blood pump is inserted. The device is synchronized to pump systole at the end of native systole; it has a maximum stroke volume of 70 ml and flows up to 10 l/min. Patients with the Novacor device do require systemic anticoagulation. Recently, the Jarvik 2000 Heart, an electrically powered, axial flow LV assist device, has been shown to provide safe circulatory assistance for heart transplant candidates.[33]

The surgical approaches differ between short- and long-term devices. Both connect the device outflow tract to the aorta. The device inflow of the short-term devices is connected to the left atrial appendage or to the right superior pulmonary vein. This keeps the myocardium intact for removal. Long-term devices receive inflow from the ventricular apex and require additional incisions in the abdomen for pumps and drive lines. Decisions to provide

right ventricular (RV) support (usually needed in 20% of patients) are based on hemodynamics following LV support. Since the short-term device operation is less complicated and can better tolerate further cardiopulmonary bypass time, there is a lower threshold to place biventricular systems to ensure early hemodynamic stability. Implantation of long-term RV support devices has a higher morbidity rate due to longer bypass times for placement and to the greater complexity of the procedure. Inotropic agents, volume infusions, and vasodilatators are used to optimize pulmonary pressures and LV flows, with right heart hemodynamic values as a guide.[23] When flows remain below 2 l/min/m^2, a RV support device should be placed, with the inflow from the right atrium and the outflow to the pulmonary artery.[34] Once a device is placed, transesophageal echocardiography is recommended to assess ventricular function and chamber pressures and volumes.[35] All patients should continue aggressive heart failure medical treatment with the goal of removal of the

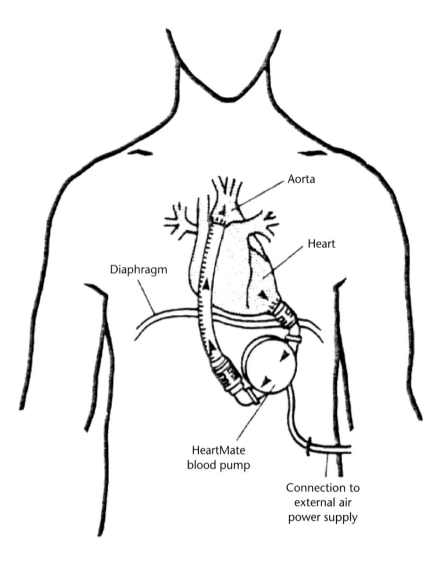

Aorta

Heart

Diaphragm

HeartMate
blood pump

Connection to
external air
power supply

Figure 24.5
Diagram of the HeartMate ventricular
assist device. (Adapted from Topol EJ.
Comprehensive Cardiovascular
Medicine. Philadelphia: Lipincott-
Raven, 1998 with permission from
Lippincott Williams & Wilkins.)

device if ventricular function returns. In particular, patients with RV support require aggressive diuretic treatment. Antibiotic prophylaxis should be administered to prevent infection.[36]

On the basis of promising results from research on left atrial to femoral artery bypass systems[37] and inherent limitations of other circulatory assist devices, a percutaneous transseptal LV assist system (TandemHeart) has recently been proposed. This is a simple, relatively inexpensive system, allowing long-term LV support, which consists of an innovative small external centrifugal pump with a specially designed transseptal inflow cannula and an outflow conduit for percutaneous femoral artery placement (Figure 24.7). It functions as a hydrodynamic bearing, with its moving surfaces suspended in saline lubricant; it is not thrombogenic and does not cause significant hemolysis. It is able to provide a cardiac output augmentation of 2.5–3.5 l/min. The TandemHeart device is believed to have several advantages over an IABP, including increased LV unloading, decreased myocardial oxygen consumption,

and enhanced coronary perfusion. It also has advantages over standard VADs: placement is simple and rapid (within 30 minutes), placement can be performed in a catheterization laboratory, eliminating the two operations required for VAD insertion and removal, it may be placed in critically ill patients, and there is a lower risk of thromboembolic events and other complications related to VAD use (mediastinitis, peritonitis, and diaphragmatic herniation). This device, however, is not applicable to patients with right heart failure in whom RV support is required and in patients with severe aortic insufficiency.

Total artificial heart insertion has lagged far behind the development of VADs. Theoretically, a total artificial heart system is necessary for patients who require both right and left ventricular support. Hemodynamic, thromboembolic, and hemostatic difficulties represent the substantial problems for successful total artificial heart development. The CardioWest and PennState are the two pneumatically driven artificial hearts currently approved by the US Food

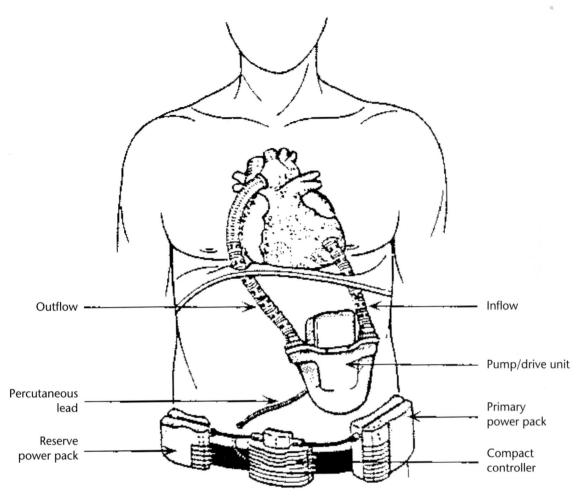

Figure 24.6
Diagram of the Novacor ventricular assist device. (Adapted from Topol EJ. Comprehensive Cardiovascular Medicine. Philadelphia: Lipincott-Raven, 1998 with permission from Lippincott Williams & Wilkins.)

and Drug Administration. The advantages of these systems are not only that they may provide biventricular support, but also that they may be placed in an orthotopic position, which obviates the need to use the abdominal cavity as a device repository.[38,39]

Conclusions

A broad spectrum of potential therapeutic strategies are available nowadays for treatment of acute heart failure. A pharmacological approach, using inotropic drugs and vasodilatators, alone or in combination, represents the initial treatment option in patients with hemodynamic compromise. Hemodynamic monitoring and overall clinical assessment of these patients is required so that med-

ical therapy can be appropriately tailored. In those patients who continue to exhibit clinical deterioration and hemodynamic compromise despite maximal pharmacological support, mechanical circulatory assistance should be considered. A broad spectrum of short- and long-term circulatory assist devices are available and can provide support in patients who are not responsive to medical treatment. This allows a more thorough diagnostic evaluation until further therapeutic options are explored. Tremendous technological progress has been made in this field in the past few years, and in the future smaller and more reliable devices with fewer complications are expected to be available. Regarding these technological advances, optimized patient selection, an individualized diagnostic and therapeutic approach, and strict clinical assessment remain the cornerstones of treatment of heart failure.

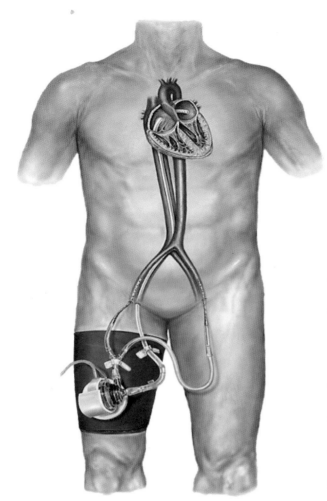

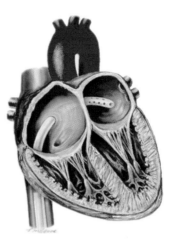

- Generate continuous flow

- Removes oxygenated blood from LA via transseptal cannula placed in the femoral vein

- Returns blood via femoral artery

- Reduces LAP and PCWP

- Reduces myocardial oxygen demand

- Increases MAP, CO

Figure 24.7
Diagram of the TandemHeart percutaneous transseptal left ventricular assist device. (Courtesy of CardiacAssist.)

References

1. Holmes DR Jr, Bates ER, Kleiman NS, et al. Contemporary reperfusion therapy for cardiogenic shock: the GUSTO-I trial experience. J Am Coll Cardiol 1995;26:688–674.

2. Anderson RD, Ohman EM, Holmes DR Jr, et al. Use of intraaortic balloon counterpulsation in patients presenting with cardiogenic shock: observations from the GUSTO-I study. J Am Coll Cardiol 1997;30:708–715.

3. Kovack PJ, Rasak MA, Bates ER, et al. Thrombolysis plus aortic counterpulsation: improved survival in patients who present to community hopitals with cardiogenic shock. J Am Coll Cardiol 1997;29:1454–1458.

4. Ohman EM, George BS, White CJ, et al. Use of aortic counterpulsation to improve sustained coronary artery patency during acute myocardial infarction: results of a randomized trial. Circulation 1994;90:792–799.

5. Stone GW, Marsalese D, Brodie BR, et al. A prospective, randomized evaluation of prophylactic intraaortic balloon counterpulsation in high-risk patients with acute myocardial infarction treated with primary angioplasty. J Am Coll Cardiol 1997;29:1459–1467.

6. Kantrowitz A, Cardona RR, Freed PS. Percutaneous intraaortic balloon counterpulsation. Crit Care Clin 1992; 8:819–837.

7. Aguirre FV, Kern MJ, Bach R, et al. Intraaortic balloon pump support during high-risk coronary angioplasty. Cardiology 1994;84:175–186.

8. van't Hof AW, Liem AL, de Boer MJ, et al. A randomized comparison of intra-aortic balloon pumping after primary coronary angioplasty in high risk patients with acute myocardial infarction. Eur Heart J. 1999;20:659–65.

9. Schreiber TL, Kodali UR, O'Neill WW, et al. Comparison of acute results of prophylactic intraaortic balloon pumping with cardiopulmonary support for percutaneous transluminal coronary angioplasty (PCTA). Cathet Cardiovasc Diagn. 1998;45:115–9.

10. Di Summa M, Actis Dato GM, Centofanti P, et al. Ventricular septal rupture after a myocardial infarction: clinical features and long term survival. J Cardiovasc Surg (Torino). 1997; 38:589–93.

11. Chen Q, Darlymple-Hay MJ, Alexiou C, et al. Mitral valve surgery for acute papillary muscle rupture following myocardial infarction. J Heart Valve Dis. 2002;11:27–31.

12. Bolooki H, Williams W, Thurer RJ, et al. Clinical and hemo-dynamic criteria for use of the intra-aortic balloon pump in patients requiring cardiac surgery. J Thorac Cardiovasc Surg. 1976;72:756–68.

13. Sezai Y. Mechanical cardiac assistance. Ann Thorac Cardiovasc Surg. 1998;4:178–87.

14. Hayakawa H, Katoh T, Nejima J, et al. Ventricular tachy-cardia associated with acute myocardial infarction–features, therapeutic effect and prognosis. Jpn Circ J 1985; 49(3):362–9

15. Christenson JT, Simonet F, Badel P, et al. Evaluation of preoperative intra-aortic balloon pump support in high risk coronary patients. Eur J Cardiothorac Surg. 1997; 11(6):1097–103.

16. Kern MJ. Intraaortic balloon counterpulsation. Coronary artery disease 1991;2:649–660.

17. Colyer WR Jr, Moore JA, Burket MW, et al. Intraaortic balloon pump insertion after percutaneous revascularization in patients with severe peripheral vascular disease. Cathet Cardiovasc Diagn. 1997;42:1–6.

18. Meharwal ZS, Trehan N. Vascular complications of intra-aortic balloon insertion in patients undergoing coronary reavscularization: analysis of 911 cases. Eur J Cardiothorac Surg. 2002;21:741–7.

19. Meco M, Gramegna G, Yassini A, et al. Mortality and morbidity from intra-aortic balloon pumps. Risk analysis. J Cardiovasc Surg (Torino). 2002;43:17–23.

20. Kumbasar SD, Semiz E, Sancaktar O, et al. Mechanical complications of intra-aortic balloon counterpulsation. Int J Cardiol. 1999;70:69–73.

21. Walls JT, Boley TM, Curtis JJ, et al. Heparin induced thrombocytopenia in patients undergoing intra-aortic balloon pumping after open heart surgery. ASAIO J 1992; 38:M574–6.

22. Bur A, Bayegan K, Holzer M, et al. Intra-aortic balloon coun-terpulsation in the emergency department: a 7-year review and analysis of predictors of survival. Resuscitation. 2002; 53:259–64.

23. Stevenson LW, Kormos RL. Mechanical cardiac support 2000: Current applications and future trial design. J Am Coll Cardiol 2001;37:340–370.

24. Mooney MR, Mooney JF, Van Tassel RA, et al. The Nimbus Hemopump: a new left ventricular assist device that combines myocardial protection with circulatory support. J Invasive Cardiol 1990;2:169–73.

25. DeBakey ME. A miniature implantable axial flow ventricular assist device. Ann Thorac Surg 1999;68:637–40.

26. Noon GP, Lafuente JA, Irwin S. Acute and temporary ventricular support with BioMedicus centrifugal pump. Ann Thorac Surg. 1999;68:650–4.

27. Curtis JJ, Walls JT, Schmaltz R, et al. Experience with the Sarns centrifugal pump in postcardiotomy ventricular fail-ure. J Thorac Cardiovasc Surg. 1992;104:554–60.

28. Bowen FW, Carboni AF, O'Hara ML, et al. Application of "double bridge mechanical" resuscitation for profound cardiogenic shock leading to cardiac transplantation. Ann Thorac Surg 2001;72:86–90.

29. Wassenberg PA. The Abiomed BVS 5000 biventricular sup-port system. Perfusion. 2000;15:369–71.

30. Farrar DJ, Hill JD. Univentricular and biventricular Thoratec VAD support as a bridge to transplantation. Ann Thorac Surg. 1993;55:276–82.

31. Hsu RB, Chu SH, Chien CY, et al. HeartMate left ventricu-lar assist device for long-term circulatory support. J Formos Med Assoc. 2000;99:336–40.

32. Loisance DY, Jansen PG, Wheeldon DR, et al. Long-term mechanical circulatory support with the wearable Novacor left ventricular assist system. Eur J Cardiothorac Surg. 2000; 18:220–4.

33. Frazier OH, Myers TJ, Gregoric ID, et al. Initial clinical experience with the Jarvik 2000 implantable axial-flow left ventricular assist system. Circulation 2002;105:2855–60.

34. Higgins RS, Elefteriades JA. Right ventricular assist devices and the surgical treatment of right ventricular failure. Cardiol Clin. 1992;10:185–92.

35. Davila-Roman VG, Barzilai B. Transesophageal Echo-cardiographic Evaluation of Patients Receiving Mechanical Assistance from Ventricular Assist Devices. Echocardiography 1997;14:505–512.

36. Grossi P, Dalla Gasperina D, Pagani F, et al. Infectious com-plications in patients with the Novacor left ventricular assist system. Transplant Proc. 2001;33:1969–71.

37. Laschinger JC, Cunningham JN Jr, Catinella FP, et al. 'Pulsatile' left atrial-femoral artery bypass. A new method of preventing extension of myocardial infarction. Arch Surg. 1983;118:965–9.

38. Pavie A, Leger P, Regan M, et al. Clinical experience with a total artificial heart as a bridge for transplantation: the pitie experience. J Card Surg 1995;10:552–8.

39. Hoenicke EM, Strange RG Jr, Weiss WJ, et al. Modifications in surgical implantation of the Penn State electric total artificial heart. Ann Thorac Surg 2001;71(3 Suppl):S150–5.

25

Groin closure devices

Manel Sabaté

Introduction

The percutaneous treatment of coronary artery disease has constantly expanded during the last two decades. Vascular access for percutaneous coronary interventions is usually obtained through the common or superficial femoral artery, employing introducer sheaths of various sizes in order to enable the positioning of different types of catheters in the coronary tree. Interventional procedures may require the use of larger sheaths than pure diagnostic procedures. Furthermore, the use of heparin and new antithrombotic agents (especially glycoprotein IIb/IIIa antagonists) during percutaneous transluminal coronary angioplasty (PTCA) makes the achievement of immediate hemostasis at the arterial puncture site challenging. Some other clinical situations, such as hypertension, aortic insufficiency, intraaortic balloon pumping, and new circulatory assist devices that require the use of large sheaths, need adequate hemostasis at the arterial puncture site. For these patients, manual or mechanical compression was until recently the only way to control bleeding, by allowing clot formation at the arterial access site. The duration of manual compression as well as the time of immobilization were in general proportional to the size of the introducer sheath and the level of anticoagulation. Manual compression techniques are in general effective with the small sheath sizes used in diagnostic procedures. However, with the employment of larger sheath sizes, prolonged surveillance time and bed rest has to be maintained.

The introduction of closure devices is aimed at increasing both patient comfort through enabling early ambulation after interventional procedures and patient safety through the reduction of puncture-related complications,

especially the development of false aneurysms and large hematomas. Additionally, reduction of patient immobilization time after the procedure may lead to a reduction of the hospitalization period and in some cases may even remove the need for hospitalization.

Closure devices can be subdivided into mechanical closure devices (suture-based closure devices, collagen-based sealing devices, and gelatin-based devices) and drug-based closure devices (Polyprolate™ and procoagulant). The aims of this chapter are to describe the procedural steps of device insertion and to review data from the literature about the safety and efficacy of those that are available in the market.

Suture-based mechanical closure devices

Among the suture-based closure devices, the Perclose system and the Suture device are currently available. The Perclose system (Figure 25.1) was first on the market. The first generation of the Perclose device comprised the Techstar and Prostar XL, which have been replaced by the Closer percutaneous vascular suture (PVS) device.

The Closer PVS device

This device was developed to deliver one or two sutures at the arterial puncture site. It presents a 'sheath-like' profile in which a sheath houses a suture loop and the

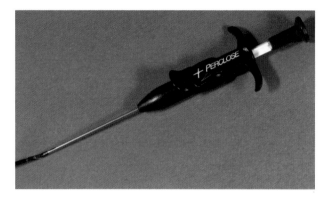

Figure 25.1
The Perclose system.

needles are positioned above the sheath in the device handle and are actuated by a plunger (Figure 25.2). A knot-tying device, the Clincher, is provided with the Closer to create a reliable and consistent sliding surgical knot.

Device insertion procedure

(Figure 25.2a–d)

1. Insert the device into the artery without subcutaneous track dissection. A pulsatile back bleed from the marker lumen indicates that the foot of the device is intraluminal (Figure 25.2a).
2. Continue to advance the device until a continuous drop of blood is evident from the marker lumen. Position the device at a 45° angle. Then deploy the foot by pulling the lever back on the top of the handle (Figure 25.2b).
3. Gently pull the device back to position the foot against the arterial wall. If correct positioning of the foot has been achieved, blood marking will cease. If marking does not stop, gently adjust the angle of the device to stop blood marking.
4. While maintaining device position, deploy the needles by pushing on the plunger of the handle (Figure 25.2b).
5. Remove the plunger of the handle with the two needles and the attached suture until the suture is pulled out (Figure 25.2c).

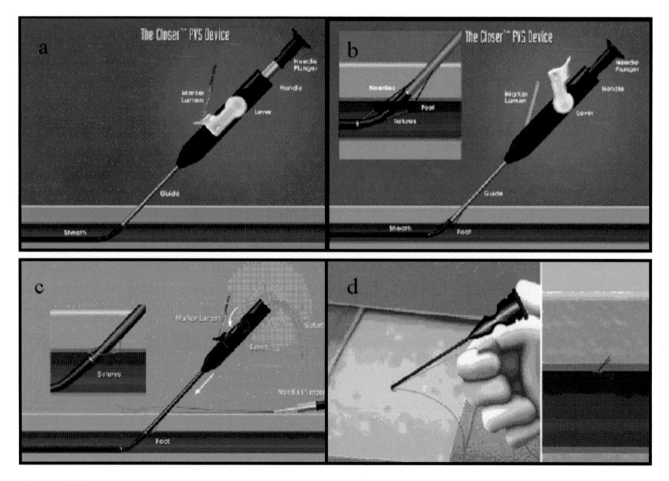

Figure 25.2
The Closer PVS device and procedural steps (a–d). See text for details.

6. Cut the suture from the needles.
7. Remove the device until the guidewire port exits the skin line. Grab the suture adjacent to the sheath and pull the suture ends through the distal end of the barrel.
8. Tie a sliding surgical knot manually or use the clincher knot tying device.
9. Once the device has been withdrawn from the puncture site, deliver the knot while pulling gently on the suture rail. Do not tighten the suture around the sheath (Figure 25.2d).
10. Once the knot is advanced to the arterial surface, use the knot pusher to complete advancement (Figure 25.2d).
11. After placing the suture in the knot pusher, tension the suture limb with the fingers of one hand while applying forward pressure to the proximal end of the knot pusher with the thumb of the same hand (Figure 25.2d).
12. To reduce resistance to knot advancement, hold the suture as vertical as possible while keeping the knot pusher coaxial to the suture. It is important to pull all of the slack out of the suture as the knot is advanced to avoid an 'air knot'. Complete hemostasis of the access site is achieved when the knot is fully advanced to the arterial surface and the tissue is in complete apposition. If hemostasis is not complete, gently advance the knot with the knot pusher with the one-handed technique while gently applying constant tension to the suture. Hold this position for 20–30 s or until hemostasis is obtained. Do not apply excessive pressure to the knot pusher or suture.
13. Once hemostasis has been achieved, trim the suture below the skin (Figure 25.2d).

Postprocedure patient management

After successful hemostasis has been achieved, an appropriate sterile pressure dressing is applied to the puncture site. Patients can be permitted to sit in their bed immediately after suture and to get up 2–4 hours after suture when no or minimal subcutaneous oozing is present. The type of catheterization procedure solely dictates the patient's recovery. The femoral access site and pulses should be monitored regularly before hospital discharge for bleeding or any other vascular complication.

Any suspected bleeding complication or incomplete hemostasis can be treated with adjunctive compression and/or prolonged application of a pressure bandage. All of these patients are to be immediately evaluated with color-coded Doppler ultrasound.

Sutura SuperStitch closer device

(Figure 25.3)

This is a recently designed suture-based closure device, developed to deliver one suture at the arterial puncture

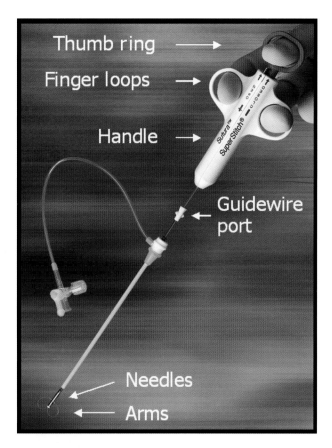

Figure 25.3
The Sutura SuperStitch closer device.

site. Operation is through the procedural sheath, eliminating arteriotomy dilatation. This device consists of a handle, a flexible nylon shaft of 'true' 6 French (Fr) and 8 Fr intrasheath design and profile, a proprietary dual-fulcrum suturing mechanism, an integral tip design, and a polypropylene monofilament suture (Figure 25.4). The insertion procedure consists of five steps (Figure 25.5): (I) insert and arm; (II) position; (III) suture; (IV) disarm; (V) withdraw and tie. Postprocedure patient management is similar to that of other suture-based closure devices.

Collagen-based mechanical closure devices

Collagen-based closure devices are bioresorbable devices that are used to seal the puncture site after arterial catheterization, thus establishing rapid hemostasis. Device application is possible through the introducer sheath without the need to extend and prepare the cutaneous access. Among this category of devices, the Angio-Seal vascular closure device and the VasoSeal system are currently available.

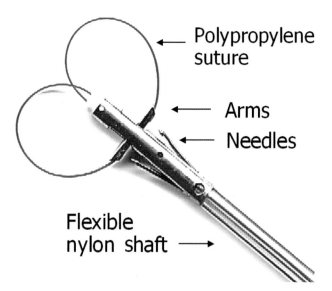

Figure 25.4
Tip of the Sutura SuperStitch closer device with the dual-fulcrum suturing mechanism and the polypropylene monofilament suture.

The Angio-Seal vascular closure device

This system consists of the Angio-Seal device itself, an insertion sheath, an arteriotomy locator (a modified dilator), and a guidewire (Figure 25.6). This device is available in 6 Fr as well as 8 Fr. The Angio-Seal device is composed of an absorbable collagen sponge and a specially designed absorbable polymer anchor that are connected by an absorbable self-tightening suture (STS) (Figure 25.7). The device seals and sandwiches the arteriotomy between its two primary members: the anchor and the collagen sponge. Hemostasis is achieved primarily by the mechanical means of the anchor–arteriotomy–collagen sandwich, which is supplemented by the coagulation-inducing properties of the collagen. The device is contained in a delivery system that stores and then delivers the absorbable components to the arterial puncture. All components are absorbed by the body in 60–90 days. Thus, repuncture at the same location as a previous Angio-Seal device is not recommended for 90 days.

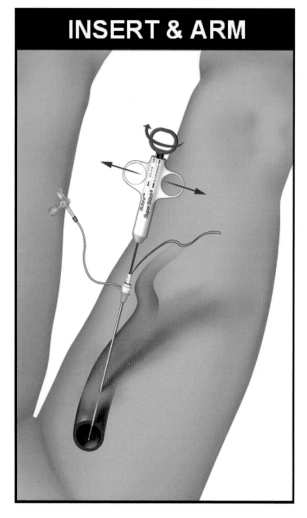

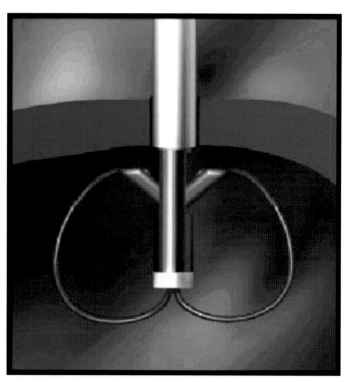

Figure 25.5
Insertion procedure of the Sutura SuperStitch closer device: insertion and arming (step I); positioning (step II); suturing (steps IIIa and IIIb); disarming (step IV); withdrawal and tying (step V).

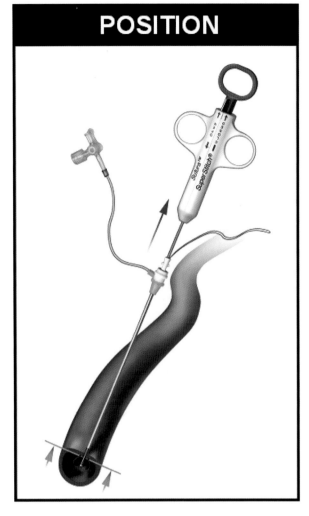

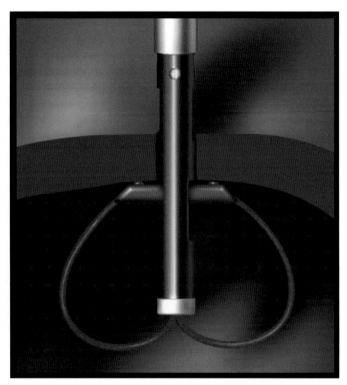

Figure 25.5 (Continued)

Device insertion procedure

The Angio-Seal procedure is composed of three stages: (A) locating the artery; (B) setting the anchor; (C) sealing the puncture.

Step I: locating the artery (Figure 25.8A)

1. Insert the arteriotomy locator into the Angio-Seal insertion sheath.
2. Insert the Angio-Seal guidewire into the procedure sheath that is currently in the patient and remove that sheath, leaving the guidewire in place to maintain vascular access.
3. Thread the Angio-Seal arteriotomy locator/insertion sheath assembly over the guidewire and insert the assembly into the puncture tract. As the tip of the insertion sheath enters the artery, blood will begin to flow from the drip hole in the locator.
4. Slowly withdraw the arteriotomy locator/insertion sheath assembly until blood slows or stops flowing from the drip hole. This indicates that the tip of the Angio-Seal insertion sheath just exited the artery.

5. From this point, advance the arteriotomy locator/insertion sheath assembly 1–2 cm into the artery using the letters of the word 'ANGIO-SEAL' on the insertion sheath as a guide (the letters are spaced 1 cm apart). Blood flow will resume from the drip hole.
6. Holding the insertion sheath steady, remove the arteriotomy locator and guidewire from the insertion sheath by flexing the arteriotomy locator at the sheath hub.

Step II: setting the anchor (Figure 25.8B)

1. Carefully grasp the Angio-Seal device at the bypass tube. Cradle the Angio-Seal carrier tube in the palm of the hand and, with the reference indicator facing up, slowly insert the bypass tube and carrier tube into the insertion sheath hemostatic valve.
2. Confirm that the reference indicator on the insertion sheath is facing up. This should align with the reference indicator on the device cap. The sheath cap and the device sleeve will snap together when properly fitted.
3. With one hand, continue to hold the insertion sheath cap steady while, with the other hand, grasping the device cap and slowly and carefully pulling back.

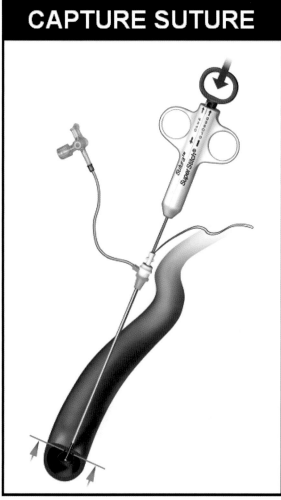

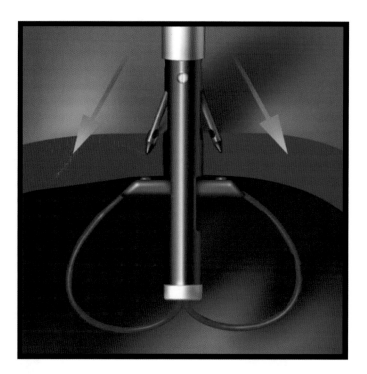

a

Figure 25.5 (Continued)

Continue pulling on the device cap until resistance from the anchor catching on the distal tip of the insertion sheath is felt.

4. After the anchor position is confirmed by proper alignment of the device cap within the colored band, while maintaining a grip on the insertion sheath, pull the device cap into the full rear locked position. The device sleeve color band should now be completely visible.

Step III: sealing the puncture (Figure 25.8C)

1. Once the previous steps have been performed correctly, slowly and carefully withdraw the device/sheath assembly along the angle of the puncture tract to position the anchor against the vessel wall.

2. When the insertion sheath clears the skin, a tamper tube will appear. At this stage, grip the tamper tube and gently advance the collagen while maintaining tension on the suture.

3. Continue to withdraw the insertion sheath and device until the clear stop on the suture appears. Continue to pull until the entire suture has been deployed (approximately 4.5 cm beyond the clear stop). The suture will then lock within the device cap where it is attached.

4. Maintain tension on the suture. Advance the collagen again with the tamper tube until resistance is felt and the black compaction marker is revealed.

5. Cut the suture below the clear stop. Remove the tamper tube using a slight twirling upward motion.

6. Gently pull up on the suture and cut it below skin level and below the black compaction marker.

Postprocedure patient management

Clean the puncture site with an antiseptic solution and apply a sterile dressing to the puncture site so that it can be easily observed during recovery. No pressure dressing is needed if the Angio-Seal has been properly inserted.

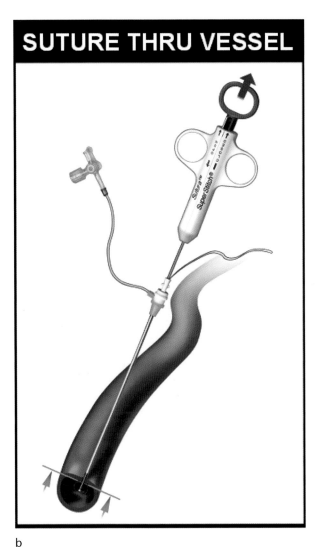

SUTURE THRU VESSEL

b

Figure 25.5 (Continued)

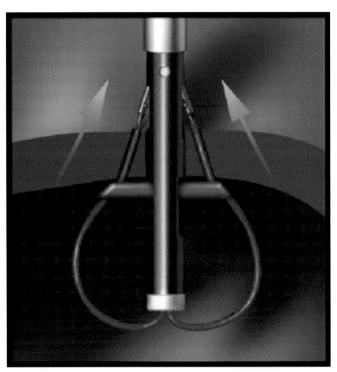

✓ **Step III(b)**

The VasoSeal system (Figure 25.9)

The VasoSeal system is a collagen-based sealing device, which is available in only one size, independently of the size of the introducer sheath employed. In contrast to the Angio-Seal system, it does not require an intravascular anchor and uses a bovine collagen plug for the sealing of the access site. The VasoSeal device consists of a localizer system, a J-segment, a dilator, the VasoSeal sheath, and a collagen syringe. After introduction of the localizer system into the sheath via a guidewire, the introducer sheath is removed completely while maintaining manual compression on the artery. The system is positioned so that the green marker becomes visible at the skin surface. The J-segment is then released and the localizer system withdrawn until a gentle resistance is felt. Now a dilator is applied over the localizer system and introduced into the access site until the white marker becomes visible. Finally the VasoSeal introducer sheath is introduced over the localizer system until the blue marker becomes visible. Before application of the collagen, the J-segment as well as the dilator are removed. Depending on the thickness of the subcutaneous tissue, one or two collagen applications are necessary. Postprocedure management is similar to that for other collagen-based closure devices.

Other mechanical closure devices

New devices based on the same technique but using different platforms are under investigation. Among them, gelatin sponge (QuickSeal) as an arterial closure device may be available in the market in the future.

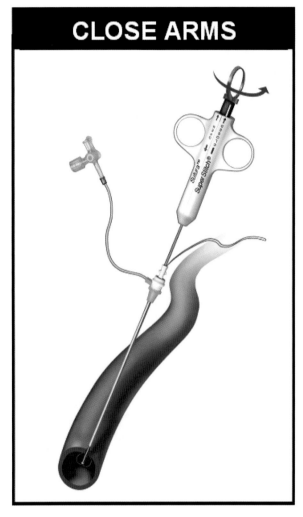

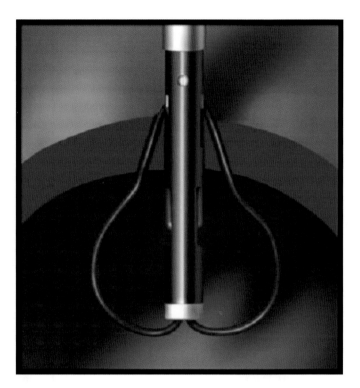

Figure 25.5 (Continued)

Drug-based closure devices

This type of system uses a drug to enhance clot formation at the puncture site. The drug is actively or passively released by means of a dedicated device.

The DUETT system (Figure 25.10)

The DUETT system can be used as a sealing device following percutaneous procedures with sheath sizes from 5 to 9 Fr and an overall length not exceeding 15 cm. This system uses a dual approach – balloon catheter and procoagulant – and is designed to rapidly seal the femoral artery puncture site, thus reducing time to hemostasis and ambulation. The DUETT sealing device works with the body's natural blood clotting process to accelerate hemostasis at the femoral artery puncture site. The system is contraindicated in patients with known sensitivity to bovine-derived materials.

Furthermore, the system should not be used in patients with suspected arterial puncture distal to the common femoral artery bifurcation, clinically severe peripheral vascular disease, or a common femoral artery estimated to be less than 6 mm in diameter. Employment of the system in these cases may lead to inadvertent intravascular delivery of the procoagulant, which typically leads to acute onset of severely diminished or absent peripheral pulses in the limb treated with the DUETT. If this is suspected, then appropriate diagnostic and therapeutic procedures for thrombus dissolution/removal need to be performed immediately.

The DUETT system should also not be used if posterior arterial wall puncture is suspected, as this may lead to incomplete sealing and bleeding complications.

The DUETT device description and procedure

The system consists of a balloon catheter device and a procoagulant. The balloon catheter is used to seal the

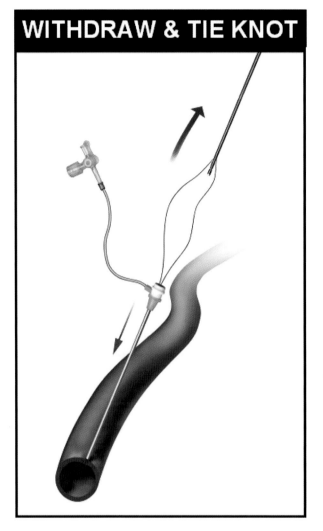

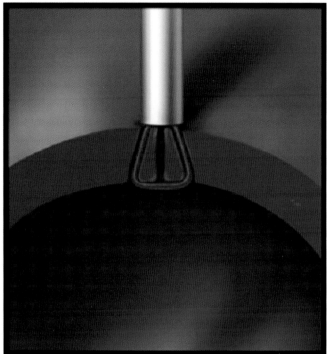

Figure 25.5 (Continued)

puncture site intraluminally to prevent the coagulant from being administered within the vessel. The actual sealing process is achieved by administering the procoagulant via the side port of the sheath to the outer surface of the vessel and the subcutaneous tract of the puncture site. When the procoagulant comes into contact with blood in the tissue tract, it accelerates the blood clotting process. The procoagulant is a flowable mixture of thrombin, collagen, and diluent.

1. The procoagulant is prepared by mixing the fluids carefully.
2. The balloon catheter is introduced into the vessel via the sheath, which is already in place.
3. The balloon is then inflated with saline solution and withdrawn until resistance is felt. At this point, the balloon should be in contact with the intravascular end of the sheath. Then, both sheath and balloon catheter are pulled back until further resistance indicates that the balloon has reached the inner wall of the arterial puncture site.

4. At this point, the draw at the balloon catheter has to be maintained throughout the entire process of procoagulant application. The sheath is withdrawn for 1–2 mm and, through aspiration via the side port, it is checked whether the tip of the sheath is still intraluminal. If it is in the appropriate position, the procoagulant can be applied gently via the side port while pulling out the sheath step by step.
5. After complete application of the procoagulant, the artery is totally compressed proximally of the puncture site, the balloon is deflated, and both system and sheath are removed completely.

Postprocedure patient management

Total compression has to be maintained for 1–2 minutes in order to allow clot formation and achievement of hemostasis at the puncture site. A pressure bandage is applied

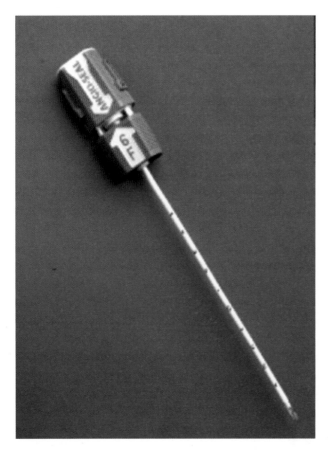

Figure 25.6
The Angio-Seal device.

for 2–6 hours, depending on the level of anticoagulation and sheath size used.

Clo-Sur P.A.D. device (Figure 25.11)

The Scion Clo-Sur P.A.D. (pressure applied dressing) device, is a soft, nonwoven hydrophilic wound dressing. The Clo-Sur P.A.D. is packed in a foil pouch and sterilized by electron-beam radiation. This device consists of the hydrophilic naturally occurring biopolymer Polyprolate™ acetate. This linear biopolymer is cationic (positively charged) in its dry state. It is the chain of positive charges that endows Polyprolate™ with its blood coagulant properties. Cationic Polyprolate™ forms a coagulum with heparinized blood, defibrinated blood, and washed red blood cells. Since there was no clot formation with serum albumin or serum globulin, it was concluded that Polyprolate™ was reacting with the cellular elements of blood and the usual clotting factors were not involved. The hemostatic property or coagulum formation of Polyprolate™ in blood is believed to involve Polyprolate™-mediated agglutination of red blood cells: the cell surface membranes carry negatively charged sialic acid residues, which react with the positively charged Polyprolate.

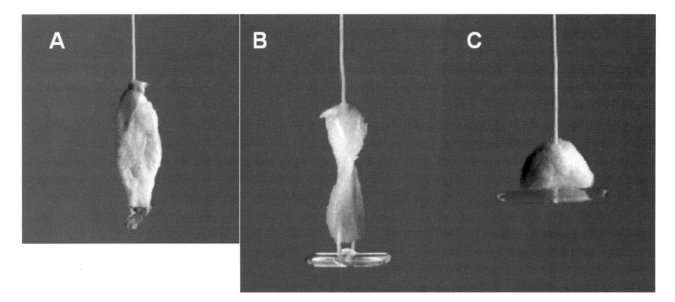

Figure 25.7
The three components of the Angio-Seal device: the absorbable collagen sponge and the absorbable polymer anchor, connected by an absorbable self-tightening suture (STS).

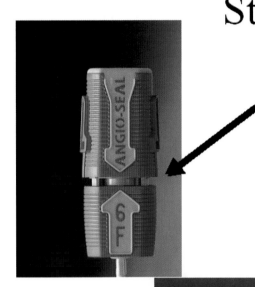

Step I : Insert the device completely into the sheath hub. An audible click indicates that the sleeves have locked into the sheath hub.

This confirms that the anchor has exited the sheath.

a

Figure 25.8
The Angio-Seal device insertion procedure (see text for details).

The Clo-Sur P.A.D. procedure

(Figure 25.11)

1. Hold pressure proximal to the puncture site.
2. Place Clo-Sur P.A.D. over the puncture site and remove the catheter.
3. After removing the catheter, release the proximal pressure.
4. Apply continuous pressure on the Clo-Sur P.A.D. until hemostasis is achieved.
5. Apply a dressing over the Clo-Sur P.A.D. and remove after 24 hours.

Discussion

Conventional treatment of the femoral access site after cardiac catheterization is associated with prolonged immo-bilization and considerable discomfort to the patient.[1] Percutaneous closure devices allow immediate sheath removal, even under a high level of anticoagulation. This may increase patient comfort after percutaneous intervention and may also reduce the length of hospital stay, thereby reducing costs.[2] Complication rates of 0.3–1.8% have been reported after diagnostic catheterization using small-bore arterial sheaths[3,4] and up to 15% after complex coronary interventional procedures under aggressive anticoagulation and large-bore femoral sheaths.[5,6]

Suture-mediated closure devices

Safety and efficacy of suture-mediated closure devices have been analyzed in large registries and several

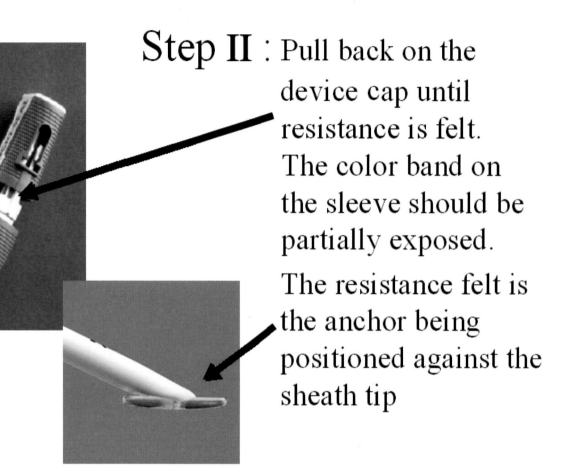

Step II : Pull back on the device cap until resistance is felt. The color band on the sleeve should be partially exposed.

The resistance felt is the anchor being positioned against the sheath tip

b

Figure 25.8 (Continued)

randomized studies. Balzer et al[7] evaluated a percutaneous vascular suture device (the Prostar and Techstar system from Perclose, Menlo Park, CA) in 930 patients with peripheral arterial occlusive disease after peripheral interventional procedures, from June 1995 to March 2000. The system was technically successful in 92.2% of cases, independently of the degree of calcification. Device malfunction or insufficient suture closure occurred in 1.7% and 2.1%, respectively. In 7%, groin-related complications occurred, most often large hematoma (>6 cm) in 4.1% and pseudoaneurysm in 0.9%. Ambulation within 2–4 hours after successful suture was possible in 96.1%. Rinder et al[8] compared, retrospectively, a cohort of 1054 patients treated by manual or mechanical (Femostop) compression with 700 treated by a suture-mediated closure device (Perclose in 6 and 8 Fr) from January 1999 to March 2000. There were no differences in most vascular complications (retroperitoneal bleed, hematoma, and arteriovenous fistula) between groups, although lower

rates of pseudoaneurysms (0.5% versus 1.8%; $p=0.02$) and transfusion requirements (8% versus 15%; $p < 0.001$) were observed in patients treated with closure devices. Kahn et al[9] compared 7783 diagnostic and 798 interventional catheterization patients treated by manual compression with 1123 diagnostic and 297 interventional catherization patients treated using the Prostar-plus device (Perclose) between 1997 and 1999. In diagnostic procedures, the compression group had a significantly lower complication rate compared with the Prostar-plus group at the expense of lower rates of small (<2 cm) and large (≥ 2 cm) hematomas, pseudoaneurysms, and surgery. However, in therapeutic patients, there were no statistical differences for either major or minor complications. Fram et al[10] assessed 1200 consecutive cases presenting for invasive cardiac procedures. The Perclose device was successfully deployed in 91.2% of cases. The complication rate was 3.4%. Complications included the development of hematoma (2.1%), the need for vascular surgery (0.6%),

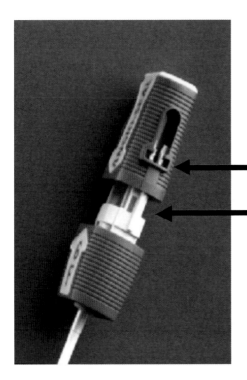

Step III : Continue to pull the device cap back into the final lock position.

The color band is now completely exposed. At this point the device cap and sheath hub can not be moved independently.

c

Figure 25.8 (Continued)

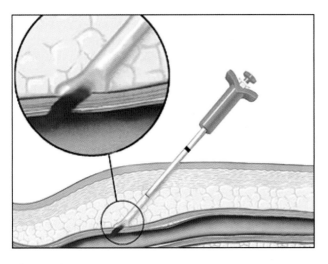

Figure 25.9
The VasoSeal system.

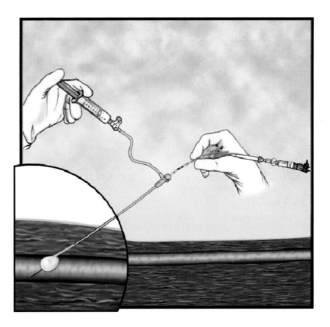

Figure 25.10
The DUETT system.

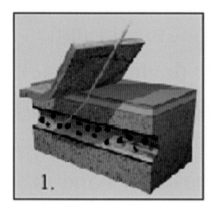 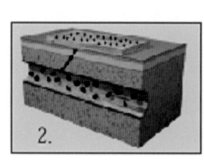 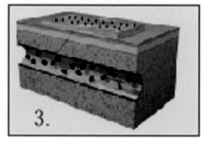

Figure 25.11
The Clo-Sur P.A.D. device and procedural steps (1–3). See text for details.

retroperitoneal hemorrhage (0.3%), blood transfusion (0.7%), local infection (0.5%) and pseudoaneurysm (0.1%). Age over 70 years, activated clotting time over 300 s, left femoral access, and the performance of primary angioplasty were independent predictors of procedural failure. In a randomized study, Gerckens et al[11] compared suture-mediated versus manual compression in 600 patients. The incidence of vascular complications was similar in the overall population (5.3% for suture-mediated versus 11.3% for compression), and in the interventional patient subset (8.4% versus 9.6%). However, the diagnostic procedure subset of the suture-mediated group experienced significantly fewer vascular complications (84.4% versus 12.1%; $p < 0.05$). Besides, hemostasis and ambulation were achieved faster with the suturing device than with manual compression (7.8 minutes versus 19.6 minutes ($p < 0.0001$) and 4.5 hours versus 17.8 hours ($p < 0.001$)). Finally, in the STAND II trial,[12] 200 patients were randomized to the 6 Fr Techstar device (Perclose) or manual compression after diagnostic or interventional procedures. Similarly, the median time to hemostasis and the time to ambulation were significantly reduced with the suture-based device, without a significant increase in the vascular complication rate.

Collagen-mediated closure devices

Sanborn et al[13] conducted a prospective randomized, multicenter trial aiming to compare the hemostasis time and the incidence of vascular complications in patients receiving a collagen vascular hemostasis device and in those receiving manual compression after diagnostic and interventional procedures. With the collagen device, the hemostasis time was significantly reduced (4.1 minutes versus 17.6 minutes; $p < 0.0001$), as was the time to ambulation, without a significant increase in peripheral vascular com-

plications. In the era of the use of glycoprotein IIb/IIIa inhibitors, VasoSeal hemostasis efficacy and safety were assessed after coronary interventions in 50 patients.[14] There were no hemorrhagic complications (hematoma, pseudoaneurysm, blood transfusion, or surgical repair) despite early activity and ambulation. The safety and efficacy of the 6 Fr Angio-Seal device were prospectively assessed in 180 patients after diagnostic or interventional coronary procedures.[15] The device was safe and effective, with a high rate of procedural success (>95%) and a low rate of vascular complications (<3%). An increased risk of complications after Angio-Seal deployment has been associated with the learning curve, 8 Fr sheaths, postprocedure heparin, and body mass index.[16]

The DUETT sealing device

A European multicenter registry using the DUETT vascular sealing device enrolled 1587 patients in 25 European countries.[17] Successful deployment was achieved in 96.2% of patients, with complete hemostasis within 2–5 minutes in 95% of patients. The total rate of complications was 2.6%, including pseudoaneurysm in 34 patients and arterial occlusions in 4. A feasibility trial in the USA[18] included 43 patients and demonstrated a 97.7% rate of procedural success, with 1 uncomplicated crossover to manual compression and the development of 1 pseudoaneurysm. A prospective, multicenter randomized trial (SEAL trial) has recently been reported.[19] At 16 sites, 630 patients who underwent diagnostic or interventional procedures were randomized 5:3 to the DUETT sealing device or standard manual compression. Time to hemostasis was significantly reduced in the DUETT group (14 minutes versus 195 minutes; $p < 0.001$), as well as time to ambulation from catheter removal (338 minutes versus 705 minutes; $p < 0.01$). No significant differences were observed between the groups in terms of vascular complications ($p=0.22$).

Comparative studies

Chamberlin et al[20] compared three different devices (Perclose, VasoSeal, and Femostop) in 185 patients receiving abciximab during percutaneous coronary interventions. VasoSeal was successful in 79% of patients, Perclose in 86%, and Femostop in 100%. Late complications were comparably low between groups. Michalis et al[21] compared the safety and efficacy of three closure devices: Angio-Seal, VasoSeal and DUETT, in a prospective and randomized fashion. In the angiography group, Angio-Seal was significantly slower in achieving hemostasis ($p=0.0001$), but resulted in earlier ambulation ($p=0.0001$). In the angioplasty patients, Angio-Seal was again slower in achieving hemostasis ($p=0.003$), but the ambulation time was comparable between the groups. Major complication rates were similar between the three devices. The incidence of peripheral embolization was lower after Angio-Seal deployment. A retrospective study[22] evaluated the outcomes of 4525 patients receiving closure devices or manual compression in the setting of the use of glycoprotein IIb/IIIa antagonists. The devices used for closure were Angio-Seal in 524 patients and Perclose in 2177, whereas manual compression was used in 1824. The success rate was 97% for Angio-Seal and 94% for Perclose. Major complications were comparably low between the three groups (1.8% for manual, 1.1% for Angio-Seal, and 1.2% for Perclose). Multivariate analysis identified only closure device failure as an independent predictor of vascular failure. Finally, two different collagen-derived devices (Angio-Seal and VasoSeal) were compared in a randomized study.[23] The times to hemostasis and to ambulation were comparable between the devices. Similarly, there were no statistical differences in deployment failure, or in major, minor, or total complication rates.

Conclusions

In randomized studies, groin closure devices are safe and effective when compared with manual/mechanical compression in interventional procedures. They work by increasing hemostasis and decreasing the period to ambulation, with comparable rates of vascular complications. Complications are usually related to large sheaths, the use of glycoprotein IIb/IIIa inhibitors, body mass index, and failure of device deployment. Additionally, there is a learning curve for the use of these devices, which has to be taken into consideration.

References

1. Silber S, Dörr R, Mülling H, König U. Sheath pulling immediately after PTCA: comparison of two different techniques for the hemostatic puncture closure device: a prospective, randomized study. Cathet Cardiovasc Diagn 1997; 41:378–83.

2. Silber S, Gershony G, Scoen B, et al. A novel vascular sealing device for closure of percutaneous arterial access sites. Am J Cardiol 1999;83:1248–52.

3. Wyman RM, Safian RD, Portway V, et al. Current complications of diagnostic and therapeutic cardiac catheterization. J Am Coll Cardiol 1988;12:1400–6.

4. Khoury M, Batra S, Berg R, et al. Influence of arterial access sites and interventional procedures on vascular complications after cardiac catheterization. Am J Surg 1992; 164:205–9.

5. Heintzen MP, Strauer BE. Local vascular complications after cardiac catheterization. Herz 1998;1:4–20.

6. Muller DW, Shamir KJ, Ellis SG, Topol EJ. Peripheral vascular complications after conventional and complex percutaneous coronary interventional procedures. Am J Cardiol 1992; 69:63–8.

7. Balzer JO, Scheinert D, Diebold T, et al. Postinterventional transcutaneous suture of femoral artery access sites in patients with peripheral arterial occlusive disease. A study in 930 patients. Cathet Cardiovasc Interv 2001;53:174–81.

8. Rinder MR, Tamirisa PK, Taniuchi M, Kurz HI, Mumm K, Lasala JM. Safety and efficacy of suture-mediated closure after percutaneous coronary interventions. Cathet Cardiovasc Interv 2001;54:146–51.

9. Kahn ZM, Kumar M, Hollander G, Frankel R. Safety and efficacy of the Perclose suture-mediated closure device after diagnostic and interventional catheterizations in a large consecutive population. Catheter Cardiovasc Interv 2002; 55:8–13.

10. Fram DB, Giri S, Jamil G, et al. Suture closure of the femoral arteriotomy following invasive cardiac procedures: a detailed analysis of efficacy, complications, and the impact of early ambulation in 1200 consecutive, unselected cases. Cathet Cardiovasc Interv 2001;53:163–73.

11. Gerckens U, Cattelaens N, Lampe EG, Grube E. Management of arterial puncture site after catheterization procedures: evaluating a suture-mediated closure device. Am J Cardiol 1999;83:1658–63.

12. Baim DS, Knopf WD, Hinohara T, et al. Suture-mediated closure of the femoral access site after cardiac catheterization: results of the Suture to Ambulate and Discharge (STAND I and STAND II) trials. Am J Cardiol 2000; 85:864–9.

13. Sanborn TA, Gibbs HH, Brinker JA, et al. A multicenter randomized trial comparing a percutaneous collagen hemostasis device with conventional manual compression after diagnostic angiography and angioplasty. J Am Coll Cardiol 1993;22:1273–9.

14. Lunney L, Karim K, Little T. VasoSeal hemostasis following coronary interventions. Cathet Cardiovasc Diagn 1998; 44:405–6.

15. Eggebrecht H, Haude M, von Birgelen C, et al. Early clinical experience with the 6 French Angio-Seal device: immediate closure of femoral puncture sites after diagnostic and interventional coronary procedures. Cathet Cardiovasc Interv 2001;53:437–42.

16. Warren BS, Warren SG, Miller SD. Predictors of complications and learning curve using the Angio-Seal closure device following interventional and diagnostic catheterization. Cathet Cardiovasc Interv 1999;48:162–6.

17. Silber S, Tofte AJ, Kjellevand TO, et al. Final Report of the European Multi-Center Registry using the DUETT™ vascular sealing device. Herz 1999;24:620–3.

18. Mooney MR, Ellis SG, Gershomy G, et al. Immediate sealing of arterial puncture sites after cardiac catheterization and coronary interventions: initial U.S. feasibility trial using the DUETT vascular closure device. Cathet Cardiovasc Interv 2000;50:96–102.

19. The Seal Trial Study Team. Assessment of the safety and efficacy of the DUETT vascular hemostasis device: final results of the Safe and Effective Vascular Hemostasis (SEAL) trial. Am Heart J 2002;143:612–19.

20. Chamberlin JR, Lardi AB, McKeever LS, et al. Use of vascular sealing devices (Vasoseal and Perclose) versus assisted manual compression (Femostop) in transcatheter coronary interventions requiring abciximab (Reopro). Cathet Cardiovasc Interv 1999;47:143–7.

21. Michalis LK, Rees MR, Pastouras D, et al. A prospective randomized trial comparing the safety and efficacy of three commercially available closure devices (Angio-Seal, VasoSeal and DUETT). Cardiovasc Interv Radiol 2002; 25:423–9.

22. Applegate RJ, Grabarczyk MA, Little WC, et al. Vascular closure devices in patients treated with anticoagulation and IIb/IIIa receptor inhibitors during percutaneous revascularization. J Am Coll Cardiol 2002;40:78–83.

23. Shammas NW, Rajendran VR, Alldredge SG, et al. Randomized comparison of VasoSeal and Angio-Seal closure devices in patients undergoing coronary angiography and angioplasty. Cathet Cardiovasc Interv 2002;55:421–5.

26

Stent retrieval

Goran Stankovic, Antonio Colombo

Introduction

Dislodgement of a stent from the delivery balloon during the deployment procedure is a rare complication of percutaneous coronary revascularization that may result in systemic or intracoronary stent embolization. While systemic embolization may cause severe cerebrovascular events,[1] intracoronary stent embolization has a high risk of coronary thrombosis and myocardial infarction.[2–4] However, stent dislodgement is not necessarily followed by stent loss. The operator still has an opportunity to retrieve the stent from the arterial system of the patient. It is therefore appropriate to define stent separation as detachment of the stent from the balloon followed by successful stent retrieval, and to define stent loss as detachment of the stent from the balloon without stent retrieval.

Stent dislodgement from the delivery system often occurs when the stent is pulled back into the guiding catheter because the target lesion either could not be reached or could not be passed.[1,4,5] Factors predisposing to inability to deliver the stent are poor support of the guiding catheter or the guidewire, vessel tortuosity proximal to the lesion, and severe vessel calcification.[5]

It is our impression that stent loss is a complication that is decreasing and almost disappearing due to the availability of more flexible stents with a lower profile and to the almost-exclusive usage of premounted stents, which appear to be more resistant to dislodgement compared with hand-mounted stents. In our experience, stent detachment and stent loss occurred 0.8% of the time in the past but now occur at least ten times less frequently. A similar incidence was reported by Eggebrecht et al[4] (1.04% for manually crimped stents, 0.24% for premounted stents, and 0.9% in total). The fact that newer stents are typically mounted on lower-profile delivery

balloons does not necessarily imply a lower likelihood for stent detachment. For example, the Medtronic beStent (Medtronic, Minneapolis, MN) experienced a higher rate of stent dislodgment than had been predicted, prompting a suspension of the beStent clinical trial in late 1997. A problem with insufficient crimping of the larger beStent iteration (BEL design) was identified and corrected, and the trial was resumed.[6]

A protective sheath should protect completely against stent dislodgment and stent loss – however, on rare occasions, these complications can occur if the operator pulls back the sheath before reaching a lesion that cannot be traversed with the sheath in place. In fact, there are only two stent delivery devices with protective sheaths that are still in use: the Radius self-expanding stent and the Magic Wall stent (both Boston Scientific, Natick, MA). Technical advances, in particular in terms of improved crimping, mean that it is now possible to obtain a very secure and stable balloon and stent retention even without a protective sheath – indeed, we do not know of any balloon-expandable stent that uses a delivery system with a protective sheath.

When stent dislodgement does occur, a number of percutaneous techniques are available for stent extraction.

Stent detachment: a problem solved by preventing its occurrence

It may appear rhetorical to say that the most effective way to deal with stent loss is to prevent its occurrence. The reality is that if the operator is careful not to force a stent through a lesion (even if this maneuver has occasionally been successful), then stent loss can be minimized. Another important point is to pay particular attention when pulling back the undeployed stent into the guiding catheter. Alignment of the stent on the balloon with the guiding catheter is very important to avoid flaring the proximal edge of the stent. If the operator is not concerned about losing the wire position, the guiding catheter and the balloon with the stent should be removed as a unit from the coronary tree until a position with good alignment is reached. In a situation where the wire position cannot be lost, this maneuver should be done over an extended guidewire if a long wire is not already in place. If the operator has not aggressively forced the stent through the lesion, then the stent will not be deformed and it will still be attached to the balloon, and stent retrieval into the guiding catheter should not be a problem.

In many of the above situations, even if appropriate care is not taken, it is quite difficult to lose a well-mounted stent. The only exception that should be kept in mind is the need to avoid entrapment of a stent while crossing another stent to proceed more distally or through the struts in order to stent a side branch. So far, we have not lost a stent even in this situation. As we all know, however, the fact that an event has not been reported in the literature does not mean that it has not happened! One of the authors had a personal communication about the removal of a stent previously placed 3 months before while pulling back a new stent that could not be advanced distally. This case is not necessarily a case of stent loss – rather it is a case of stent gain!

Stent retrieval when the stent is no longer firmly secured on the balloon

When the operator realizes that the stent has become mobile on the balloon, a number of maneuvers should be used to prevent total separation of the stent from the balloon. In our series of 17 stents partially dislodged from the balloon, only 8 were successfully retrieved from the patient. With more experience and with the availability of new retrieval devices such as the Amplatz Goose Neck (Microvena Corp., White Bear Lake, MN) (Figure 26.1), the success rate can now be higher. In nine of our patients with stent embolization, there were no clinical consequences, and there is generally little information in the literature on clinical sequelae following stent embolization.[7] Kozman et al[7] have reported the long-term outcome (36±13 months) of 23 patients having either stent embolization or misdeployment, and have found a higher incidence of adverse events in those in whom the stent remained in the coronary circulation. However, extracoronary stent embolization was associated with minimal

long-term sequelae. Figure 26.2 shows immediate and 5-year follow-up angiographic images of our patient in whom a Palmaz biliary stent 10 mm long embolized to the right popliteal artery.[8] The stent did not migrate from its original position, and normal vessel patency and distal flow were observed in the right popliteal artery. During that time period, the patient had been free of any symptom related to peripheral vascular disease.

Despite a favorable outcome following stent loss, we believe that stent retrieval should be actively pursued, especially with the increase in usage of long stents. In order to avoid stent embolization to the brain, any attempt to retrieve a mobile stent into the guiding catheter should be done below the diaphragm.

Several techniques and devices have been developed for the retrieval of damaged or misplaced stents, including loop snares,[1,4] myocardial biopsy or biliary forceps,[4,9–11] multipurpose baskets,[9] two twisted guidewires,[12] and balloon catheters.[4,13,14] The Amplatz Goose Neck snare has a shaft diameter of 0.018 inch and is tipped by a closed wire loop angulated at 90° to the shaft axis (Figure 26.1). Retraction or advancement of the wire within an outer plastic catheter of 2.3 French (Fr) (the 'Wanderer') permits the snare to be opened or closed. For stent retrieval, the snare is passed over the distal end of the detached stent and cinched tightly. The snare and the stent are then withdrawn as a whole. Use of this approach is advocated in cases of inadvertent loss of the guidewire position. Snares can be fashioned in the laboratory from a 300 cm coronary wire and a 5 Fr diagnostic catheter. Commercial loop snares are, however, available with loops that either extend in the direction of the long axis of the guiding catheter or are folded to open at a 90° angle from the delivery catheter. Myocardial bioptomes and long alligator forceps have both been used for stent retrieval.[10,11] The main limitations on the use of forceps devices are too large a shaft diameter, device rigidity, and catheter length (often 80–90 cm). The thinner, softer, and longer disposable bioptomes may offer advantages. The biliary stone forceps device consists of a set of curved, fingerlike projections that can be expanded/extended or contracted/retracted. By manipulating the 'fingers' of this device, an operator can grab hold of lost or retained components. This device is most useful in recovering partially expanded stents or in situations in which a portion of a stent has become separated from the delivery system. Biliary forceps are available with catheter bodies of 4 or 5 Fr, and in lengths of 130 cm. The alligator forceps devices have distal tip modifications that allow grasping of structures through a 'biting jaws' action. The basket retrieval device consists of a set of helically arranged loops that can be expanded or collapsed. It can be used to catch a stent from the side and pull it free of a deployment balloon.

When the stent is mobile on the balloon or deformed, we suggest the use of the Amplatz Goose Neck 4 mm loop to anchor the stent further to the shaft of the balloon in order to retrieve it. The balloon shaft should be used as

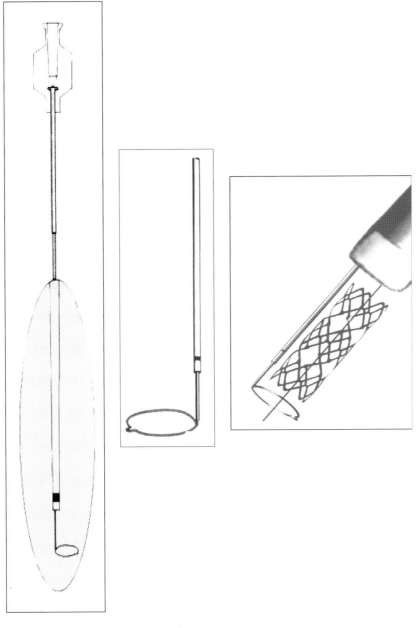

Figure 26.1
The Amplatz Goose Neck
(Microvena Corp., White Bear Lake,
MN).

a 'wire' on which the snare is advanced. In order to get the loop of the snare on the balloon shaft, it may be necessary to cut the hub of the balloon. When the snare reaches the stent, tightening the snare at the proximal edge of the stent will allow the operator to secure the stent on the balloon and help retrieval into the femoral sheath.

Another approach to retrieve a stent from the iliac artery is to use a large peripheral balloon to wrap in the stent partially and then remove the balloon from the same sheath.[13] When retrieval through the vascular sheath seems impossible, some authors suggest that the retrieved stent be deployed in the iliac artery and anchored with the peripheral stent.[15]

A device that we have found to be effective in retrieving a stent located in a large vessel is the 3 Fr Cook Retrieval System (Cook Inc., Bloomington, IN)

(Figure 26.3). As shown in the figure, this device has a guidewire attached to its distal end, similar to a fixed-wire angioplasty balloon catheter. An articulating arm operable from the proximal hub is used to grasp and retrieve fractured fragments. The device is available in 80 cm and 145 cm lengths. On some occasions, this device can be used to retrieve a 'U-shaped' deformed stent without the need for a contralateral approach. The 3 Fr size of this device may allow its introduction into the same guiding catheter in which the deformed stent cannot be entered. Snaring the stent at one edge allows its retrieval into the guiding catheter or into the sheath.

The last resort, especially when a slotted tubular stent has been severely deformed (Figure 26.4), is the use of a contralateral approach. In this situation a 10 Fr sheath should be inserted in the other femoral artery, and a 10 Fr

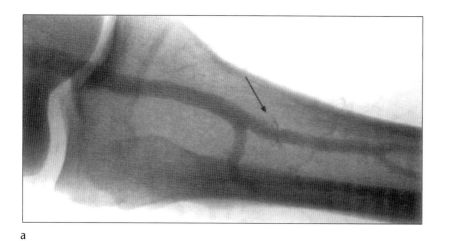

a

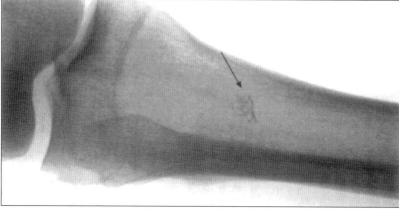

b

Figure 26.2
(a) Immediate angiographic image of the Palmaz biliary stent embolized to the right popliteal artery (arrow). There is normal vessel patency and brisk distal flow. (b) Five-year follow-up angiographic image. As in the immediate angiogram, there is normal vessel patency and brisk distal flow.

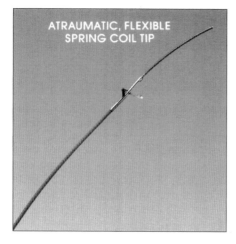

ATRAUMATIC, FLEXIBLE
SPRING COIL TIP

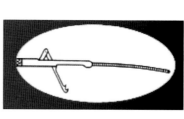

Figure 26.3
Cook Retrieval System (Cook Inc., Bloomington, IN).

right coronary or multipurpose guiding catheter is then negotiated from the contralateral iliac artery into the iliac artery where the deformed stent is present (Figure 26.5). The stent is then retrieved into this large guide with a snare (Figure 26.6).

If the contralateral approach is not possible, an attempt can be made to upsize the introducer already present in the original groin. This procedure is reformed by inserting a new 0.035 inch or smaller wire into the current introducer, placing a second larger introducer over this sec-

ond wire, and removing the first introducer. What will happen in this case is that there will be one large introducer in place, with the shaft of the stent balloon or its wire on the side. The stent can now be retrieved with a Goose Neck from the new introducer. It is important to cut any hypotube or other hard part in the system still attached to the stent, because on pulling back the stent into the new introducer, the wire or the balloon still attached will make a 180° revolution to come fully back into the artery and then into the sheath.

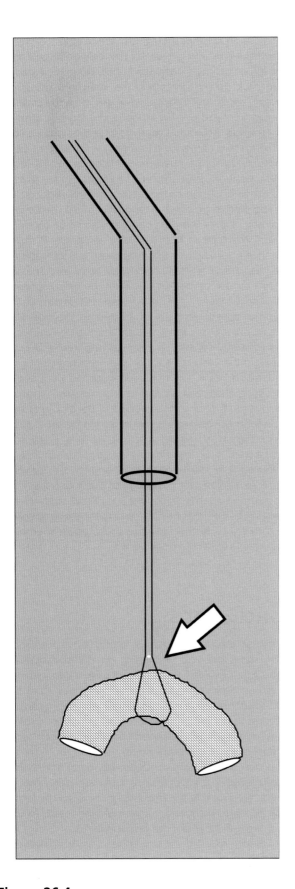

Figure 26.4
A 'U-shaped' deformed slotted tubular stent: stent retrieval with the lasso in the center.

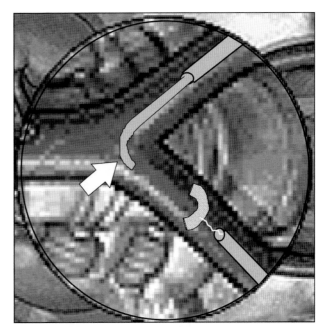

Figure 26.5
Initial step of the contralateral stent retrieval approach.

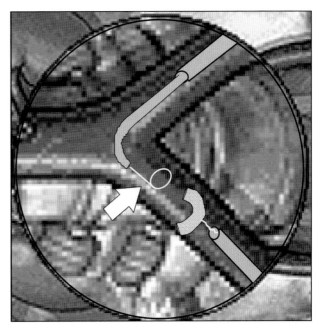

Figure 26.6
Final step of the contralateral stent retrieval approach.

Stent retrieval from the coronary tree

Stent dislodgment usually tends to occur when negotiating a tortuous artery with a balloon-mounted stent, especially if the artery is irregularly calcified or when applying a rigid stent. The approach in situations of misplaced or embolized stents within the coronary artery is primarily oriented towards minimizing the consequences of the event and not necessarily retrieving the stent. In the event of stent embolization in a coronary vessel, the operator should consider stent deployment versus stent retrieval. If the stent is a coil stent, stent retrieval is almost always successful. We favor the use of the Amplatz Goose Neck 2 or 4 mm loop, which should be advanced over the wire if wire access is still there.

A number of different approaches have been used successfully or suggested:

- is the absence of a dedicated snare, a custom snare can be constructed using conventional coronary guidewires;[16]
- biopsy forceps (Cordis J & J Corp., Miami, FL);[11]
- biliary forceps or a multipurpose basket (Meditech, Watertown, MA);[9]
- two coronary wires can be used to tangle the stent;[12,17,18]
- an angioplasty guidewire incorporating a distal occlusion balloon (PercuSurge);[19]
- a small balloon (1.5 or 2 mm) can be advanced over the coaxial stent wire distally to the stent, with subsequent inflation of the balloon to retrieve the stent into the guiding catheter;[20]
- a fixed wire system can be passed on the side of the stent[14] or in a coaxial position to the stent.[21]

Other retrieval devices that can be employed and are particularly delicate are the Retriever-18 and Retriever-10 Endovascular snares (Target Therapeutics, Freemont, CA) (Figure 26.7).

If a slotted tubular stent has been used, the operator should evaluate the possibility of removing the stent from the coronary tree without dissecting the vessel against the risk of deploying the stent in a specific location. An important aspect is to try to preserve the coaxial guidewire position inside the stent.

Initially, an attempt should by made to advance over the guidewire a very low-profile 1.5 mm balloon distally to the stent. When properly positioned, the balloon is inflated and pulled back slowly to retrieve the stent into the guiding catheter ('retrieve'). If the retrieval fails, then the small balloon can be partially inflated inside the stent (2 atm) and used to advance the stent gently to a location more suitable for deployment ('advance plus deploy'). If the stent cannot be advanced and the operator is forced to deploy it in its current position, then the small balloon can be used for progressive dilatation of the stent and then replaced with the appropriately sized balloon for final deployment ('deploy'). In any event, the operator should be careful not to force the balloon into the stent, especially if there is resistance – a maneuver that may cause balloon rupture.

If the coaxial wire position has been lost and stent retrieval cannot be performed, then the only approach is to plaster the stent against the vessel wall (Figure 26.8). A balloon of appropriate size is inflated on the side of the stent to deploy the stent against the wall of the vessel. Another stent (or stent graft[22]) is implanted in a coaxial position in the vessel to exclude the plastered stent only if an adequate result has not been obtained or a residual obstructing dissection is present. Intravascular ultrasound interrogation facilitates this process of decision-making.

Under no circumstance should a stent be left as such in the coronary tree without at least plastering it against the wall. If a stent is left free-floating in a large branch, then the chances of late occlusion of the branch are significant (Figure 26.9). The only exception to this rule is a situation where the stent has been lost in a small and terminal branch. In fact, one of the last resorts in dealing with stent loss is to try to further advance and purposely embolize the stent in a small terminal branch.

Conclusions

Thanks to the availability of a new generation of premounted stents, stent loss is a decreasing or almost-disappearing complication. Avoiding the forcing of a stent into a lesion or through another stent, and thereby preventing stent damage, is the best approach for successful retrieval. In particular situations, the operator should consider using an absolutely safe system, such as a stent with partial protection such as the Radius self-expandable stent with sheath system. A variety of snaring devices of other systems are now available to help remove a stent from a coronary tree. The best retrieval technique to use depends primarily on the location of the damaged stent and the type of stent used. As a last resort, stent deployment can be considered.

Clinically relevant consequences for the patient are extremely rare following this type of complication. The operator should never forget that sometimes leaving a stent behind may be less dangerous for the patient than relentless fruitless attempts to remove it.

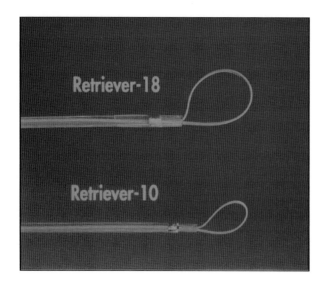

Figure 26.7
The Retriever-18 and -10 endovascular snares (Target Therapeutics, Freemont, CA).

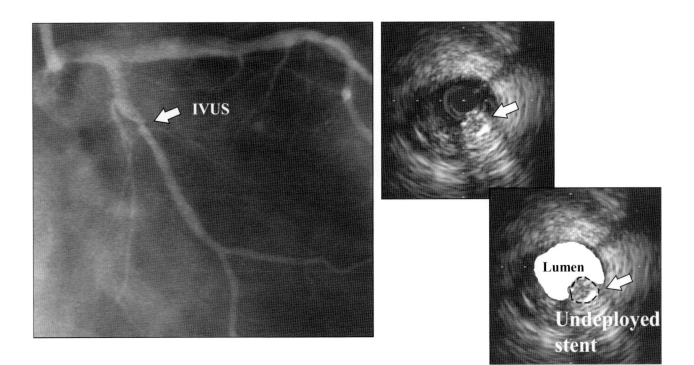

Figure 26.8
Angiographic and intravascular ultrasound (IVUS) images of a plastered stent.

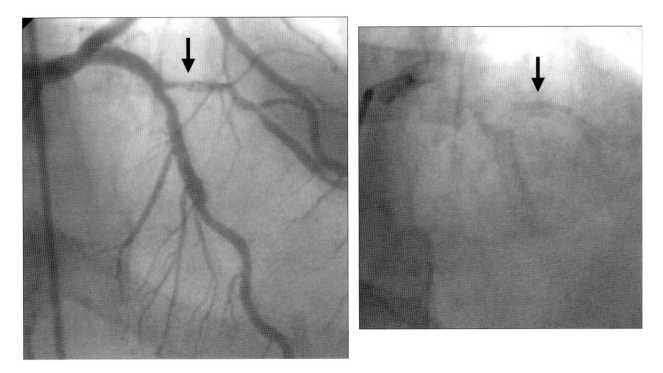

Figure 26.9
A case of subacute thrombosis of a stent dislodged in a diagonal branch.

References

1. Elsner M, Peifer A, Kasper W. Intracoronary loss of balloon-mounted stents: successful retrieval with a 2 mm-'Microsnare'-device. Cathet Cardiovasc Diagn 1996; 39:271–6.

2. Colombo A, Maiello L, Almagor Y, et al. Coronary stenting: single institution experience with the initial 100 cases using the Palmaz–Schatz stent. Cathet Cardiovasc Diagn 1992;26:171–6.

3. Shiojima I, Ikari Y, Abe J, et al. Thrombotic occlusion of the coronary artery associated with accidental detachment of undeployed Palmaz–Schatz stent. Cathet Cardiovasc Diagn 1996;38:360–2.

4. Eggebrecht H, Haude M, von Birgelen C, et al. Nonsurgical retrieval of embolized coronary stents. Cathet Cardiovasc Interv 2000;51:432–40.

5. Holmes DR Jr, Garratt KN, Popma J. Stent complications. J Invasive Cardiol 1998;10:385–95.

6. Garratt KN. Coronary stent retrieval: devices and techniques. In: Strategic Approaches in Coronary Intervention (Ellis SG, Holmes DR Jr, eds). Baltimore: Williams & Wilkins, 2000:441–51.

7. Kozman H, Wiseman AH, Cook JR. Long-term outcome following coronary stent embolization or misdeployment. Am J Cardiol 2001;88:630–4.

8. Briguori C, Kobayashi N, De Gregorio J, Colombo A. Palmaz–Schatz stent embolization: long-term clinical and angiographic follow-up. Int J Cardiovasc Interv 1999;2:247–8.

9. Foster-Smith KW, Garratt KN, Higano ST, Holmes DR. Retrieval techniques for managing flexible intracoronary stent misplacement. Cathet Cardiovasc Diagn 1993; 30:63–8.

10. Eeckhout E, Stauffer JC, Goy JJ. Retrieval of a migrated coronary stent by means of an alligator forceps catheter. Cathet Cardiovasc Diagn 1993;30:166–8.

11. Berder V, Bedossa M, Gras D, et al. Retrieval of a lost coronary stent from the descending aorta using a PTCA balloon and biopsy forceps. Cathet Cardiovasc Diagn 1993; 28:351–3.

12. Veldhuijzen FL, Bonnier HJ, Michels HR, et al. Retrieval of undeployed stents from the right coronary artery: report of two cases. Cathet Cardiovasc Diagn 1993;30:245–8.

13. Cishek MB, Laslett L, Gershony G. Balloon catheter retrieval of dislodged coronary artery stents: a novel technique. Cathet Cardiovasc Diagn 1995;34:350–2.

14. Rozenman Y, Burstein M, Hasin Y, Gotsman MS. Retrieval of occluding unexpanded Palmaz–Schatz stent from a saphenous aorto-coronary vein graft. Cathet Cardiovasc Diagn 1995;34:159–61.

15. Meisel SR, DiLeo J, Rajakaruna M, et al. A technique to retrieve stents dislodged in the coronary artery followed by fixation in the iliac artery by means of balloon angioplasty and peripheral stent deployment. Cathet Cardiovasc Interv 2000;49:77–81.

16. Pan M, Medina A, Romero M. Peripheral stent recovery after failed intracoronary delivery. Cathet Cardiovasc Diagn 1992;27:230–3.

17. Wong PH. Retrieval of undeployed intracoronary Palmaz–Schatz stents. Cathet Cardiovasc Diagn 1995;35:218–23.

18. Bogart DB, Jung SC. Dislodged stent: a simple retrieval technique. Cathet Cardiovasc Interv 1999;47:323–4.

19. Webb JG, Solankhi N, Carere RG. Facilitation of stent retention and retrieval with an emboli containment device. Cathet Cardiovasc Interv 2000;50:215–17.

20. Iyer SS, Roubin GS. Nonsurgical management of retained intracoronary products following coronary interventions. In: Interventional Cardiovascular Medicine: (Roubin GS, ed). Edinburgh: Churchill Livingstone, 1994:635–41.

21. Eisenhauer AC, Piemonte TC, Gossman DE. Extraction of fully deployed coronary stents. Cathet Cardiovasc Diagn 1996;38:393–401.

22. Lotze U, Ferrari M, Dannberg G, et al. Unexpanded, irretrievable stent in the proximal right coronary artery: successful management with stent graft implantation. Catheter Cardiovasc Interv 1999;46:344–9.

27

Percutaneous atrial septal defect, patent foramen ovale closure and patent ductus arteriosus closure

David McGaw, Richard Harper

Introduction

Percutaneous transvenous closure of atrial septal defects (ASDs), patent foramen ovale (PFO), and patent ductus arteriosus (PDA) has become feasible in recent years. Later-generation devices have largely overcome initial difficulties and may now be deployed with high procedural success and low complication rates. The advent of a non-surgical therapeutic option for a wide range of atrial septal and ductal pathology has lowered the threshold for intervention, and such procedures are now commonplace.

This chapter will give a brief overview of percutaneous closure of ASDs, PFO, and PDA, including clinical indications, patient selection, and technical details, as well as potential pitfalls and their solutions. There have been a series of devices in use for percutaneous closure of congenital pathologies. The Amplatzer range of devices was not the first, and may not be the last; however, it is currently in the most widespread use due to several advantageous design features. For the sake of simplicity and to reflect current clinical practice, discussion will be limited to these devices.

Amplatzer occluder devices

The Amplatzer Septal Occluder (ASO) device, Amplatzer Patent Foramen Ovale Occluder (PFO Occluder) device and Amplatzer Duct Occluder (ADO) device (AGA Medical Inc., Golden Valley, MN) are self-expanding paired discs made from nitinol woven wire mesh (Figure 27.1). Nitinol is a nickel alloy with a strong shape memory. This allows it to be factory-set in the desired conformation, to which it returns after being elongated and passed through a sheath during percutaneous delivery.

Amplatzer Septal Occluder device

With the ASO, the left and right atrial discs are joined by a waist in a continuous weave of the same material (Figure 27.1a). A polyester patch is sewn within both discs and the waist, which serves to occlude blood flow through the device. The devices are screwed to a delivery cable and delivered into position across the septum through a 6–12 French (Fr) preshaped delivery sheath, where they are released.

The ASO ranges in size from 4 to 40 mm, as measured by the diameter of the central waist, which stents the defect. This 4 mm-long waist also serves to center the device in the defect, which is a great advantage of this design. The left atrial disc overhangs the waist by 6–8 mm and the right by 4–5 mm, depending on the size of the device. These flanges serve to grip the septum and provide stability for the waist within the defect.

Amplatzer Patent Foramen Ovale Occluder

The PFO Occluder differs from the ASO in two features (Figure 27.1b). Firstly, the central waist is only a few millimeters in diameter and is flexible. It serves to connect the atrial discs, but does not stent the defect, and therefore does not self-center the device. Secondly, the right atrial disc is larger than the left atrial disc. The PFO Occluder has two sizes, 25 and 35 mm, which refer to the size of the larger right atrial disc. The smaller left atrial discs are 18 and 25 mm in diameter, respectively.

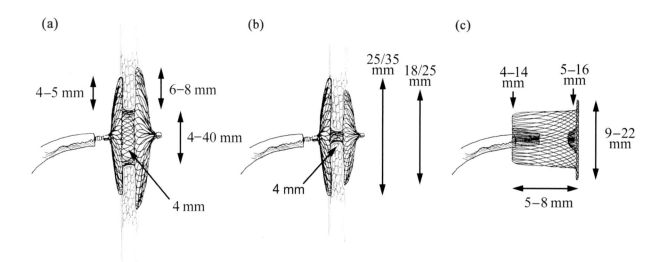

Figure 27.1
(a) The Amplatzer Septal Occluder (ASO) device, sized by the diameter of the waist. (b) The Amplatzer Patent Foramen Ovale Occluder (PFO Occluder) device, sized by the diameter of the larger right atrial disc. (c) The Amplatzer Duct Occluder (ADO) device, sized by the diameter of the device body.

Amplatzer Duct Occluder

The ADO differs from the septal occluding devices in that it has only one larger retention disc on the aortic side (Figure 27.1c). The device is described in terms of the dimensions of the body of the device, which tapers away from the retention disc by 1–2 mm. For example, a 10/8 mm device has a retention disc of 14 mm, and a body that tapers from 10 mm to 8 mm over its 7 mm length. The sizes of the device are from 5/4 to 16/14 mm, with lengths 5–8 mm. The aortic retention discs are 4–6 mm larger in diameter than the body.

Another difference in the ADO is that the delivery cable attachment screw is seated within the device, sited on the pulmonary artery end. The device is therefore deployed through a delivery sheath from the pulmonary artery. The device is stabilized in the ductus by the aortic retention disc and by oversizing the body of the ADO such that it is gripped in the ductus in the shape of a 'champagne cork'.

Atrial septal pathologies

Suitability of ASDs for closure

An ASD is a pathological congenital communication between the left and right atria. The indications for closure of ASDs have widened over recent years. Historically, when open heart surgery was the only corrective treatment, the indication was a pulmonary-to-systemic shunt of 2 : 1 or greater. As surgery has become less invasive and percutaneous closure has become a

viable option, the indications now include a shunt of 1.5 : 1 or echocardiographic evidence of right heart volume overload.

The ideal ASD for percutaneous closure is the small secundum defect. This provides a complete rim of tissue for ease of device deployment and an adequate margin of tissue to avoid encroachment on adjacent structures (Figure 27.2). However, many ASDs fall outside this ideal description. Primum atrial ASDs are unsuitable due to their involvement of and proximity to the atrioventricular valves. Similarly, sinus venosus ASDs are unsuitable due to the over-riding nature of the superior vena cava and high frequency of anomalous pulmonary drainage.

Although a small ideal secundum defect may be closed by any available device, if a device does not self-center the atrial discs must be approximately twice the diameter of the defect to ensure that the defect is covered. With a self-centering device such as the ASO, this degree of overlap is not necessary, as the stenting waist ensures that the central position of the device in the defect (Figure 27.3). This feature permits closure of larger defects with smaller margins to adjacent structures.

In practice, the ASO may be used to close defects up to 40 mm in diameter that have a 5 mm margin to the mitral valve, the orifices of the venae cavae, and the right upper pulmonary vein. A margin of only 2–3 mm to the coronary sinus is acceptable, as the orifice is sufficiently large for some overlap not to significantly limit flow. The anterosuperior (aortic) rim is frequently deficient in secundum ASDs. Fortunately, the woven wire nitinol frame of the ASO demonstrates enough flexibility to mould around and 'grip' the aorta. Aneurysmal and fenestrated atrial septa raise other challenging decisions and technical issues that will be addressed in detail later in this chapter.

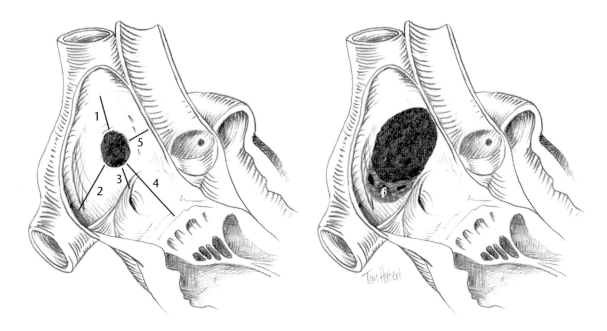

Figure 27.2
Atrial septal defect with optimal (a) and suboptimal (b) characteristics for percutaneous closure. (1–5) Rims to the superior vena cava (1), inferior vena cava (2), coronary sinus (3), tricuspid valve (4), and aorta (5). (6) A fenestrated inferoposterior rim. (Reproduced from Harper et al. Cathet Cardiovasc Interv 2002;57:508–24.[48] This material is used by permission of Wiley-Liss, Inc., a subsidiary of John Wiley & Sons, Inc.)

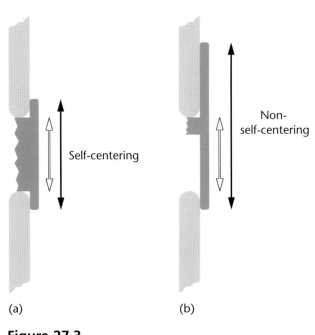

Figure 27.3
Comparison of a non-self-centering device (a) and a self-centering device (b).

Technique of ASD closure

Preprocedure

Preprocedural assessment of suitability for percutaneous closure of ASDs is best done by transthoracic echocardiography (TTE) and transesophageal echocardiography (TEE).[1] Three-dimensional echocardiography constructed from TEE images may improve the evaluation of complex defects;[2–4] however, these reconstructions are not widely available, are time-consuming, and do not provide information novel to the underlying TOE.

Procedure

Intraprocedural echocardiography is essential in guiding the deployment of the closure device. This may be provided either through TEE or intracardiac echocardiography (ICE) from the femoral vein.[5] These imaging modalities are interchangeable for most procedures; however, ICE does permit better visualization of the inferoposterior region near the inferior vena cava. Additionally, ICE enables the operator to gather the images directly rather than through a third party. Unfortunately, ICE probes are disposable and this expense limits the availability of this technology.

General anesthesia is administered routinely to all pediatric patients and to those undergoing intraprocedural TEE to provide airway protection in the supine position. Venous access is obtained via the femoral vein, and there is rarely any difficulty in negotiating a multipurpose diagnostic catheter across the defect. Left atrial angiography adds little information to TEE, and so it is not routinely performed. It is greatly advantageous for the operator to have a clear view of both the fluoroscopic and echocardiographic images, as the deployment procedure is guided by both. All patients receive pretreatment with 48 hours of low-dose aspirin and low-dose intravenous heparinization at the commencement of the procedure. In addition, intravenous antibiotics are administered for endocarditis prophylaxis.

Sizing the defect

Accurate sizing is of the utmost importance in avoiding both embolization of the device and the expense of changing to a device of another size. The defect is sized by the use of inflated sizing balloons, using either a 'dynamic' measurement passing the balloon through the defect or a 'static' measurement of the balloon within the defect.[6]

The multipurpose catheter across the defect is replaced with an exchange length 0.035 inch J-tipped guidewire, which is ideally positioned in the left upper pulmonary vein for stability. A sizing balloon larger than the anticipated defect size is chosen and passed across the defect using a sheath-less technique.

The 'dynamic' balloon sizing is performed with a spherical Meditech balloon (Boston Scientific Corporation, Waterdown, MA), which is inflated with a 30% contrast,

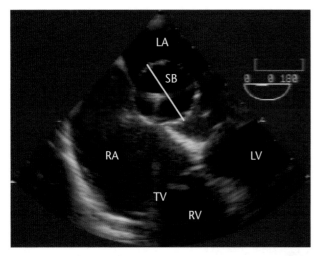

a

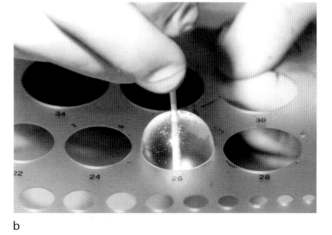

b

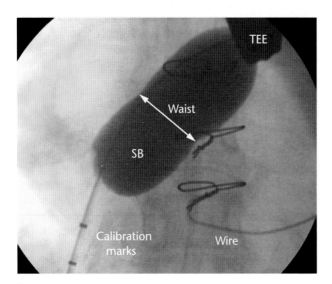

c

Figure 27.4
(a,b) Meditech sizing balloon shown at the size that crossed the defect (a) and at confirmation of size with a sizing plate (b). (c) Amplatzer sizing balloon with indentation by a defect. SB, sizing balloon; LA, left atrium; RA, right atrium; TV, tricuspid valve; RV, right ventricle; LV, left ventricle; TEE, transesophageal probe. (Reproduced from Harper et al. Cathet Cardiovasc Interv 2002;57:508–24.[48] This material is used by permission of Wiley-Liss, Inc., a subsidiary of John Wiley & Sons, Inc.)

70% saline solution. The balloon is inflated free in the body of the left atrium to a size larger than the defect and then firm traction is placed on the balloon catheter to appose it to the septum. TEE is reviewed to ensure that there is no persistent color flow across the defect and that there is no color flow from additional defects.

The balloon is slowly deflated with firm but not undue traction until it 'pops' through the defect into the right atrium. The diameter at which this occurs is the 'stretched balloon diameter' (SBD) and it is carefully measured by TEE (Figure 27.4a). TEE measurement correlates well with fluoroscopic measurement and subsequent confirmation with a sizing plate (Figure 27.4b). If there is more than a 1 mm difference, the balloon is reinserted and the measurements repeated.

The 'static' balloon measurement is performed using the Amplatzer balloon (AGA Medical Inc., Golden Valley, MN). This balloon is cylindrical and highly compliant. It is inflated across the defect such that a waist is formed (Figure 27.4c). The diameter of the waist can then be measured with TEE and radiologically using calibration markers on the balloon catheter. The advantages of this balloon are that it has a short inflation/deflation cycle and that it distorts the septum less than the 'dynamic' maneuver of the Meditech balloon; however, it is more expensive and tends to 'melon seed' in larger defects. Furthermore, distortion of the septum with the Meditech balloon probably more closely resembles what actually occurs with the ASO than does the cylindrical Amplatzer balloon. Familiarity with both balloon sizing techniques is advisable.

In some patients, the atrial septum has a flap valve-like anatomy where a larger Meditech balloon can be pushed through the defect into the left atrium than can be pulled back into the right atrium. This may be recognized by the way in which the septum forms a flap, bowing into the left atrium (Figure 27.5). In these cases, the reverse push size can be used or a 'static' measurement can be made.

Choice of device size

Postmortem[7] and three-dimensional echocardiographic studies[8] have shown that most ASDs are not circular in shape, and indeed change shape during the cardiac cycle.[9] However, irregular and oval defects conform to the circular cross-section of the sizing balloon during the SBD measurement. Therefore, the SBD accurately reflects the size that the defect will be under the radial stress of the waist of the ASO once in position. The SBD is always larger than the preprocedural TOE assessment, which is not performed under stretch. The disparity between the two measurements depends upon the nature of the defect rims, as flimsier rims are more easily pushed aside by the balloon and the device (Figure 27.6).

For most ASDs, a device of 1–4 mm diameter greater than the SBD is chosen to ensure device stability. Factors that influence this decision are the defect shape, the resistance to 'dynamic' balloon measurement and the

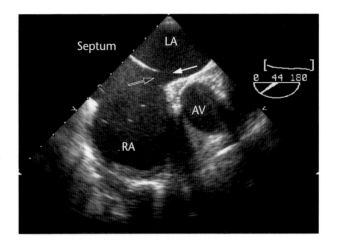

Figure 27.5
Flap valve-like atrial septum. This septal anatomy permits a larger sizing balloon to push from the right to left atrium (hollow arrow) than to pull from the left to right atrium (solid arrow). Such anatomy requires a 'dynamic' 'reverse' push or a 'static' balloon sizing technique. LA, atrium; RA, right atrium; AV, aortic valve. (Reproduced from Harper et al. Cathet Cardiovasc Interv 2002;57:508–24.[48] This material is used by permission of Wiley-Liss, Inc., a subsidiary of John Wiley & Sons, Inc.)

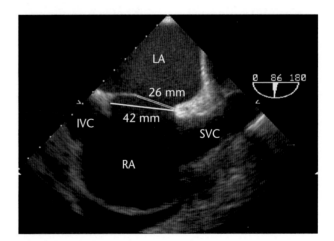

Figure 27.6
Preprocedural transesophageal echocardiogram illustrating the disparity between atrial septal defect sizing at rest (solid line) and with balloon stretch (hollow line). LA, left atrium; RA, right atrium; IVC, inferior vena cava; SVC, superior vena cava. (Reproduced from Harper et al. Cathet Cardiovasc Interv 2002;57:508–24.[48] This material is used by permission of Wiley-Liss, Inc., a subsidiary of John Wiley & Sons, Inc.)

appearance of the rims, particularly the aortic rim. When the aortic rim is absent, the device is more oversized to ensure that the atrial flanges are well splayed around the aorta. This presents the flat segment of the flange rather than its edge to the vessel wall, which is thought to minimize risk of subacute perforation.

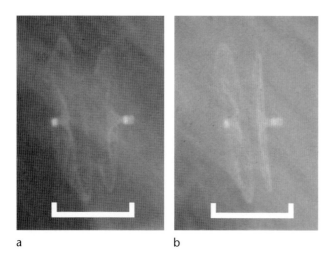

a   b

Figure 27.7
Oversizing of the device causes incomplete expansion of the waist and prevents the atrial discs from flattening, leading to 'mushrooming' (a). This conformation resolves with time (b). (Reproduced from Harper et al. Cathet Cardiovasc Interv 2002;57:508–24.[48] This material is used by permission of Wiley-Liss, Inc., a subsidiary of John Wiley & Sons, Inc.)

If an ASO is oversized in relation to the ASD, the waist will not be permitted to fully expand to its remembered shape. The continuous weave of the nitinol wires results in the atrial discs also not achieving their flat remembered shape, and the device remains somewhat bulky, or 'mushroomed'. This is of little consequence if there is no compromise of adjacent structures, as with time the atrial septum accommodates the waist and the device flattens (Figure 27.7).

Deployment

Once the device size has been selected, the right atrial screw pin is attached to the delivery cable with a clockwise motion. Care should be taken that the device can spin freely on the thread before tightening, to ensure that it is not 'cross-threaded'. It is important that the device be attached firmly enough to avoid premature release but not so firm as to prevent subsequent unscrewing. It is worth noting the appearance of the attachment. The thin threaded portion of the delivery cable screw is entirely drawn into the right atrial pin. If this becomes visible radiologically during manipulation, the device has loosened and is at risk of premature release (Figure 27.8).

The device is then loaded backwards into the delivery tube while providing some tension on the device by hand to aid in its elongation. This helps to prevent the delivery tube flaring, which hinders later connection to the delivery sheath. It is essential to appreciate the degree of elongation that the device undergoes when drawn into the sheath. This is most dramatic with the larger sizes, and must be understood in order to later safely deploy the

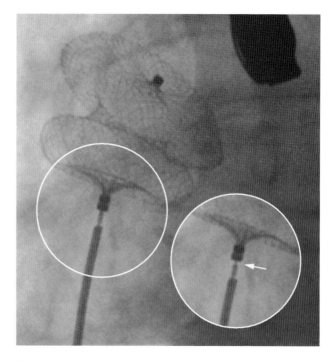

Figure 27.8
Outline of the delivery cable and right atrial pin with the device firmly attached, and the appearance of the thin delivery cable screw with loosening of the device. Note the visible thread (arrow).

device in the desired position across the septum. The device is loaded under heparinized saline to avoid air entrapment within the device and is left there while the delivery sheath is positioned.

Each device has a recommended delivery sheath ranging from 6 to 12 Fr in size. The preshaped delivery sheath and dilator are inserted over the exchange wire only as far as the right atrium. The dilator is then removed, which entrains air into the delivery sheath. The sheath is then permitted to generously back-bleed, prior to advancing the tip into the left atrium and again after the guidewire is removed. Air that is inadvertently released into the left atrium in the supine position preferentially passes anteriorly into the right coronary artery and may result in transient inferior ST-segment elevation with assorted arrhythmias.[10–12] There are reports in the literature of transient cerebrovascular ischemic events possibly related to air embolism.[13,14]

The delivery sheath is filled with contrast immediately prior to attaching the delivery tube, which enables excellent opacification of the delivery sheath tip. The delivery tube must therefore be connected efficiently to avoid loss of opacification through back-bleeding at this point. It is worth noting that the delivery cable should be permitted to rotate clockwise freely as the delivery tube is attached. Until the deliberate act of device release, any rotational movement of the device relative to the delivery cable should be fastidiously avoided. Once the delivery tube has been attached, the device is delivered through into the delivery sheath, with some initial resistance. It is desirable to select a generously sized sheath to avoid unnecessary force on the device and possible rotation.

The device is advanced until it reaches the tip of the delivery sheath. It is essential to ensure that the tip of the sheath is free in the body of the left atrium or at the junction of the left upper pulmonary vein and the left atrium. This is observed on TEE and also by the way in which the contrast is displaced out of the sheath as the device advances. Advancing the device out of a sheath abutting the left atrial wall has been reported to perforate the atrium, leading to tamponade and necessitating emergency surgery. Advancing the device into the left atrial appendage or deep into a pulmonary vein can prevent the device from unwinding into its remembered shape, leading to twisting of the device (see the discussion of twisting deformation of the device later in this chapter). This is reversible, but requires device removal and reloading.[15]

The significant elongation of the device in the delivery sheath (Figure 27.9:A) demands a careful balance of movement between retraction of the delivery sheath and advancement of the delivery cable during deployment (Figure 27.9:B). If deployment is performed only with delivery cable advancement, the device will be positioned entirely in the left atrium against the free wall, which may risk perforation (Figure 27.9:C). If deployment is performed with only delivery sheath retraction, the device will be positioned proximally – as low as the inferior vena cava with large devices (Figure 27.9:D).

The left atrial disc is opened in the body of the left atrium under fluoroscopic and echocardiographic guidance by gentle retraction of the delivery sheath and advancement of the delivery cable (Figure 27.10B). The waist of the device is then opened, so that it may act to self-center the device in the defect (Figure 27.10C). The delivery sheath and cable are then retracted as a unit to bring the waist through the defect and the left atrial disc into apposition with the septum. Once septal resistance is encountered, the right atrial disc is deployed by further retraction of the delivery sheath. Modest tension must be maintained on the delivery cable, as this holds the left atrial disc apposed to the septum; however, as the disc deploys and shortens longitudinally, the delivery cable will need to be advanced somewhat. Consistent modest tension on the delivery cable is the key to correct deployment of the right atrial disc (Figure 27.10D).

Once the device has been deployed, it is essential to confirm by TEE or ICE that both discs have opened and flattened on the correct side of the defect.[1,16] Direct

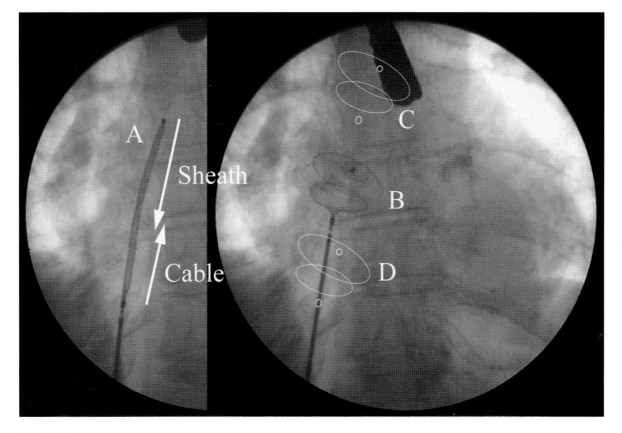

Figure 27.9
Correct deployment of the device (A) requires a balanced retraction of the delivery sheath and advancement of the delivery cable. (B) Balanced deployment. (C) Predominant delivery cable advancement. (D) Predominant delivery sheath retraction.

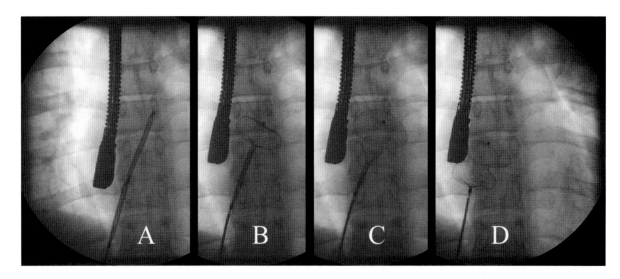

Figure 27.10
Sequence of device deployment. (A) Device within sheath before deployment. (B) Left atrial disc opened. (C) Left atrial disc and waist opened and retracted onto the septum. (D) Right atrial disc opened in the right atrium.

observation of septal tissue between the discs in all planes is ideal. Careful assessment of adjacent structures is carried out to ensure that the device offers no interference.

A small amount of shunting through the center of the device is usually seen immediately after deployment, because the polyester patches do not seal completely while the patients are heparinized. Such shunting may persist for a few days.

Shunting around the periphery of the device needs more careful assessment. It is most commonly due to the angular tension that the delivery cable maintains on the device, which distorts the septum from its normal plane (Figure 27.11a). This type of shunting resolves with release of the device (Figure 27.11b). Septal angulation of greater than 60° suggests that the device is not correctly aligned, and redeployment should be considered.[16]

Shunting through additional defects will have been identified during balloon sizing; however, small perforations in the margins of the defect rim (Figure 27.2:6) are likely to be covered by the released device and to be

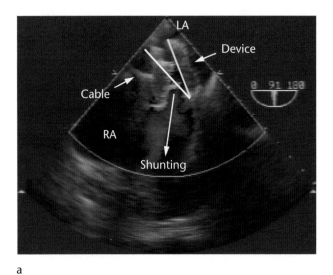
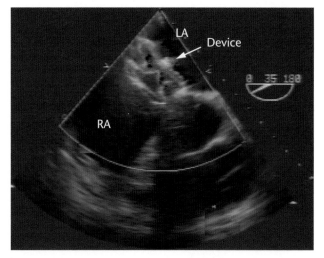

a

b

Figure 27.11
(a) Extreme septal distortion by the tension of the delivery cable, resulting in left-to-right interatrial shunting through the device. (b) Resolution of septal distortion after delivery cable release and elimination of shunting. Solid line: plane of septum under delivery cable tension. Hollow line: plane of septum after release of tension. LA, left atrium; RA, right atrium. (Reproduced from Harper et al. Cathet Cardiovasc Interv 2002;57:508–24.[48] This material is used by permission of Wiley-Liss, Inc., a subsidiary of John Wiley & Sons, Inc.)

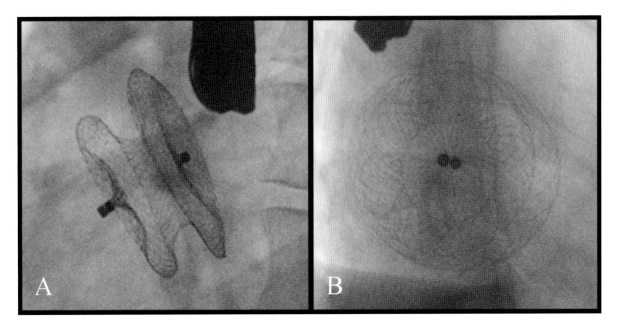

Figure 27.12
Deployed and released Amplatzer Septal Occluder device in profile (A) and en face (B).

sealed with subsequent endothelialization and fibrotic response.

Once the echocardiographic assessment of the position is complete, the stability of the device is tested. The delivery cable is firmly pushed forward to ensure that the right atrial disc does not prolapse into the left atrium, and is then pulled back to ensure that the left atrial disc does not prolapse into the right atrium. This to-and-fro maneuver is known as the 'Minnesota wiggle'.[17] Once this has been performed, the device is released by a counter-clockwise rotation of the delivery cable. Upon release of the delivery cable tension, the device springs superiorly and leftward as the septum returns to its natural position (Figure 27.12).

Anatomical challenges

Large ASDs

There are two difficulties in closing ASDs that are larger than 30 mm. Firstly, large defects are more likely to approach adjacent structures. A device large enough to close the defect securely occupies a great proportion of the septal area and may encroach on the atrioventricular valves or venae cavae (Figure 27.13).

Secondly, it is more difficult to deliver a device correctly into a large defect when the rims are less substantial. It is common for the inferoposterior rim to be flimsy and the anterosuperior (aortic) rim entirely deficient. The delivery sheath arises from the inferior vena cava and, despite its curve, approaches the septum from an inferior

oblique angle. The left atrial disc therefore tends to open across the septum into both atria rather than exclusively in the left (Figure 27.14). Fortunately, the ASO may be retracted and redeployed multiple times until a satisfactory position is achieved, although after four or five

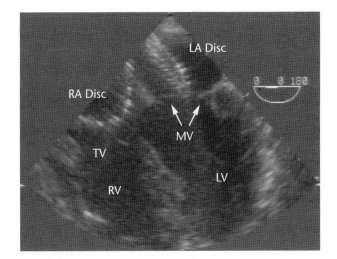

Figure 27.13
Successful deployment of a 40 mm Amplatzer Septal Occluder in a large atrial septal defect with deficient anterosuperior rim. Unfortunately, the left atrial (LA) disc encroached into the mitral valve, necessitating removal. RA, right atrial; MV, mitral valve; TV, tricuspid valve; LV, left ventricle; RV, right ventricle. (Reproduced from Harper et al. Cathet Cardiovasc Interv 2002;57:508–24.[48] This material is used by permission of Wiley-Liss, Inc., a subsidiary of John Wiley & Sons, Inc.)

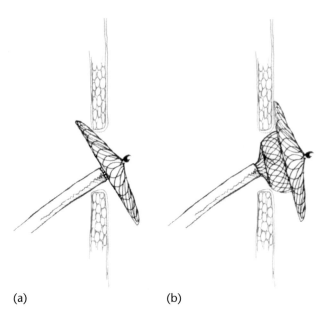

(a)   (b)

Figure 27.14
Alignment of the device with the septum may be difficult in large atrial septal defects due to the inferior oblique angle of the delivery sheath from the inferior vena cava (a). Alignment is often aided by early deployment of the waist (b).

unsuccessful attempts it is prudent to withdraw the device to clean, resecure, and then redeploy it.

Maneuvers to reposition the delivery sheath are often of great assistance where it is difficult to achieve coaxial alignment of the device with the septum. Commencing deployment from different regions of the left atrium by rotating the entire delivery sheath to the left atrial appendage (counterclockwise) or to the right upper pulmonary vein (clockwise), may enable the left atrial disc to 'catch' on the septum and remain on the left atrial side. Deploying the waist after the device has been apposed to the septum may also assist. Finally, increasing the curve of the delivery sheath and dilator by moulding it out of the body may permit the necessary angle of approach. These difficulties are particularly found in the common setting where the anterosuperior (aortic) rim is deficient and the device must grip the aorta itself (Figure 27.15). Such defects can be the most technically challenging.

Multiple ASDs

Multiple ASDs are not uncommon,[18] and range from small perforations in flimsy rims of a defect through a spectrum to multiple distinct defects. As mentioned previously, closely adjacent small defects are managed incidentally in the placement of a device in the primary defect. The device will embrace them between the discs as it stents the defect, and the secondary endothelialization and fibrotic reaction will abolish them.

Defects that are larger and more distinct from one another require careful assessment.[2] When the intervening rim is narrow or flimsy, it is not possible to ensure a secure position for devices. However, when the separating rim is significant, the defects can be addressed with two devices, which may or may not overlap, depending upon the size and proximity of the defects. The technique is a variation on the standard procedure, whereby two venous punctures are made to enable the defects to be addressed simultaneously. The catheter will often favor one defect as it crosses the septum, and it may be useful to occlude the first defect as the second is crossed. The defects are sized

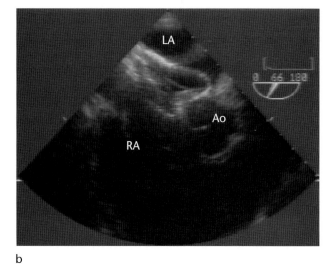

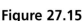

a   b

Figure 27.15
Atrial septal defect (ASD) with deficient aortic rim prior to device deployment (a) and post deployment with the Amplatzer Septal Occluder device splayed around the aortic root (b). LA, left atrium; RA, right atrium; AV, aortic valve; TV, tricuspid valve; RV, right ventricle; Ao, aorta. (Reproduced from Harper et al. Cathet Cardiovasc Interv 2002;57:508–24.[48] This material is used by permission of Wiley-Liss, Inc., a subsidiary of John Wiley & Sons, Inc.)

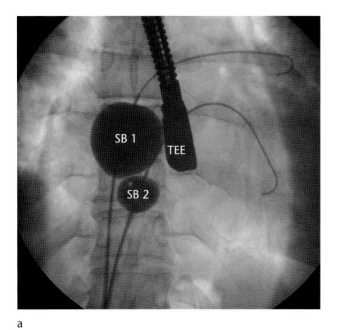

a

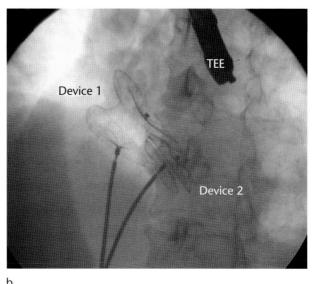

b

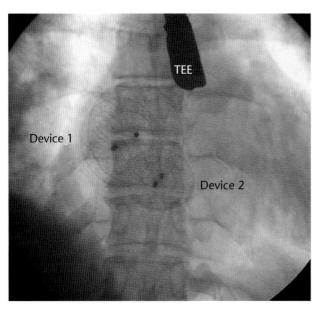

c

Figure 27.16
Closure of two defects with two Amplatzer Septal Occluder (ASO) devices. (a) Simultaneous sizing of the two defects. SB, sizing balloon. (b) Deployment of overlapping ASO. (c) After release. (Reproduced from Harper et al. Cathet Cardiovasc Interv 2002;57:508–24.[48] This material is used by permission of Wiley-Liss, Inc., a subsidiary of John Wiley & Sons, Inc.)

simultaneously to exclude further defects on colour flow (Figure 27.16a), before the devices are sequentially deployed (Figure 27.16b) and released (Figure 27.16c). Where the devices will overlap, it may be easier to inter-lock them if the smaller device is deployed first.[2] The first device should not be released until the security of both devices has been confirmed by echocardiography and the 'Minnesota wiggle'.

Aneurysmal/fenestrated atrial septum

Population-based studies widely estimate the prevalence of atrial septal aneurysms (ASAs) as between 2% and 13%

(using a definition of 15 mm aneurysmal excursion and basal diameter) (Figure 27.17).[19,20] They are commonly associated with PFO, ASDs, or multiple septal fenestra-tions, which impart a higher risk of stroke than PFO alone.[21,22] In addition to their association with PFO, ASAs have been implicated as an independent risk factor for stroke, possibly due to in situ left atrial thrombus forma-tion.[23] Therefore, the indication for percutaneous closure of ASAs includes both shunt reduction and stroke risk reduction. Ideally, closure of the defect will achieve both aims of abolishing interatrial shunting and eliminating the ASA.[24]

There are several treatment options for aneurysmal septa, depending upon the position and size of associated defects (Figure 27.17).[24] In the case of a large ASD, a

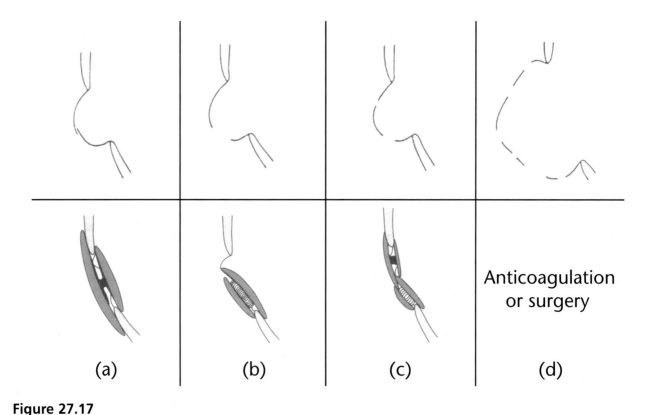

(a)   (b)   (c)   (d)

Anticoagulation
or surgery

Figure 27.17
Anatomical variation of the aneurysmal/fenestrated atrial septum and potential percutaneous closure options. (Adapted from Ewert et al. Heart 2000;84:327–31[24] with permission from the BMJ Publishing Group.)

single ASO device may be able to capture the aneurysmal septum within the discs and achieve both aims. In the setting of a PFO and an aneurysmal septum, this may be achieved with a PFO Occluder. For all but the smallest of aneurysms, the larger PFO Occluder device is advised.

Large aneurysmal septa with multiple perforations are less amenable to percutaneous treatment and require careful echocardiographic assessment and planning to achieve both aims. One option is to perform a balloon septostomy through a central defect to make it large enough to accommodate the desired ASO.[25] This procedure is straightforward due to the flimsy nature of a fenestrated aneurysmal septum. Merely oversizing an ASO may be sufficient. Another option is to place a PFO Occluder (usually the larger) through a central defect to encompass the remaining defects. Finally, a combination of devices may be used to provide appropriate cover. These may be either ASOs or PFO Occluders, or a combination of both. The devices will not assume their final position until the delivery cables are released, since there is often little septal structure to resist the tension of the delivery cables. This can make it difficult to predict the final outcome until the last step of commitment is taken.

Suitability of PFOs for closure

A PFO is a communication between the right and left atria that occurs as a result of incomplete fusion of the septum primum with the septum secundum (Figure 27.18a). As these two structures overlap, the communication is of a flap valve type rather than a discrete hole. Under normal physiological conditions, the higher pressure in the left atrium keeps the flap valve shut. However, if the right atrial pressure exceeds the left atrial pressure either permanently or transiently, such as with straining, the flap valve will open, allowing shunting of venous (desaturated) blood and its constituents into the systemic circulation (Figure 27.18b).

A PFO is present in approximately 25% of the adult population.[26,27] Its incidence declines with age, suggesting that PFOs may close late in life, probably in response to an increase in left atrial pressure. In contrast, the incidence rises in conditions such as chronic pulmonary disease,[28] suggesting that a persistently high right atrial pressure may in some cases render a previously closed foramen ovale patent.

In vivo, a PFO is best diagnosed by contrast TEE.[29,30] Agitated saline is injected into a peripheral vein during a Valsalva maneuver. When the microbubbles appear in the right atrium, the Valsalva is released. The appearance of microbubbles in the left atrium within three cardiac cycles

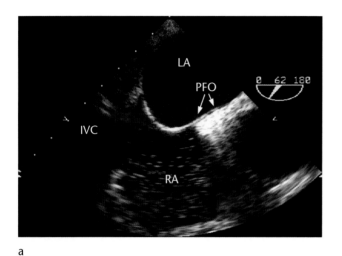
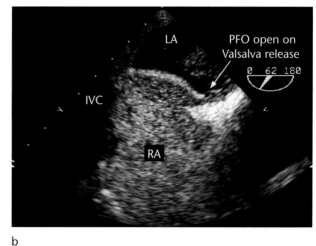

a

b

Figure 27.18
(a) Patent foramen ovale (PFO) seen as a flap valve structure during Valsalva as the right atrium (RA) fills with microbubble echo contrast from the superior vena cava. (b) PFO open with contrast passage into the left atrium (LA) upon Valsalva release. IVC, inferior vena cava.

of Valsalva relief is diagnostic of a PFO. The amount of contrast (number of microbubbles) correlates reasonably closely with the size of the PFO. The size of a PFO may vary from less than 2 mm (small) to greater than 5 mm (large), and is measured by the maximum separation of the two septa during Valsalva.[31] Likewise, the length of the PFO may also vary considerably.

In the vast majority of instances, a PFO is a benign finding, but the anomaly is associated with some pathological entities. For example, the presence of a PFO significantly worsens the prognosis in both major pulmonary embolism[32] and fat embolism.[33] It can cause arterial desaturation in chronic lung disease,[28] it increases the risk of decompression sickness and brain injury in deep sea divers[34,35] and astronauts,[36] it has a significant association with migraine with aura,[37,38] and it is responsible for the rare but disabling platypnea/orthodeoxia syndrome.[39,40] In this latter syndrome, which most commonly occurs after pneumonectomy or in the setting of serious lung disease, patients become markedly hypoxic when assuming the upright posture.

The most serious complication of a PFO is paradoxical embolism of venous thrombus to the systemic circulation. The potential for emboli to pass through a PFO has been demonstrated by over 40 case reports where thrombotic material was observed within a PFO, usually by echocardiography.[41] Unfortunately, thrombus is rarely caught in the act, and identifying which PFOs are responsible for embolic events is difficult since the etiology of systemic embolism is multifactorial. Potential sites of origin include the peripheral arteries and the left atrium and ventricle, in addition to the deep venous system via a paradoxical route through a PFO. Embolic events most commonly include transient ischemic attacks and cerebrovascular accidents, but also include peripheral systemic emboli.

The incidence of PFO in the general population is 25%;[26,27] however, in young (<55 years) people with stroke of unknown origin (cryptogenic), it is as high as 50%.[42,43] This association suggests an etiological role for PFO. On the other hand, 50% of these patients do not have a PFO and therefore must have an alternative cause of stroke (Figure 27.19). It is reasonable to assume that

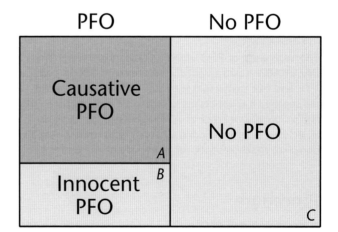

Figure 27.19
Etiology of cryptogenic stroke in young patients. While 25% of the general population have a PFO, 50% of young cryptogenic stroke patients do so: $(A + B)/(A + B + C)$. Of these stroke patients, 50% must have an alternative cause: $C/(A + B + C)$. Assuming that patients with alternative causes for stroke are similar to the general population, 25% will have an incidental innocent PFO: $B/(B + C)$. Therefore of those with cryptogenic stroke and a PFO, only 66% will have a causative PFO: $A/(A + B)$; and 33% will have an innocent PFO: $B/(A + B)$. (Reproduced from McGaw D and Harper R. Intern Med J 2001;31:42–7[44] with permission from Blackwell Publishing.)

25% of those with strokes from an alternative cause will, like the general population, have innocent PFOs. Therefore, one-third of young cryptogenic stroke patients with a PFO will have an innocent PFO and an alternative cause for stroke and the remainder a causative PFO.[44]

In the setting of ischemic stroke, distinguishing an innocent from a causative PFO is difficult. Clinical features such as the presence or absence of overt venous thrombosis is generally unreliable.[44] Small PFOs (<2 mm with <5 microbubbles of shunt) are likely to be innocent. On the other hand, large PFOs (>5 mm), those associated with shunting during normal respiration, and those associated with an atrial septal aneurysm or a highly mobile interatrial septum are likely to be causative.[20,45,46]

Even when a likely causative PFO has been identified, the most appropriate treatment has yet to be defined. Randomized trials comparing medical treatment (warfarin or aspirin) with percutaneous device closure are in progress. Until such data are available, it is reasonable to confine percutaneous closure to patients who have an associated ASA, to those who are intolerant of medical therapy, and to those who have experienced recurrent events despite such therapy. Closure of a PFO is recommended as a preventive measure in deep sea divers and for treatment of the platypnea/orthodeoxia syndrome.

Technique of PFO closure

Preprocedure

The technique of PFO closure is essentially the same as that of ASD closure with the ASO device. Preprocedural TTE and TEE are essential to assess the characteristics of the septum. It is important to assess the nature of the PFO and to identify whether an ASA is present. Performance of an echocardiographic contrast study with normal respiration and Valsalva maneuver is important for comparison with subsequent follow-up studies.

Procedure

A straightforward PFO may be closed easily without the need for an intraoperative TEE, whereas a long tunnel-like PFO or one accompanied by an ASA is better closed under TEE or ICE imaging. General anesthesia should be administered routinely to those requiring intraprocedural TEE. The PFO is almost invariably crossed with a standard multipurpose catheter, but probing the foramen with a sheathed Brockenborough needle can be performed.

Choice of device size

The PFO does not need to be sized, as there is no need to accurately stent the defect with the waist of a device. The thin waist of the PFO Occluder device passes through the defect, and it captures the septum with the two large atrial discs. For this reason, it is also much less common for a PFO Occluder to embolize.

For most PFOs, the smaller PFO Occluder device (25 mm right atrial disc) is sufficient to occlude the defect. In more complex septa, the larger 35 mm device has a particular role to play, as discussed above in the context of aneurysmal/fenestrated atrial septum.

Deployment

The technique of loading and deploying a PFO Occluder device through a delivery sheath is the same as for an ASO device, with the exception that the waist is not deployed as a separate identity. Closure of a simple PFO is more straightforward than that of an ASD, as there is rarely any question whether the discs are appropriately deployed on either side of the septum. If the device is radiologically flattened and the 'Minnesota wiggle' is secure, the device is unlikely to embolize. Similar to the ASO device, shunting immediately post deployment through the device will diminish over the next few days as the polyester patches occlude.

Anatomical challenges

Tunnel PFOs

The anatomy of PFO varies from a short flap to a long tunnel-like structure (Figure 27.20). It is possible that a long tunnel-like PFO may distort the waist of a closure device, resulting in device distortion and malapposition of the atrial discs to the septum. This problem has been described with an umbrella-type device, where a recommendation was made to perform a transseptal puncture through the foramen ovale.[47] In this way, the device could be preferentially deployed through a short iatrogenic defect rather than the long native PFO. Although this has also been described for the Amplatzer PFO Occluder,[48] the flexible waist of the PFO Occluder accommodates all but the longest tunnel-like PFO adequately (Figure 27.21).

Technical challenges

Entrapment of right atrial structures

The eustachian valve is found at the junction of the inferior vena cava and the right atrium, where in utero it directs oxygenated blood from the placenta across the foramen ovale. In some patients, this structure is redundant or even forms a mobile fibrillary structure termed a Chiari network (Figure 27.22). It has been described as becoming

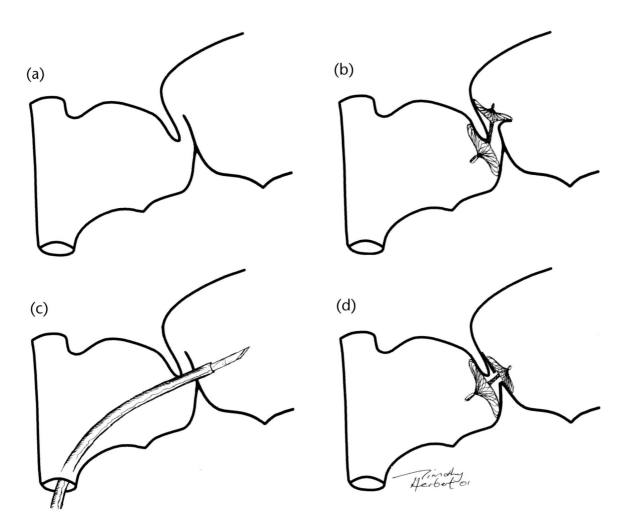

Figure 27.20
(a) Schematic of a 'tunnel' patent foramen ovale (PFO). (b) Malalignment of a PFO closure device after deployment through the 'tunnel'. (c) Transseptal puncture through the foramen ovale region permitting satisfactory deployment (d). (Adapted from Ruiz CE et al. Cathet Cardiovasc Interv 2001;53:369–72.[47] This material is used by permission of Wiley-Liss, Inc., a subsidiary of John Wiley & Sons, Inc.)

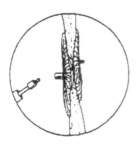

Figure 27.21
Amplatzer Patent Foramen Ovale Occluder waist flexing through a 'tunnel-like' patent foramen ovale. From AGA Medical.

tangled with the delivery sheath and protruding across an ASD into the left atrium during ASO deployment.[49,50] Obviously, if not recognized, this may serve as a nidus for thrombus formation. Withdrawing the delivery sheath and recrossing the defect,[49] or using a steerable electrophysi-ology catheter inserted from a separate venous puncture to displace it laterally, have been described.[50]

Twisting deformation of the device

During deployment of an ASO, the left atrial disc rotates counterclockwise as it exits the delivery sheath and returns to its remembered shape. In a similar way, the central waist and right atrial disc also rotate. If this rotation is impeded by the device being opened in the orifice of the left atrial appendage or a pulmonary vein, then the device may become twisted and assume a 'cobra head' appearance (Figure 27.23). This does not damage the device; however, the twist must be manually corrected, which requires extraction from the patient prior to redeployment.[15,51–53] This deformity is most common with the left atrial disc, but has also been described in the right atrial disc.

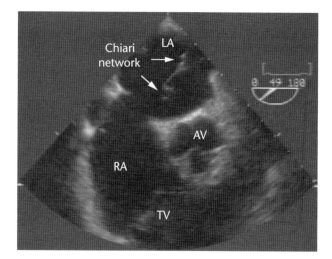

Figure 27.22
A prominent eustachian valve or Chiari network arising from the inferior vena cava–right atrial junction may become entangled by the delivery sheath and advanced into the left atrium (LA). RA, right atrium; AV, aortic valve; TV, tricuspid valve. (Reproduced from Harper et al. Cathet Cardiovasc Interv 2002;57:508–24.[48] This material is used by permission of Wiley-Liss, Inc., a subsidiary of John Wiley & Sons, Inc.)

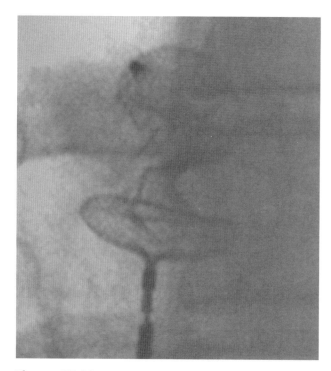

Figure 27.23
Benign 'cobra head' malformation caused by limiting the natural untwisting of the device as it exits the delivery sheath. (Reproduced from Harper et al. Cathet Cardiovasc Interv 2002;57:508–24.[48] This material is used by permission of Wiley-Liss, Inc., a subsidiary of John Wiley & Sons, Inc.)

Inability to release a device after deployment

There are two potential reasons why it may not be possible to release a device from the delivery cable after it has been deployed. Firstly, the device may be too firmly attached to the cable or 'cross-threaded'. This leads to an increase in the torque felt on the delivery cable during attempted release. Secondly, the device may not have enough purchase on the septum to prevent it from rotating freely with the cable. This problem is more likely to occur with the nonstenting waist of the PFO Occluder, and is differentiated by the absence of increasing torque on the delivery cable. In either case, the device must be retracted into the delivery sheath and removed. Ideally, the sheath tip is advanced back into the left atrium after the right atrial disc has been captured, so that access across the defect is not lost. The removed device is then examined and attached more loosely for redeployment, or replaced if 'cross-threaded'.

Inability to withdraw a device into the delivery sheath

One of the great strengths of the Amplatzer Occluder devices is the ease with which they can be recaptured in the delivery sheath and redeployed multiple times. However, difficulty in withdrawing a fully deployed device into the delivery sheath has been described.[48] This is invariably due to damage of the delivery sheath tip such

that the device no longer collapses down and enters smoothly. Unfortunately, the delivery sheath also has a tendency to kink and concertina when undue force is applied in retracting a device. For this reason, selection of a generously sized delivery sheath is advised. If retraction of the device is not possible, then the sheath may be exchanged for a larger one over a dockable delivery cable extension produced by AGA Medical for this purpose.

Retrieval of a device after release from the delivery cable

Embolization of a closure device is one of the more serious complications, but fortunately is rare and is usually confined to more difficult closures of larger defects. Careful defect sizing, postdeployment echocardiographic examination, and the 'Minnesota wiggle' are important steps to minimize this risk.

Embolization of a device may occur as a result of inadvertent premature release before correct placement has been achieved or after deliberate release of a device thought to be correctly placed but in fact not sufficiently secure in the septum. In the latter instance, such displacement may occur in the first 24 hours after deployment and may be asymptomatic. Most cases reported in the literature have embolized to the right heart or pulmonary circulation, but some have embolized to the left ventricle or aortic bifurcation.[54]

Retrieval of a displaced release device is technically difficult and can only be achieved successfully by snaring the right atrial pin and pulling the device into a large sheath. Depending on the site of embolization, movement of the device can render this task difficult. In these circumstances, the device may be sufficiently stabilized to enable the right atrial pin to be captured by first snaring a guidewire through the device via a separate puncture.[55]

Success

Procedural success in device deployment is now extremely high. With improved understanding of the importance of the stretched balloon diameter in ASO sizing and the management of defects with deficient rims.

Studies also show that the rate of immediate complete abolition of shunting is 97.4%, which rises to 99.1% by 12 months,[54] and the rate of device embolization has fallen to 0.4%.[54]

Complications

The most serious complication reported so far is one case of fatal subacute perforation of the aorta. This complication is thought to be more likely to occur when the edge of a closure device has pressed against the aorta. Compared with most ASD closure devices, the flexible rounded nature of the Amplatzer device makes this complication less likely – hence, it is recommended to slightly oversize the device when the aortic rim is deficient so as to allow the device to mould to the shape of the aorta. Other complications include atrial arrhythmias, which are rare and easily treated with medical therapy or electrical cardioversion.[54] Thromboembolic events have been reported in four patients.[54] Adequate heparinization at the time of procedure and preprocedural aspirin is thought to minimize this small risk.

Follow-up

Routine postprocedural follow-up is important, since both underlying atrial septal pathology and device embolization are frequently asymptomatic. Routine chest X-ray and TTE should be performed on day 1 post procedure and repeated within a few months. TEE is required to exclude residual shunting, which, once abolished, probably renders further investigations redundant.

These devices are reported to be fully endothelialized by 6 months, and until this time patients should receive at least antiplatelet therapy with low-dose aspirin. Similarly, they should receive antibiotic prophylaxis for any procedures that would warrant it over this time period.

Patent ductus arteriosus

Suitability of PDAs for closure

A PDA is a persistent communication between the pulmonary artery and the proximal descending aorta. Like the foramen ovale, the ductus arteriosus forms an integral part of the fetal circulation but is pathological in the adult circulation. The indication for closure of PDA in the child and adult is universal. A persistently patent ductus should be closed because of the long-term risks of right heart volume overload and infective arteritis. Traditionally, PDA has been closed by placement of thrombogenic coils, which remain an economic means of closure. However, the use of coils is limited to only some of the anatomical variations of PDA.

Technique of PDA closure

Preprocedure

Preprocedural assessment of suitability for percutaneous closure of PDA is best done by TTE and TEE. The duct itself is seen poorly by TEE, although TTE is adequate; however, other associated congenital abnormalities requiring surgical correction need to be excluded. PDA is classified anatomically[56] according to the narrowest part of the ductus (Figure 27.24), which may be found at the junction with the pulmonary artery (type A), aorta (type B), neither (type C), or both (Type D). Others are more bizarre in their anatomy (type E). Almost all PDAs may be closed with an ADO, although type C are, not surprisingly, at most risk of device embolization.

Procedure

Fluoroscopic guidance of PDA closure is possible, since opacification of the ductus with contrast affords adequate anatomical assessment. Intraprocedural echocardiographic guidance is not required, and therefore general anesthesia is unnecessary. Intravenous antibiotics are administered for infective arteritis prophylaxis; however, aspirin therapy is not routinely given.

Vascular access is required via both the femoral arterial and venous routes. A pigtail catheter is placed in the proximal descending aorta and an aortogram is performed in a steep left anterior oblique projection. This opens the aortopulmonary window and allows visualization of the ductus arteriosus (Figure 27.25a). A selective image of the

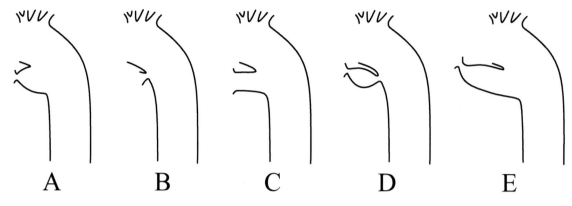

Figure 27.24
Classification of patent ductus arteriosus according to anatomical variation. (Adapted from Krichenko et al. Am J Cardiol 1989;63:877–80.[56])

ductus is then performed using a Judkins left coronary catheter. This image best defines the anatomy of the ductus (Figure 27.25b).

A multipurpose catheter is then passed from the pulmonary artery into the ductus and down the descending aorta (Figure 27.25c). The use of a straight guidewire may facilitate this maneuver. If localization of the ductus is difficult, passage of a guidewire through the Judkins catheter from the aorta to the pulmonary artery through

the ductus may serve as a guide. Once in the descending aorta, the multipurpose catheter is then replaced by an exchange-length J-curve guidewire, and a balloon-tipped catheter (Berman Angiographic Catheter, Arrow International Inc., Reading, PA) is advanced into the ductus for ductus sizing. The balloon is filled with the contrast/saline mix and a standard 'dynamic' balloon sizing is performed (Figure 27.25d). This is an essential step, as the duct often stretches to a much greater diameter than that

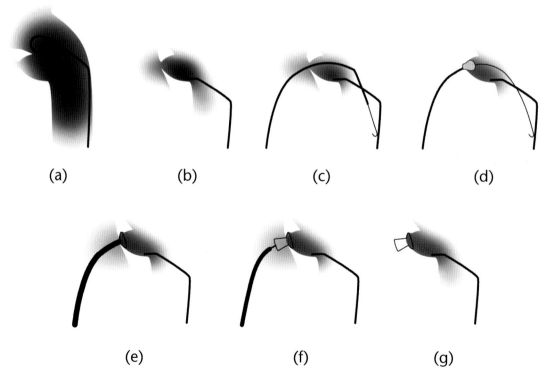

Figure 27.25
Schematic sequence of Amplatzer Ductal Occluder deployment in a patent ductus arteriosus: (a) aortogram; (b) selective ductal angiogram; (c) passage of multipurpose catheter from pulmonary artery to aorta; (d) balloon sizing of ductus; (e) deployment of aortic retention disc; (f) deployment of device body; (g) final selective ductal angiogram.

measured radiologically. Reliance on the radiologically measured diameter may result in the insertion of a device that is too small, thus compromising stability or resulting in an incomplete occlusion. The device size should be 1–2 mm larger than the stretched balloon size to ensure that it is firmly held by the ductus.

An Amplatzer PDA delivery catheter is exchanged for the balloon, and the device is loaded and advanced using the standard Amplatzer techniques. The aortic retention disc is opened in the ampulla or free in the aorta (Figure 27.25e) before the device and sheath are drawn into the ductus and the body of the device is unsheathed. The device should adopt a 'champagne cork' appearance as its neck is compressed by the ductus (Figure 27.25f). The retention disc should sit flat outside in the ampulla, with the body in the neck of the ductus.

A 'Minnesota wiggle' confirms device security prior to release by anticlockwise rotation of the delivery cable. Immediately after release, a selective ductus angiogram demonstrates flow from the aorta to the pulmonary artery; however, this ceases within a few minutes (Figure 27.25g). This sequence is also illustrated with cine images (Figure 27.26).

Technical challenges

Inability to cross the ductus

It is invariably possible to cross the ductus arteriosus from the aorta to the pulmonary artery. In general, this is most easily performed with a more curved catheter such as a Judkins left coronary catheter. Deployment of the ADO device requires access across the duct from the pulmonary artery side. If it is not possible to cross directly with the above techniques, then a snare must be used. This is best done by passing an exchange-length guidewire from the aorta through the ductus into a waiting snare in the pulmonary artery. The snare with captured exchange-length guidewire can then be drawn out of the venous sheath to provide pulmonary artery-to-aortic access.

Success

The success rate of immediate complete closure is reported as 93–95%,[57,58] which increases toward 100% by 1 month.[59] Closure may be confirmed by immediate TTE in addition to the final ductus angiogram.

Complications

Potential complications such as mechanical hemolysis have been described, but fortunately are rare and have been treated percutaneously with subsequent insertion of occlusive coils.[60,61] Device embolization also is fortunately rare, although it has occurred in early series in undersized devices. The device may embolize into the pulmonary bed or down the descending aorta.[62,63] The risk of embolization is greater in type C PDA, where the retention disc may be simply indenting the tubular ductus (Figure 27.24). Encroachment into the aortic lumen is possible in infants. It this occurs, then the device should be removed prior to release.

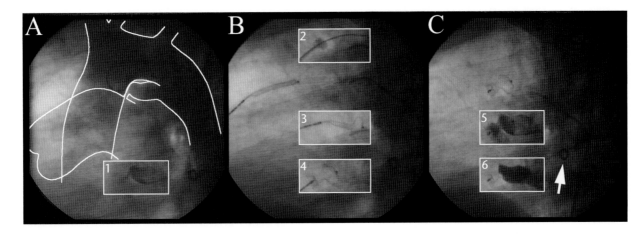

Figure 27.26
Cine image sequence of Amplatzer Ductal Occluder deployment in a patent ductus arteriosus. (A) Aortogram with selective ductal angiogram (insert 1). (B) Deployment of device with balloon sizing (insert 2), aortic retention disc deployment (insert 3), and deployment of the device body (insert 4). (C) Postrelease images showing 'champagne cork' appearance and contrast passage through the device immediately post deployment (insert 5), with complete occlusion after 10 minutes (insert 6).

Conclusions

Percutaneous transvenous closure of ASDs, PFO, and PDA is now feasible using safe and practical later-generation closure devices. Short- and intermediate-term follow-up data have demonstrated high success and low complication rates. Although definitive data regarding long-term follow-up and late complications are not yet available, a viable alternative to surgery has been achieved.

References

1. Cooke JC, Gelman JS, Harper RW. Echocardiologists' role in the deployment of the Amplatzer Atrial Septal Occluder device in adults. J Am Soc Echocardiogr 2001;14:588–94.
2. Cao Q, Radtke W, Berger F, et al. Transcatheter closure of multiple atrial septal defects. Initial results and value of two- and three-dimensional transoesophageal echocardiography. Eur Heart J 2000;21:941–7.
3. Acar P, Saliba Z, Bonhoeffer P, et al. Influence of atrial septal defect anatomy in patient selection and assessment of closure with the Cardioseal device; a three-dimensional trans-oesophageal echocardiographic reconstruction. Eur Heart J 2000;21:573–81.
4. Zhu W, Cao QL, Rhodes J, Hijazi ZM. Measurement of atrial septal defect size: a comparative study between three-dimensional transesophageal echocardiography and the standard balloon sizing methods. Pediatr Cardiol 2000;21:465–9.
5. Hijazi Z, Wang Z, Cao Q, et al. Transcatheter closure of atrial septal defects and patent foramen ovale under intracardiac echocardiographic guidance: feasibility and comparison with transesophageal echocardiography. Cathet Cardiovasc Interv 2001;52:194–9.
6. Hijazi ZM. Measurement of the stretched diameters of atrial septal defects. Catheter Cardiovasc Interv 1999;46:58.
7. Ferreira SM, Ho SY, Anderson RH. Morphological study of defects of the atrial septum within the oval fossa: implications for transcatheter closure of left-to-right shunt. Br Heart J 1992;67:316–20.
8. Marx GR, Fulton DR, Pandian NG, et al. Delineation of site, relative size and dynamic geometry of atrial septal defects by real-time three-dimensional echocardiography. J Am Coll Cardiol. 1995;25:482–90.
9. Franke A, Kuhl HP, Rulands D, et al. Quantitative analysis of the morphology of secundum-type atrial septal defects and their dynamic change using transesophageal three-dimensional echocardiography. Circulation 1997;96: II-323–7.
10. Formigari R, Santoro G, Rossetti L, et al. Comparison of three different atrial septal defect occlusion devices. Am J Cardiol 1998;82:690–2.
11. Chan KC, Godman MJ, Walsh K, et al. Transcatheter closure of atrial septal defect and interatrial communications with a new self expanding Nitinol double disc device (Amplatzer Septal Occluder): multicentre UK experience. Heart 1999;82:300–6.
12. Demkow M, Ruzyllo W, Konka M, et al. Transvenous closure of moderate and large secundum atrial septal defects in adults using the Amplatzer Septal Occluder. Cathet Cardiovasc Interv 2001;52:188–93.
13. Godart F, Rey C, Prat A, et al. Atrial right-to-left shunting causing severe hypoxaemia despite normal right-sided pressures. Report of 11 consecutive cases corrected by percutaneous closure. Eur Heart J 2000;21:483–9.
14. Windecker S, Wahl A, Chatterjee T, et al. Percutaneous closure of patent foramen ovale in patients with paradoxical embolism: long-term risk of recurrent thromboembolic events. Circulation 2000;101:893–8.
15. Cooke JC, Gelman JS, Harper RW. Cobrahead malformation of the Amplatzer Septal Occluder device: an avoidable compilation of percutaneous ASD closure. Cathet Cardiovasc Interv 2001;52:83–5; discussion 86–7.
16. Salaymeh KJ, Taeed R, Michelfelder EC, et al. Unique echocardiographic features associated with deployment of the Amplatzer atrial septal defect device. J Am Soc Echocardiogr 2001;14:128–37.
17. Masura J, Gavora P, Formanek A, Hijazi ZM. Transcatheter closure of secundum atrial septal defects using the new self-centering Amplatzer Septal Occluder: initial human experience. Cathet Cardiovasc Diagn 1997;42:388–93.
18. Podnar T, Martanovic P, Gavora P, Masura J. Morphological variations of secundum-type atrial septal defects: feasibility for percutaneous closure using Amplatzer Septal Occluders. Cathet Cardiovasc Interv 2001;53:386–91.
19. Agmon Y, Khandheria BK, Meissner I, et al. Frequency of atrial septal aneurysms in patients with cerebral ischemic events. Circulation 1999;99:1942–4.
20. Homma S, Di Tullio MR, Sacco RL, et al. Characteristics of patent foramen ovale associated with cryptogenic stroke. A biplane transesophageal echocardiographic study. Stroke 1994;25:582–6.
21. Cabanes L, Mas JL, Cohen A, et al. Atrial septal aneurysm and patent foramen ovale as risk factors for cryptogenic stroke in patients less than 55 years of age. A study using transesophageal echocardiography. Stroke 1993;24:1865–73.
22. Mas JL, Arquizan C, Lamy C, et al. Recurrent cerebrovascular events associated with patent foramen ovale, atrial septal aneurysm, or both. N Engl J Med 2001;345:1740–6.
23. Berthet K, Lavergne T, Cohen A, et al. Significant association of atrial vulnerability with atrial septal abnormalities in young patients with ischemic stroke of unknown cause. Stroke 2000;31:398–403.
24. Ewert P, Berger F, Vogel M, et al. Morphology of perforated atrial septal aneurysm suitable for closure by transcatheter device placement. Heart 2000;84:327–31.
25. Carano N, Hagler DJ, Agnetti A, Squarcia U. Device closure of fenestrated atrial septal defects: use of a single Amplatzer atrial septal occluder after balloon atrial septostomy to create a single defect. Cathet Cardiovasc Interv 2001;52:203–7.
26. Hagen PT, Scholz DG, Edwards WD. Incidence and size of patent foramen ovale during the first 10 decades of life: an autopsy study of 965 normal hearts. Mayo Clin Proc 1984;59:17–20.
27. Meissner I, Whisnant JP, Khandheria BK, et al. Prevalence of potential risk factors for stroke assessed by transesophageal echocardiography and carotid ultrasonography: the SPARC study. Stroke Prevention: Assessment of Risk in a Community. Mayo Clin Proc 1999;74:862–9.
28. Soliman A, Shanoudy H, Liu J, et al. Increased prevalence of patent foramen ovale in patients with severe chronic obstructive pulmonary disease. J Am Soc Echocardiogr 1999;12:99–105.

29. Belkin RN, Pollack BD, Ruggiero ML, et al. Comparison of transesophageal and transthoracic echocardiography with contrast and color flow Doppler in the detection of patent foramen ovale. Am Heart J 1994;128:520–5.

30. Baguet JP, Besson G, Tremel F, et al. Should one use echocardiography or contrast transcranial Doppler ultrasound for the detection of a patent foramen ovale after an ischemic cerebrovascular accident? Cerebrovasc Dis 2001;12:318–24.

31. Kerut EK, Norfleet WT, Plotnick GD, Giles TD. Patent foramen ovale: a review of associated conditions and the impact of physiological size. J Am Coll Cardiol 2001;38:613–23.

32. Konstantinides S, Geibel A, Kasper W, et al. Patent foramen ovale is an important predictor of adverse outcome in patients with major pulmonary embolism. Circulation 1998;97:1946–51.

33. Forteza AM, Koch S, Romano JG, et al. Transcranial Doppler detection of fat emboli. Stroke 1999;30:2687–91.

34. Moon RE, Camporesi EM, Kisslo JA. Patent foramen ovale and decompression sickness in divers. Lancet 1989;i:513–14.

35. Knauth M, Ries S, Pohimann S, et al. Cohort study of multiple brain lesions in sport divers: role of a patent foramen ovale. BMJ 1997;314:701–5.

36. Bendrick GA, Ainscough MJ, Pilmanis AA, Bisson RU. Prevalence of decompression sickness among U-2 pilots. Aviat Space Environ Med 1996;67:199–206.

37. Anzola GP, Magoni M, Guindani M, et al. Potential source of cerebral embolism in migraine with aura: a transcranial Doppler study. Neurology 1999;52:1622–5.

38. Wilmshurst PT, Nightingale S, Walsh KP, Morrison WL. Effect on migraine of closure of cardiac right-to-left shunts to prevent recurrence of decompression illness or stroke or for haemodynamic reasons. Lancet 2000;356:1648–51.

39. Waight DJ, Cao QL, Hijazi ZM. Closure of patent foramen ovale in patients with orthodeoxia-platypnea using the Amplatzer devices. Cathet Cardiovasc Interv 2000;50:195–8.

40. Rao PS, Palacios IF, Bach RG, et al. Platypnea–orthodeoxia: management by transcatheter buttoned device implantation. Cathet Cardiovasc Interv 2001;54:77–82.

41. Aboyans V, Lacroix P, Ostyn E, et al. Diagnosis and management of entrapped embolus through a patent foramen ovale. Eur J Cardiothorac Surg 1998;14:624–8.

42. Lechat P, Mas JL, Lascault G, et al. Prevalence of patent foramen ovale in patients with stroke. N Engl J Med 1988; 318:1148–52.

43. Webster MW, Chancellor AM, Smith HJ, et al. Patent foramen ovale in young stroke patients. Lancet 1988;ii:11–12.

44. McGaw D, Harper R. Patent foramen ovale and cryptogenic cerebral infarction. Intern Med J 2001;31:42–7.

45. Hausmann D, Mugge A, Daniel WG. Identification of patent foramen ovale permitting paradoxic embolism. J Am Coll Cardiol 1995;26:1030–8.

46. Steiner MM, Di Tullio MR, Rundek T, et al. Patent foramen ovale size and embolic brain imaging findings among patients with ischemic stroke. Stroke 1998;29:944–8.

47. Ruiz CE, Alboliras ET, Prophal SG. The puncture technique: a new method for transcatheter closure of patent foramen ovale. Cathet Cardiovasc Interv 2001;53:369–72.

48. Harper R, Mottram P, McGaw D. Closure of secundum atrial septal defects with the Amplatzer Septal Occluder device: techniques and problems. Cathet Cardiovasc Interv 2002;57:508–24.

49. Cooke JC, Gelman JS, Harper RW. Chiari network entanglement and herniation into the left atrium by an atrial septal defect occluder device. J Am Soc Echocardiogr 1999;12:601–3.

50. McMahon CJ, Pignatelli RH, Rutledge JM, et al. Steerable control of the eustachian valve during transcatheter closure of secundum atrial septal defects. Cathet Cardiovasc Interv 2000;51:455–9.

51. Arora R, Kalra GS, Singh S, et al. Transcatheter closure of atrial septal defect using self-expandable septal occluder. Indian Heart J 1999;51:289–93.

52. Taeed R, Shim D, Kimball TR, et al. One-year follow-up of the Amplatzer device to close atrial septal defects. Am J Cardiol 2001;87:116–18.

53. Waight DJ, Hijazi Z. Amplatzer devices: benign cobrahead formation. Cathet Cardiovasc Interv 2001;52:86–7.

54. Omeish A, Hijazi ZM. Transcatheter closure of atrial septal defects in children and adults using the Amplatzer Septal Occluder. J Interv Cardiol 2001;14:37–44.

55. Peuster M, Boekenkamp R, Kaulitz R, Fink C, Hausdorf G. Transcatheter retrieval and repositioning of an Amplatzer device embolized into the left atrium. Cathet Cardiovasc Interv 2000;51:297–300.

56. Krichenko A, Benson LN, Burrows P, et al. Angiographic classification of the isolated, persistently patent ductus arteriosus and implications for percutaneous catheter occlusion. Am J Cardiol 1989;63:877–80.

57. Thanopoulos BD, Hakim FA, Hiari A, et al. Further experience with transcatheter closure of the patent ductus arteriosus using the Amplatzer Duct Occluder. J Am Coll Cardiol 2000;35:1016–21.

58. Masura J, Walsh KP, Thanopoulous B, et al. Catheter closure of moderate- to large-sized patent ductus arteriosus using the new Amplatzer Duct Occluder: immediate and short-term results. J Am Coll Cardiol 1998;31:878–82.

59. Ebeid MR, Masura J, Hijazi ZM. Early experience with the Amplatzer Ductal Occluder for closure of the persistently patent ductus arteriosus. J Interv Cardiol 2001; 14:33–6.

60. Godart F, Rodes J, Rey C. Severe haemolysis after transcatheter closure of a patent arterial duct with the new Amplatzer Duct Occluder. Cardiol Young 2000;10:265–7.

61. Joseph G, Mandalay A, Zacharias TU, George B. Severe intravascular hemolysis after transcatheter closure of a large patent ductus arteriosus using the Amplatzer Duct Occluder: successful resolution by intradevice coil deployment. Catheter Cardiovasc Interv 2002;55:245–9.

62. Bilkis AA, Alwi M, Hasri S. The Amplatzer Duct Occluder: experience in 209 patients. J Am Coll Cardiol 2001; 37:258–61.

63. Simoes LC, Pedra CA, et al. Percutaneous closure of ductus arteriosus with the Amplatzer prosthesis. The Brazilian experience. Arq Bras Cardiol 2001;77:520–31.

28

Carotid and peripheral angiography and intervention

Gishel New, Sriram S Iyer, Jiri J Vitek, Gary S Roubin

Cerebral angiography and carotid artery stenting

The growing use of carotid stenting as an alternative to carotid endarterectomy by interventionalists from a number of different specialty areas (cardiology, radiology, neurology, and vascular surgery) requires an understanding of the entire vascular tree from the aortic arch to the intracranial arteries. Selective angiography of the supraaortic vessels with intracranial views is imperative in order for a rational decision to proceed with carotid stenting (CS) can be made. Intracranial anomalies as well as incidental pathological findings are also important to diagnose. For example, intracranial stenoses, cerebral aneurysms, arteriovenous malformations, and neoplasms need to be identified and may preclude CS. The most common cerebrovascular disease affecting the supraaortic vessels is atherosclerosis; however, fibromuscular dysplasia and traumatic abnormalities may also require stenting. In addition, knowledge of the collateral routes in the cerebral circulation is important for stroke-risk stratification and selection of distal protection devices used during carotid stenting.

Clinical approach

Patients are usually referred with symptoms and/or with carotid duplex and/or magnetic resonance angiography (MRA) or CT angiography (CTA) studies suggesting evidence of either unilateral or bilateral carotid bifurcation disease. Patients should be assessed for the presence of atherosclerotic vascular disease with a thorough history and physical examination. A history of prior stroke, tran-

sient ischemic attack, amaurosis fugax, or carotid endarterectomy (CEA) should prompt a detailed assessment for carotid disease. Clinical examination should document the presence or absence of carotid bruits and evidence of coronary and peripheral vascular disease. The ubiquitous nature of atherosclerosis should raise suspicion in patients with coronary disease or peripheral vascular disease, and should prompt carotid duplex ultrasound studies. If there is a history of stroke or transient ischemic attack or if there is an abnormality on neurological examination, then a computed tomography (CT) or magnetic resonance imaging (MRI) scan of the brain to document baseline cerebral abnormalities should be performed. All patients should be referred for formal assessment by a neurologist to document the pre- and postprocedural clinical neurological status.

The risks and benefits of carotid stenting, and the availability of alternative surgical and medical therapy, should be discussed in detail with all patients. In particular, it should be explained to patients that major complications in experienced operators are rare. The risk of minor stroke is in the 2–4% range.[1] It should be explained to patients and relatives that a minor stroke means either minor weakness or numbness of a limb, vision loss, or dysphasia, that will completely resolve within 1 month. The risk of a major stroke – one that would leave the patient with a permanent disability – is around 0.75% and the risk of a fatal stroke or death is 0.5% (authors' data). These results have improved from previous published data due to the introduction of neuroprotection devices. For patients over 80 years of age, the risks are slightly higher.

Patients are commenced on antiplatelet therapy, soluble aspirin 300 mg daily and clopidogrel (Plavix/Iscover) 75 mg daily, preferably for 4 days prior to the procedure. In all cases, patients should have received a *total* dose of at

Table 28.1   Carotid stenting equipment

Equipment	Diameter	Length	Manufacturer
VTK Torocon Advantage	5 Fr	100 cm	Cook Inc.
Terumo Glidewire – angled tip, stiff	0.038 inch	190 cm	Meditech
Amplatz wire – extra stiff	0.038 inch	260 cm	Cook Inc.
Shuttle sheath	6 and 7 Fr	90 cm	Cook Inc.
Wallstent	10 mm	24 mm	Boston Scientific Corp.
Smart stent	10 mm	20–40 mm	Cordis Endovascular
Predilatation balloon (monorail)	4 mm	40 mm	
Cross-Sail			Guidant Inc.
Postdilatation balloon (monorail)	5.0–5.5 mm	20 mm	
Cross-Sail			Guidant Inc.
Gazelle			Boston Scientific Corp.

least 300 mg of clopidogel prior to the intervention. Antihypertensive medications are withheld on the day of the procedure. Patients should be well hydrated with intravenous saline prior to the procedure.

No premedication, sedation, or general anesthesia is used. Local anesthesia is infiltrated at the femoral access site as for standard angiography. Patients spend one night in hospital and are discharged the next day. The four-vessel cerebral angiogram and carotid stenting can be performed in the same procedure. The patient's head is cradled in a commercially available foam head constraint. The patient is asked to remain as still as possible and focus on the ceiling. A three-lead electrocardiogram monitors the heart rate. Arterial pressure is monitored via a transducer attached to the injection syringe (manifold). Dentures and eyeglasses are removed. Intravenous drugs such as atropine (for bradycardia), aramine (for hypotension), and dopamine (rarely required) and nitroglycerin (for hypertension and arterial spasm) should be available.

Single-plane angiographic equipment with 9″, 7″ and 5″ image magnification is the minimum requirement. Ideally, the catheterization laboratory should have roadmapping and digital subtraction capability to allow detailed examination of intracranial vessels and to minimize contrast load. A variety of subtracted and 'cine' mode ($7\frac{1}{2}$ frames) modalities are utilized. In a routine procedure, initial four-vessel cerebral angiography takes approximately 15–20 minutes and the stenting procedure is completed within another 20–30 minutes.

Postprocedure, the patient should be monitored with hemodynamic (heart rate and blood pressure), groin, peripheral pulses, and neurology observations every 15 minutes for the first hour, and half-hourly for the next 4 hours, then hourly observations for the next 6 hours. Sheaths should be removed as soon as possible, or a closure device can be used. A neurologist should see the patient approximately 24 hours postprocedure to assess neurological status.

Carotid stenting: technique (Table 28.1 and 28.2)

Our current technical approach can best be discussed in the following terms:

1. Four-vessel cerebral angiography
2. Carotid sheath/guide placement
3. Neuroprotection device delivery and deployment
4. Predilatation
5. Stent deployment
6. Postdilatation
7. Neuroprotection device retrieval

Table 28.2   Ten steps to carotid stenting

Step 1	Cannulate CCA with VTK catheter over Glide Wire.
Step 2	Acquire angiogram of carotid bifurcation or 'roadmap' to display origin of ECA.
Step 3	Advance Glidewire into ECA and follow with VTK catheter
Step 4	Replace Glidewire with Amplatz wire
Step 5	Advance sheath into CCA to just below bifurcation
Step 6	Remove Amplatz wire and VTK, 'back bleed', and flush carefully. Heparinize patient via sheath
Step 7	Acquire 'guiding' images of lesion by injecting through sheath side arm
Step 8	Advance neuroprotection device across lesion. Deploy neuroprotection device
Step 9	Advance predilatation balloon across lesion
Step 10	Advance stent across lesion and deploy
Step 11	Postdilate conservatively (size and pressure), depending on ICA diameter
Step 12	Retrieve neuroprotection device
Step 13	Perform final carotid angiogram and AP and lateral intracranial views

Four-vessel cerebral angiography

For most cases, the 5 French (Fr) VTK catheter (Cook Inc.; Figure 28.1) and a 0.038 inch Glidewire (Meditech) can catheterize all brachiocephalic arteries. The distal end of the catheter can be shaped into a double curve with the tip, and when located in the aortic arch it points upward. The proximal curve of this catheter can be opened; this facilitates advancement of the Glidewire into brachiocephalic arteries. The sequence of catheterization of brachiocephalic vessels is usually from left to right, but depends on which side is the most likely to be intervened upon. First, the left subclavian artery, then the left common carotid artery (CCA), and finally the innominate artery are cannulated in the straight anteroposterior (AP) fluoroscopic projection. The catheter can be advanced into the left subclavian artery. Then, slight, slow advancing movements are required to enter the left CCA and to slip the catheter into the innominate artery. After finding the origin of the vessel, the 0.038 inch Glidewire is advanced into the left CCA or the innominate artery. Slight rotation of the catheter within the innominate artery often helps to guide the wire into the right CCA if it tends to select the right subclavian artery. The catheter should never be advanced into the artery alone – only via advancing it over the wire. With difficult and angulated origins of vessels, the catheter should be advanced into the artery over the wire slowly, using a slow, 'push–pull' technique. Deep inspiration and turning of the head of the patient maybe helpful in advancing the catheter over the wire in order to prevent the wire from prolapsing back into the aorta. Occasionally, in extremely dilated aortic arches, a sidewinder-curved catheter is needed (Simmons 3 curve). Some operators prefer less-shaped 5F H$_1$, HINK, or Berenstein diagnostic catheters to perform angiography. The HN$_5$ curve is occasionally useful in the left CCA or left subclavian artery.

Cerebrovascular anatomy

In children and young adults, the aortic arch is a symmetrically curved vascular structure tilted from the right anterior to the left posterior upper mediastinal compartment. The origins of the brachiocephalic arteries are nicely aligned in straight lines and course superiorly. The aging process and especially the atherosclerotic degenerative process elongate the aortic arch, displace the aortic knob more superiorly and posteriorly, and shift the ostia of brachiocephalic arteries. The most common congenital anomaly of the aortic arch is a joint origin of the left CCA and innominate artery. The second is a left CCA originating from the innominate artery itself. In young adults, the left CCA courses superiorly, but with the aging process, it can become elongated and then course to the left with a sharp superior turn. This anatomical variation can make selective catheterization of the left CCA very difficult.

The bifurcation of the CCAs is usually located at the level of the C3 and C4 vertebral bodies; however, higher or lower bifurcations can occur. Within the common carotid bifurcation, the origin of the internal carotid artery (ICA) usually points medially and posterior. The origin of the external carotid artery (ECA) points anteriorly and laterally. For these anatomical reasons, the best projections to separate origins of the ICA and ECA are lateral oblique and pure lateral projections (Figure 28.2). The ECA supplies the facial and meningeal structures. It can also become an important source of collateral blood supply to the brain if the ICA is occluded (via the ophthalmic artery).

The ICA can have kinks, coils, and tortuosities. These are exaggerated by the aging process, atherosclerosis, and shortening of the cervical spine. All of these conditions are prone to produce spasm from guidewire or catheter manipulation and may make delivery and deployment of a distal protection device difficult (Figure 28.3). The cervical segment of the ICA does not have any branches. The cavernous segment of the ICA can be straight or very tortuous. The intracranial segment of the ICA is divided into the clinoidal and supraclinoidal segments. The ophthalmic artery is the first intracranial branch of the ICA from within the clinoidal segment. The posterior communicating and

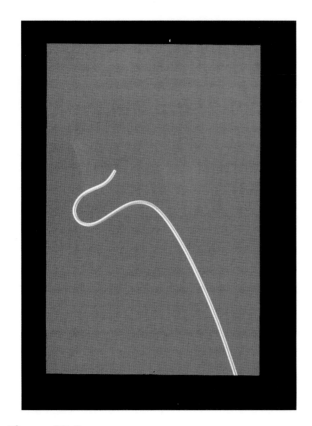

Figure 28.1
The 5 Fr VTK catheter.

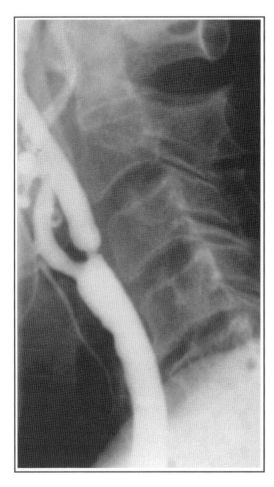

Figure 28.2
A 90° lateral view separates the internal and external carotid arteries.

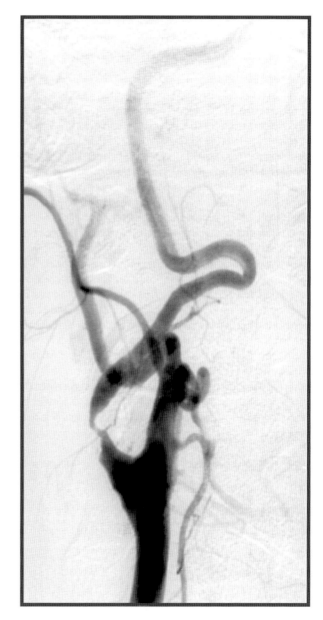

Figure 28.3
Severe kinking and tortuosity of the distal internal carotid artery making delivery of neuroprotection device a challenge.

anterior choroidal arteries originate more distally. The posterior communicating artery can be absent or developed to a degree that it may exclusively supply the posterior cerebral artery. The supraclinoidal segment terminates in a bifurcation where the ICA divides into smaller anterior and larger middle cerebral arteries (Figure 28.4). The horizontal segments of the anterior cerebral arteries (the AI segments) can communicate across the midline through the anterior communicating artery. The horizontal segment of the middle cerebral artery (the MI segment) terminates within the trifurcation in the proximal Sylvian fissure. The distal branches of the middle cerebral artery are the ascending frontoparietal artery, the parietal artery, and the anterior temporal artery. The most important collateral pathways are through the anterior and posterior communicating arteries. These, with the anterior, middle, posterior cerebral, and basilar arteries, form the circle of Willis. This collateral channel can readily compensate for an occluded internal carotid or vertebral arteries. The circle of Willis is not developed in all people. Both anterior and posterior communicating arteries can be hypoplastic or absent. The hemispheric blood supply can

be completely isolated, and can depend only on the ipsilateral ICA in this situation. Even a short, temporary occlusion of this ICA, such as with the use of a balloon occlusion neuroprotection device, can result in significant clinical symptoms. Another, but somewhat less important, brain collateral supply is through the leptomeninges. The small branches of the anterior, middle, and posterior cerebral arteries are connected within the pia mater and can supply peripheral branches of these vessels through retrograde flow. The collateral brain supply through the ECA artery has been mentioned previously.

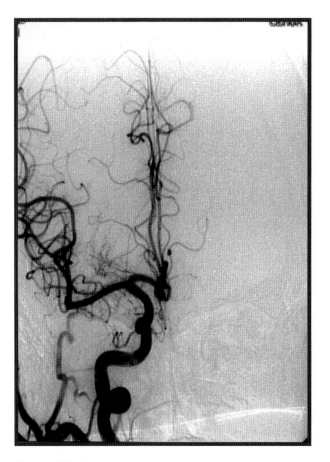

Figure 28.4
Intracranial view of the right internal carotid artery. Note the patency of the anterior communicating artery supplying the contralateral anterior cerebral artery.

Techniques

The catheter is placed in the junction of the aortic arch and the upper thoracic aorta, with its tip pointing to the left. By advancing the catheter into the aortic arch, the catheter reshapes and attains its double curve, with the tip pointing cephalad. In most instances, the tip of the catheter first enters the left subclavian artery. If the catheter does not reshape, folds, or twists to the right, then the Glidewire is used to reposition it. The wire can also be used to 'stiffen' the catheter. The wire should not be advanced beyond the distal tip of the catheter, as this may prevent the tip of the catheter from entering the vessel ostium and may disturb and distend the preshaped catheter curve. After placing the catheter within the proximal left subclavian artery, this vessel is studied. It is essential to carefully aspirate the catheter every time the Glidewire is removed in order to withdraw blood from the catheter to prevent air embolism. A hand injection is performed using a 6 ml control syringe, with the speed of injection adjusted so that the catheter is not ejected from the subclavian artery. This

arteriogram shows the origin of the left vertebral artery. The Glidewire is then used to enter the left vertebral artery. The wire should always enter the artery first, followed by the catheter. To change the direction in which the wire is advanced, the catheter can be rotated, pushed forward, or slightly retracted. These movements with rotation of the angled Glidewire give innumerable possibilities to change direction and angulation in advancing the wire (roadmapping is useful). Once the wire has entered the vertebral artery, the catheter is slipped cephalad over the wire, holding the wire and advancing the catheter. When the wire starts to slip proximally, it is advanced cephalad. Advancement of the catheter (pushing the catheter over the wire) is done slowly, whilst taking advantage of pulsating blood flow. This movement is performed several times until the catheter is securely placed in the vertebral artery. If there is tortuosity of the proximal vertebral artery, it often straightens with the Glidewire. The same technique is used to catheterize both the CCA and the right vertebral artery. After the catheter has entered the desired artery, a slow hand injection is done to confirm the position of the catheter, and to make sure that good blood flow is maintained and that there is no subintimal entry of the contrast agent. The intracranial vasculature is then studied in the AP and lateral projections. Injections of contrast agent into all brachiocephalic arteries should be done by hand and with small amounts of contrast ($\leq$ 6 ml per injection, diluted 50/50 with saline). After completion of the vertebral artery study, the catheter is withdrawn into the proximal subclavian artery, but not into the aortic arch. By keeping the catheter in the subclavian artery, the shape of the catheter is reformed. At this point, the catheter is gently advanced forward up to the moment when it slips into the ostium of the left CCA. Slow injections of contrast agent can be used to confirm the catheter position. Once the origin of the left CCA has been found, the same technique as described for catheterizing the left vertebral artery is employed. The trick is to advance the catheter slowly over the Glidewire while maintaining the wire deep inside the carotid artery. The left wall of the upper thoracic aorta can be used to support advancement of the catheter into the carotid artery. It is important to learn to recognize 'favourable' and 'bad' curves of the catheter that form within the aortic arch while the catheter is advanced into the CCA. If the wire is deep in the carotid artery, the catheter can also be rotated while being advanced to straighten out a 'bad' curve. Whether clockwise or counterclockwise rotation is used depends on the curve formation in the aortic arch.

The catheter is withdrawn proximally, so that the tip is still in the left CCA and the curve of the catheter has reformed. It is then advanced up to the point where it enters into the innominate artery. Again, a small injection of contrast agent confirms the position. The same technique as described in catheterizing the left vertebral artery and left CCA is used to selectively catheterize the right CCA, right subclavian artery, and the right vertebral artery.

AP and lateral projections of both bifurcations and intracranial views of the ICA and its branches should be imaged.

Carotid sheath/guide placement

Once the diagnostic study has been completed and the stenotic internal carotid artery identified, the 5 Fr catheter is advanced, using the 0.038 inch Glidewire, into the ipsilateral ECA (Figure 28.5). Roadmapping can be very useful in identifying the ECA. This is best performed in the lateral projection, as this angle usually demonstrates the maximum separation of the ECA from the ICA. If the stenosis involves the distal CCA, then the wire is kept in the CCA and not advanced past the lesion. The Glidewire is then withdrawn and replaced with an extra stiff 0.038 inch exchange-length Amplatz wire (Cook Inc.; Figure 28.6). The 6 or 7 Fr 90 cm Shuttle sheath (Cook Inc.) is then advanced into the CCA over the Amplatz wire (Figure 28.7). The sheath is slipped over the VTK catheter into the

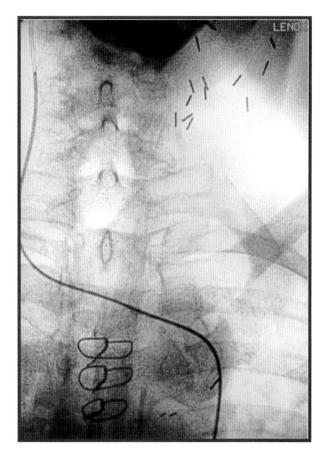

Figure 28.6
The Amplatz exchange wire is advanced in the VTK catheter into the external carotid artery.

CCA and positioned just below the stenosis. The radiopaque band is incorporated in the distal end for accurate positioning. The proximal end of the sheath has an open-ended Tuohey–Bourst manual-adjusting valve seal that permits unimpeded catheter or guidewire introduction. After withdrawing the inner dilator and Amplatz wire simultaneously from the sheath, the sheath can be carefully flushed. Heparin (5000 units) is administered via the sheath.

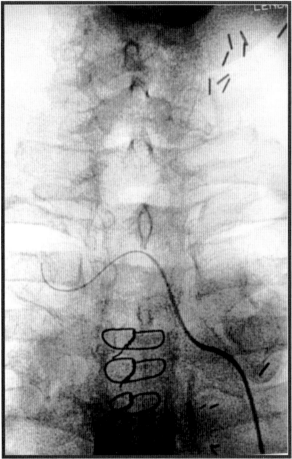

Figure 28.5
The Glidewire is advanced into the innominate, common carotid, and external carotid arteries.

Insertion of the neuroprotection device

Arteriography through the sheath, in the appropriate angulation, is performed to maximize the 'opening' of the bifurcation and the angulation of the lesion and to view the distal ICA for positioning of a neuroprotection device (Figure 28.8). The neuroprotection device is prepared. A number of devices are available. They are in the form of balloon occlusion devices or filters (Figure 28.9). Each device has its unique preparation, mode of deployment,

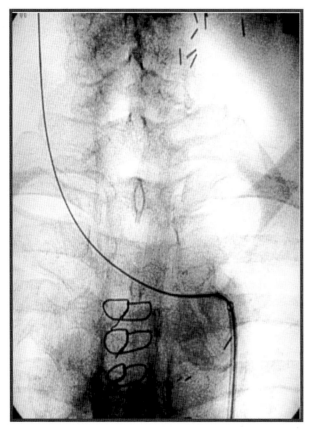

Figure 28.7
The Shuttle sheath is advanced over the Amplatz wire into the common carotid artery.

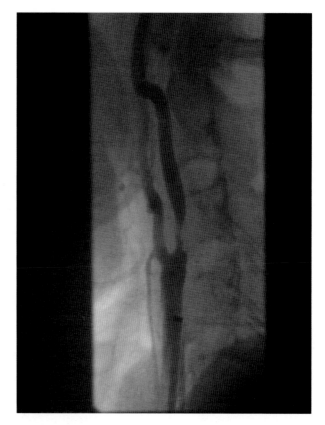

Figure 28.8
Preprocedure angiogram displaying the carotid bifurcation and site for distal protection placement.

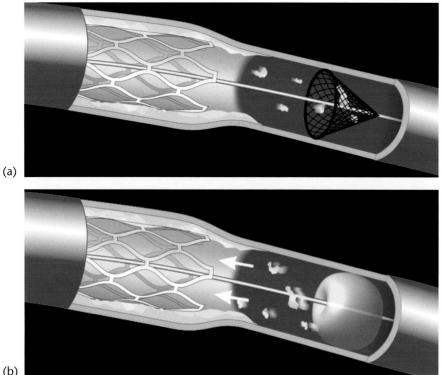

(a)

(b)

Figure 28.9
(a) Diagram of a filter device.
(b) Diagram of a balloon occlusion device.

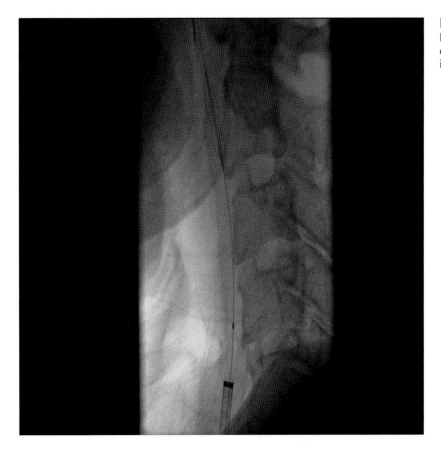

Figure 28.10
Deployment of the neuroprotection device in a distal straight portion of the internal carotid artery.

and retrieval. The techniques involved is the use of each device are beyond the scope of this chapter. Essentially, the stenotic lesion is crossed with a neuroprotection device and delivered to the distal ICA for deployment. Ideally, a straight part of the distal ICA not near a bend or kink should be used. The neuroprotection device is then deployed (Figure 28.10).

Predilatation

If the neuroprotection device cannot cross the stenosis (due to severe tortuosity and/or pre-occlusion) and/or cannot be adequately advanced distal enough to the stenosis, the lesion may be crossed with a 0.014 or 0.018 inch coronary wire and used as a buddy wire to 'straighten-out' the ICA. If this does not allow the neuroprotection device to be advanced easily, then the stenosis can be predilated using a 0.014 inch coronary guidewire and a 2.0 mm × 40 mm coronary balloon. It has been shown that predilatation with a small balloon rarely results in clinically significant emboli. I After deployment of the neuroprotection device, predilatation of the stenosis with a larger (4 mm × 40 mm) coronary balloon is performed (Figure 28.11). The greater length of this balloon has the advantage of preventing it from 'melon-seeding' during the inflation. This predilatation balloon is usually sufficient to

pass the stent smoothly, without encountering major resistance, through the stenosis. One should be mindful of the position of the neuroprotection device and the distal end of the guidewire at all times, ensuring minimal movement during the procedure to avoid distal ICA spasm.

Stent deployment

Self-expanding stents such as the Wallstent (Boston Scientific Corp., Watertown, MA, USA), Memotherm, X-act, Acculink, and Precise stent are most commonly used (Figure 28.12). These stents have several advantages over balloon-expandable stents. First, only one stent is usually required. Second, they are easily deployed using vertebral bodies as landmarks (the distal end of the stent can be deployed from the non-atheromatous of the ICA distal to the stenosis, while the proximal end of the stent will end up across the bifurcation and in the distal CCA). The unconstrained diameter of the self-expanding stent to be deployed should be at least 1–2 mm larger than the largest vessel segment to be covered by the stent. Usually, we use 10 mm × 20 mm stents. Stents can be deployed completely in the ICA with suitable 6 and 8 mm diameters. If the stent is to be deployed across the bifurcation, then an 8–10 mm stent should be utilized. If the self-expanding stent delivery system will not pass through a calcified,

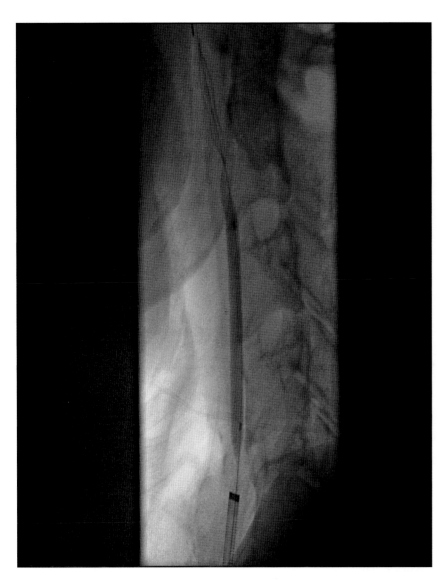

Figure 28.11
Predilatation with a 4.0 mm × 40 mm balloon.

'recoiling' lesion, forcing the current high-profile delivery systems is not advised, as they may break off plaque and cause distal embolization. In this situation, a short 5 mm balloon-expandable stent is deployed to hold the lesion open before passing a definitive self-expanding stent.

Postdilatation

The self-expandable stent is postdilated with either 5.0 mm or 5.5 mm × 20 mm balloon, depending on the size of the internal carotid artery. It is safer to underdilate than overdilate. Overdilatation may squeeze the athero-sclerotic material through the stent mesh and cause cerebral emboli. A 10% residual stenosis has not been shown to cause any problems or increase the rate of restenosis.[1] Furthermore, it is not necessary to dilate the stent to oblit-

erate segments of contrast-filled ulcerated areas external to the stent. This angiographic appearance poststenting is of no prognostic significance, and follow-up angiography has documented complete healing of these 'pockets' over time. Covering the ECA with a stent may cause some 'jail-ing' of the ECA. However, on follow-up arteriograms, the ECA usually remains patent, with only rare exceptions. The ECA is only dilated if it becomes preocclusive and there is TIMI < 3 flow or if it is completely occluded after postdilatation of the stent and the contralateral ECA is also occluded. (Radiologists have for years been coiling or embolizing the ECA for the treatment of severe epistaxis.) The ECA can be accessed through the stent mesh with a 0.014 inch wire and reopened with a 2–4.0 mm coronary balloon. After postdilatation, the neuroprotection device should be retrieved according to protocol. Final angio-grams of the carotid bifurcation and intracranial views are performed prior to removal of the sheath (Figure 28.13).

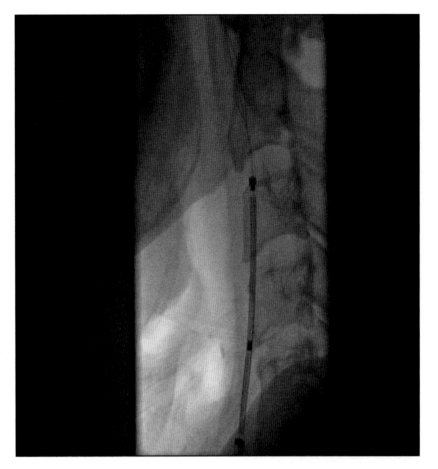

Figure 28.12
Stent deployment.

Procedural monitoring

All carotid angiograms and interventions are performed under only local anaesthesia so that the neurological status of the patient can be continuously monitored. A 'squeeze toy' is placed in the contralateral hand to monitor upper extremity motor functions after each step in the procedure. In addition, the patient is asked to speak and move the contralateral foot to confirm that they are neurologically intact. Continuous monitoring of the heart rate and blood pressure throughout the intervention is mandatory. Bradycardia and even asystole are not uncommon, especially when the bulb of the internal carotid artery is stretched, exerting pressure on the carotid sinus. Atropine (0.6–1 mg) is given prophylactically. Hypotension is managed aggressively with fluid boluses, metaraminol boluses (100–200 μg by push injection), and rarely a dopamine infusion. Loss of consciousness can occur with balloon inflation when the ipsilateral hemispheric blood supply is isolated or if the contralateral carotid artery is occluded. This recovers spontaneously after immediate deflation of the balloon. Occasionally, spasm can develop, especially after placement of the neuroprotection device. This usually resolves with removal of the wire, intraarterial nitroglycerin (100–200 μg), and retraction of the sheath into the arch.

Renal angiography and renal artery stenting

Renal artery stenosis (RAS) can cause two clinical syndromes: renovascular hypertension and ischemic renal failure. RAS can be unilateral or bilateral. If it is unilateral, renal function is not impaired, as the contralateral kidney generally compensates. Three etiologies can cause RAS: atheromatous disease, fibromuscular dysplasia, and rarely Takayasu's arteritis. Atheromatous disease is the most common, and may be associated with disease in other vascular beds (Figure 28.14). Fibromuscular dysplasia is often seen in childhood and young adults and has a characteristic 'string of beads' appearance at angiography (Figure 28.15). RAS can be asymptomatic, and so its prevalence is unclear. Estimates suggest that 10% of patients with coronary heart disease (CHD) for angiography will have RAS. RAS should be looked for in unexplained cases of flash pulmonary edema. It is usually located in the proximal portion of the renal artery and in 80% of cases it involves the ostium. The natural history of RAS is unclear. There have been no prospective angiographic studies.

The clinical manifestations of RAS can be subtle. Progression to occlusion can even be silent and not

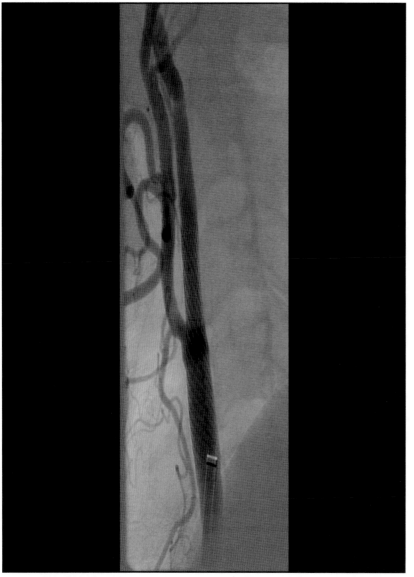

Figure 28.13
Postprocedure angiogram.

associated with impaired renal function. Clinical suspicion should be raised in patients who give a history of recent onset of hypertension, onset at an early or late age, recent deterioration in hypertension, severe or difficult-to-control hypertension, retinopathy, abdominal bruit, and elevation in creatinine after institution of an angiotensin-converting enzyme (ACE) inhibitor (suggestive of bilateral disease). One must consider and exclude the diagnosis in any patient presenting with acute or chronic renal failure.

Screening for RAS can be done using a number of non-invasive tests. These include plasma renin levels, renal Doppler ultrasound, renal captopril studies, and CT or MRI of the renal arteries. Renal arteriography remains the gold standard for the diagnosis of RAS. Clinical assessment of the patient prior to angiography should focus on cardio-vascular risk factors, evidence of end-organ disease from hypertension, and other vascular disease. Investigations should include urea and electrolytes, creatinine, full blood

evaluation, and prothrombin time. Informed consent and the risks and complications associated with renal angiography and stenting should be discussed with the patient. These involve a small risk of renal failure, perforation, hemorrhage, allergy to contrast, and arterial access complications. It should be emphasized to patients that an improvement in their hypertension and renal impairment may occur but a cure obviating the need for antihypertensive medication is unlikely.

The technique of renal angiography first requires an abdominal angiogram in the AP projection. Between 20% and 30% of people will have an accessory renal artery, which can be missed if non-selective renal angiography is not performed. A pigtail catheter with sideholes (5 or 6 Fr) can be used. The catheter is placed just above the origin of the renal arteries (lower border of the L1 vertebral body). Accessory renal arteries are usually more distal; therefore, it is unlikely that they will be missed if this technique is

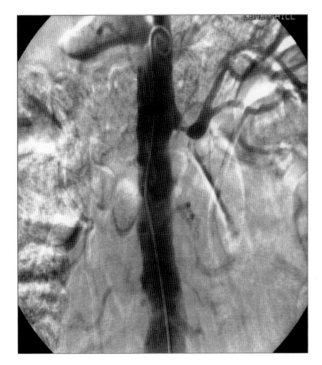

Figure 28.14
Renal artery stenosis due to atherosclerosis.

applied. Oblique views may also be required, as the origin of the right renal artery is more anterior than that of the left, which comes from the posterolateral wall of the aorta. Digital subtraction should be used if available, as it reduces contrast volume (12–15 ml at rates between 6 and 20 ml/s). If an abnormality is noted or if there is uncertainty as to the degree of stenosis, selective renal arteriography may be performed. This allows better visualization but increases

the risk of dissection. A JR4, IMA, Cobra, or Simmons diagnostic catheter can be used with small-volume hand injections of contrast. The angiogram should be performed using the smallest frame size to ensure that the entire kidney parenchymal outlines can be seen on the angiogram.

Renal angioplasty and stenting is performed using femoral or brachial (in caudal angulation of the proximal renal artery) arterial access. A short sheath is inserted into the artery, cannulated in the usual fashion. Heparin is administered to achieve an activated clotting time (ACT) above 250 s. A method whereby a diagnostic catheter is inserted into a guiding catheter is often used to nontraumatically engage the ostium of the renal artery. Guide catheters specially designed for renal artery cannulation are available. A Hockey-Stick coronary guide also has a suitable angle. A 5 Fr diagnostic catheter (IMA or JR4) with a Touhey–Bourst is inserted into the guiding catheter. The ostium of the renal artery is engaged with the diagnostic catheter. A 0.014 inch floppy coronary wire inside an exchange balloon catheter is advanced through the diagnostic catheter, which itself is inside the guiding catheter. The lesion is then crossed with the floppy coronary wire. A hydrophilic wire may be required for preocclusive lesions. The balloon (usually 2.0 mm × 20 mm) is then advanced across the stenosis. Predilatation should be gentle, just to eliminate the waste in the balloon to allow passage of the stent but not aggressive (to avoid atheroembolization). The over-the-wire balloon can then be advanced distal in the renal artery, and the 0.014 inch floppy wire is exchanged for a more supportive wire (Iron Man [Guidant Inc., Temecula, CA, USA] or an 0.018 inch wire). We do not advocate using a 0.035 inch wire, as this increases the risk of perforation and embolization, and the 0.035 inch wire can also distort the lesion and cause spasm. After a supportive wire has been advanced into the

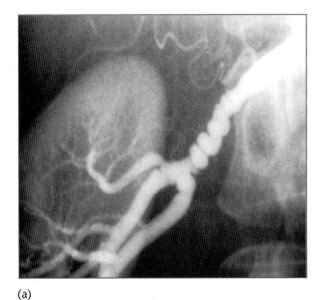

(a)

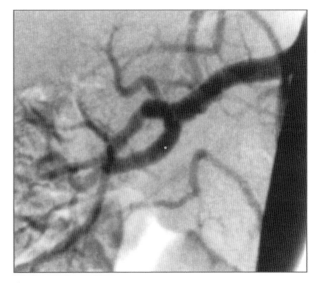

(b)

Figure 28.15
Renal artery stenosis due to fibromuscular dysplasia: (a) pre- and (b) post-stenting.

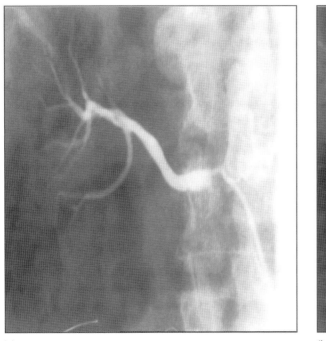
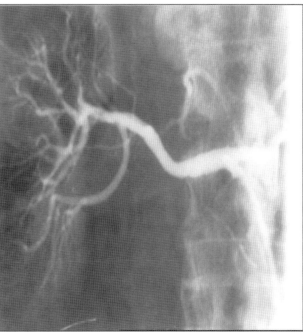

(a)   (b)

Figure 28.16
Pre (a) and post (b) renal angioplasty and stenting of angiograms.

renal artery, the balloon catheter and diagnostic catheter are removed, and in the same step the guiding catheter is advanced and seated in the ostium of the renal artery. This step is important for support during insertion and for accurate positioning and deployment of the stent. Stenting is usually mandatory, as it is necessary if heavily calcified or ostial lesions are to be adequately eliminated. It also reduces restenosis rates. Some operators have used distal protection devices; however, significant embolization of atheroma is rare when coronary wire and balloon systems are employed. Balloon-expandable stents are advised. Stent and balloon sizing should be in a 1 : 1 ratio with arterial diameter (usually 6 mm) and length should be according to the lesion. High-pressure balloon dilatation, as in the coronary circulation, is not advised. Back pain during balloon dilatation is of concern, and should alert the operator to a perforation if it persists. Stent positioning is critical, and care should be taken to cover the ostium by hanging the stent out into the aorta by 1–2 mm. Because of the location of the ostium, oblique views may be required. The guide catheter must be adequately seated in the ostium of the renal artery before the stent exits the guide. If this is not ensured, it may be very difficult to advance the stent across the stenosis. The stent on the balloon catheter with the guide catheter is then advanced across the stenosis. The guide catheter is retracted to cover just the proximal part of the stent. A contrast injection should be performed to identify the renal ostium. Minor foreshortening of the stent should be factored into its positioning. The guide catheter should be retracted out of the ostium without moving the position of the stent. The

stent is then expanded by inflating the balloon to nominal pressure. The guide catheter is reinserted into the stent in order to easily retract the balloon catheter after deflation Postdilatation is rarely necessary. Overdilatation can cause perforation. A final contrast injection is performed (Figure 28.16).

Patients are usually premedicated with aspirin and clopidogrel. The clopidogrel is prescribed (300 mg loading and 75 mg maintenance) for at least 1 month and aspirin is lifelong. Glycoprotein IIb/IIIa inhibitors are not recommended. Postoperative care is as per other interventional procedures. Marked changes in blood pressure are not usually noted. Using this or similar techniques, the technical success rate for renal stenting is over 90%. Restenosis rates vary according to published series.

Abdominal/lower limb angiography and iliac/lower limb artery stenting

Although there are now many noninvasive tests that are excellent for screening, including Doppler ultrasound, CT, and MRA, abdominal and peripheral angiography remains the 'gold standard' for evaluating the patency and distribution of blood vessels and for planning interventions. Angiography is also useful in evaluating aneurysms, vascular malformations, arteriovenous fistula, traumatic abnormalities, graft and stent patency, and thromboembolic disease. The procedure is usually performed via a femoral or brachial artery approach, and 4–6 Fr sheaths and catheters are used as in coronary procedures. Digital subtraction angiography (DSA), where background tissues and structures are subtracted and contrast in the vessels appears black, is preferred. This allows for better definition of the arterial tree, which may be obscured by bony structures if coronary cine angiography is employed. With the patient holding their breath, abdominal structures do not move, and contrast outlining the arterial tree can be clearly visualized. A variety of postprocessing capabilities and 'roadmapping' facilities are now available in standard angiography suites, allowing operators to adjust images after acquisition. Complications from angiography are usually very low (<1%), and include hematoma, pseudoaneurysm, arteriovenous fistula, spasm, retroperitoneal hemorrhage, and arterial occlusion. Knowledge of the arterial anatomy of the lower limbs is imperative prior to learning this procedure.

The simplest technique for abdominal and peripheral angiography is to gain arterial access and insert a short sheath via retrograde femoral artery cannulation. A standard 0.035 inch angled or J wire (an alternative is a Glidewire [Boston Scientific Corp., Watertown, MA, USA] or a Wholey [Mallinckrodt, St Louis, MO, USA]) is used to advance a pigtail catheter into the abdominal aorta. The pigtail end of the catheter is placed at the level of the renal arteries and the wire is removed. An upper abdominal and renal angiogram is the first angiogram that is acquired (see the discussion of renal angiography above). After this image, the pigtail catheter should be pulled back to where the aorta bifurcates into the common iliac vessels near the bottom of the screen. A useful trick is to put the first image up on the fixed screen and to not move the image intensifier down until the pigtail is in position. This allows one to see where the bifurcation is from the previous image. The image intensifier is then moved down so that the pigtail is at the top of the screen and the image will include the common iliac bifurcation and internal and external iliac vessels. If this procedure is performed for each angiogram, no section of the arterial tree will be missed. This second angiogram should also be performed in the AP projection with a similar amount of contrast as used in the first angiogram.

With a large 15° image intensifier, simultaneous bilateral lower extremity imaging can be performed. This allows the entire length of both legs to be imaged with one bolus of contrast. This technique appears to be time- and contrast-saving. However, it has some limitations. First, opacification of distal vessels may be reduced with the catheter in the aorta. If there is more disease in one limb, there may also be discrepancies between contrast transit times in the two limbs, impairing vessel opacification. Second, the patient may find it difficult to remain still for the longer period of time required for this technique. Finally, disease at the distal bifurcation of the common iliac

and at the bifurcation of the femoral artery may not be appreciated if oblique views are not obtained. There are two alternative techniques involving bilateral selective catheterization of the common iliac that avoid these problems mentioned above.

The first technique is to take multiple-injection single-field lower extremity filming. In all the subsequent angiograms of the lower limbs, the shutters can be used to narrow the field range and to improved visualization of the artery. From 5 to 10 ml of half-strength contrast, either via an injector, pump or hand injection, can be used. The pigtail catheter is pulled back into the common iliac of the side of arterial access. To open up and view the common iliac distal bifurcation into external and internal iliac arteries, a 15° contralateral oblique view is required. In this way, a stenosis at the common iliac bifurcation may be identified that may have not been appreciated in the AP view. Similarly, an ipsilateral 30° angle with 30° caudal is used to open up the femoral artery bifurcation into the superficial femoral and the profunda arteries.

If there is no disease in the external iliac and femoral arteries, the pigtail catheter can be pulled back into these vessels to improve opacification of the lower limb images. The patient's legs should be placed in an inverted ('pigeon-toed') position so as to expose the origin of the anterior tibial artery. The AP projection is used for the following angiograms of the lower limb, Approximately 4–6 subsequent angiograms, depending on the size of the image intensifier, will be required to completely visualize the lower limb. Lower limb DSA is the preferred filming modality and patients must keep their legs still but are not required to hold their breath for these images. The image intensifier is moved down the leg to film the entire lower limb down to the ankles. Using the second screen to view the prior image and noting bony landmarks will prevent missing any portion of the artery. To acquire similar pictures of the contralateral limb, one must pass a slippery wire (Glidewire or Wholey) in the pigtail catheter up into the abdominal aorta. With the wire ahead of the catheter, the pigtail shape can be straightened. Then, as one pulls the catheter back proximal to the bifurcation, the pigtail curve can reform and slip over the horn, and the wire can be advanced down the contralateral iliac artery. This is a skill that requires some practice. A 5 Fr IMA, JR4, or SOS catheter may be helpful in cases where the angle of the common iliac bifurcation is very acute. The slippery wire should be advanced down the contralateral femoral artery and the catheter advanced as distal in the femoral artery as possible (providing there is no disease in the artery). After this has been done, the catheter can be attached to an injector pump or hand injections of contrast can be used. Images of the contralateral limb are obtained in exactly the same way as described for the first leg.

An alternative to this single-field film technique of imaging below the femoral artery is known as a 'bolus chase' examination. After the pigtail catheter has been placed in the external iliac or femoral artery, a bolus of contrast is injected. The image intensifier is positioned at the uppermost position (lower abdomen). As the bolus of contrast agent transits and begins to fill the femoral arteries, the operator moves the table while the image intensifier remains in a fixed position. The operator must ensure that the image intensifier is as caudal as possible, to allow for the distal portion of the lower limb to be visualized. The table movement must be synchronized with the flow of contrast. The speed of motion of the table can be slowed to coincide with areas where opacification is delayed. An angiogram of the entire leg can be obtained in this manner. The contralateral leg is imaged in a similar way after access has been obtained via the method mentioned above.

Angioplasty and stenting of the lower limb arterial tree below the aortic bifurcation is an increasing alternative to operative intervention. The low morbidity, reduced recovery time, and low complication rate have led to its increasing utilization. The use of vascular stents has expanded the indications and enabled improved angiographic success rates. However, debate still exists regarding the long-term restenosis rates for stents versus angioplasty alone. Standard doses of heparin, aspirin, and clopidogrel are used. Angioplasty and stenting of the iliac vessels is a relatively simple technique. In contrast, femoral artery angioplasty is preferred over stenting to preserve the femoral artery for future arterial access.

Retrograde femoral artery access with a short sheath on the ipsilateral side is one technique used. No guiding catheter is required. A 0.035 inch wire system (SuperCore [Guidant, Temecula, CA, USA], Wholey, or Glidewire) can be used to cross the stenosis. If a lesion is preocclusive, then a 0.018 or 0.014 inch wire can be used on a balloon catheter for support. Predilatation with an undersized balloon (usually 6.0″) is recommended. Heavily calcified stenoses may require a noncompliant balloon. It is recommended that balloon-expandable stents be used for lesions at the aorto-iliac bifurcation. Self-expanding stents are usually used for lesions distal to the bifurcation (Figure 28.17). Postdilatation with a balloon no larger than a 1 : 1 ratio can be used. Balloon inflations are usually prolonged. However, care must be taken to not overinflate a balloon in an iliac vessel, as perforation, often heralded by back or loin pain, can lead to fatal retroperitoneal hemorrhage. Occasionally, simultaneous femoral and brachial arterial access may be required when attempting to cross complex lesions. Kissing balloon and stent techniques with bilateral femoral artery access have also been described for complex aorto-iliac stenoses.

Angioplasty and stenting of the superficial femoral artery (SFA) and popliteal artery can be performed via contralateral retrograde or antegrade femoral artery access. In the contralateral retrograde technique, a long sheath is inserted (going up and over the horn and down the contralateral iliac) after angiography (using a stiff wire such as 0.035 inch SuperCore) with the distal end in the contralateral femoral artery. This provides the extra support required to advance a stent 'up and over' the iliac bifurcation. Stenoses or occlusions can also be crossed with 0.035 inch wires (SuperCore or Glidewire). Intimal

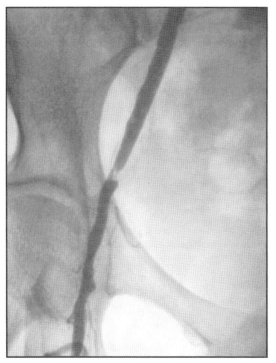

(a)

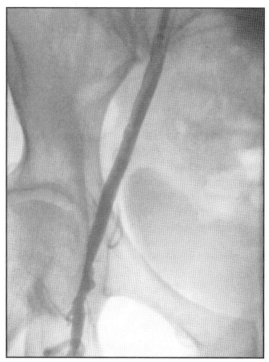

(b)

Figure 28.17
Pre (a) and post (b) angioplasty and stenting of the right external iliac artery.

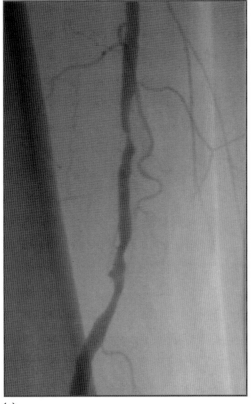

(a)

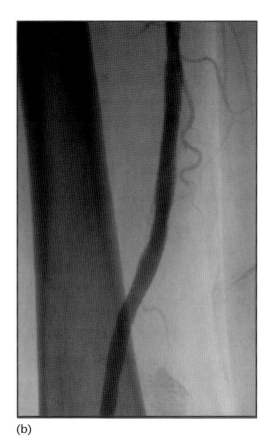

(b)

Figure 28.18
Pre (a) and post (b) angioplasty and stenting of the right superficial femoral artery.

dissection is common but is rarely of clinical consequence. Recannalization of the SFA can actually be achieved via intimal dissection and re-entry of the arterial lumen. Antegrade ipsilateral arterial access can also be used. This technique requires more skill and care, especially with postoperative management of the groin, to avoid complications. If an SFA occlusion cannot be crossed, then popliteal artery access via the popliteal fossa may be required. The value of stenting over angioplasty, apart from improved angiographic appearance, has not been demonstrated in the SFA. Consequently, a shift back to balloon angioplasty alone (despite the presence of an intimal dissection) if an adequate lumen is obtained is the preferred approach. Again, an undersized balloon is used to predilate lesions. A self-expanding stent is usually used. Postdilatation balloon sizing is also conservative

(Figure 28.18). Promising data are emerging regarding the use of brachytherapy and drug-eluting stents to reduce the high restenosis rate in the SFA.

Angioplasty and stenting of the vessels below the knee is a relatively new technique. Coronary wires, balloons, and stents are utilized. There are few data on long-term patency rates and clinical outcomes; however, this technique is sometimes performed for the purpose of limb salvage.

Reference

New G, Roubin GS, Iyer SS, et al. Low stroke rate during carotid artery stenting with neuroprotection. J Am Coll Cardiol 2003; 41:50A.

29

The importance of echocardiography to the interventionalist

Michael JA Williams

Introduction

Echocardiography allows both anatomic evaluation and noninvasive assessment of the severity of valvular disease, providing complementary information to the hemodynamic and angiographic information obtained in the catheterization laboratory. The widespread availability and noninvasive nature of echocardiography has made it the predominant technique for diagnosis, serial evaluation, and presurgical assessment of valvular disease.

Valvular disease more commonly affects left heart valves than right-sided valves. Stenosis of the atrioventricular valves leads to atrial dilatation and elevated pulmonary and/or systemic venous pressure. Significant atrioventricular valvular regurgitation results in volume overload and ventricular dilatation. Stenosis of the semilunar valves produces pressure overload, ventricular hypertrophy, and ultimately ventricular dilatation and failure. Mixed valvular disease causes variable volume and pressure overload, depending on the severity of the lesions. Evaluation of the most common valvular lesions is considered in the following sections.

Mitral valve

The normal mitral valve is a scalloped bileaflet structure supported by chordae tendineae, papillary muscles and their underlying myocardium, and the fibromuscular annulus.[1,2] The anterior leaflet is a longer semicircular-shaped structure than the posterior leaflet, which is shorter, although with a greater length of attachment to the mitral annulus. The normal mitral valve diastolic orifice area is 4–6 cm^2.

Mitral stenosis

Mitral stenosis is predominantly secondary to rheumatic fever, less commonly as a result of calcification of the mitral annulus and leaflets[3] and rarely congenital valvular disease. With increasing stenosis, there is a progressive increase in the transvalvular gradient from mild stenosis (valve area of 2 cm^2), through moderate to severe stenosis (1.5–1 cm^2). Left atrial pressure increases to maintain cardiac output, and left atrial enlargement occurs. With increasing severity of valvular obstruction, left atrial pressure increases further and pulmonary venous and arterial pressures are increased. Pulmonary vascular disease subsequently develops secondary to prolonged elevation of pulmonary arterial pressure. Right ventricular systolic function is usually preserved until pulmonary arterial pressure exceeds 80 mmHg, when right ventricular failure may ensue. About 25% of patients with rheumatic heart disease have pure mitral stenosis, while approximately 40% have mixed mitral stenosis and mitral regurgitation.[4] Most patients with rheumatic mitral stenosis have some degree of aortic regurgitation.

Mitral stenosis: echocardiography

Echocardiographic evaluation provides much of the information required to fully assess and plan management for mitral stenosis. Two-dimensional echocardiographic assessment of mitral stenosis allows evaluation of thickened mitral valve leaflets and chordal structures, fusion of the valve commissures, reduced mitral orifice area, and abnormal diastolic leaflet motion. The long-axis parasternal view allows assessment of leaflet and chordal thickening and also the typical restriction of anterior leaflet

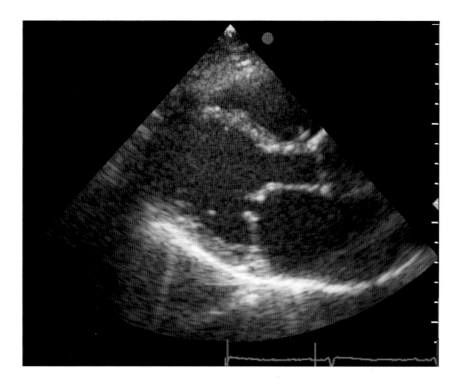

Figure 29.1
Long-axis parasternal view of mitral stenosis showing doming of the mitral valve leaflets due to restricted motion of the leaflet tips during diastole.

motion. While the anterior leaflet remains pliable, 'doming' of the mitral valve in diastole is observed (Figure 29.1); however, this may not be evident with extensive calcification of the leaflet. The parasternal short-axis view with appropriate angulation allows planimetry of the mitral valve area in over 90% of patients.[5] The accuracy of this method has been compared with direct measurement of surgically excised valves, and was within 0.3 cm^2 in 86% of patients.[6] Planimetry of the mitral valve area also correlates well ($r = 0.95$) with valve area determined at cardiac catheterization.[7]

The four-chamber view is used for two-dimensional assessment of the mitral valve and also Doppler assessment of transmitral flow and severity of mitral stenosis. The instantaneous peak pressure gradient can be calculated using the modified Bernoulli equation

$$P = 4v^2,$$

where v is the peak transvalvular velocity measured by continuous-wave Doppler. The mean gradient is calculated as the sum of the squares of the velocities divided by the number of velocity measurements. On echocardiography machines, the mean gradient is automatically calculated after manual tracing of the transmitral time–velocity profile (Figure 29.2). The Doppler-calculated mean mitral gradient has a good correlation with the mean gradient measured at cardiac catheterization.[8]

Mitral valve area is calculated using the continuity equation, which states that constant flow is equal to the product of mean velocity and cross-sectional area. The mitral valve area (A_m) can therefore be calculated as

$$A_m = \frac{A_a \times TVI_a}{TVI_m},$$

where A_a is the aortic valve area, TVI_a is the time–velocity integral across the aortic valve, and TVI_m is the time–velocity integral across the mitral valve. A_a is calculated as $\pi(r_a)^2$, where r_a is half the diameter of the aortic valve annulus. Studies comparing mitral valve area calculated using the continuity equation have shown a good correlation ($r = 0.91$) with catheterization measurements, irrespective of the presence of aortic regurgitation.[9]

Pulmonary arterial pressure can be evaluated by estimating the pressure difference between the right ventricle and right atrium by measuring the time–velocity profile of the tricuspid regurgitant jet when present. Transesophageal echocardiography provides superior images of the mitral valve compared with transthoracic imaging, and detailed evaluation for the presence of left atrial and left atrial appendage thrombus is possible.

Mitral stenosis: cardiac catheterization

The information required from cardiac catheterization includes peak and mean valve gradient derived from left ventricular diastolic and left atrial (pulmonary capillary wedge) pressures, valvular area derived from cardiac output, heart rate, and transvalvular pressure, and pulmonary arterial pressure. A right heart study is performed to determine pressure measurements. The left atrial pressure trace may have a prominent a wave with elevation of

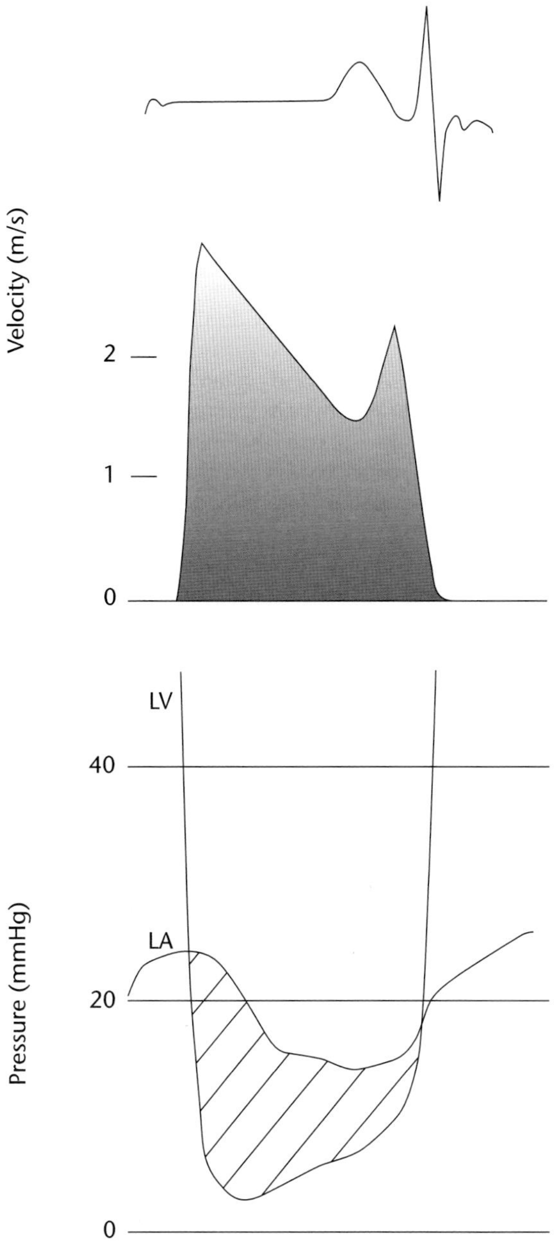

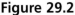

Figure 29.2
Mitral stenosis continuous-wave Doppler transvalvular
time–velocity profile (shaded). Simultaneous left
ventricular (LV) and left atrial (LA) pressure tracings are
shown in the lower panel, illustrating the pressure
gradient across the stenotic mitral valve. The mean mitral
valve pressure gradient is calculated by planimetry of the
area of the diastolic transmitral gradient (lined).

mean atrial pressure. In mild to moderate mitral stenosis,
pulmonary arterial pressure is usually normal. With more
severe stenosis, pulmonary arterial pressure is increased
and there is a progressive increase in pulmonary vascular
resistance. Pulmonary capillary wedge pressure is measured simultaneously with left ventricular diastolic pressure
to evaluate the transmitral gradient. Left ventricular dias-

tolic pressure is normal in patients with pure mitral stenosis. Cardiac output is determined immediately after assessment of the mitral transvalvular gradient.

Mitral valve area is determined using the Gorlin
formula:[10,11]

$$A = \frac{CO / (DFP)(HR)}{37.7\sqrt{\Delta P}},$$

where A is the mitral valve area in cm^2, CO is the cardiac
output in ml/min, DFP is the diastolic filling period in
s/beat, HR is the heart rate in beats/min, and ΔP is the
mean transmitral gradient in mmHg.

The diastolic filling period is calculated as the interval
during which the mitral valve is open. The mean transmitral gradient is determined by planimetry of the area of the
diastolic transmitral gradient (Figure 29.2). An increase in
heart rate shortens the diastolic filling interval and increases the transvalvular gradient, making subjects with mitral
stenosis vulnerable to tachycardia. The transvalvular gradient for any orifice area is a function of the square of the
transvalvular flow rate. Increases in cardiac output associated with exercise or stress will therefore markedly
increase left atrial pressure in those with significant mitral
stenosis.

Mitral stenosis: angiography

Cine angiography of the left ventricle allows assessment of
mitral valve motion and left ventricular systolic performance. Left ventricular systolic performance and end-
diastolic volume are normal in the majority of patients with
mitral stenosis. Up to 25% have an impaired ejection fraction and regional hypokinesis.[12] Left atrial angiography
allows assessment of left atrial size and reduced motion of
the mitral valve leaflets. Injections of contrast into the main
pulmonary artery potentially allows visualization of left-
sided structures as contrast enters the left heart.

Mitral regurgitation

Abnormalities of the mitral annulus, mitral valve leaflets,
chordae tendineae, or papillary muscles may result in
mitral regurgitation. An important cause of mitral regurgitation is myxomatous degeneration of the mitral valve
(mitral valve prolapse). Ischemia-related dysfunction of the
mitral valve and rheumatic disease also commonly result in
mitral regurgitation. Mitral regurgitation related to annular
dilatation occurs with dilatation of the left ventricle in all
forms of heart disease, including dilated cardiomyopathy.

Regurgitation begins during isovolumetric contraction
and continues through ventricular ejection. The regurgitant volume is influenced by the size of the regurgitant
orifice, the pressure gradient between left ventricle and
left atrium, left atrial compliance, duration of systole, and
afterload.[13] With chronic regurgitation, there is an increase

in end-diastolic volume, which leads to an increase in wall tension related to the increase in ventricular radius. Dilatation of the left ventricle in turn leads to mitral annular dilatation and apical displacement of the papillary muscles, with decreased apposition of the mitral valve leaflets and worsening mitral regurgitation. With more severe degrees of mitral regurgitation, ejection fraction falls, end-systolic volume progressively increases, and there is a progressive increase in pulmonary arterial pressure resulting in right heart failure.

Mitral regurgitation: echocardiography

Two-dimensional echocardiography commonly defines the etiology of mitral regurgitation and the associated left atrial and left ventricular dilatation. Mitral valve prolapse is best assessed in the long-axis parasternal view as systolic displacement of the mitral leaflet/s into the left atrium past a line connecting the annular hinge points[5] (Figure 29.3). Classic mitral valve prolapse is characterized by diffuse leaflet thickening ($\geq$ 5 mm) and redundancy of the leaflets secondary to myxomatous degeneration of the mitral valve leaflets.[14] Other etiologies for mitral regurgitation identifiable with echocardiography include ruptured chordae, ruptured papillary muscles, rheumatic valvular disease, and vegetations.

Color Doppler is used to qualitatively assess the severity of mitral regurgitation (Figure 29.4). The area of the color Doppler flow is expressed as a percentage of left atrial area, with jet areas less than 20% corresponding to mild regurgitation, areas between 20% and 40% to moderate regurgitation, and areas greater than 40% to severe regurgitation.[15] The percentage jet area has a modest correlation ($r = 0.72$) with regurgitant fraction determined angiographically. This method of estimating mitral regurgitation severity is only valid for free jets. Eccentric or wall jets have less jet area than free jets, and estimation of jet area in these cases will significantly underestimate the severity of mitral regurgitation. Other methods, such as measurement of the width of the regurgitant jet[16] and regurgitant orifice area,[17] provide more accurate estimations of mitral regurgitation severity.

Regurgitant fraction and volume can be estimated echocardiographically by calculating the difference between diastolic flow across the mitral valve and systolic flow across the aortic valve in the absence of aortic regurgitation. The flows are determined using the continuity equation described above, with forward flow calculated by integrating the Doppler velocity over the period of antegrade flow and multiplying the annular cross-sectional area.[18] Although these methods have demonstrated accuracy, they are rarely performed clinically because of the multiple measurements required and their time-consuming nature.

Pulsed Doppler evaluation of systolic reversal of flow in the pulmonary veins (akin to v wave) is an insensitive method (60%) of determining the presence of severe mitral regurgitation.[19] The best echocardiographic predictors of survival and left ventricular function after mitral valve surgery are preoperative echocardiographic ejection fraction[20] and an end-systolic diameter of <40–45 mm.[21] Serial evaluation of these parameters in patients with moderate–severe

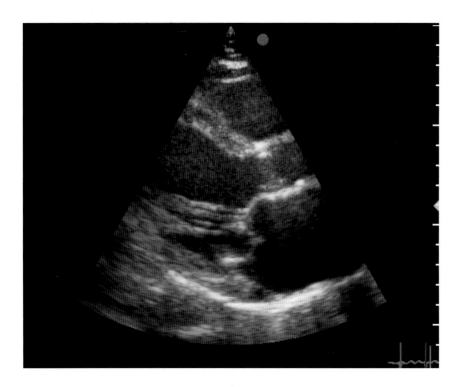

Figure 29.3
Long-axis parasternal view of posterior mitral valve leaflet prolapse.

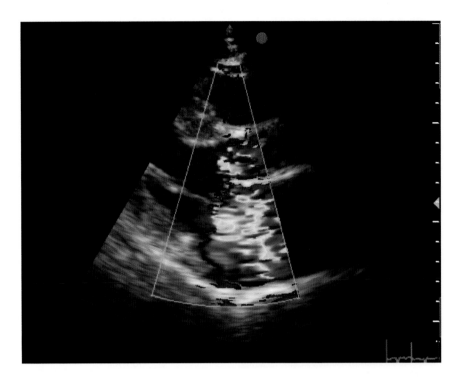

Figure 29.4
Posterior mitral leaflet prolapse
with severe mitral regurgitation.

mitral regurgitation allows prompt referral for surgery in those with progressive change. Transesophageal echocardiography is the best modality to assess the etiology of mitral regurgitation and is especially valuable in the assessment of patients suitability for mitral valve repair. This evaluation has important implications for patient outcome, as mitral valve repair is associated with superior long-term survival compared with mitral valve replacement.[22]

Mitral regurgitation: cardiac catheterization

A right heart study is performed to measure right heart pressures and cardiac output. The total left ventricular output is usually increased with a reduced effective cardiac output through the aorta. The normal v wave is produced by left atrial filling during ventricular systole. The influence of mitral regurgitation on the size of the v wave is determined by left atrial compliance. When the left atrium has normal compliance, as in acute mitral regurgitation, there is marked elevation of left atrial pressure, with giant v waves. In chronic severe mitral regurgitation, there may be considerable left atrial dilatation with increased compliance, and the v wave may be small or absent. There may also be v waves present in the absence of mitral regurgitation, such as in acute left ventricular failure with a distended noncompliant atrium. These presence or absence of v waves is therefore of limited diagnostic utility.[23]

Mitral regurgitation: angiography

A left heart study is performed to measure left heart pressures and perform angiographic assessment of the severi-

ty of mitral regurgitation. Qualitative assessment grades the mitral regurgitation according to the degree of opacification of the left atrium. Grade 1+ (mild) regurgitation clears with each beat and does not opacify the left atrium. Opacification of the entire left atrium after several beats is seen with 2+ (moderate) regurgitation. In 3+ (moderately severe) regurgitation, the left atrium is equally opacified with the left ventricle (Figure 29.5). Complete opacification of the left atrium in one beat denotes 4+ (severe) regurgitation.

Regurgitant fraction can also be calculated angiographically by measuring total left ventricular stroke volume. Total stroke volume is the difference between left ventricular end-diastolic volume and end-systolic volume. The forward stroke volume can be determined by estimation of cardiac output, with the regurgitant volume calculated as the difference between total stroke volume and forward stroke volume. The regurgitant fraction (RF) is calculated as

$$RF = \frac{(EDV - ESV) - FSV}{EDV - ESV}$$

where EDV is the end-diastolic volume, ESV is the end-systolic volume, and FSV is the forward stroke volume. Calculation of the regurgitant fraction relies on selecting an average representative beat to calculate the total stroke volume. This is not possible in atrial fibrillation or with extrasystoles during ventriculography. Inaccuracies will also be introduced if hemodynamic conditions change between the measurement of cardiac output to calculate FSV and the measurement of total stroke volume. A study comparing qualitative assessment of mitral regurgitant grade and regurgitant fraction showed wide variation in

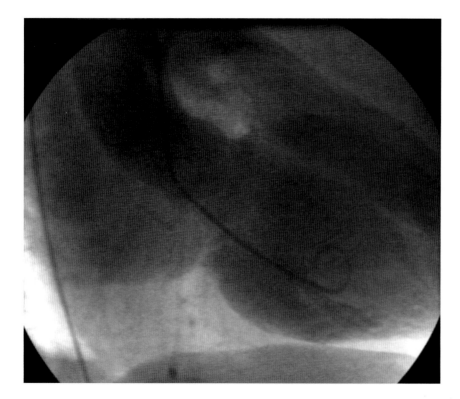

Figure 29.5
Cine angiography of severe mitral regurgitation secondary to mitral valve prolapse. There is equal contrast opacification of the left atrium and left ventricle.

regurgitant fraction in grades 3+ and 4+ mitral regurgitation, implying significant limitations on the qualitative assessment of mitral regurgitation.[24] The advent of improved echocardiographic assessment of mitral regurgitation severity has meant invasive assessment of mitral regurgitant fraction is performed less commonly.

Assessment of left ventricular ejection fraction and end-systolic volume as described above are an important part of the assessment of mitral regurgitation, as both of these parameters are important determinants of long-term outcome.[25,26]

Aortic valve

The components of the normal aortic valve include the three leaflets, the sinuses of Valsalva, and the fibrous interleaflet triangles.[27] The sinuses support the leaflets at their superior margins. A three-leaflet configuration allows opening of the valve to the full dimensions of the aortic annulus, with a normal valve area of 3–4 cm^2.

Aortic stenosis

Valvular stenosis is the most common form of obstruction to left ventricular outflow. Calcific degenerative aortic stenosis is the most common cause of stenosis in the elderly. Rheumatic disease is now a less common cause of aortic stenosis, and is often associated with aortic regurgitation or other valvular involvement. A bicuspid aortic valve is one of the most common congenital cardiac anomalies, and is often associated with progressive stenosis in middle age. Obstruction may also occur at a subvalvular level due to discrete membranes or dynamic obstruction, as occurs with hypertrophic obstructive cardiomyopathy. Supravalvular obstruction is generally congenital and rare.

The severity of aortic stenosis has generally been graded using aortic valve area.[28] In mild aortic stenosis, the valve area is greater than 1.5 cm^2 and in moderate aortic stenosis it ranges from 1 to 1.5 cm^2. With severe aortic stenosis, there is usually a mean transvalvular aortic gradient of 50 mmHg or more, with a valve area of 1 cm^2 or less. Chronic obstruction of left ventricular outflow results in progressive hypertrophy of the left ventricle. Left ventricular output is usually maintained for prolonged periods before the onset of symptoms or evidence of left ventricular failure. Left ventricular diastolic pressure increases – initially as a consequence of left ventricular hypertrophy with its associated diastolic dysfunction and subsequently secondary to systolic dysfunction. Atrial pressure rises to maintain left ventricular filling and prominent *a* waves appear in the left atrial pressure trace. End-stage aortic stenosis is associated with dilatation of the ventricle and a fall in the ejection fraction and transvalvular gradient. Pulmonary venous and arterial pressures are then increased, with elevation of right ventricular and right atrial pressures and clinical evidence of right heart failure.

Aortic stenosis: echocardiography

Transthoracic echocardiography is the dominant technique used for the diagnosis and serial evaluation of aortic stenosis. Two-dimensional parasternal views allow evaluation of

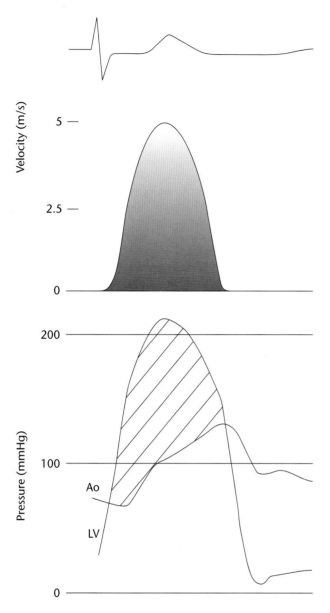

Figure 29.6
Aortic stenosis continuous-wave Doppler transvalvular
time–velocity profile (shaded). Simultaneous left
ventricular (LV) and aortic (Ao) pressure tracings are
shown in the lower panel, illustrating the pressure
gradient across the stenotic aortic valve (lined).

the number of leaflets, leaflet thickening/calcification, and
leaflet motion. In congenital aortic stenosis, there is commonly systolic leaflet 'doming'. There is decreased leaflet
motion in degenerative calcific aortic stenosis. Planimetry
of the aortic valve area is difficult with transthoracic studies, but can be accurately determined with transesophageal echocardiography.

The apical views are used with Doppler echocardiography to determine velocities across the level of obstruction to left ventricular outflow (Figure 29.6). The peak and
mean transaortic valve gradients are calculated using the
modified Bernoulli equation. Measurements of left ven-

tricular outflow tract diameter and Doppler velocities
allow calculation of aortic valve area (A_a) using the continuity equation:

$$A_a = \frac{A_{lvot} \times TVI_{lvot}}{TVI_a},$$

where A_{lvot} is the left ventricular outflow tract area, TVI_{lvot}
is the time–velocity integral just below the aortic valve,
and TVI_a is the maximal time–velocity integral across the
aortic valve determined using continuous-wave Doppler.
A_{lvot} is calculated as πr_{lvot}^2, where r_{lvot} is half the diameter of
the left ventricular outflow tract just below the aortic valve
annulus.

Calculation of the aortic valve area is especially valuable in the presence of markedly impaired left ventricular
systolic function, where transvalvular gradients may
underestimate the severity of aortic stenosis. Dobutamine
echocardiography can be used to increase cardiac output
and allow sequential assessment of aortic valve area at
increasing flows.[29] In patients with severe aortic stenosis,
an unchanged or slightly increased aortic valve area with
increased cardiac output implies true valvular stenosis,
with the potential for improved ventricular function and
survival after aortic valve replacement. In those with
severe impairment of left ventricular function and apparent severe stenosis, an increase in calculated valve area
(≥ 0.3 cm^2) implies aortic pseudostenosis, with uncertain
benefits (if any) after aortic valve replacement.[30]

Aortic stenosis: cardiac catheterization

Coronary angiography is an essential part of the assessment of patients with significant aortic stenosis where surgical intervention is being considered. In straightforward
severe aortic stenosis, satisfactory hemodynamic information can be obtained with Doppler echocardiography, and
invasive hemodynamic studies are seldom required. In
cases where there is a discrepancy between the clinical
and echocardiographic data, right and left heart catheterization may be indicated. The right heart study is performed to determine right heart pressures and pulmonary
arterial pressures, followed by determination of cardiac
output. The left heart study is performed to determine left
ventricular end-diastolic pressure and the mean gradient
across the aortic valve, and to calculate the aortic valve
area using the Gorlin formula:[10,11]

$$A = \frac{CO / (SEP)(HR)}{44.3\sqrt{\Delta P}},$$

where A is the aortic valve area in cm^2, CO is the cardiac
output in ml/min, SEP is the systolic ejection period in
s/beat, HR is the heart rate in beats/min, and ΔP is the
mean transaortic gradient in mmHg. The systolic ejection
period is calculated as the interval during which the
aortic valve is open. The mean transaortic gradient is
determined by planimetry of the area of the systolic

gradient (Figure 29.6). A pigtail catheter and standard 0.35 inch J guidewire are used to cross the stenotic aortic valve. In difficult cases, a straight guidewire via pigtail, right Judkins, or left Amplatz catheter can assist in crossing an eccentric aortic valve orifice.

Aortic stenosis angiography

Fluoroscopy will often demonstrate calcification of the aortic valve leaflets and adjacent aortic root. Cine angiography of the left ventricle may be poorly tolerated in patients with severe aortic stenosis and is rarely justified in echocardiographically proven severe aortic stenosis. In occasional cases where echocardiography has not satisfactorily evaluated left ventricular systolic function or mitral valve function, the risks and benefits of this procedure must be determined before proceeding. Ascending aortography demonstrates poststenotic dilatation and assessment of any aortic regurgitation that may be present.

Aortic regurgitation

Abnormalities of the aortic valve leaflets or dilatation of the aortic root result in aortic regurgitation. Rheumatic fever is the most common cause of aortic valve regurgitation. Other causes include aortic regurgitation associated with calcific degenerative aortic stenosis, infective endocarditis, and a bicuspid aortic valve. Aortic root disease with dilatation of the ascending aorta is an increasingly common cause of aortic regurgitation. Hypertension, Marfan syndrome, cystic medial necrosis, and spondyloarthropathies may lead to progressive aortic dilatation with separation of the aortic leaflets and consequent aortic regurgitation.

Aortic regurgitation: echocardiography

The parasternal views allow detailed evaluation of aortic leaflet morphology and, in particular, evaluation of any leaflet prolapse. Measurements of the aortic diameter at sinus, sinotubular, and ascending aorta levels are performed to determine if aortic dilatation is contributing to the presence of aortic regurgitation. Serial measurements of left ventricular end-diastolic dimension, end-systolic dimension and calculation of ejection fraction are undertaken. An end-systolic dimension greater than 55 mm or subnormal ejection fraction are considered as indications for surgery in asymptomatic patients. Aortic regurgitation may result in high-frequency diastolic flutter of the anterior mitral leaflet or blunting of the early-diastolic opening of the leaflet.

Short-axis views with color Doppler will usually determine whether there is central or eccentric aortic regurgitation. Estimating the area of the regurgitant color Doppler jet is an inaccurate method of assessing the severity of aortic regurgitation. The height or area of the regurgitant color Doppler jet can be used to estimate the size of the regurgitant orifice, and are reasonable predictors of the angiographic grade of aortic regurgitation.[31] A ratio of jet height to left ventricular outflow height of 47–64% indicates moderate regurgitation, and a ratio of 65% or more indicates severe regurgitation. The rate of decline of the regurgitant diastolic flow velocity has been used to estimate aortic regurgitation severity,[32] but slope values may not discriminate between different grades of angiographically defined aortic regurgitation. In chronic aortic regurgitation, measurement of end-diastolic velocity in the descending thoracic aorta provides a good estimate of the severity of aortic regurgitation as determined by magnetic resonance-calculated aortic regurgitant fraction.[33]

Echocardiographic quantification of aortic regurgitant volume and regurgitant fraction can be performed in several ways. Aortic forward flow can be calculated as the product of the systolic velocity integral and the left ventricular outflow tract area. The cardiac output can similarly be calculated using a competent cardiac valve. The regurgitant volume is calculated as the difference between these two measures.[34] The limitations of this technique are the fact that flows are calculated from measurements with inherent errors and the time-consuming nature of the calculations.

Aortic regurgitation: cardiac catheterization

Generally cardiac catheterization is not required in chronic aortic regurgitation unless there are significant questions persisting after clinical assessment and noninvasive testing.[28] Coronary angiography is performed in those at risk for coronary artery disease prior to planned aortic valve replacement. In some cases, hemodynamic and angiographic assessment of the severity of aortic regurgitation and left ventricular function may be indicated. Chronic aortic regurgitation is associated with an increased pulse pressure and increased end-diastolic and end-systolic ventricular volumes. In acute aortic regurgitation, the increased pulse pressure is absent and stroke volumes are smaller.[35] A high left ventricular end-diastolic pressure exceeding left atrial pressure may lead to premature closure of the mitral valve. Right heart catheterization is performed for measurement of pressures and cardiac output. Left heart catheterization is then undertaken for measurement of left ventricular diastolic pressure and evaluation of aortic transvalvular gradients and aortic pulse pressure.

Aortic regurgitation: angiography

Angiography may be indicated to assess the severity of regurgitation or left ventricular function when noninvasive tests are inconclusive or discordant with clinical findings.[28]

Aortic regurgitation severity is assessed qualitatively using opacification of the left ventricle. Grade 1+ (mild) regurgitation partially opacifies the ventricle and is cleared with each beat. Faint opacification of the entire left ventricle occurs with 2+ (moderate) regurgitation. In 3+ (moderately severe) regurgitation, the left ventricle is equally opacified compared with the ascending aorta. Complete opacification of the left ventricle in one beat denotes 4+ (severe) regurgitation. Calcification of the aortic valve leaflets, leaflet number and motion, and aortic dilatation are also assessed in the left anterior oblique view. Left ventriculography is performed to assess ventricular volumes and ejection fraction. Regurgitant fraction can also be calculated using the method described on page 411 for mitral regurgitation.

References

1. Lam JHC, Ranganathan N, Wigle ED, et al. Morphology of the human mitral valve: I. Chordae tendineae: a new classification. Circulation 1970;41:449–58.
2. Ranganathan N, Lam JHC, Wigle ED, et al. Morphology of the human mitral valve: II. The valve leaflets. Circulation 1970;41:459–67.
3. Osterberger LE, Goldstein S, Khaja F, et al. Functional mitral stenosis in patients with massive mitral annular calcification. Circulation 1981;64:472–6.
4. Kumar A, Sinha M, Sinha DN. Chronic rheumatic heart diseases in Ranchi. Angiology 1982;33:141–5.
5. Weyman AE. Left ventricular inflow tract I. In: Principles and Practice of Echocardiography, 2nd edn (Weyman AE, ed). Malvern: Lea & Febiger, 1994: 391–470.
6. Henry WL, Griffith JM, Michaelis LL, et al. Measurement of mitral orifice area in patients with mitral valve disease by real-time, two-dimensional echocardiography. Circulation 1975;51:827–31.
7. Nichol PM, Gilbert BW, Kisslo JA. Two-dimensional echocardiographic assessment of mitral stenosis. Circulation 1977;55:120–8.
8. Stamm RB, Martin RP. Quantification of pressure gradients across stenotic valves by Doppler ultrasound. J Am Coll Cardiol 1983;2:707–18.
9. Nakatani S, Masuyama T, Kodama K, et al. Value and limitations of Doppler echocardiography in the quantification of stenotic mitral valve area: comparison of the pressure half-time and the continuity equation methods. Circulation 1988;77:78–85.
10. Gorlin R, Gorlin SG. Hydraulic formula for calculation of the area of the stenotic mitral valve, other cardiac valves, and central circulatory shunts. Am Heart J 1951;41:1–29.
11. Cohen MV, Gorlin R. Modified orifice equation for the calculation of mitral valve area. Am Heart J 1972;84:839–40.
12. Gash AK, Carabello BA, Cepin D, et al. Left ventricular ejection performance and systolic muscle function in patients with mitral stenosis. Circulation 1983;67:148–54.
13. Braunwald E. Valvular heart disease. In: Heart Disease, 6th edn (Braunwald E, Zipes DP, Libby P, eds). Philadelphia: WB Saunders, 2001: 1643–722.

14. Marks AR, Choong CY, Sanfilippo AJ, et al. Identification of high-risk and low-risk subgroups of patients with mitral-valve prolapse. N Engl J Med 1989;320:1031–6.
15. Helmcke F, Nanda NC, Hsiung MC, et al. Color Doppler assessment of mitral regurgitation with orthogonal planes. Circulation 1987;75:175–83.
16. Hall SA, Brickner ME, Willett DL, et al. Assessment of mitral regurgitation severity by Doppler color flow mapping of the vena contracta. Circulation 1997;95:636–42.
17. Vandervoort PM, Rivera JM, Mele D, et al. Application of color Doppler flow mapping to calculate effective regurgitant orifice area: an in vitro study and initial clinical observations. Circulation 1993;88:1150–6.
18. Enriquez-Sarano M, Bailey KR, Seward JB, et al. Quantitative Doppler assessment of valvular regurgitation. Circulation 1993;87:841–8.
19. Enriquez-Sarano M, Dujardin KS, Tribouilloy CM, et al. Determinants of pulmonary venous flow reversal in mitral regurgitation and its usefulness in determining the severity of regurgitation. Am J Cardiol 1999;83:535–41.
20. Enriquez-Sarano M, Tajik AJ, Schaff HV, et al. Echocardiographic prediction of survival after surgical correction of organic mitral regurgitation. Circulation 1994;90:830–37.
21. Wisenbaugh T, Skudicky D, Sareli P. Prediction of outcome after valve replacement for rheumatic mitral regurgitation in the era of chordal preservation. Circulation 1994;89:191–7.
22. Mohty D, Orszulak TA, Schaff HV, et al. Very long-term survival and durability of mitral valve repair for mitral valve prolapse. Circulation 2001;104(Suppl):11–7.
23. Fuchs RM, Heuser RR, Yin FC, et al. Limitations of pulmonary wedge V waves in diagnosing mitral regurgitation. Am J Cardiol 1982;49:849–54.
24. Croft CH, Lipscomb K, Mathis K, et al. Limitations of qualitative angiographic grading in aortic or mitral regurgitation. Am J Cardiol 1984;53:1593–8.
25. Crawford MH, Souchek J, Oprian CA, et al. Determinants of survival and left ventricular performance after mitral valve replacement. Circulation 1990;81:1173–81.
26. Borow KM, Green LH, Mann T, et al. End-systolic volume as a predictor of postoperative left ventricular performance in volume overload from valvular regurgitation. Am J Med 1980;68:655–63.
27. Angelini A, Ho SY, Anderson RH, et al. The morphology of the normal aortic valve as compared with the aortic valve having two leaflets. J Thorac Cardiovasc Surg 1989;98:362–7.
28. Bonow RO, Carabello B, de Leon AC Jr, et al. ACC/AHA Guidelines for the Management of Patients with Valvular Heart Disease: a report of the American College of Cardiology/American Heart Association Task Force on Practice Guidelines (Committee on Management of Patients with Valvular Heart Disease). J Am Coll Cardiol 1998;32:1486–588.
29. deFilippi CR, Willett DL, Brickner ME, et al. Usefulness of dobutamine echocardiography in distinguishing severe from nonsevere valvular aortic stenosis in patients with depressed left ventricular function and low transvalvular gradients. Am J Cardiol 1995;75:191–4.
30. Carabello BA. Ventricular function in aortic stenosis: How low can you go? J Am Coll Cardiol 2002;39:1364–5.
31. Perry GJ, Helmcke F, Nanda NC, et al. Evaluation of aortic insufficiency by Doppler color flow mapping. J Am Coll Cardiol 1987;9:952–9.

32. Labovitz AJ, Ferrara RP, Kern MJ, et al. Quantitative evaluation of aortic insufficiency by continuous wave Doppler echocardiography. J Am Coll Cardiol 1986;8:1341–7.

33. Reimold SC, Maier SE, Aggarwal K, et al. Aortic flow velocity patterns in chronic aortic regurgitation: implications for Doppler echocardiography. J Am Soc Echocardiogr 1996;9:675–83.

34. Kitabatake A, Ito H, Inoue M, et al. A new approach to non-invasive evaluation of aortic regurgitant fraction by two-dimensional Doppler echocardiography. Circulation 1985;72:523–9.

35. Mann T, McLaurin L, Grossman W, et al. Assessing the hemodynamic severity of acute aortic regurgitation due to infective endocarditis. N Engl J Med 1975;293:108–13.

30

Percutaneous mitral valvuloplasty

Gerard T Wilkins

Introduction

The role of percutaneous balloon valvuloplasty (PMV) has continued to develop since Inoue et al[1] described the technique nearly 20 years ago. Progressive improvements in equipment, operator experience, and case selection have contributed to the emergence of PMV as the management procedure of choice for patients with important mitral stenosis. Numerous large series suggest that the most important predictor of success is careful case selection.[2–7]

Present guidelines from the American Heart Association (AHA)/American College of Cardiology (ACC) state: 'In centers with skilled, experienced operators, PMV should be considered the initial procedure of choice for symptomatic patients with moderate to severe mitral stenosis who have a favorable valve morphology in the absence of significant mitral regurgitation or left atrial thrombus. In asymptomatic patients with favorable valve morphology, PMV may be considered if there is evidence of a hemodynamic effect on left atrial pressure (new-onset atrial fibrillation) or pulmonary circulation (pulmonary artery pressure >50 mmHg at rest or >60 mmHg with exercise)' (Table 30.1).[8]

Case selection

Age

With advancing years, the process of rheumatic inflammation, scarring, and reactivation due to repeated bouts (clinical or subclinical) of streptococcal pharyngitis will frequently lead to increased scarring, deformity, and calcification of the mitral leaflets. Age alone therefore predicts that PMV will be less likely to succeed. However, studies show that the predictive effects of age are accounted for by examining the valve echocardiographically.[7,9] Despite advanced years, patients with suitable anatomy will achieve very satisfactory results. It is also noted that elderly patients with multiple comorbidities who are high-risk candidates for valvular surgery and who possess valve morphology that is less than ideal for PMV can still have an increase in valve area with PMV that would generally be considered suboptimal but can lead to substantial clinical improvement, making PMV a reasonable choice in this group.

Valve morphology

No other factor has been as closely studied in case selection for PMV. From the earliest days of closed surgical valvotomy, surgeons observed a correlation between valve pliability and the degree of thickening with subsequent outcome from their intervention.[10,11] These observations hold true also when the intervention is performed percutaneously.[2–5,7] A simple echocardiographic score, now widely used, noting leaflet mobility, leaflet thickening, leaflet calcification, and the extent of subvalvular disease has proven to be highly effective in predicting both immediate and long-term outcome from PMV[12–14] (Table 30.2). Large patient series with long-term follow-up suggest that patients with valve scores of 8 or less will usually achieve a superior result and significantly greater survival and freedom from combined events than patients with echo scores greater than 8 (representing increasing scarring and rigidity in the valve mechanism) (Figures 30.1 and 30.2).[4,7]

Table 30.1a Consensus recommendations for percutaneous mitral balloon valvotomy from the ACC/AHA Guidelines for the Management of Patients with Valvular Heart Disease

Indication	Class
1. Symptomatic patients (NYHA functional Class II, III, or IV), moderate or severe MS (mitral valve area ≤1.5 cm²),* and valve morphology favorable for percutaneous balloon valvotomy in the absence of left atrial thrombus or moderate to severe MR.	I
2. Asymptomatic patients with moderate or severe MS (mitral valve area ≤1.5 cm²)* and valve morphology favorable for percutaneous balloon valvotomy who have pulmonary hypertension (pulmonary artery systolic pressure >50 mmHg at rest or 60 mmHg with exercise) in the absence of left atrial thrombus or moderate to severe MR.	IIa
3. Patients with NYHA functional Class III-IV symptoms, moderate or severe MS (mitral valve area ≤1.5 cm²),* and a nonpliable calcified valve who are at high risk for surgery in the absence of left atrial thrombus or moderate to severe MR.	IIa
4. Asymptomatic patients, moderate or severe MS (mitral valve area ≤1.5 cm²)* and valve morphology favorable for percutaneous balloon valvotomy who have new onset of atrial fibrillation in the absence of left atrial thrombus or moderate to severe MR.	IIb
5. Patients in NYHA functional Class III-IV, moderate or severe MS (MVA ≤1.5 cm²), and a nonpliable calcified valve who are low-risk candidates for surgery.	IIb
6. Patients with mild MS.	III

* The committee recognizes that there may be variability in the measurement of mitral valve area and that the mean transmitral gradient, pulmonary artery wedge pressure, and pulmonary artery pressure at rest or during exercise should also be taken into consideration.
Reproduced from J Am Coll Cardiol 1998;32:1486–588.[8]

Patients with valve scores greater than 8 are more likely to be older, have mitral calcification under fluoroscopy, be in atrial fibrillation, and have a history of previous surgical mitral commissurotomy. In the initial 5-year period after PMV, the incidence of adverse clinical events is low in the group with optimal valve morphology (low echo score). At 8 years of follow-up, 50% of patients with echo score of 8 or less are free of combined events, whereas only 38% are free of events at 12 years of follow-up.[7] Patients with

Table 30.1b Summary of the definitions for 'class of evidence' referred to in Table 30.1a

Class I:	Conditions for which there is evidence and/or general agreement that a given procedure or treatment is useful and effective.
Class II:	Conditions for which there is conflicting evidence and/or a divergence of opinion about the usefulness/efficacy of a procedure or treatment.
IIa.	Weight of evidence/opinion is in favor of usefulness/efficacy.
IIb.	Usefulness/efficacy is less well established by evidence/opinion.
Class III:	Conditions for which there is evidence and/or general agreement that the procedure/ treatment is not useful and in some cases may be harmful.

higher echo scores do considerably worse, particularly those with scores of 12 or more (Figure 30.3).[7] However, in clinical practice, an abrupt threshold in case selection should not be adopted.[9] No absolute contraindications based on echocardiographic morphology alone should be applied, with the score usefully acting as a predictor of outcome and event-free survival.[15] Generally, PMV should always be applied in patients with a score of 8 or less, while those with a score of 12 or more should generally undergo mitral valve replacement. On an individual basis, commissural and subvalvular factors may override the numerical score in decision making. Several small studies have highlighted the importance of commissural calcification, and its role in the development of complications of PMV.[16–18]

Since the mechanism of dilatation is splitting along fused commissures,[12] calcification at this point may hinder separation and encourage tearing through the leaflet. If dense calcification of commissures is suspected on transthoracic echocardiography, a thorough transesophageal study is indicated, with careful attention to the commissures and subvalvular apparatus. If commissural separation appears unlikely, a surgical approach may be indicated.

Mitral regurgitation

The presence of significant mitral regurgitation (MR) is a contraindication to PMV, as a successful balloon procedure will still leave the patient with a significant hemodynamic lesion (MR) and there is a general tendency for MR to worsen after dilatation.[2–4] The best results are those obtained in patients with no or minimal regurgitation. Although the quantitative assessment of MR is imprecise by either contrast angiography or echocardiography, it is generally recommended that valve regurgitation greater than grade 2 should be considered a contraindication to

Table 30.2 Grading of mitral valve characteristics from the echocardiographic examination

Grade	Mobility	Subvalvar thickening	Thickening	Calcification
1	Highly mobile valve with only leaflet tips restricted	Minimal thickening just below the mitral leaflets	Leaflets near normal in thickness (4–5 mm)	A single area of increased echo brightness
2	Leaflet mild and base portions have normal mobility	Thickening of chordal structures extending up to one third of the chordal length	Mid-leaflets normal, considerable thickening of margins (5–8 mm)	Scattered areas of brightness confined to leaflet margins
3	Valve continues to move forward in diastole, mainly from the base	Thickening extending to the distal third of the chords	Thickening extending through the entire leaflet (5–8 mm)	Brightness extending into the mid-portion of the leaflets
4	No or minimal forward movement of the leaflets in diastole	Extensive thickening and shortening of all chordal structures extending down to the papillary muscles	Considerable thickening of all leaflet tissue (>8–10 mm)	Extensive brightness throughout much of the leaflet tissue

The total echocardiographic score was derived from an analysis of mitral leaflet mobility, valvar and subvalvar thickening, and calcification which were graded from 0 to 4 according to the above criteria. This gave a total score of 0 to 16.
Reproduced from Wilkins GT. Br Heart J 1988;60:229–308[12] with permission from the BMJ Publishing Group.

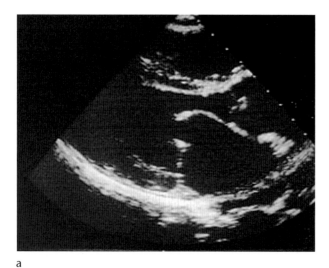
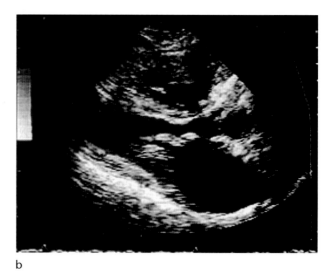

a   b

Figure 30.1
(a) Transthoracic echocardiographic parasternal long-axis view showing a highly mobile, 'doming' anterior mitral valve leaflet with thickening of anterior and posterior leaflet tips only. There is no evidence of subvalvular thickening. The echo score is 4. (b) The mitral valve leaflets in a parasternal long axis view are thickened, and this thickening extends below the leaflet tips and into the subvalvular apparatus. The echo score is 11.

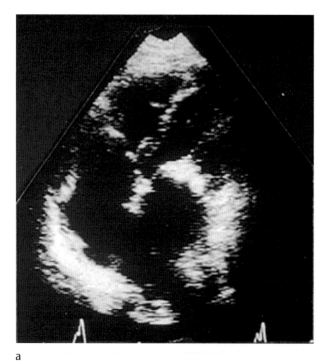
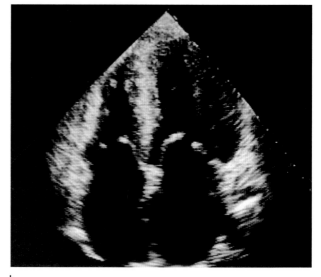

                                                                                       b

a

Figure 30.2
(a) Transthoracic echocardiographic apical four-chamber view showing doming of the mitral valve with slight thickening of the margins of the anterior and posterior leaflets. The echo score is 4. (b) Apical four-chamber view with marked thickening extending throughout the leaflets. A marked increase in echo density suggests the presence of calcification. The echo score is 11.

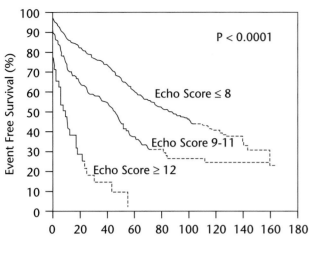

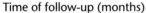

Figure 30.3
Kaplan–Meier event-free survival estimates (alive and free of mitral valve replacement or redo PMV) for patients with echo scores of 8 or less, 9–11, and 12 or more, in 879 patients who underwent percutaneous mitral balloon valvuloplasty. Lower echo scores predict a higher likelihood of an event-free survival over the next 10 years. (Reproduced from Palacios IF, et al. Circulation 2002;105:1465–71.)

attempts at PMV. The development of severe MR as a result of PMV (one of the major immediate complications) can occur in those with no pre-existing MR (see the section below on complications).[18]

Left atrial thrombus

Since PMV requires instrumentation and manipulation of catheters within the left atrium (LA), the presence of LA thrombus is considered a contraindication, as systemic emboli may be readily produced in this situation. Patients in atrial fibrillation would generally be on warfarin for the management of embolic risk, but a period of 4–6 weeks treatment is usually indicated prior to undertaking PMV if this is not the case. For those in sinus rhythm, the likelihood of atrial thrombus is lower, but a period of anticoagulation may also be appropriate in this group, particularly if there is severe stenosis, a markedly enlarged LA, and spontaneous echo contrast noted on transesophageal examination. Transesophageal echocardiography (TEE) is the most effective tool for identifying atrial thrombus (in either the body or appendage), and is recommended as part of the routine preprocedural workup of all patients. If thrombus is identified, a 4- to 6-week period of anticoagulation (for those not already on therapy) or intensified therapy with an International Normalized Ratio (INR) of around 3–3.5 is recom-

mended, before repeat TEE. If thrombus has resolved, PMV should proceed as planned.[19] If thrombus remains (particularly mobile thrombus attached to the interatrial septum or near the valve), a surgical approach is recommended. Successful PMV has been reported in patients with small, fixed thrombus in the LA appendage, with a low rate of complications.[20]

Patients with previous surgical commissurotomy or PMV

PMV can be performed effectively in patients who have previously undergone surgical commissurotomy or previous PMV.[7,21,27] It is noted that valve morphology is generally less favorable in this group (generally higher echo scores), with the echo score correctly predicting outcome when applied in the usual manner. Repeated PMV at short intervals has been used in children with active rheumatic disease and rapid occurrence of restenosis in order that valve replacement can be avoided at an early age.

Pregnancy

PMV has been performed commonly in pregnant women with severe mitral stenosis since the procedure was first reported.[22] Since pregnancy can provoke severe heart failure due to increases in circulating blood volume and cardiac output, intervention can be necessary when heart failure becomes refractory to medical therapy. The risks of radiation to the fetus are substantially reduced after 14 weeks, making PMV more appropriate if delayed till after that time. A minimal screening approach with radiation shielding of the pelvic and abdominal area is undertaken. The use of echocardiographic guidance for transseptal puncture and transmitral balloon positioning can assist further in reducing radiation exposure. In experienced centers, PMV is the procedure of choice in this difficult situation.[8]

Combined valve lesions

Since rheumatic fever affects mitral, aortic, and tricuspid valve tissue, it is not uncommon to assess patients with combined valve lesions. PMV is recommended in those with dominant mitral stenosis. The presence of significant other valvular lesions makes a surgical approach more appropriate. Successful balloon dilatation of severe tricuspid stenosis has been reported using a similar approach to that for the mitral valve.[23]

Mitral valvuloplasty techniques

Several approaches have been described and have evolved since the procedure was first performed. The original concept described by Inoue using a single multistage balloon has become the dominant technique. Double-balloon techniques, using either two separate balloons positioned over wires or a double balloon on a single catheter and wire, have been widely used (Figure 30.4). Comparative studies have demonstrated a consistently larger orifice area with a double-balloon approach, but no difference in outcome.[24–26] More recently, a rapid exchange double-balloon, single-shaft catheter approach has been developed (Bonhoeffer), as has a percutaneous metallic valvulotome (Cribier) (Figure 5a,b). The Inoue technique will be described in detail, as this has emerged as the approach with a consistently low risk of complications.

Inoue mitral valvuloplasty technique

Set-up

Patients are minimally sedated only and the procedure is conducted via the right femoral vein in most. Arterial puncture is performed, usually 5 French (Fr) in the left groin (to keep this catheter away from the Inoue catheter during manipulation), a pigtail catheter is positioned in the left ventricle (LV) for arterial pressure monitoring, transmitral gradient measurements, and left ventriculography, and to act as a landmark during balloon dilatation. If the patient has been on oral anticoagulant, this should be stopped 3–5 days prior to the procedure such that the INR is approximately normal. Prior to transseptal puncture, we give no systemic heparin but use heparin in all pressure bags and saline flushes. The in-dwelling LV pigtail should be flushed frequently with heparinized saline, particularly if the transseptal puncture is time-consuming.

Prior to PMV, routine coronary angiography is recommended in patients older than 40 years. Right heart pressures and contrast ventriculography may be indicated when the suitability of the patient for PMV is equivocal, particularly when more than trivial MR is present.

We have abandoned the routine positioning of a Swan–Ganz thermodilution catheter in the pulmonary artery for pressures and cardiac output measurements, preferring in-lab echocardiography as the best judge of progress during mitral balloon dilatation.

Transseptal puncture

In order to introduce the Inoue balloon through the stenotic mitral valve orifice in an antegrade manner along the direction of blood flow, transseptal puncture and instrumentation of the LA is necessary. Transseptal catheterization is associated with serious complications of pericardial tamponade, perforation of the aorta, and death, so that a safe, systematic approach is necessary to minimize risk. Numerous approaches have been described. A simple approach is outlined here:

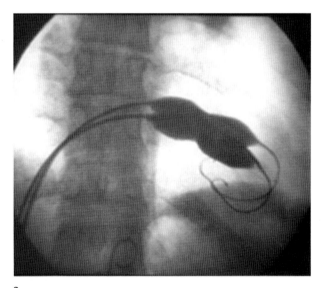

a

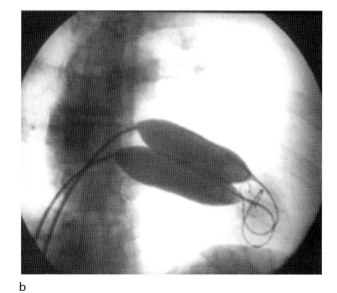

b

Figure 30.4
Double-balloon approach for percutaneous mitral valvuloplasty, with (a) demonstrating the waist as the balloons are inflated across the stenotic orifice and (b) showing the fully inflated profile.

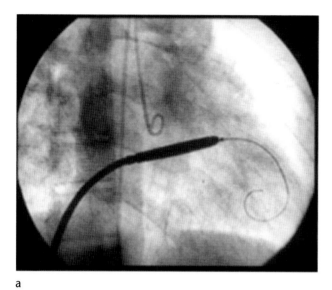
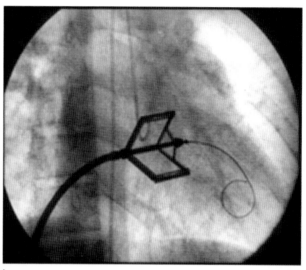

a   b

Figure 30.5
Cribier valvulotome for percutaneous mitral valvuloplasty (commissurotomy) showing (a) the device positioned across the mitral orifice and (b) the valvulotome opened.

1. Right femoral vein puncture is performed and a 0.0032 inch J wire is positioned across the right atrium (RA) into the superior vena cava (SVC).
2. In a 40–45° right anterior oblique (RAO) position, a contrast left ventriculogram is performed to assess the degree of preprocedural mitral regurgitation and the position of landmarks to guide in transseptal puncture. In this rotated position, the posterior curve formed by wall of the LA adjacent to the vertebrae can usually be seen under fluoroscopy. The interatrial septum (IAS) is viewed en face in this projection. With contrast in the LV and aorta, these structures can be clearly visualized. The mitral annulus is viewed 'side-on' in this view. It is therefore relatively simple to establish an approximate position for the center of the IAS, and this position can be related to some adjacent bony structure and the pigtail catheter for later guidance of the transseptal needle (Figure 30.6).
3. After returning to the standard anteroposterior (AP) screening position, a Mullins transseptal dilator (without the 7 Fr sheath) is positioned using the wire into the SVC. It is helpful to position the tip with its natural curve posteriorly. This can be facilitated by marking the hub of the catheter in such a way that the position of the curve can be recognized after insertion.
4. A standard curved Brockenbrough needle, is flushed and connected to a second pressure transducer. The needle is then slowly introduced along the Mullins dilator and the tip of the needle held in the posterior position approximately 1–2 cm from the tip of the dilator. This position can be safely maintained by placing a finger between the two hubs. The position of the needle point is indicated by the direction indicator on

the needle hub. The indicator will now be pointing toward the bed (in the 6 o'clock position).
5. While still in the AP screening position, the direction indicator is rotated anticlockwise to 4 o'clock and the tip pulled downwards from the SVC to the mid RA. The tip is seen to move medially onto the IAS, and with further downward movement can sometimes be felt to 'click' into the foramen ovale.
6. The original 40–45° RAO position is again selected, while continuing to hold the transseptal needle and dilator in the same position. The position of the ascending aorta, the posterior extent of the LA, and the level of the mitral annulus have already been established. Viewed from this position, the needle and dilator are curving away from the observer toward the IAS so that the curve is often not apparent. If the tip is too anterior toward the aorta, more clockwise rotation is applied. If it is toward the posterior edge of the LA more anticlockwise rotation is applied. The tip should be at the level of the midpoint of the mitral annulus so that the puncture will generally penetrate through the thinner tissue of the foramen ovale (Figure 30.6).
7. The RA pressure is noted (it can be damped at this point) and the needle advanced out from its covered position and hence across the IAS. An LA pressure tracing should now be seen, and 'bright' oxygenated blood is aspirated. Injected contrast confirms placement in the LA (Figure 30.7). The needle and dilator are advanced approximately 2 cm across the IAS, and then the needle is held stationary and the dilator alone advanced a further 2 cm before the needle is withdrawn.
8. A transmitral gradient is measured using the LV pigtail and the Mullins dilator.

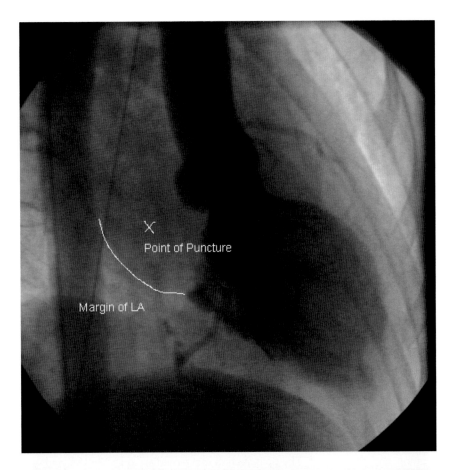

Figure 30.6
Left ventricular angiogram in the 45° left anterior oblique position is performed prior to transseptal puncture and PMV. In this view, the interatrial septum is viewed en face. The posterior margin of the left atrium (LA) can usually be seen on screening, and the aorta visualized. The Mullins dilator and needle are positioned with the curve directly away from the observer in this view, usually in the midpoint (marked ×) on the figure, and at the same level as the mitral valve orifice. Such a view ensures that the puncture is not made too posteriorly (through the back of the right atrium) or too high and anteriorly (through the aorta).

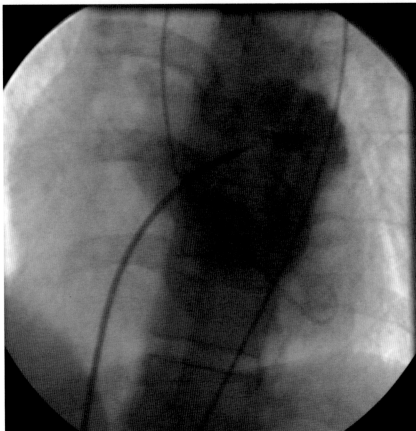

Figure 30.7
After transseptal puncture, the dilator is advanced over the needle into the left atrium. Here an injection of contrast through the dilator (after the needle has been withdrawn) confirms placement in the left atrium in an anteroposterior screening projection.

9. The patient is now heparinized at 100 u/kg as a bolus. Heparin is withheld until this point to prevent serious bleeding if atrial perforation occurs during attempted transseptal puncture.

Balloon preparation

The Inoue balloon comes with a number of associated pieces of equipment (Figure 30.8). The balloon has both an inflation port and a vent port. With the vent open, the balloon is flushed with markedly diluted contrast. Concentrated contrast slows inflation/deflation and is not necessary, as the balloon is so visible. Using the marked syringe and measurement gauge provided, at each step, it is checked that the balloon inflates to the correct size. A metal balloon-stretching tube is inserted down the center lumen and locked into place. This elongates the balloon and lowers the profile for ease in crossing the femoral entry point puncture and IAS. The balloon is now ready to use (Figure 30.9).

Balloon insertion

With the Mullins dilator in the left atrium, the 0.025 inch Inoue balloon guidewire is now inserted. This firm wire has a specially designed floppy coil forming its proximal end. As the wire is advanced into the LA, the coil forms in the body of the LA. If it does not, some manipulation may be required (usually modest, with drawing of the Mullins dilator to prevent the tip of the wire entering either the LA appendage or pulmonary vein. The top of the coil should be against the roof of the LA. After removing the Mullins dilator from the wire, a large 14 Fr dilator is used to enlarge the femoral vein puncture site and the IAS puncture site. The wire position in the LA should be maintained carefully by screening. The dilator is passed to the uppermost extent of the coil, confirming passage across the IAS, and then removed from the wire. The 'stretched' balloon is now inserted

along the wire in a similar manner. Initially, the tip of the 'stretched' balloon is taken to the top of the curve (the roof of the LA), without bending the guidewire. At this point, the stretching tube is released and withdrawn 2–3 cm, and the balloon is advanced further. The flexible balloon will now follow the curve of the wire into the LA. With the stretching tube removed completely, it can be fully advanced around the coiled wire so that it forms a loop looking down toward the mitral valve. The 0.025 inch guidewire is now removed fully. A pressure line can be used on the balloon hub for LA pressure measurements.

Crossing the mitral valve

This is generally accomplished in the 40–45° LAO view, where the positions of the mitral valve and annulus have already been identified from angiography. The Inoue balloon has two very useful features to aid in crossing: the 'nose' of the balloon can be partially inflated to give 'flow guidance', and a cleverly designed stylet directs the balloon toward the orifice.

A few milliliters of contrast are used to inflate the tip or nose of the balloon, and the stylet is inserted. Once in place, the balloon–stylet assembly usually needs to be withdrawn a few centimeters and rotated counterclockwise, lining it up with the long-axis plane of the LV and the mitral orifice. In some cases, this maneuver alone will guide the balloon across the valve, but generally it is aided by rapid withdrawal of 4–5 cm while applying counterclockwise rotation of the stylet.

An alternative technique is to form a large loop in the LA. This approach can be very helpful if the transseptal puncture is not central in the IAS. A loop can be formed by pulling the stylet back 3–5 cm and advancing the balloon to the roof of the LA. The assembly is now rotated a complete turn (360°) so that the balloon can now be advanced as a large loop counterclockwise around the LA and across to the mitral orifice.

Description	Use
① Inoue balloon catheter	Dilation of mitral valve
② Balloon-stretching tube	Elongation of balloon
③ Dilator	Dilation of insertion areas
④ Guidewire	Guiding the balloon catheter and dilator
⑤ Stylet (spring)	Directing balloon to mitral valve
⑥ Syringe	Inflation of balloon
⑦ Ruler	Measurement of balloon diameter

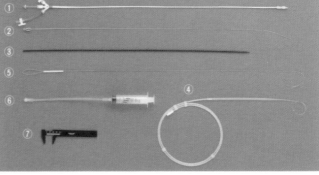

Figure 30.8
The Inoue mitral balloon comes as a kit with a number of essential components, including a guidewire, a dilator for the interatrial septum, and a preshaped stylet to aid in positioning the balloon across the mitral orifice.

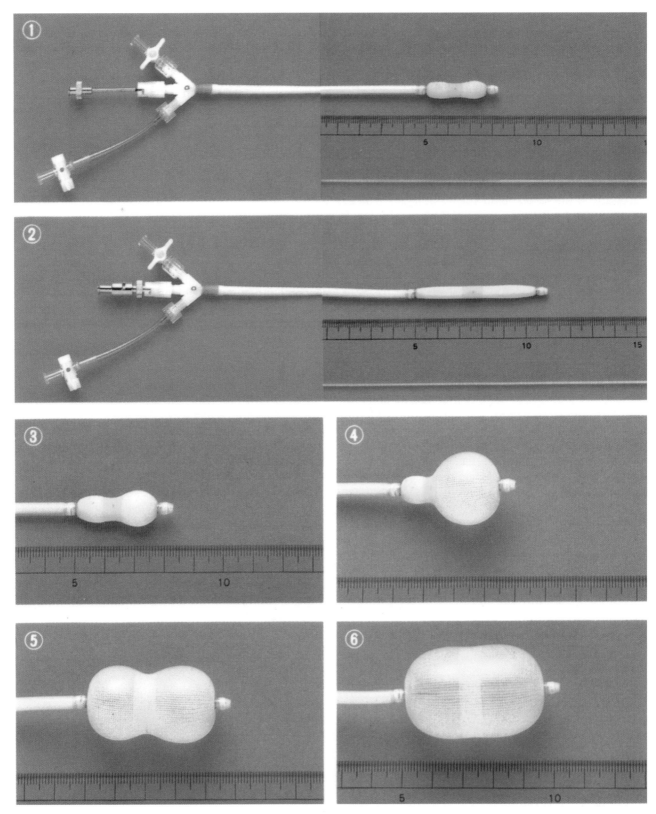

Figure 30.9
The Inoue balloon can be elongated with the use of a metal stretching tube that lowers the profile of the balloon and aids during insertion through the skin and across the interatrial septum (1 and 2). On inflation, the balloon inflates in a unique stepwise manner: initially, only the tip inflates (3), with further contrast, the tip inflates fully (4), allowing positioning against the leaflets. Next, the balloon inflates as a 'dumbbell' (5), maintaining its position until full inflation (6).

Stepwise dilatation of the mitral valve

Once the balloon is across the mitral orifice, its unique three-stage shape assists in positioning and dilatation of the valve (Figure 30.9).

The catheter should move freely toward the apex. It is now partially withdrawn and more volume is pushed into the balloon by an assistant, until the distal end inflates more fully. With very gentle traction, the balloon will now rest against the mitral orifice (Figure 30.10). When movement toward the LA stops, the balloon is fully inflated. It will initially inflate as a dumbbell shape. A 'waist' is often seen centrally in the balloon at this point where the valve is being dilated. As soon as the balloon is taken to its predetermined size, it is immediately deflated. Since all transmitral flow has been halted briefly, the blood pressure will often fall dramatically. A short inflation time usually means that this is well tolerated. The balloon is now withdrawn into the LA.

Assessing the result

Using the Inoue balloon central lumen and the LV pigtail, a transmitral gradient is measured and compared with the initial recordings before dilatation. The use of echo-Doppler to visualize the valve has proven to be most helpful at this time. Parasternal long- and short-axis views, as well as apical two- and four-chamber views, can usually be obtained. Using these views, it is possible to determine the adequacy of commissural splitting, the orifice area by direct visualization, the presence of increased MR, and the transmitral gradient by continuous-wave Doppler. The Doppler half-time should be avoided as a measure of mitral valve area at this time, as it has been shown to be inaccurate with acute changes in hemodynamic conditions.[28]

If positioning of the balloon has been difficult or uncertain, direct echocardiographic visualization is very helpful in confirming the correct balloon placement (Figure 30.11).

Dilatation of the valve is performed in a stepwise manner with the balloon gradually increased in diameter and careful assessment of the valve between each progressively larger inflation diameter. Generally, the initial inflation is carried out with an initial diameter 4 mm below the nominal balloon size (for example, with a 26 mm balloon, the initial inflation would be at 22 mm). If a sufficient drop in gradient or increase in valve area fails to occur, a further inflation is performed with the balloon 1 mm larger, provided there is no significant increase in MR. If MR increases by one grade on color Doppler assessment, further dilatation should not be performed. Assessment of the commissures is possible in subjects with reasonable echocardiographic windows. Stepwise assessment can be helpful in guiding the inflation strategy. If both commissures show evidence of separating evenly, in the absence of increasing MR, progressive dilatation can be attempted

until both are separated. If only one commissure splits, further dilatation by one step can be cautiously undertaken, provided MR has definitely not increased. Caution should be exercised if there is thickening or calcification of the remaining fused commissure. If both commissures remain fused, the decision to attempt a further step should be based in part upon knowledge of the valve morphology. If the valve has a low echo score and homogeneous thickening, a further step should be undertaken in the absence of increasing MR. If the valve is unevenly thickened, or if any evidence of increasing MR or tearing into the body of the leaflet is seen, no further dilatation should be performed. The most important complication of mitral valvuloplasty is the development of severe MR (see below).

An 'adequate' result should be considered in the clinical context. A less-than-ideal result may be appropriate in patients who are poor surgical candidates, particularly those with a high echo score. For most, success is defined as a valve area of 1.5 cm^2 or more and no significant increase in MR.[2] Usually, this is readily demonstrated by echocardiography, with good separation of the commissures and a significant reduction in the measured gradient (Figure 30.12).

Removal of the balloon catheter

The balloon is withdrawn through the atrial septum with minimal damage, by again reducing it to a low profile with the balloon-stretching tube inserted over the 0.025 inch guidewire. It is important to insert the guidewire first, as the tube alone can fail to align with the tip of the balloon after the balloon has been used for dilatation. Once reduced to a low profile, the device is pulled gently back through the IAS and femoral vein. Although the device leaves a 14 Fr puncture, the venous site makes this easy to control.

Complications of PMV

Generally, mitral valvuloplasty can be expected to have a low complication rate and low chance of technical failure.[2–5] Several well-documented complications are recognized as directly related to the procedure.

Mitral regurgitation

This is the commonest serious adverse event during mitral valvuloplasty (Figure 30.13).[2–7,29,30] In a recently published large series by Palacios et al,[7] severe MR (defined as Sellers' grade 3 or higher) occurred in 9.4% of patients with Sellers grade 3 (6%) and Sellers grade 4 (3.4%). The development of severe MR led to in-hospital mitral valve replacement in 3.3% of patients, with a higher incidence

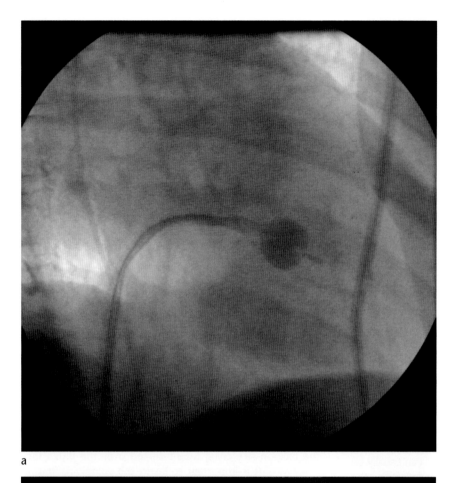

a

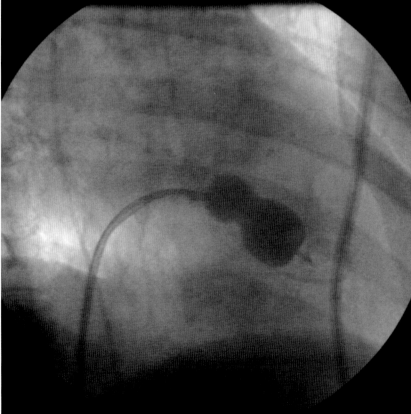

b

Figure 30.10
(a) The distal end of the Inoue balloon is inflated, and with gentle traction the balloon rests against the mitral orifice. (b) The balloon is more fully inflated, and its 'waist' allows centering across the orifice.

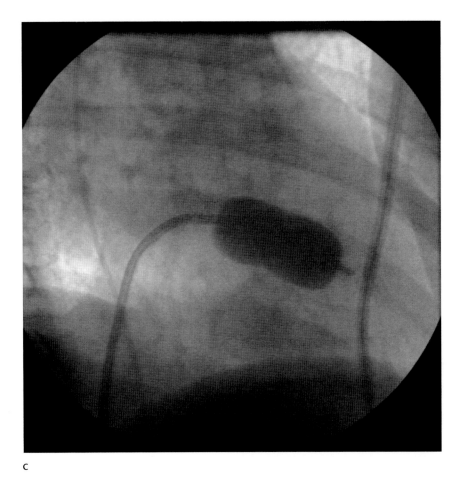

Figure 30.10 (Continued)
(c) The balloon is then fully inflated.

c

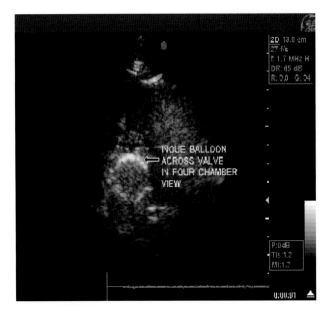

Figure 30.11
An echocardiographic apical four-chamber view performed during balloon inflation can be helpful in confirming correct placement in the mitral orifice. Parasternal and subcostal views can also be helpful.

in patients with an echo score higher than 8. Emergent mitral valve replacement was required in 1.4% of patients.

The mechanism of severe MR has been reported from surgical or postmortem examination of valves.[6,18,31] Rupture of chords to the anterior or posterior leaflet accounted for more than 50% of regurgitation in a large registry series.[31] This was followed by tearing into the body of the leaflet or overdilatation of the commissures. Kaul et al[6] have found that very severe MR requiring emergent mitral replacement has been more associated with leaflet tearing or rupture (72% of cases) (Figure 30.14).

Unfortunately, prediction of patients in whom severe MR will occur has proven to be difficult. Although the echo score predicts those who will have significant improvement in valve area, it has not been shown to accurately predict those who will develop severe MR.[18] It has been noted that the presence of pre-existing MR does not predict the occurrence of severe MR. A careful analysis of the distribution of valve thickening (homogenous versus inhomogenous), commissural calcification, and subvalvular thickening has been used to create an echocardiographically derived MR valve score. The study demonstrates that severe MR is more likely to occur in valves where there is considerable variability in leaflet thickness, calcification of

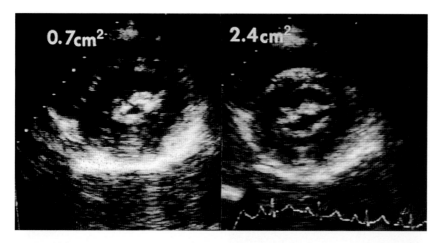

Figure 30.12
Short-axis parasternal echocardiographic views of the mitral valve (a) before and (b) after PMV, demonstrating an initial valve area (by planimetry) of 0.7 cm² and a post-PMV area of 2.4 cm². Note that the mechanism of valve area increase is cleavage along the medial and lateral commissures, which had previously appeared as densely scarred areas.

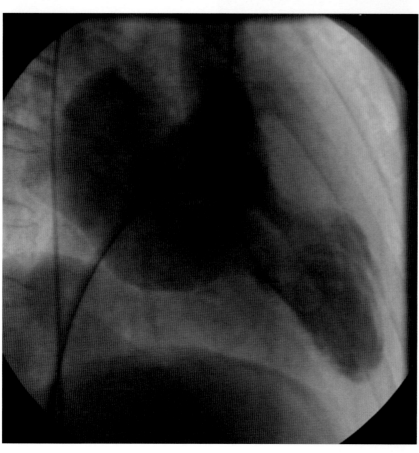

Figure 30.13
A left ventricular cine angiogram (45° LAO) performed in a patient who has developed severe mitral regurgitation (MR) immediately after balloon valvuloplasty. Contrast has been injected through a pigtail catheter into the left ventricle, outlining its shape in systole. Severe MR results in the left atrium and proximal pulmonary veins being densely opacified also (4+ MR). Note the deflated Inoue balloon still in position in the left atrium.

commissures, and marked subvalvular involvement.[18] Thus, a dilating force applied to a mitral valve orifice where the commissures cannot easily split due to calcification leads to leaflet rupture, particularly if there is more variation in leaflet thickness with thinner (or weaker) areas present.

Pericardial tamponade

Pericardial tamponade during mitral valvuloplasty is a rare complication, occurring in 1% of patients in a large series.[7]

This complication can occur as a result of attempted transseptal puncture entering the pericardial space, or from manipulation of balloon and guidewires. The latter complication is more likely to occur when a technique requiring a stiff guidewire (double-balloon approach) into the left ventricular apex is used. Perforation of the left ventricle with the wire or nose of the balloon can more readily occur than with the Inoue approach, where there is no wire and the balloon has a soft, blunt end. Prompt pericardial drainage is usually necessary. Tamponade can be managed conservatively in some cases by reversing anticoagulation and leaving an indwelling pericardial catheter in place once bleeding has ceased.

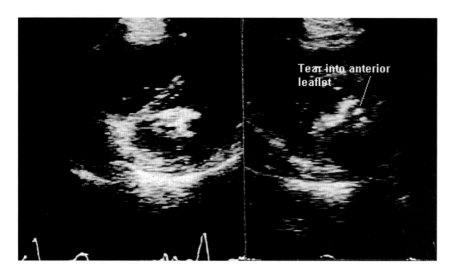

Figure 30.14
Echocardiographic short-axis views of the same patient (a) before and (b) after PMV. A small central slit-like orifice can be seen in (a). After PMV (b), the orifice appears to be a much broader slit, but there is also a split into the lateral side of the anterior mitral leaflet. This complication usually results in severe mitral regurgitation.

Thromboembolic events

Thromboembolic complications are rare during PMV, occurring only 1.8% of the time in a large recently published series.[7] Prediction of this complication has been difficult, although the presence of left atrial thrombus has generally been considered a contraindication to intervention.[19,20]

Iatrogenic atrial septal defect

Passage of a dilator through the IAS and subsequent manipulation of the balloon creates an atrial septal defect, which can persist. These defects are generally small, and close over a period of approximately 6 months.[32] Larger defects may be more likely to occur with double-wire techniques. A left-to-right shunt of >1.5 : 1 has been noted in 5.3% of patients in a large single-center experience.[7]

Late outcome

Many large series now demonstrate that balloon valvuloplasty is effective in producing immediate haemodynamic and clinical improvement and that this is associated with a good intermediate and long-term result.[2–7] Studies have compared the results of PMV versus open or closed surgical mitral commissurotomy, with generally comparable results between open surgical commissurotomy and PMV.[33–36] Hemodynamic improvement, in-hospital complications, long-term restenosis rate, and the need for re-intervention were superior for patients treated with either PMV or open surgical commissurotomy than for those treated with closed commissurotomy.[36]

Most studies show that adverse clinical events are unlikely in patients during the initial years after PMV, especially for those with favorable valve morphology. Palacios and co-workers have shown that event rates in the first 5 years after PMV are low, with a gradual increase in clin-

ical events (mostly mitral valve replacement surgery) beyond this time. The echo score predicts event-free survival throughout the follow-up period.[7] In 879 patients who underwent 939 PMV procedures, and who were followed for a mean of 4.2±3.7 years (range 0.5–15 years), actuarial survival was better in patients who had an echo score of 8 or less compared with those with scores above 8. Survival rates were 82% for patients with echo score of 8 or less and 57% for those patients with scores above 8 at a follow-up time of 12 years ($p < 0.001$) (Figure 30.15).[7]

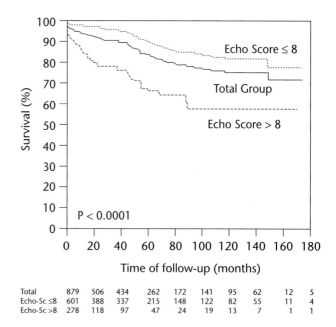

Total	879	506	434	262	172	141	95	62	12	5
Echo-Sc ≤8	601	388	337	215	148	122	82	55	11	4
Echo-Sc >8	278	118	97	47	24	19	13	7	1	1

Figure 30.15
Kaplan–Meier survival estimates for a group of patients who underwent PMV. The data are presented for the total group ($n = 879$), those with echo scores of 8 or less ($n = 601$) and those with echo scores above 8 ($n = 278$). Patients with a higher echo score (which represents a thicker, less mobile valve and the presence of subvalvular involvement) have a lower survival following PMV. (Reproduced from Palacios IF, et al. Circulation 2002;105:1465–71.)

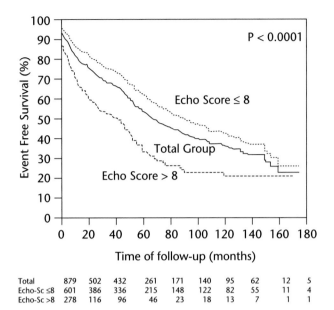

Total	879	502	432	261	171	140	95	62	12	5
Echo-Sc ≤8	601	386	336	215	148	122	82	55	11	4
Echo-Sc >8	278	116	96	46	23	18	13	7	1	1

Figure 30.16
Kaplan–Meier event-free survival estimates for a group of patients who underwent PMV (alive and free of mitral valve replacement or redo PMV). The data is presented for the total group (*n* = 879), those with echo scores of 8 or less (*n* = 601) and those with echo scores above 8 (*n* = 278). A lower rate of further intervention is seen in the group with low echo scores. (Reproduced from Palacios IF, et al. Circulation 2002;105:1465–71.)

Event-free survival (freedom from death, mitral valve replacement, and redo PMV) at 12 years (38% versus 22%, respectively, for a score of 8 or less and a score above 8; *p* < 0.001) was also significantly influenced by valve morphology (Figure 30.16).

It is noted that patients with higher echo scores tend to be older, to have valve calcification on fluoroscopy, to be in atrial fibrillation, and to be more likely to have a history of previous surgical mitral commissurotomy. The less favorable outcome of this group is therefore multifactorial and, although best accounted for by the echo score, still mandates that clinical judgment and decision making should play a role in considering the best long-term interests of each patient.

PMV has therefore become the procedure of choice for the treatment of rheumatic mitral stenosis in patients who are younger and who have ideal mitral valve morphology. The procedure has a role, albeit more palliative, in patients who have less favorable characteristics, particularly those who are not surgical candidates.

References

1. Inoue K, Owaki T, Nakamura T, et al. Clinical application of transvenous mitral commisurotomy by a new balloon catheter. J Thorac Cardiovasc Surg 1984;87:394–402.

2. Palacios IF, Block PC, Wilkins GT, Weyman AE. Follow-up of patients undergoing percutaneous mitral balloon valvotomy. Circulation 1989;79:573–9.

3. Vahanian A, Michel PL, Cormier B, et al. Results of percutaneous mitral commissurotomy in 200 patients. Am J Cardiol 1989;63:847–52.

4. Hernandez R, Banuelos C, Alfonso F, et al. Circulation 1999;99:1580–6.

5. Palacios IF. Farewell to surgical mitral commissurotomy for many patients. Circulation 1998;97:223–6.

6. Kaul UA, Singh S, Kalra GS, et al. Mitral regurgitation following percutaneous tranvenous mitral commissurotomy: a single-center experience. J Heart Valve Dis 2000;9:262–8.

7. Palacios IF, Sanchez PL, Harrell LC, et al. Which patients benefit from percutaneous mitral balloon valvuloplasty? Prevalvuloplasty and postvalvuloplasty variables that predict long-term outcome. Circulation 2002;105:1465–71.

8. Bonow RO, Carabello B, de Leon AC Jr, et al. ACC/AHA Guidelines for the Management of Patients with Valvular Heart Disease. A report of the American College of Cardiology/American Heart Association Task Force on Practice Guidelines (Committee on Management of Patients with Valvular Heart Disease). J Am Coll Cardiol 1998; 32:1486–588.

9. Abascal VM, Wilkins GT, O'Shea JP, et al. Prediction of successful outcome in 130 patients undergoing percutaneous balloon mitral valvotomy. Circulation 1990;82:448–56.

10. Harken DE, Ellis LB, Ware PF, Norman LF. The surgical treatment of mitral stenosis. N Engl J Med 1948; 239:801–9.

11. Sellors TH, Bedford DE, Somerville W. Valvotomy in the treatment of mitral stenosis. BMJ 1953;ii:1059–67.

12. Wilkins GT, Weyman AE, Abascal VM, et al. Percutaneous balloon dilatation of the mitral valve: an analysis of echocardiographic variables related to outcome and the mechanism of dilatation. Br Heart J 1988;60:299–308.

13. Abascal VM, Wilkins GT, Choong CY, et al. Echocardiographic evaluation of mitral valve structure and function in patients followed for at least 6 months after percutaneous balloon mitral valvuloplasty. J Am Coll Cardiol 1988; 12:606–15.

14. Hung JS, Chern MS, Wu JJ, et al. Short and longterm results of catheter balloon percutaneous transvenous mitral commissurotomy. Am J Cardiol 1991;67:854–62.

15. Post JR, Feldman T, Isner J, Herrman HC. Inoue balloon mitral valvotomy in patients with severe valvular and subvalvular deformity. J Am Coll Cardiol 1995;25:1129–36.

16. Fatkin D, Roy P, Morgan JJ, Feneley MP. Percutaneous balloon mitral valvotomy with the Inoue single balloon catheter: commissural morphology as a determinant of outcome. J Am Coll Cardiol 1993;21:390–7.

17. Cannan CR, Nishimura RA, Reeder GS, et al. Echocardiographic assessment of commissural calcium: a simple predictor of outcome after percutaneous mitral balloon valvotomy. J Am Coll Cardiol 1997;29:175–80.

18. Padial LR, Freitas N, Sagie A, et al. Echocardiography can predict which patients will develop severe mitral regurgitation after percutaneous mitral valvotomy. J Am Coll Cardiol 1996;27:1225–31.

19. Hung JS, Lin FC, Chiang CW, Successful percutaneous transvenous catheter balloon commissurotomy after warfarin therapy and resolution of left atrial thrombus. Am J Cardiol 1989;64:126–8.

20. Chen WJ, Chen MF, Liau CS, et al. Safety of percutaneous transvenous balloon commissurotomy in patients with mitral stnosis and thrombi in the left atrial appendage. Am J Cardiol 1992;70:117–19.

21. Rediker DE, Block PC, Abascal VM, Palacios IF. Mitral balloon valvuloplasty for mitral re-stenosis after surgical commissurotomy. J Am Coll Cardiol 1988;11:252–6.

22. Palacios IF, Block PC, Wilkins GT, et al. Percutaneous mitral balloon valvotomy during pregnancy in a patient with severe mitral stenosis. Cathet Cardiovasc Diagn 1988;15:109–11.

23. Orbe LC, Sobrino N, Arcas R, et al. Initial outcome of percutaneous balloon valvuloplasty in rheumatic tricupid valve stenosis. Am J Cardiol 1993;71:353–4.

24. Abdullah M, Halim M, Rajendran V, et al. Comparison between single (Inoue) and double balloon mitral valvuloplasty: immediate and short term results. Am Heart J 1992,123:1581–8.

25. Park SJ, Kim JJ, Park SW, et al. Immediate and one year results of mitral balloon valvuloplasty using Inoue and double balloon techniques. Am J Cardiol 1993;71:938–43.

26. Ruiz CE, Zhang HC, Macaya C, et al. Comparison of Inoue single-balloon versus double-balloon techniques for percutaneous mitral valvuloplasty. Am Heart J 1992;123:942–7.

27. Herman HC, Wilkins GT, Abascal VM, et al. Percutaneous balloon mitral valvotomy for patients with mitral stenosis : analysis of factors influencing early results. J Thorac Surg 1988;96:33–8.

28. Thomas JD, Wilkins GT, Choong CYP, et al. Inaccuracy of mitral valve pressure halftime immediately after percutaneous mitral valvotomy. Dependence on the transmitral gradient and the left atrial and left ventricular compliance. Circulation 1988;78:980–93.

29. Hung JS, Chern MS, Wu JJ, et al. Short and long-ter, results of catheter balloon percutaneous trasvenous mitral commissurotomy. Am J Cardiol 1991;67:854–62.

30. Chen CR, Cheng TO, Chen JY, et al. Long-term results of percutaneous mitral valvuloplasty with the Inoue balloon catheter. Am J Cardiol 1992;70:1445–8.

31. Hermann HC, Lima JA, Feldman T, et al. Mechanisms and outcome of severe mitral regurgitation after Inoue balloon valvuloplasty. North American Inoue Balloon Investigators. J Am Coll Cardiol 1993;22:783–9.

32. Yoshida K, Yoshikawa J, Akasaka T, et al: Assessment of left-to-right shunting after percutaneous mitral valvuloplasty by transesophageal color Doppler flow-mapping. Circulation 1989;80:1521–6.

33. Arora R, Nair M, Kalra GS, et al. Immediate and long term results of balloon and surgical closed mitral valvotomy: a randomised comparitive study. Am Heart J 1993;125;1091–4.

34. Turi ZG, Reyes VP, Raju BS, et al. Percutaneous balloon versus surgical closed commissurotomy for mitral stenosis: a prospective, randomised trial. Circulation 1991;83:1179–85.

35. Reyes VP, Raju BS, Wynne J, et al. Percutaneous balloon valvuloplasty compared with open surgical commissurotomy for mitral stenosis. N Engl J Med 1994;331:961–7.

36. Farhat MB, Aayari M, Maatouk F, et al. Percutaneous balloon versus surgical closed and open mitral commissurotomy: seven-year follow-up results of a randomised trial. Circulation 1998;97:245–50.

Index